Musculoskeletal Ultrasound

Musculoskeletal Ultrasound

Ian Beggs, FRCPE, FRCR

Consultant Musculoskeletal Radiologist
Department of Radiology
Royal Infirmary of Edinburgh
Edinburgh, United Kingdom

Wolters Kluwer | Lippincott Williams & Wilkins
Health

Philadelphia • Baltimore • New York • London
Buenos Aires • Hong Kong • Sydney • Tokyo

Senior Executive Editor: Jonathan W. Pine, Jr.
Product Manager: Amy G. Dinkel
Production Project Manager: Alicia Jackson
Senior Manufacturing Coordinator: Beth Welsh
Senior Marketing Manager: Kimberly Schonberger
Designer: Stephen Druding
Production Service: S4Carlisle Publishing Services

First Edition

Library of Congress Cataloging-in-Publication Data

9781451144987
1451144989

Care has been taken to confirm the accuracy of the information presented and to describe generally accepted practices. However, the authors, editors, and publisher are not responsible for errors or omissions or for any consequences from application of the information in this book and make no warranty, expressed or implied, with respect to the currency, completeness, or accuracy of the contents of the publication. Application of the information in a particular situation remains the professional responsibility of the practitioner.

The authors, editors, and publisher have exerted every effort to ensure that drug selection and dosage set forth in this text are in accordance with current recommendations and practice at the time of publication. However, in view of ongoing research, changes in government regulations, and the constant flow of information relating to drug therapy and drug reactions, the reader is urged to check the package insert for each drug for any change in indications and dosage and for added warnings and precautions. This is particularly important when the recommended agent is a new or infrequently employed drug.

Some drugs and medical devices presented in the publication have Food and Drug Administration (FDA) clearance for limited use in restricted research settings. It is the responsibility of the health care provider to ascertain the FDA status of each drug or device planned for use in their clinical practice.

To purchase additional copies of this book, call our customer service department at (800) 638-3030 or fax orders to (301) 223-2320. International customers should call (301) 223-2300.

Visit Lippincott Williams & Wilkins on the Internet: at LWW.com. Lippincott Williams & Wilkins customer service representatives are available from 8:30 am to 6 pm, EST.

10 9 8 7 6 5 4 3 2 1

DEDICATION

To Jean, Simon, and Paul

Ronald S. Adler PhD, MD
Professor of Radiology
Department of Radiology
NYU Langone Medical Center
and Hospital for Joint Diseases
Center for Musculoskeletal Care
New York, New York

**Gina M Allen BM, DCH, MRCGP,
MRCP, FRCR, MFSEM, DipSEM**
Consultant Radiologist
Department of Radiology
Saint Luke's Hospital
Oxford, United Kingdom
Teaching Associate and Teaching Advisor Green
Templeton College
University of Oxford, Oxford University Hospitals
Oxford, United Kingdom

Tom Anderson MSc
Senior Research Fellow
Department of Medical Physics
University of Edinburgh
Edinburgh, United Kingdom

Ian Beggs FRCPE, FRCR
Consultant Musculoskeletal
Radiologist
Department of Radiology
Royal Infirmary of Edinburgh
Edinburgh, United Kingdom

Stefano Bianchi MD
Director
CIM SA
Cabinet Imagerie Médicale
Geneva, Switzerland

Jean-Louis Brasseur MD
Praticien Consultant
Service de Radiologie
GH Pitié-Salpêtrière
Paris, France

Guilio Comin FRANZCR (Hons)
Consultant Radiologist
Saint Vincent's Hospital
Sydney, Australia

David A. Connell FRANZCR, FFSEM
Associate Professor
Department of Medicine
Monash University
Clinical Director
Imaging at Olympic Park
AAMI Stadium
Melbourne, Australia

Michel Court-Payen MD, PhD
Head of Department
Department of Musculoskeletal Radiology
Gildhøj Private Hospital
Brøndby, Denmark

Nicole C. Fernandes MD
Radiologist
Department of Radiology
Leiden University Medical Center
Leiden, Netherlands

David P. Fessell MD
Associate Professor
Department of Radiology
University of Michigan
Ann Arbor, Michigan

**James F. Griffith MB, BCh, BAO, MD (CUHK),
MRCP (UK), FRCR, FHKCR, FHKAM (Radiology)**
Professor
Department of Imaging and Internventional Radiology
The Prince of Wales Hospital
The Chinese University of Hong Kong
Shatin, Hong Kong

Jon A. Jacobson MD
Professor of Radiology
University of Michigan
Director
Division of Musculoskeletal Radiology
Department of Radiology
University of Michigan
Ann Arbor, Michigan

Ryan Ka Lok Lee FRCR
Clinical Tutor
Department of Imaging and Internventional Radiology
The Prince of Wales Hospital
The Chinese University of Hong Kong
Shatin, Hong Kong

Dien Hung Luong MD
Assistant Clinical Professor
Department of Medicine
Montreal University
Active Member
Department of Physical Medicine
& Rehabilitation
Montreal University Health Center
Montreal, Quebec, Canada

Paul I. Mallinson MBChB, FRCR
Department of Musculoskeletal Radiology
Leeds Teaching Hospitals
Chapel Allerton Hospital
Leeds, United Kingdom

Carlo Martinoli MD
Associate Professor of Radiology
Department of Health Sciences
DISSAL
University of Genoa
Genoa, Italy

Norman McDicken PhD
Emeritus Professor
Department of Medical Physics
University of Edinburgh
Edinburgh, United Kingdom

Theodore T. Miller MD
Professor of Radiology
Weill Cornell Medical College
Attending Radiologist
Department of Radiology and Imaging
Hospital for Special Surgery
New York, New York

Gerard Morvan MD
Musculoskeletal Radiologist
Imagerie Léonard de Vinci
Paris, France

Lionel Pesquer MD
Co-Chief
Department of Radiology
Clinique du Sport de Bordeaux
Merignac, France

Monique Reijnierse MD
Head of Musculoskeletal Radiology
Department of Radiology
Leiden University Medical Center
Leiden, Netherlands

Philip Robinson MB ChB, FRCR
Honorary Clinical Associate Professor
Department of Musculoskeletal Diseases
University of Leeds
Consultant Musculoskeletal Radiologist
Radiology
Leeds Teaching Hospitals
Leeds, United Kingdom

Marcin Szkudlarek MD, PhD
Consultant Rheumatologist
Dept. of Rheumatology
University of Copenhagen Hospital at Koge
Koge, Denmark

Alberto Tagliafico MD
Istituto di Anatomia
Department of Experimental Medicine
DIMES
Università di Genova
Genoa, Italy

David J. Wilson MBBS, BSc, MFSEM, FRCP, FRCR
Senior Clinical Lecturer
University of Oxford
Consultant Radiologist
Oxford University Hospital and Saint Luke's Hospital
Oxford, United Kingdom

Ultrasound has become increasingly important in diagnosis and treatment across a wide range of musculoskeletal conditions in recent years, driven by a combination of technical advances, increased understanding of disease processes, and new and effective therapies.

Appreciation of anatomy, pathophysiology, clinical presentation, and ultrasound technique are essential for successful practice. Ultrasound and MRI are complementary—not competing—modalities. Understanding their relative strengths and weaknesses is vital. All these, together with tricks of the trade, are presented in this book by contributors who are internationally acknowledged experts in musculoskeletal imaging. The aim is to provide a comprehensive and concise account of musculoskeletal ultrasound, a book that shows you how to do it and explains what you see.

ACKNOWLEDGMENTS

To the patients, colleagues, and friends from whom I have learned.

CONTENTS

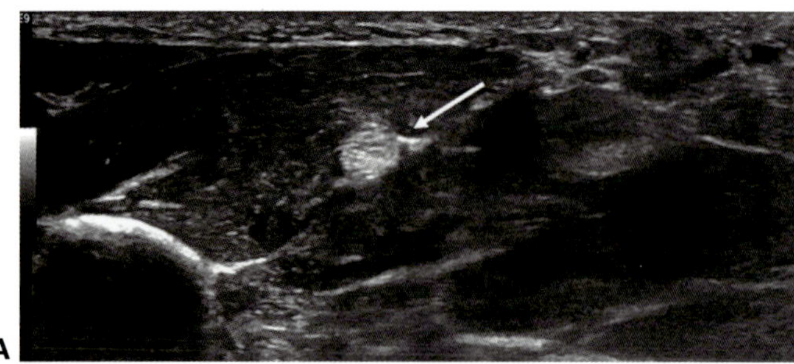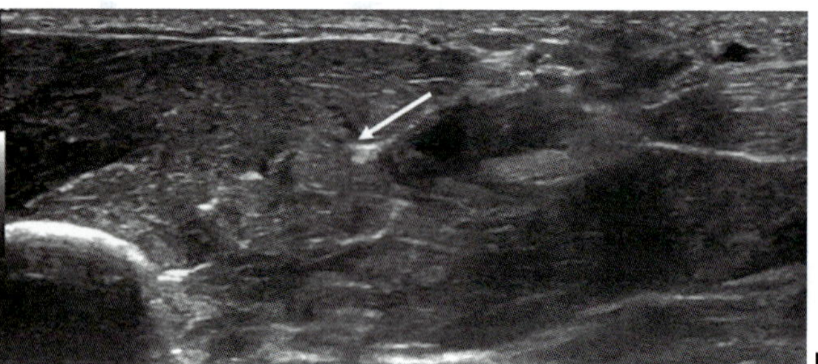

Figure 1.1. **A:** Transverse scan of the thenar eminence. The angle of insonation is 90° to the flexor pollicis longus tendon *(arrow)*, which appears echogenic. **B:** The angulation of the transducer has been altered by about 5°, and the tendon *(arrow)* is no longer visible.

perpendicular, the sound will be reflected away from the transducer and the loss of reflected sound will result in a hypoechoic appearance. Tendons are the most important specular reflectors (**Fig. 1.1**), but ligaments, nerves, and muscles (**Fig. 1.2**) are also specular reflectors, and it is essential to ensure that the transducer is always perpendicular to these structures. Anisotropy is a particular problem with tendons that curve, for example, supraspinatus at the shoulder and tibialis posterior and the peroneal tendons at the ankle. Compound imaging produces sound waves at different angles and helps to overcome the problem of anisotropy and reduces noise and speckle.[5]

Beam steering also assists, although most experienced sonologists simply angle the transducer. Tissue harmonic imaging, which utilizes frequencies that arise within the tissue examined, helps to reduce other artifacts and improve contrast resolution.[6]

The effect of anisotropy can be harnessed profitably if a tendon is difficult to locate because it is surrounded by echogenic fat, for example, at the ankle. Altering transducer angulation to make the tendon hypoechoic (**Fig. 1.3**) will help locate the tendon. Then transducer angulation is corrected to examine the tendon.

Beam edge artifact (**Fig. 1.4**) is another artifact that can affect tendons, particularly large tendons. Loss of definition of the tendon edge and distal acoustic shadowing may simulate or obscure fluid in the tendon sheath.

Extended field-of-view imaging (**Fig. 1.5**) may improve diagnostic accuracy, for example, in assessing atrophy of the rotator cuff muscles, and has a valuable role in teaching and presenting findings.

Doppler examination is essential in assessing tendinopathy[7] and detecting (**Fig. 1.6**) or monitoring synovitis.[8] Neovascularity has been correlated with pain in tendinopathy (although the relationship between tendinopathy and neovascularity is controversial) and with active synovitis in inflammatory joint disease. Power Doppler is usually employed using low pulse repetition frequency, medium persistence, small color box, low wall filter, and appropriate color velocity scale. Doppler signal (**Fig. 1.7**) may be reduced or abolished by pressing too hard or if a tendon is under tension; therefore, a light touch should be employed and tendons should be relaxed while being examined.

The role of contrast-enhanced ultrasound (CEUS) is yet to be established. However, CEUS improves diagnostic

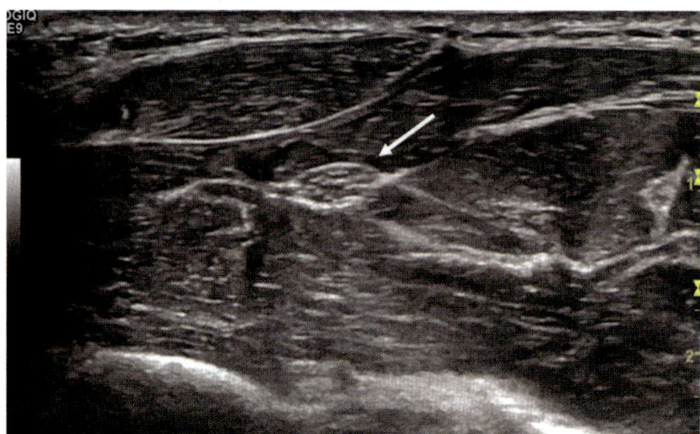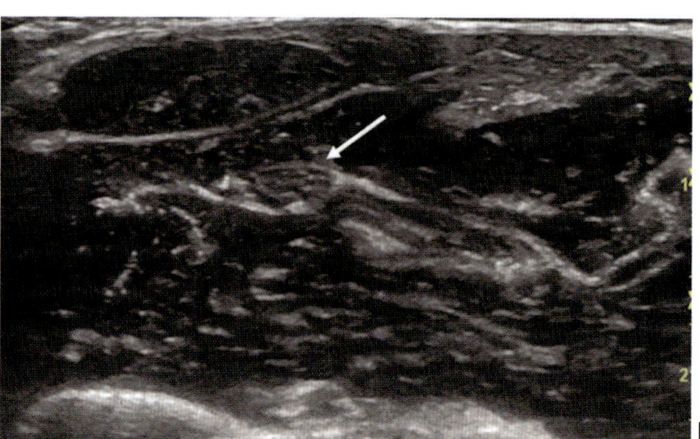

Figure 1.2. **A:** Transverse scan of the forearm showing the median nerve *(arrow)* between the flexor digitorum superficialis and flexor digitorum profundus muscles. The transducer is perpendicular to the muscles and nerve. **B:** The transducer is no longer perpendicular, and all structures, including the median nerve *(arrow)*, are now poorly seen and appear hypoechoic.

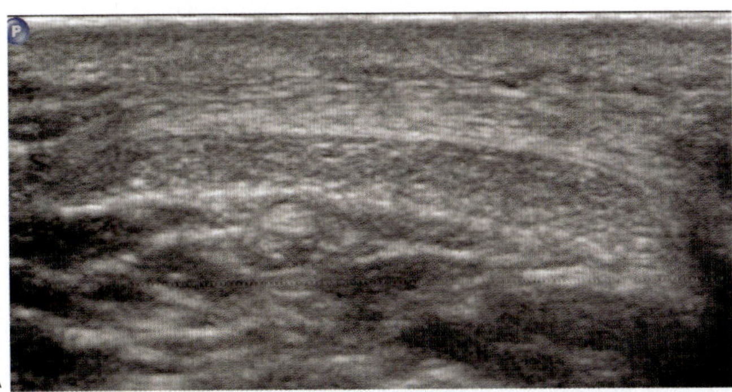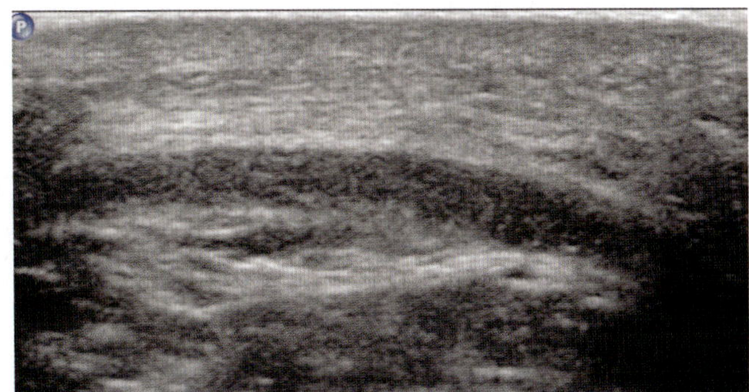

Figure 1.3.   **A:** Short-axis scan of patellar tendon, with the angle of insonation at 90°. The tendon is correctly imaged and is echogenic, but the echogenicity is similar to that of the overlying subcutaneous fat. **B:** The altered angle of insonation results in a hypoechoic tendon that is clearly distinguished from the subcutaneous fat.

sensitivity in inflammatory joint diseases, shows areas of relatively low vascularity that might predispose to tendinopathy, and demonstrates age-related changes in vascularity in the rotator cuff.[9,10]

Elastography (**Fig. 1.8**) assesses tissue softening by measuring tissue displacement before and after compression, and has shown promising results in epicondylitis at the elbow and in Achilles tendinopathy.[1,11,12]

TENDON

Tendons are part of the musculotendinous unit and transmit force from muscle to bone to produce movement at joints. They are subject to tensile and compressive forces. Tendon strength depends on the size, number, and orientation of collagen fibers, thickness, and internal organization.[13]

Tendons are composed of collagen fibers, ground substance, and tenocytes. Collagen provides tensile strength.

Ground substance provides structural support for collagen fibers and regulates collagen production. Tenocytes are scattered among collagen fibers and produce collagen precursors and ground substance. Collagen is arranged hierarchically and has a uniform appearance, which is distorted in tendinosis (**Fig. 1.9**). Tropocollagen, a triple-helix polypeptide chain, forms fibrils, which coalesce to form fibers, which in turn form the primary, secondary, and tertiary bundles that comprise the tendon. Most collagen fibers are parallel and run in the direction of the long axis of the tendon with a spiral element, but some fibers run transversely.[13]

Tendons are covered by the epitenon, a loose connective tissue sheath that contains vessels, nerves, and lymphatics that supply the tendon. The epitenon extends deeply as endotenon between tertiary bundles of collagen, and blends externally with the paratenon or deep fascia when tendons have a straight course. Some tendons that alter direction with joint movement, typically those that run in osteofibrous tunnels at the ankle and wrist, have double-layered tendon sheaths that are lined by synovial cells and contain a thin film of fluid. Vessels cross the tendon sheath at the mesotendon. Curved tendons are held in position by fibrous retinacula (e.g., at the wrist and ankle) or pulleys (e.g., the flexor tendons of the fingers).

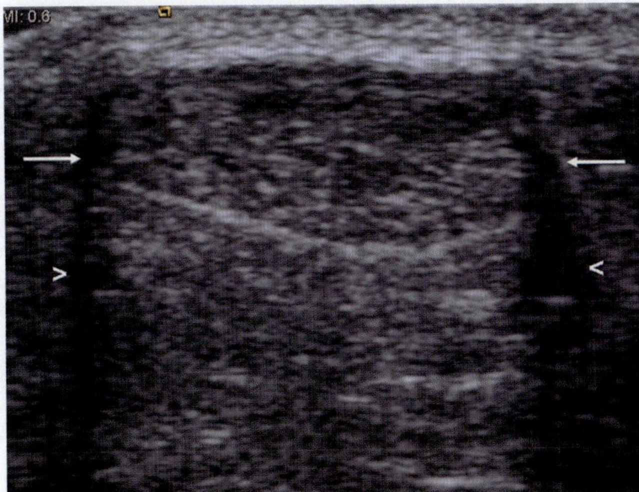

Figure 1.4.   Transverse scan of tendo Achilles. Edge artifact *(arrows)* obscures the margins of the tendon and results in acoustic shadowing *(arrowheads)*.

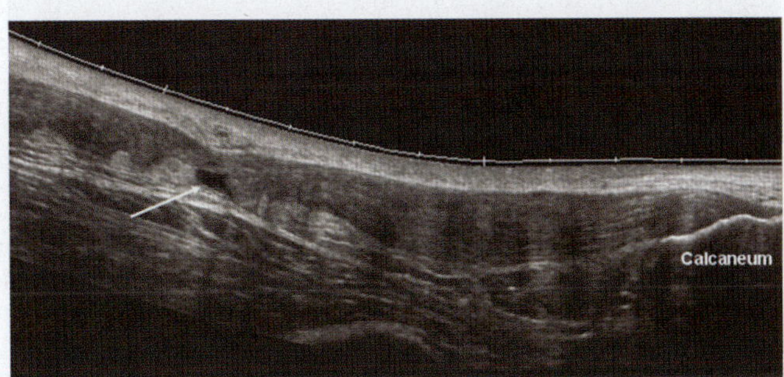

Figure 1.5.   Extended field-of-view image showing partial tear *(arrow)* in tendo Achilles. The tendon distal to the tear is swollen.

Figure 1.6.   Power Doppler longitudinal scan of volar aspect of the fifth metacarpophalangeal joint. The proximal recess is distended and contains echogenic synovium and neovascularity in keeping with synovitis.

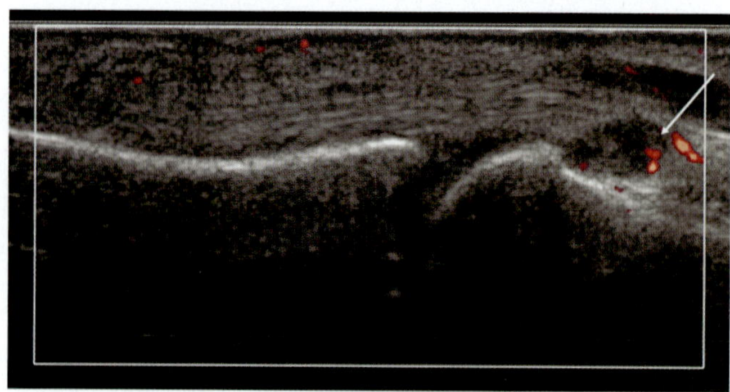

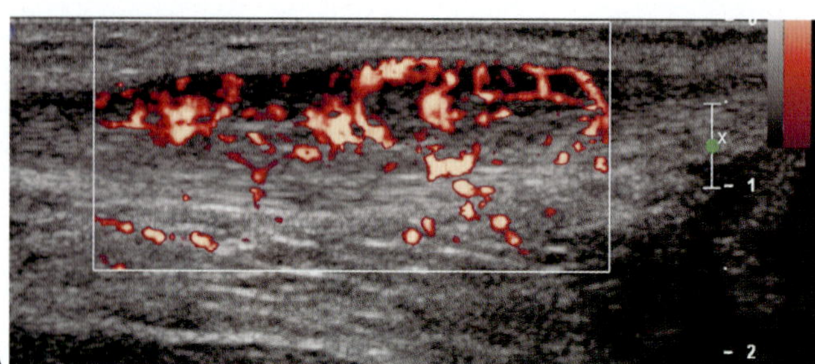

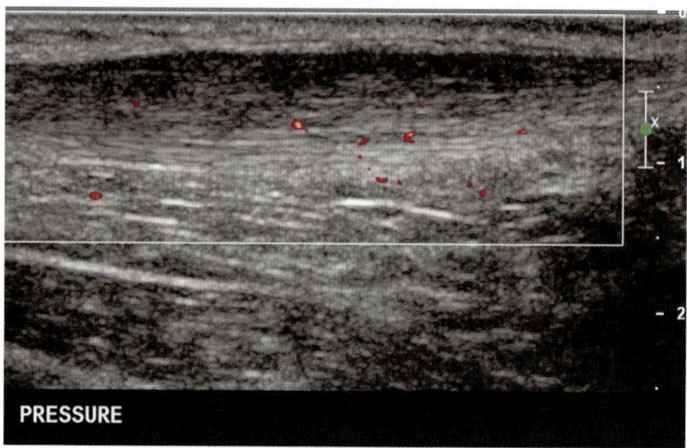

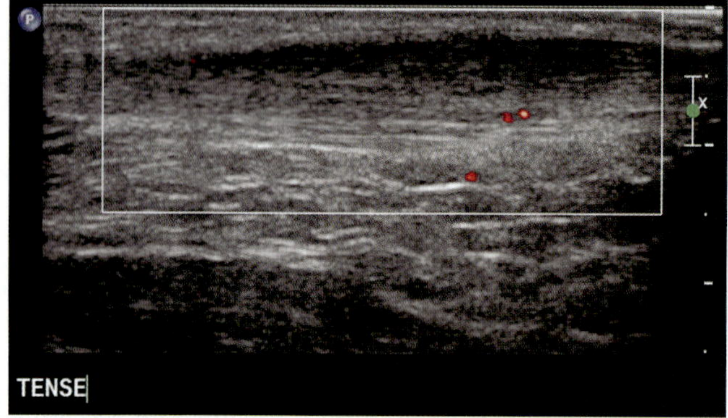

Figure 1.7.   **A:** Power Doppler longitudinal scan showing typical Achilles tendinosis. There is fusiform thickening of the tendon, its superficial fibers are hypoechoic, and there is extensive neovascularity in the tendon and adjacent soft tissues. **B:** Heavy pressure has obliterated the Doppler signal. **C:** Putting the tendon under tension by dorsiflexing the foot has also abolished the Doppler signal.

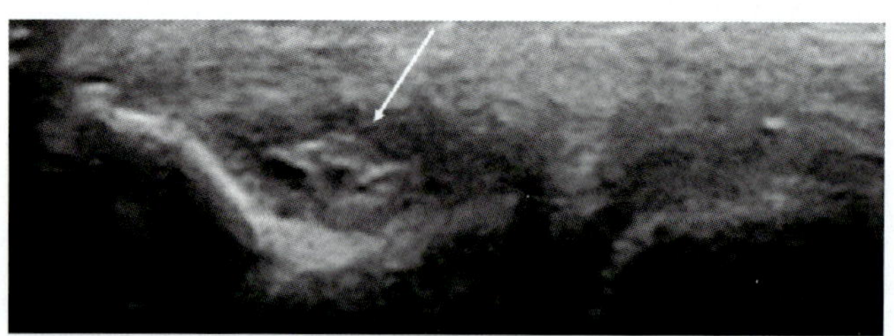

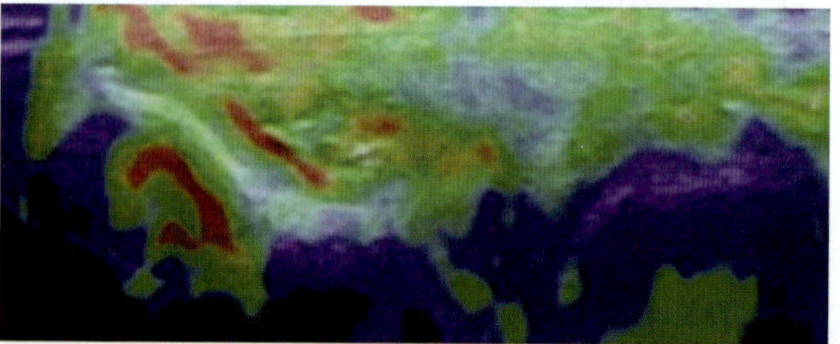

Figure 1.8.   **A:** Swelling, reduced echogenicity, and cystic areas *(arrow)* in common extensor origin at elbow, consistent with lateral epicondylitis. **B:** Elastography of the same area shows red areas due to softening. The green areas are normal. (Both images courtesy of Professor A. Klauser.)

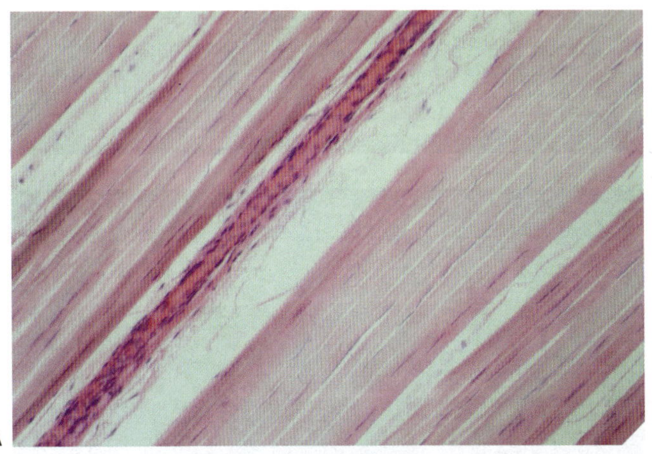 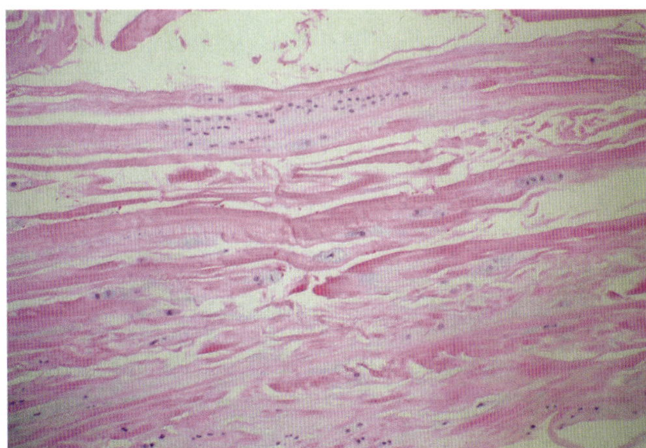

Figure 1.9. **A:** H&E preparation of normal tendon showing the highly uniform linear pattern. (Courtesy of Dr. F. Bonar. Reproduced with permission from Klein MJ, Bonar SF, eds. *Fascicle 9: Non-neoplastic Disease of Bone and Joints.* Silver Springs, MD: ARP Press; 2011.) **B:** H&E preparation of severe tendinosis showing disruption of the normal pattern and chondroid lacunae. (Courtesy of Dr. F. Bonar.)

Ultrasound (**Fig. 1.10**) demonstrates the internal architecture of tendons in greater detail than most conventional MRI scanners. Tendons have an echogenic, fibrillar pattern in long-axis scans and a speckled, echogenic appearance in short-axis scans, caused by the interfaces between the echogenic collagen bundles and the endotenon. Both tendon texture and caliber should be uniform, although some tendons narrow (e.g., supraspinatus) and others expand (e.g., distal patellar tendon) as they run to their insertions. Tendons normally show no flow on color or power Doppler scans, although contrast-enhanced scans can show vascularity. Epitenon, paratenon, and synovial sheath all appear echogenic, although a thin layer of anechoic fluid may be present in a tendon sheath. Pulleys and retinacula are usually thin and hypoechoic,[14,15] although the extensor retinaculum at the wrist is an exception and is thick (**Fig. 1.11**).

As tendons are highly anisotropic, the transducer must be maintained at 90° to the tendon at all times. Altering the angle of insonation by as little as 5° may make a tendon hypoechoic and apparently abnormal.

MUSCLE

Muscles account for up to 50% of body weight. Muscle fibers are elongated structures (**Fig. 1.12**) that are uniform in size within a muscle, but vary from muscle to muscle. Groups of muscle fibers form fascicles. Aggregations of fascicles form muscles. Muscle fibers are surrounded by strands of connective tissue called the endomysium, fascicles are surrounded by a thicker perimysium, and muscles are surrounded by epimysium.

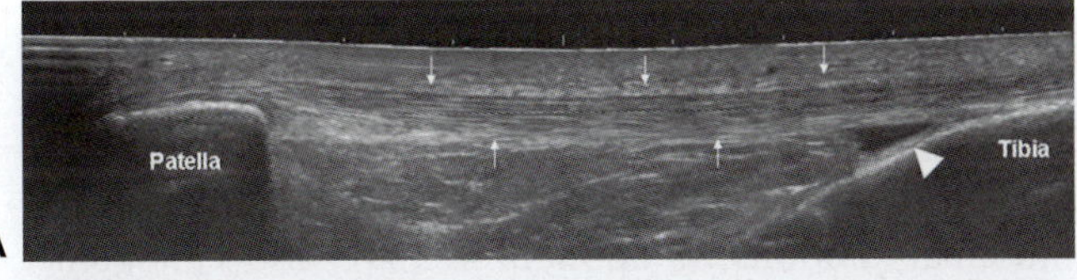

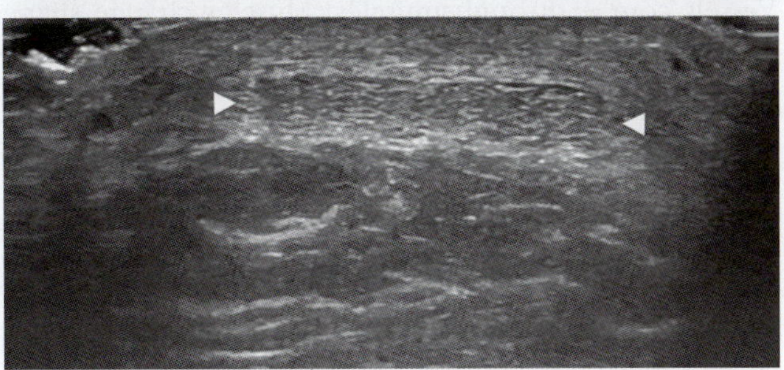

Figure 1.10. **A:** Long-axis scan of patellar tendon *(arrows).* The tendon has a fibrillar pattern and uniform caliber and texture. There is a small bursa *(arrowhead)* deep to the distal tendon. This is normal. **B:** Short-axis scan of the patellar tendon *(between the arrowheads).* The tendon has a speckled appearance and is well-defined and homogeneously echogenic.

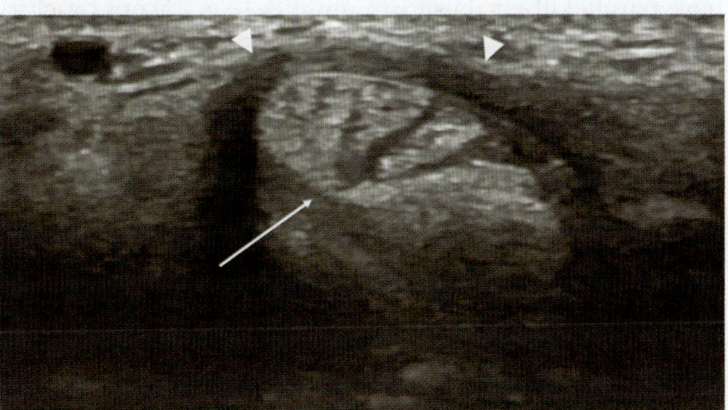

Figure 1.11. Thick (normal) retinaculum *(arrowheads)* overlying the extensor digitorum longus tendons *(arrow)* at the wrist.

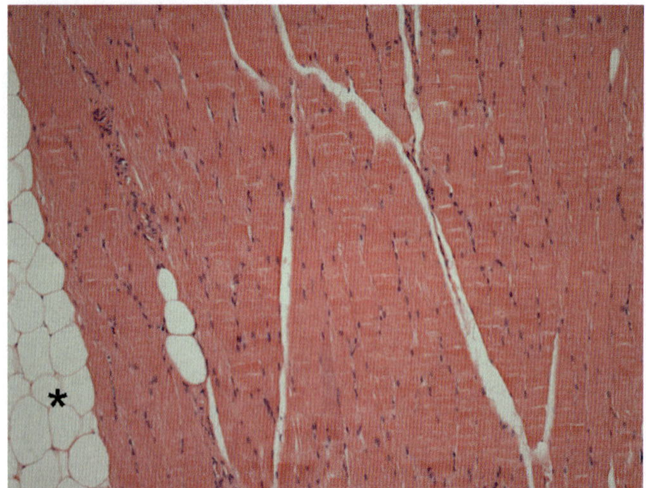

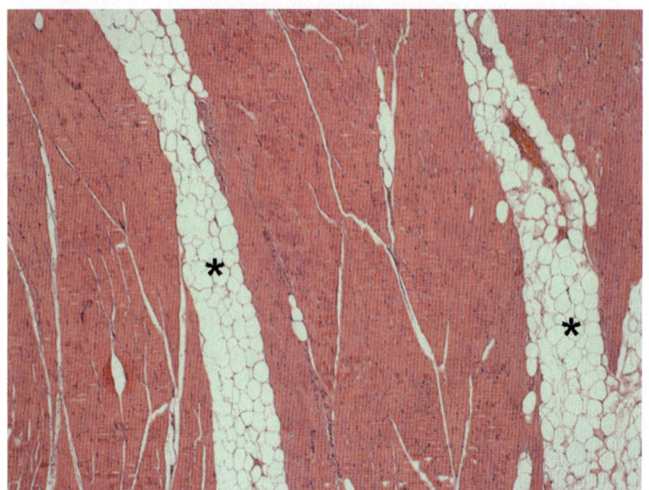

Figure 1.12. **A:** H&E preparation of normal muscle at high power showing the uniform distribution of the elongated muscle cells. Contraction of muscle cells results in contraction of the muscle. There is a fibroadipose septum *(asterisk)* at the edge of the image. **B:** Lower-powered H&E preparation showing fibroadipose septa *(asterisks)* separating muscle bundles. (Both images courtesy of Professor D. Salter.)

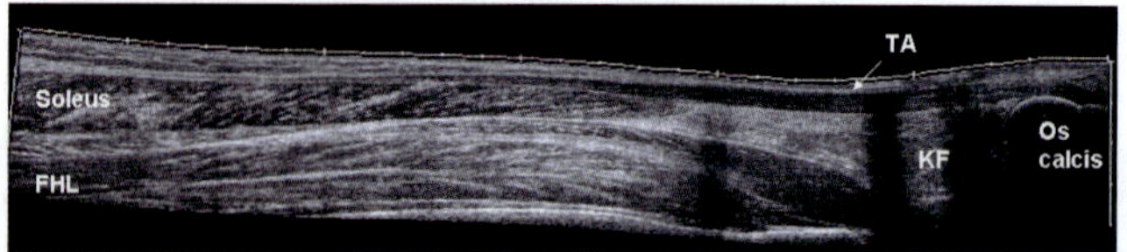

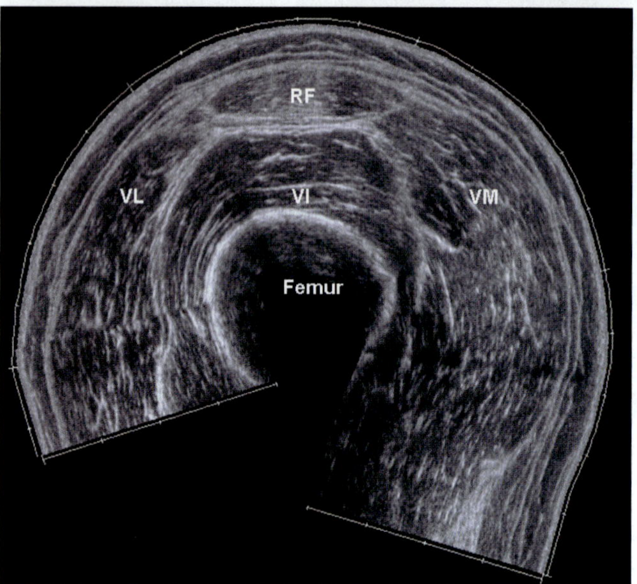

Figure 1.13. **A:** Longitudinal ultrasound scan of the lower calf showing the soleus and FHL muscles. The muscle boundaries are demarcated by echogenic fascia. Echogenic fibroadipose septa lie between hypoechoic muscle bundles and are oblique to the long axes of the muscles. FHL, flexor hallucis longus; KF, Kager's fat; TA, tendo Achilles. **B:** EFOV transverse scan of mid-thigh. Echogenic fascia outlines the muscle boundaries (of RF and VI, VM, and VL muscles). The fibroadipose septa are seen in cross section as echogenic dots and dashes. RF, rectus femoris; VL, vastus lateralis; VI, vastus intermedius; VM, vastus medialis.

There are several muscle patterns. Flat (e.g., pronator quadratus) or strap-like (e.g., rectus abdominis) muscles have parallel fibers. Fusiform muscles (e.g., biceps brachii) have parallel fibers mid-muscle that converge on the tendon. Pennate muscles have oblique fibers and a feathery appearance and may be triangular (e.g., trapezius). In unipennate muscles (e.g., flexor pollicis longus), all fibers run obliquely in the same direction, while in bipennate muscles (e.g., rectus femoris), they converge on the aponeurosis, or intramuscular tendon, from two separate directions. Multipennate muscles (e.g., subscapularis) have several tendons. Spiral arrangements (e.g., pectoralis major) also occur.

Ultrasound (**Fig. 1.13**) reflects the anatomy of muscles: Muscle bundles and fascicles are hypoechoic, while the connective tissue structures are echogenic. In long-axis scans, fleshy, hypoechoic muscle bundles are separated by the parallel echogenic lines of fibroadipose septa or perimysium. In short-axis scans, the fibroadipose septa produce echogenic dots and dashes scattered uniformly between the muscle fascicles. The outer epimysium is echogenic in both long-axis and short-axis scans. Intramuscular tendons or aponeuroses are also echogenic. Vessels course through muscles. Muscles change shape and become hypoechoic on contraction, and the obliquity of the fibroadipose septa increases.[16]

Muscles are anisotropic structures, and the appearance of a muscle will change with the angle of insonation. An individual muscle tends to be uniformly echogenic, but different muscles vary in echogenicity. Muscle echogenicity can be altered by pathology (e.g., fatty infiltration and infection cause increased echogenicity).

LIGAMENTS

Ligaments are very similar to tendons in structure, appearance, and acoustic properties. They consist of tightly

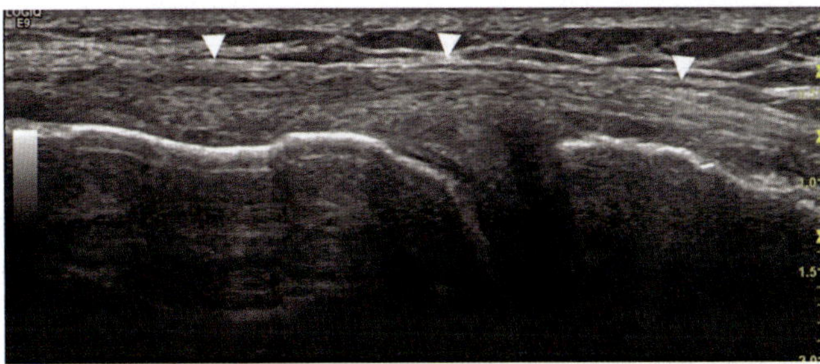

Figure 1.14.   Long-axis scan of the medial collateral ligament of the knee *(arrowheads).*

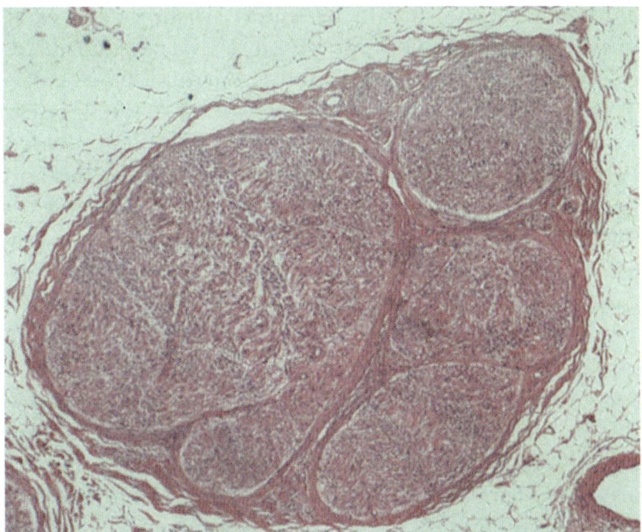

Figure 1.15.   H&E axial section of peripheral nerve at high power. The plump nerve fascicles are surrounded by the connective tissue epineurium, and the whole nerve is enveloped by perineurium. (Courtesy of Professor D. Salter.)

bound parallel collagen bundles arranged hierarchically, although ligaments have slightly less collagen and more proteoglycan matrix than do tendons. Ligaments are covered by the vascular epiligament, which is indistinguishable from the ligament and merges with the periosteum where the ligament attaches to bone.[17] Ligaments are intra-articular (such as the cruciate ligaments at the knee), capsular (such as the glenohumeral ligaments at the shoulder), or extra-articular and extracapsular (such as the lateral collateral ligament at the knee).[16]

Ultrasound (**Fig. 1.14**) shows echogenic, fibrillar structures, uniform in caliber and texture, running between bony joint margins and merging with the adjacent periosteum. Ligaments are echogenic and lamellar in long-axis scans and speckled in short-axis scans. The echogenic areas are the collagen bundles, and the hypoechoic areas are the supporting structures. Ligaments are anisotropic. Therefore, the incident sound beam should be at 90° to the ligament to demonstrate it adequately. This is best achieved if the ligament is stretched; for example, the calcaneofibular ligament is concave and not well seen with the ankle in neutral, but straightens and is well-demonstrated in dorsiflexion.

NERVES

Nerves are composed of multiple nerve fibers or axons, both myelinated and nonmyelinated, which are surrounded by the supporting connective tissue endoneurium. Nerve fibers are bundled together in fascicles, which are surrounded by connective tissue perineurium (**Fig. 1.15**). The nerve is enveloped by a sheath of connective tissue epineurium that may be focally thickened in fibro-osseous tunnels where the nerve is compressed or stretched. The connective tissue contains elastic fibers and vessels, but Doppler signal is not normally identified, and the Doppler signal in nerves is generally considered pathologic. Nerve caliber diminishes from proximal to distal as branches leave the nerve.

The ultrasound (**Fig. 1.16**) and histologic appearances of nerves are closely correlated.[18–20] The neural elements are hypoechoic or anechoic, whereas the supporting

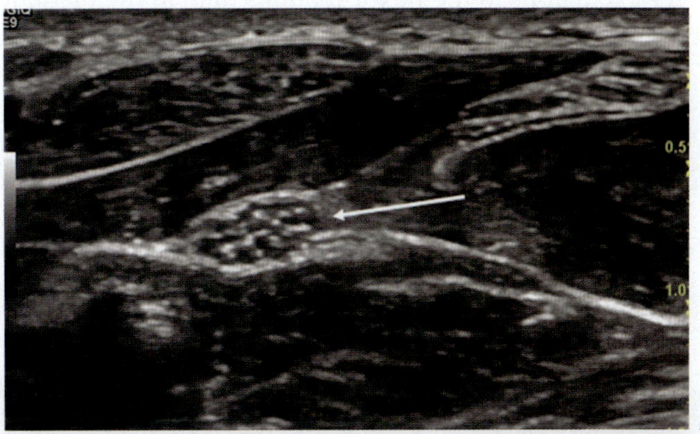

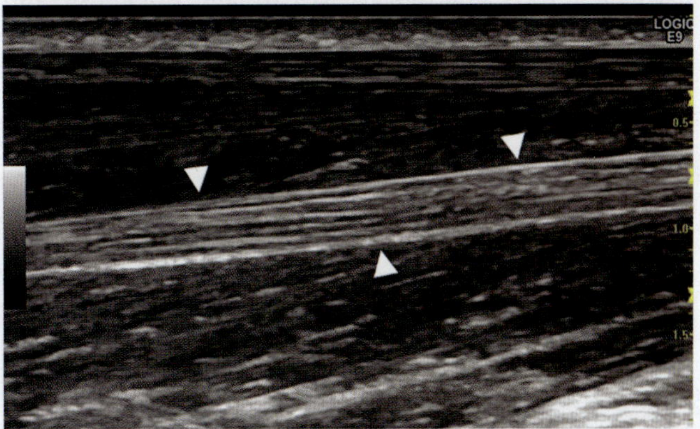

Figure 1.16.   **A:** Short-axis scan of median nerve *(arrow).* The nerve is well-defined. The neural elements are hypoechoic, whereas the surrounding connective tissues are echogenic. **B:** Long-axis scan of median nerve *(arrowheads).* The nerve is of uniform thickness and texture. The neural elements are hypoechoic and continuous.

connective tissues are hyperechoic. In short-axis scans, nerves appear well-defined, round or oval, and speckled; the round hypoechoic fascicles are surrounded by echogenic connective tissue. In long-axis scans, nerves appear well-defined and tubular and contain alternating hyperechoic and hypoechoic lines. In contrast to tendons and ligaments, the hypoechoic components are much thicker and continuous in nerves. Loss of echogenicity and fibrillar pattern may occur where nerves are subject to pressure in fibro-osseous tunnels.

Nerves are easily examined on transverse images. Once the nerve is identified in an axial scan, an "elevator" technique may be employed, sweeping the transducer to and fro, proximally and distally, following the course of the nerve over quite long distances. Nerves are anisotropic structures, although not as strongly as tendons, and a nerve may appear hypoechoic if the incident sound beam is not perpendicular. Although nerves and tendons are not dissimilar in appearance, the distinction between them is easy. Anatomical position helps. Nerves are less echogenic and contain plumper hypoechoic areas than tendons. Nerves move, but not as much as tendons. This can be seen at the wrist when flexion and extension of the fingers produce much longer excursions in the flexor tendons than in the median nerve.

CARTILAGE

Normal hyaline or articular cartilage appears homogeneously hypoechoic on ultrasound (**Fig. 1.17**) and has a smooth superficial margin. A thin echogenic line may appear on the surface of the cartilage especially if fluid is present in the joint. The subchondral bone at the deep margin is echogenic and casts an acoustic shadow. Conventional ultrasound does not show the histological layers of cartilage. However, ultrasound can demonstrate cartilage ulcers, alterations in cartilage thickness, and increased echogenicity in and on the surface of the cartilage in crystal deposition disease.

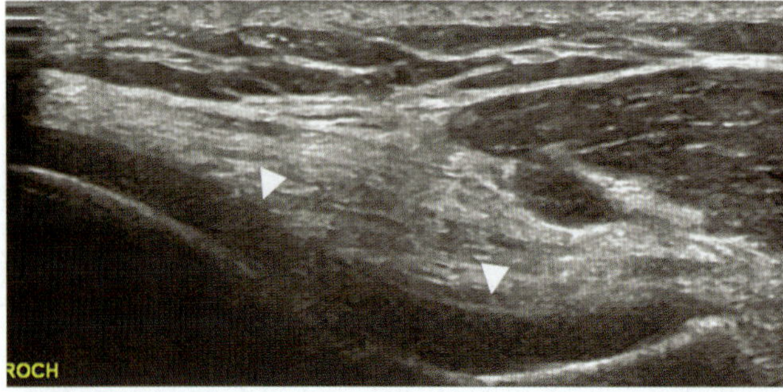

Figure 1.17. The articular cartilage *(arrowheads)* in the patellar sulcus is anechoic.

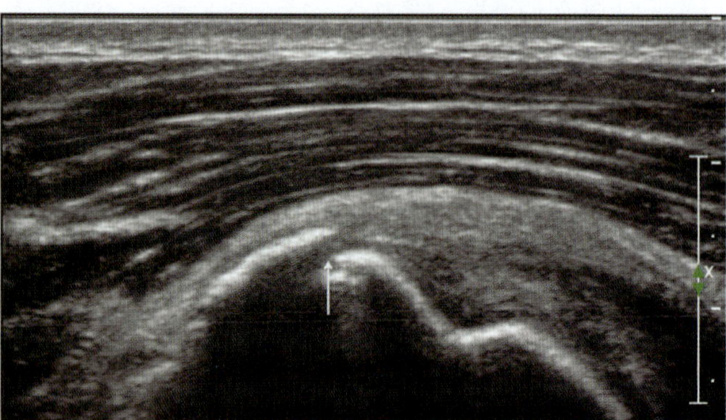

Figure 1.18. Sagittal oblique scan of shoulder showing a radiographically occult greater tuberosity fracture *(arrow)*. The fracture fragment is elevated by <1 mm.

Fibrocartilage structures, such as the menisci at the knee or the glenoid labrum at the shoulder, are echogenic.

SYNOVIUM

Normal synovium is one to two cells thick, too thin to be seen with ultrasound.

JOINT CAPSULE

Joint capsules are thin and hyperechoic and merge with surrounding soft tissues.

BONE

Bone is highly echogenic and casts an acoustic shadow. Small depressions or pits in articular surfaces are frequently seen as normal variants and should be distinguished from erosions, which frequently show Doppler signal. Hyperostosis at tendon insertions is common and may be a manifestation of tendinosis. Periosteum is not usually distinguished separately from bone cortex, but ultrasound may show periosteal elevation early in infection, stress fracture, or tumor. Lytic tumors may destroy the cortex and extend into adjacent soft tissues. Fractures result in cortical defects, elevation, or depression that may not be visible in radiographs (**Fig. 1.18**). Ultrasound can also show echogenic areas typical of early osteogenesis or cystic changes that prevent bone healing following limb-lengthening surgery.

CONCLUSION

Ultrasound has a wide and increasing range of diagnostic and therapeutic roles in the musculoskeletal system. Careful attention to technique and good knowledge of anatomy and pathology are critical to success and develop with experience.

REFERENCES

1. Klauser AS, Peetrons P. Developments in musculoskeletal ultrasound and clinical applications. *Skeletal Radiol.* 2010;39:1061–1071.
2. Jamadar DA, Jacobson JA, Caoili EM, et al. Musculoskeletal sonography technique: focused versus comprehensive evaluation. *AJR Am J Roentgenol.* 2008;190(1):5–9.
3. Murphy C, Russo A. *An Update on Ergonomic Issues in Sonography.* Report. http://www.sdms.org/pdf/sonoergonomics.pdf.
4. Sunley K. *Prevention of Work-Related Musculoskeletal Disorders in Sonography.* http://www.sor.org/public/document-library/sor_prevention_work_related_musculoskeletal.pdf.
5. Lin DC, Nazarian LN, O'Kane PL, et al. Advantages of real-time spatial compound sonography of the musculoskeletal system versus conventional sonography. *AJR Am J Roentgenol.* 2002;179(6):1629–1631.
6. Strobel K, Zanetti M, Nagy L, et al. Suspected rotator cuff lesions: tissue harmonic imaging versus conventional US of the shoulder. *Radiology.* 2004;230(1):243–249.
7. Zanetti M, Metzdorf A, Kundert H-P, et al. Achilles tendons: clinical relevance of neovascularization diagnosed with power Doppler US. *Radiology.* 2003;227(2):556–560.
8. Farrant JM, O'Connor PJ, Grainger AJ. Advanced imaging in rheumatoid arthritis. Part 1: synovitis. *Skeletal Radiol.* 2007;36(4):269–279.
9. Adler RS, Fealy S, Rudzki JR, et al. Rotator cuff in asymptomatic volunteers: contrast-enhanced US depiction of intratendinous and peritendinous vascularity. *Radiology.* 2008;248(3):954–961.
10. Rudzki JR, Adler RS, Warren RF, et al. Contrast-enhanced ultrasound characterization of the vascularity of the rotator cuff tendon: age- and activity-related changes in the intact asymptomatic rotator cuff. *J Shoulder Elbow Surg.* 2008;17(suppl 1):96S–100S.
11. De Zordo T, Lill SR, Fink C, et al. Real-time sonoelastography of lateral epicondylitis: comparison of findings between patients and healthy volunteers. *AJR Am J Roentgenol.* 2009;193(1):180–185.
12. De Zordo T, Fink C, Feuchtner GM, et al. Real-time sonoelastography findings in healthy Achilles tendons. *AJR Am J Roentgenol.* 2009;193(2):W134–W138.
13. O'Brien M. Anatomy of tendons. In: Maffulli N, Renström P, Leadbetter WB, eds. *Tendon Injuries: Basic Science and Clinical Medicine.* London: Springer-Verlag; 2005:3–4.
14. Martinoli C, Derchi LE, Pastorino C, et al. Analysis of echotexture of tendons with US. *Radiology.* 1993;186(3):839–843.
15. Adler RS, Finzel KC. The complementary roles of MR imaging and ultrasound of tendons. *Radiol Clin North Am.* 2005;43(4):771–807.
16. Erickson SJ. High-resolution imaging of the musculoskeletal system. *Radiology.* 1997;205(3):593–618.
17. Frank CB. Ligament structure, physiology and function. *J Musculoskelet Neuronal Interact.* 2004;4(2):199–201.
18. Silvestri E, Martinoli C, Derchi LE, et al. Echotexture of peripheral nerves: correlation between US and histologic findings and criteria to differentiate tendons. *Radiology.* 1995;197(1):291–296.
19. Martinoli C, Bianchi S, Derchi LE. Tendon and nerve sonography. *Radiol Clin North Am.* 1999;37(4):691–711.
20. Bianchi S. Ultrasound of the peripheral nerves. *Joint Bone Spine.* 2008;75(6):643–649.

CHAPTER

2

Physics

Norman McDicken
Tom Anderson

This chapter provides an introduction to the physics of medical ultrasound (US). Several books exist that can be consulted to extend the material presented here.[1-4] Values are quoted for physical quantities related to ultrasound in tissues, such as speed of sound and attenuation. This will enable a better qualitative and quantitative understanding of musculoskeletal scanning. A detailed knowledge of these quantities is not required; indeed, it is often not available, but a working knowledge helps in the production and interpretation of ultrasound images and Doppler blood flow measurements. Some knowledge of the physics is also helpful for an appreciation of safe usage. However, safety is not a major concern in musculoskeletal work since most tissues examined are not sensitive to ultrasound energy of the levels encountered in clinical scanning.

ULTRASOUND

Ultrasound Propagation

Ultrasound vibrations are generated by a very small rapid push–pull action of a transducer held against a medium such as tissue. The ultrasound then passes through ("propagates" through) the tissue. A transducer converts electrical signals to ultrasound vibrations for transmission and conversely for detection. The vibrations are so small that they cannot be observed by eye. Vibration rates of a pitch too high to be heard by the human ear are called ultrasound. Vibration rates in the range 1,000,000 to 50,000,000 cycles per second are found in different applications of medical ultrasound. The term "frequency" is employed rather than vibration rate, and the unit is hertz (Hz) rather than cycles per second. Frequencies in the range 5 to 15 megahertz (MHz) are used in musculoskeletal ultrasound.

In medicine, ultrasound is transmitted when one or more piezoelectric crystals (element) in a transducer are driven to vibrate by an applied fluctuating voltage. Ultrasound is detected when vibrations strike a piezoelectric crystal, producing a small voltage signal across it. That the same piezoelectric crystal can generate large amplitude vibrations and detect extremely small ones has been central to the development of medical ultrasound technology. Piezoelectric properties occur naturally in some materials, for example, quartz, but today specially developed ceramics

are employed. Medical ultrasound scanners often generate short bursts (pulses) of vibration, for example, each of three or four cycles in duration. **Figure 2.1** illustrates pulsed and continuous ultrasound. For a continuous wave (CW), an alternating (oscillating) voltage is applied continuously, whereas for a pulsed wave (PW) it is applied for a short time. As the ultrasound from the transducer travels through the subject, echoes are generated by reflection or scattering of the transmitted ultrasound at changes in tissue structure within the body. The returning low-amplitude echoes are used to create images of these structures.

The vibration of the transducer elements, a push–pull action, causes regions of compression and rarefaction to pass from the transducer face into the tissue. A waveform can be drawn to represent these regions of increased and decreased pressure **(Fig. 2.2)**. The distance between equivalent points on the waveform is called the wavelength, and the maximum pressure fluctuation is the wave amplitude **(Fig. 2.3)**. Waves or wavefronts are said to have been transmitted from the transducer face. They can be focused by making the transducer face concave or by attaching a lens to it, but focusing is much more commonly achieved electronically by driving a large number of elements at slightly different times.

Ultrasound waves pass through tissue at very high speed, around 1540 m per second for most soft tissues. This is extremely useful since pulses can be transmitted and echoes collected in a fraction of a millisecond after

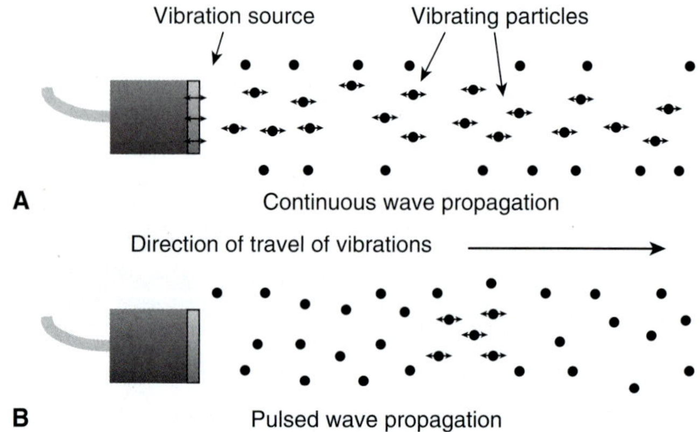

Figure 2.1.   The generation of continuous **(A)** and pulsed wave **(B)** ultrasound by a vibrating source in contact with a propagating medium.

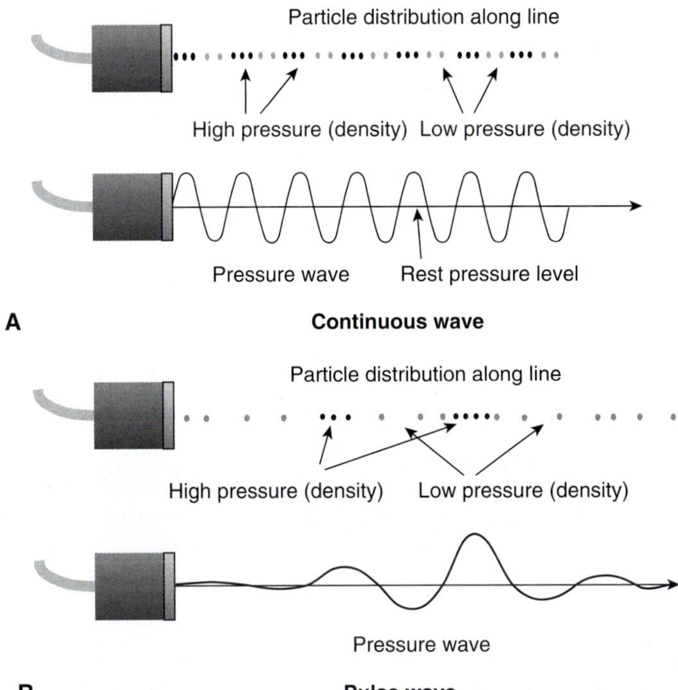

Figure 2.2. Waveform patterns related to pressure variations in ultrasound fields **(A)** Continuous wave, **(B)** Pulsed wave.

the instant of transmission and hence many images can be produced in a second. If 50 images are presented per second, the frame rate is said to be 50 per second. The speed of sound is simply related to the frequency and the wavelength by the formula:

$$c = f - \lambda$$

where c is the speed of sound, f is the frequency, and λ is the wavelength.

In most ultrasound waves used in medicine, oscillations of the particles of the medium are in the same direction as wave travel. Such waves are called longitudinal or compressional waves since they give rise to regions of increased and decreased pressure. Waves in which oscillations are perpendicular to the direction of travel, like ripples on

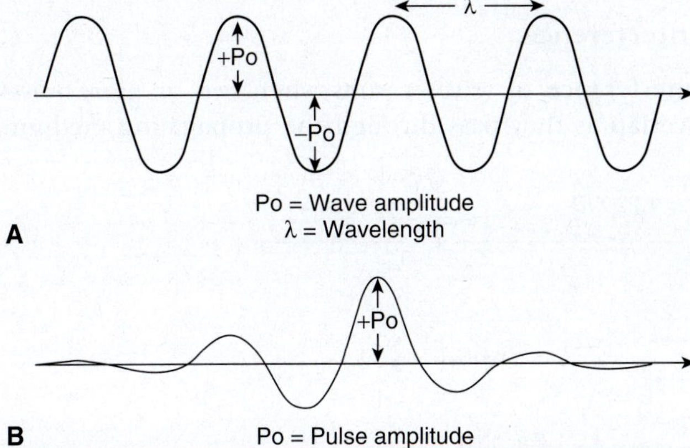

Figure 2.3. Definition of ultrasound wavelength and amplitude **(A)** Continuous wave, **(B)** Pulsed wave.

TABLE 2.1.	Speed of Ultrasound (m/s) in Tissue
Blood	1457
Water	1480
Fat	1450
Liver	1550
Muscle	1580
Skin	1600
Cartilage	1660
Tendon	1750
Bone	3500
Air	330
Soft tissue (average)	1540

a pond, are called transverse or shear waves. At megahertz frequencies, shear waves are rapidly attenuated in tissue and fluids and hence are not used at present in medical ultrasound. Developments at lower frequencies aim to utilize them in elastography (see later).

Speed of sound in a material depends on its rigidity and density (**Table 2.1**); the more rigid a material, the higher the speed. Diagnostic instruments measure the time of echo return to the transducer after the instant of pulsed ultrasound transmission and then use the average speed to convert this time into the depth in tissue of the reflecting structure. For a mixture of soft tissues along the pulse path, an accurate measure of depth is obtained by assuming an average speed of 1540 m per second for conversion of time into depth. As noted later, the speed of sound in bone can cause severe problems due to refraction of ultrasound. If possible, bone is best avoided during ultrasound examinations. The speed of ultrasound in tissues is independent of frequency over the diagnostic range, that is, 1 to 50 MHz.

Tip:
- Ultrasound is vibration of frequency (pitch) above that which can be heard by the human ear.
- Ultrasound is high-frequency vibration that travels through tissue at high speed, close to 1540 m per second in soft tissue.
- The frequency range used in musculoskeletal applications is 5 to 15 MHz.
- Ultrasound vibration travels as a pressure waveform.
- Ultrasound can be generated and detected by piezoelectric crystals contained in small handheld transducers.
- Echoes produced by reflection of transmitted ultrasound pulses at tissue interfaces are the basic source of information in diagnostic ultrasound.

Ultrasound Intensity and Power

When vibrations travel into tissue, energy passes from the transducer to the tissue. The intensity at a point in the

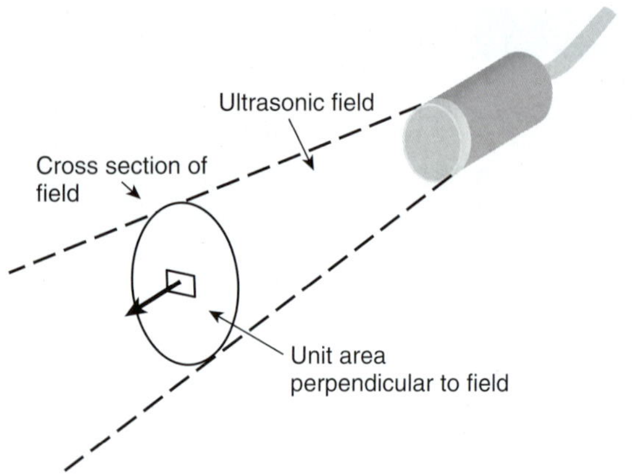

Figure 2.4. Power is the rate of flow of energy through the whole cross section of the field. Intensity at a point is the rate of flow of energy through unit area perpendicular to the field at that point.

tissue is the rate of flow of energy through unit area at that point (**Fig. 2.4**); for example, the intensity may be 100 mW per cm^2. The region of tissue in front of the transducer subjected to the vibrations is referred to as the ultrasound field or beam. For safety studies, intensity needs to be precisely defined. For a PW beam, ISPTA is the intensity at its spatial peak (often the focus) averaged over time, and ISPPA is the intensity at the spatial peak averaged over the pulse length. Intensities are not used in routine scanning, but it is useful to know their definitions when the safety literature is being considered. Later we will consider two quantities of interest to optimize safety: thermal index (TI) and mechanical index (MI). The energy of a pulsed or continuous wave is related to amplitude. It is not a quantity that is widely used in clinical practice.

The power output of a machine is the rate of flow of energy through the cross-sectional area of the field (**Fig. 2.4**). The output power is related to possible biological effects, due to heating. Effects may also be due to cavitation, which is the violent response of bubbles when subjected to the pressure fluctuations of an ultrasound wave. The TI and MI are related to heating and cavitation, respectively, and are displayed on screen.

Ultrasonic intensity is normally measured with a hydrophone, a small probe containing a piezoelectric element. Ultrasonic power is measured with a radiation pressure balance whose pan is placed in the beam. Associated with the flow of energy in a beam there is a flow of momentum.

When this momentum is interrupted by the pan, a force is experienced that is directly related to the power of the beam. This radiation force is small, for example, 0.135 mg per mW. Later it will be seen that radiation force is employed to generate shear waves in an elastography technique designed to measure tissue elasticity.

> **Tip:**
> - The ultrasound field or beam is the region in front of the transducer that is affected by the transmitted vibration.
> - The vibration produced by the transducer is a flow of energy through the tissue.
> - Intensity and power are related and are of particular interest with regard to safety.
> - Radiation force is experienced when the transmitted energy strikes a target and is reflected or absorbed.

Diffraction

Diffraction is the spreading out of a wave as it passes through a medium. The pattern of spread depends on the size of the source relative to the wavelength. The diffraction pattern of a disc-shaped crystal as found in basic transducers is approximately cylindrical for a short distance, after which it diverges at a small angle (**Fig. 2.5**). The diffraction pattern from a small element of an array transducer is divergent at a large angle from close to the transducer (**Fig. 2.6A**). A diffraction pattern may exhibit fluctuations in intensity, particularly close to the transducer. Diffraction also occurs beyond a small obstacle or a slit aperture (**Fig. 2.6B**). The narrowness of a beam or the sharpness of a focus is determined by diffraction. The small wavelengths of high-frequency ultrasound enable the generation of well-focused beams. This is one of the most important facts in medical ultrasound technology. The higher the frequency, the narrower the beam, and hence finer detail is achieved in an image. Absorption increases with frequency, which puts an upper limit on the frequency that can be used.

Interference

Interference of waves results when two or more waves overlap as they pass through the propagating medium.

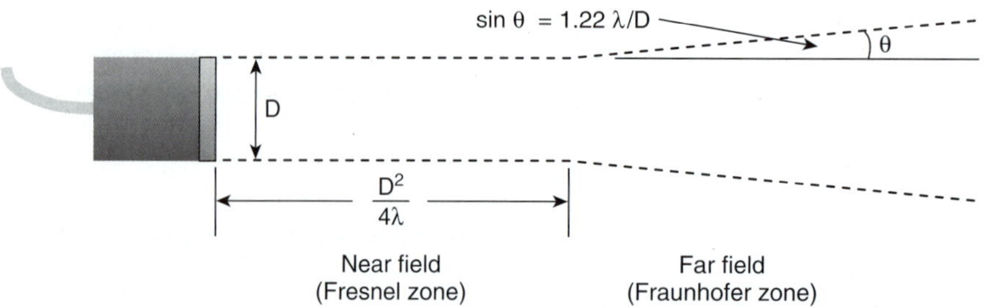

Figure 2.5. Idealized field for a disc-shaped source generating a continuous wave.

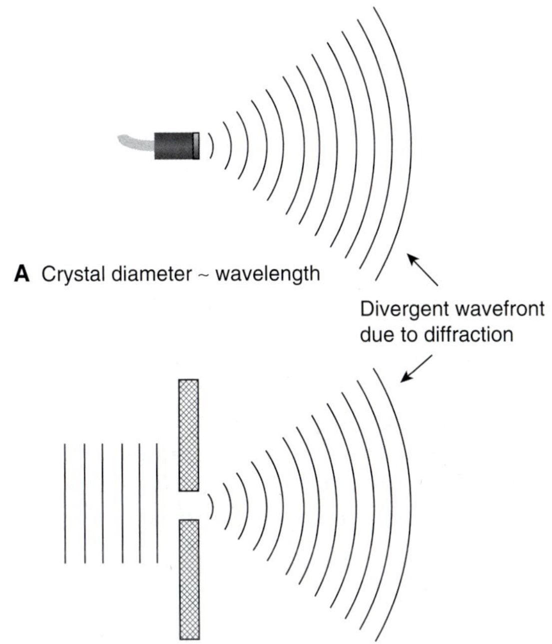

Figure 2.6. Diffraction of ultrasound from (**A**) a small source or on passing through (**B**) a small aperture.

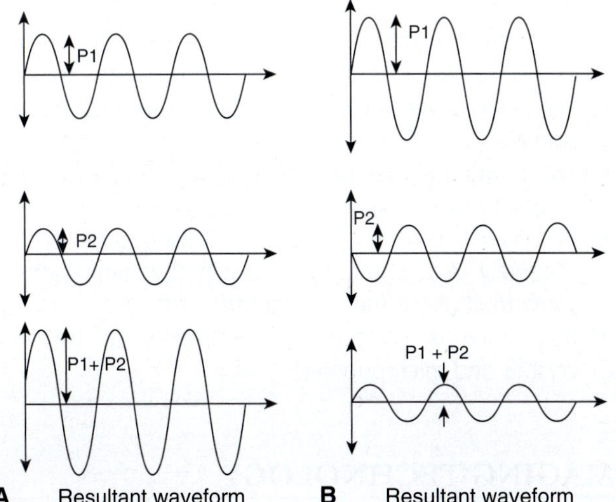

Figure 2.7. Examples of (**A**) constructive and (**B**) destructive interference.

The resultant wave pressure amplitude at any point is determined by adding the pressure amplitudes from each wave at the point (**Fig. 2.7A**). When waveforms are in step, they add to produce constructive interference, giving an increase in amplitude. Out of step they add destructively, resulting in a lower amplitude (**Fig. 2.7B**).

Image Speckle

Small echoes from tissue overlap and interfere, both constructively and destructively, to produce a fluctuating resultant signal at the transducer (**Fig. 2.8A,B**). The transducer signal is presented in the display as

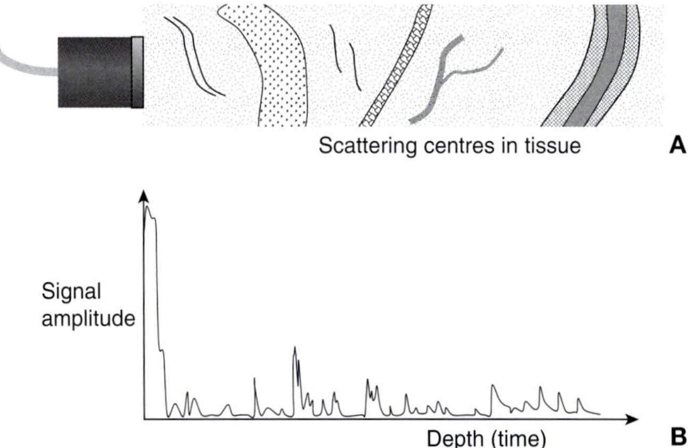

Figure 2.8. The fluctuating echo pattern produced by large and small structures lying along the beam.

fluctuations in gray shades. The resultant tissue image is a speckle pattern. In practice, overall image speckle is often a combination of "true speckle" from very small parenchymal tissue structures and "coarser speckle" from bigger, more distinct echoes from structures such as small blood vessels or muscle fibers. The "true" speckle does not depict the very small tissue structures, but is the result of their echoes interfering. The overall speckled appearance of an image may help to identify a tissue and its state. The patterns generated by muscle, tendon, and nerve are examples of this. Comparison of speckle patterns between machines is problematic, as transducer design and signal processing affect the pattern. Tissue motion may be measured by tracking the speckle pattern, for example, in myocardial velocity imaging or elastography.

The true speckle image of blood can be observed with a sensitive high-frequency B-mode scanner. The complex pattern relates to the motion of cells or groups of cells.

Frequency (Fourier) Analysis

When two waves or signals overlap, the resultant wave pattern has a shape different from either of the two original waves (see Interference section). If two or more waves of different frequencies overlap, complex resultant waveforms can be produced (**Fig. 2.9A–C**). The opposite process of breaking a complex waveform down into its frequency components is called frequency or Fourier analysis. A CW of pure sinusoidal shape has one frequency component (Fourier component). A pulse has a range of frequency components, its bandwidth (**Fig. 2.10**). A transducer is able to handle a specific range of frequencies (the transducer bandwidth). Frequencies outside this range are lost to further processing. A Doppler blood flow signal is often analyzed into its frequency components since they relate directly to the velocities of blood cells (see Spectral Doppler).

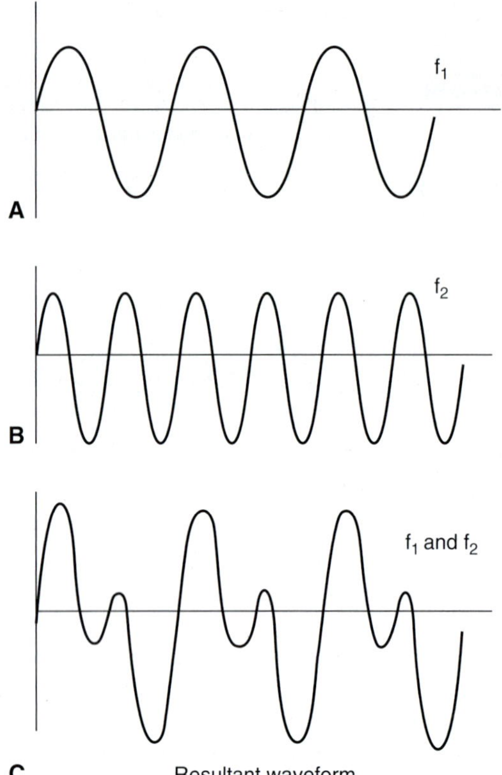

Figure 2.9.   Overlapping signals of different frequencies producing a complex signal.

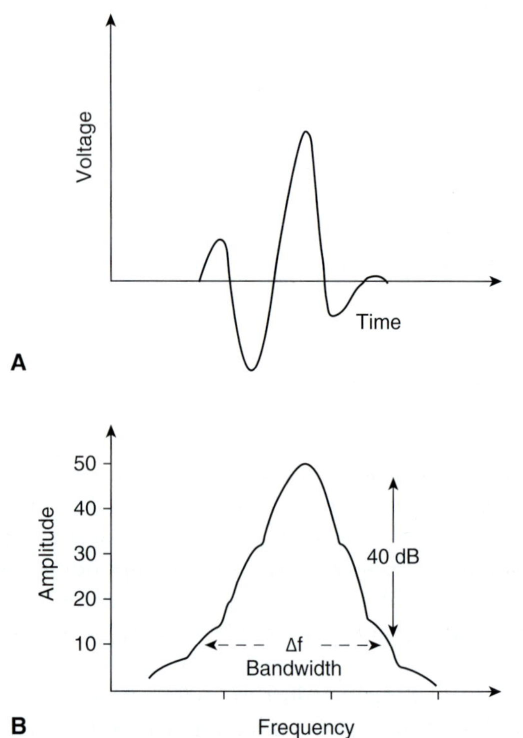

Figure 2.10.   **A:** A short pulsed signal. **B:** The spectrum of frequencies in the pulse and the pulse bandwidth.

Resonance

When a wave bounces around within a structure, there can be a buildup of wave amplitude (resonance) due to interference if the dimensions of the structure are simply related to the wavelength. Piezoelectric transducer elements are made equal in thickness to one half of the wavelength of the desired operating frequency. This gives efficient generation and detection of ultrasound. Continuous wave Doppler transducers have little or no damping and resonate at their operating frequency. Imaging and pulsed wave Doppler transducers have some damping, which spreads their sensitivity over a frequency range; that is, they have a wide bandwidth. Another interesting example is microbubbles of a particular size resonating in an ultrasound field. This resonance is exploited to improve their detection in blood when they are used as contrast agents.

Tip:
- Waves diffract and interfere. At high frequencies, and hence small wavelengths, diffraction can be controlled to produce directional beams.
- High frequencies produce narrow beams.
- Image speckle is produced by interference of echoes from small structures within tissue.
- Complex waveforms (ultrasonic or electronic) can be broken down into frequency components. Frequency analysis is a very powerful technique for characterizing signals.
- The frequency spectrum of a signal is important when Doppler blood flow detection is employed.
- Resonance can occur when ultrasound is reflected internally in a structure in which the dimensions are some multiple of the wavelength.
- Resonance is commonly encountered in transducer crystals and microbubbles.

IMAGING TECHNOLOGY

Transducers

The transducer most suited to a particular application is chosen at the start of an examination, usually by referring to the literature. The highest frequency that will give the required tissue penetration is selected. The size and shape are chosen to couple well with the patient surface and provide good acoustic access to the site of interest. **Figure 2.11** shows transducer shapes. Linear arrays are most commonly employed in musculoskeletal work. It is worth noting that modern transducers contain many active elements, for example, 256, which are under computer control during both transmission and reception. Computer control also governs both focusing and steering of the beam. Indeed, several beams may be manipulated simultaneously, provided there is clarity as to the

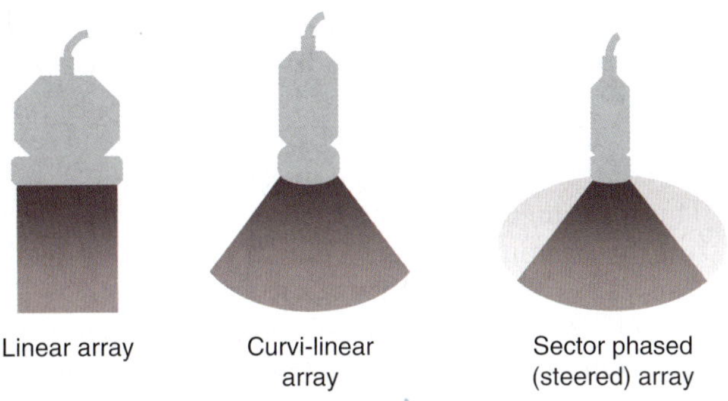

Figure 2.11. Common transducers and fields of view employed in musculoskeletal scanning.

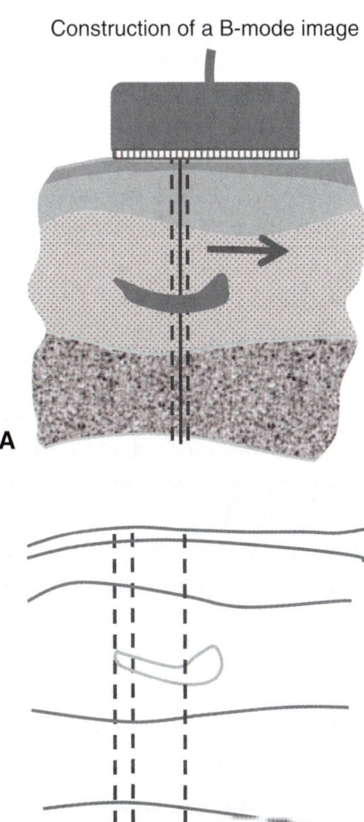

Figure 2.12. **A:** The production of an ultrasound image by sweeping a beam in a scan plane. **B:** For each beam step, a line of echoes is displayed on the screen.

sources of echoes. As mentioned earlier, the piezoelectric property exhibited by the elements is very well-suited to transmitting large pulses and then switching quickly to receive weak echoes.

Basic 2D B-Mode Imaging

To produce an image, a very short ultrasound pulse, say of length 0.5 mm and frequency 10 MHz, is transmitted along a narrow beam into the body. The beam may be regarded as the acoustic analogue of a light beam of width 1 mm from a small torch, which can be directed along different paths through the tissue. When a pulse passes through small or large discontinuities within the tissue, echoes are produced, which travel back to the transducer, where they are converted into electronic signals for the production of an image. In addition to echoes, two further pieces of information are required, namely, the beam direction and the return time of each echo after the instant of transmission. Using these times and the known speed of sound in tissue, the distance along the beam of each discontinuity can be calculated. Using a number of beam directions in a 2D plane, say 128, echo information (position and echo amplitude) can be presented in the appropriate pixels on the image display **(Fig. 2.12)**. Beam directions are determined by using neighboring groups of elements (say 16 at a time) across the transducer face. Different echo amplitudes are presented in different shades of gray, which can be related to the magnitude of the tissue discontinuities that produced the echoes. Since the speed of ultrasound is very high (1540 m per second), echo information is gathered rapidly, allowing many images to be presented per second, for example, at frame rates of 100 per second. At such high frame rates, tissue motion can be observed in the image and the scanning is said to be performed in real time. The small size of the transducer and the real-time nature of the images make ultrasound well-suited to examinations involving patient manipulation. The effects on the images of some physical processes such as attenuation, reflection, refraction, scattering, and non-linear propagation are discussed later to provide a fuller understanding of the generation of image data and the factors that are relevant for image interpretation.

Compound Imaging

In most scanners, tissue is interrogated from one beam direction. It is possible to scan the tissues from several directions. Effectively, the image is produced by adding (compounding) simple images from different directions. Compound imaging can provide more complete images, especially of smooth surfaces, which may reflect echoes away from the transducer at some beam directions. Compounding also lowers noise by averaging the echoes from different directions for each structure.

Extended Field-of-View (Panoramic) Imaging

In situations where there is interest in having wide images, the field of view may be extended by moving the transducer in a lateral direction. As this is done, the computer matches and links neighboring images. Extended images suit the requirements of limb and vascular imaging.

3D Imaging

Just as the beam transmission and echo collection can be performed in a 2D plane to produce a 2D image, the scanning can be performed throughout a 3D volume to produce a 3D image. Image presentation is more problematic in 3D. It is also worth noting that once a 3D volume data set has been collected, a 2D image can be presented of any section through the 3D volume. Imaging rates are slower in 3D than in conventional 2D since many more echoes have to be collected.

M-Mode Imaging

M-mode imaging is a simple technique in which a single beam is held fixed in a direction so as to interrogate a moving structure. Lines of consecutive echo data are displayed in parallel lines of adjacent pixels across the display. Traces of the tissue motions are produced. This mode is primarily used to record the motion of cardiac structures. Since the pulsing rate can be very high, for example, 1000 lines per second, fine temporal detail can be seen in the traces. These traces can also be readily recorded along with other simultaneous physiological data.

Needle Guidance

A needle tip can be imaged as it passes through a tissue. The real-time nature of the images makes them well-suited to interactive procedures such as biopsy, aspiration, and injection. Care should be taken to ensure that the needle tip is being imaged and not the needle body.

Internal Imaging

Small transducers can be manufactured that are suitable for endoscopy and inserting into arteries.

Scanner Controls

The controls of a scanner can be somewhat daunting when first encountered; however, they are quickly mastered if approached in a systematic way. The control panels of different machines can look quite different, but controls can be grouped under headings that describe their function.

1. Sensitivity controls govern the number and size of the echoes presented on the display. They are power, receiver gain, time gain compensation (TGC) (or depth gain compensation (DGC)), and frequency. Power and receiver gain have similar effects on the echoes. Frequency is determined by the transducer selected and has a large effect on the penetration. All of the sensitivity controls have an effect on the image resolution; for example, if the gain or power is too high, the displayed echoes will appear larger and coarser than optimum. TGC increases the gain after the instant of transmission and so compensates for attenuation of echoes from deeper structures. Some machines offer the option of putting the sensitivity largely under computer control (adaptive control). Here the computer senses whether echo magnitudes are close to what might be expected from each depth in tissue. There are attractions to this when the tissue or transducer is moving since the operator cannot continually alter the controls to optimize the image quality.

2. The transducer is selected from several available to suit the examination. Selection is determined by the size, shape, and frequency of the transducer.

3. The effect of display controls is usually obvious, but their impact on the final result is very significant. Image processing options are sometimes offered but are usually fixed when a technique is first being worked up.

4. Velocity range, whether in Doppler spectrograms or color flow images, should be set to show maximum image detail (see later).

5. To get the most from the versatile technology incorporated in a scanner, the user's manual should be studied.

ULTRASOUND IN TISSUE

Reflection

Reflection of ultrasound occurs at a boundary between two tissues where there is a change in density or compressibility (**Fig. 2.13A**). More formally stated, reflection occurs at a change in acoustic impedance (ρc), where ρ is the density and c is the speed of ultrasound. The speed of ultrasound in a medium is related to its compressibility. The size of an echo in an image (the shade of gray) relates to the size of the change in acoustic impedance. Shades of gray are therefore related to the properties of the tissues; however, signal processing in the scanner also plays an important part. Large changes in acoustic impedance at bone/soft tissue and gas/soft tissue interfaces can cause problems since the transmitted pulse is then greatly reduced or even totally blocked. An indication of the percentage energy reflected at some typical tissue interfaces is presented in **Table 2.2**. Properties of tissue are usually not well known, so these examples should be regarded as a rough guide. The high reflection at gas tissue boundaries should be

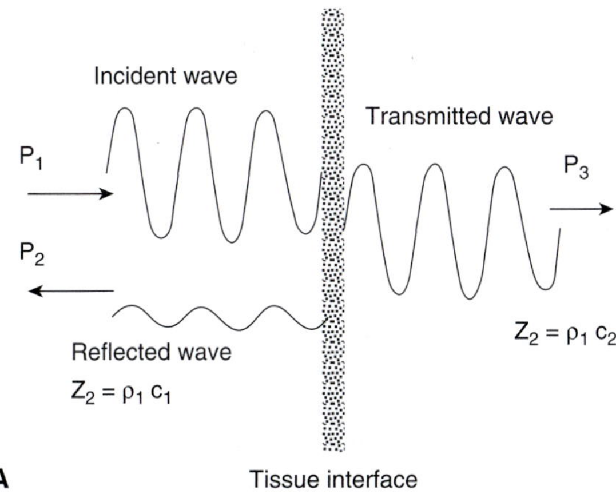

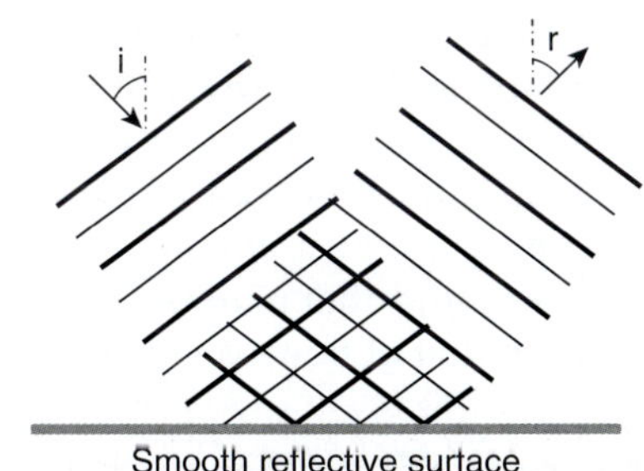

Figure 2.13. **A:** The reflection of ultrasound at a flat interface between two media of different acoustic impedance. **B:** The reflection of ultrasound at a smooth interface.

noted. It is important to use an adequate amount of coupling gel between the transducer and the skin since even a slightly dry patch greatly attenuates the beam. In this situation there is little to be gained by pressing harder; indeed, this may compress blood vessels. Reflection of ultrasound at a smooth surface is similar to light reflecting at a mirror or glass plate (specular reflection) **(Fig. 2.13B).**

Scattering

Ultrasound traveling through tissue interacts with many small structures of size similar to or less than its wavelength. Some of the wave energy is scattered in many directions **(Fig. 2.14).** Scattering is important. It provides most of the echo information for both B-mode imaging and Doppler blood flow techniques. Echo signals from scattering produce the speckled patterns depicted in

TABLE 2.2.	Percentage Energy Reflected at Tissue Interfaces
Fat/muscle	1.1
Muscle/blood	0.1
Bone/fat	48.9
Bone/muscle	41.2
Soft tissue/water	0.2
Soft tissue/air	99.9

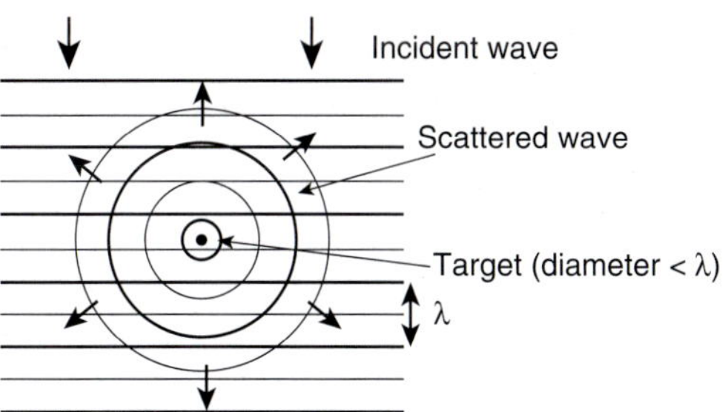

Figure 2.14. Scattering of ultrasound at a target smaller than the wavelength.

images. Red cells in blood are the scattering centers that produce the echoes used in Doppler techniques (see later). Scattering at a nonsmooth tissue interface enables it to be imaged more easily than a smooth interface since echoes are detected over a wide range of angles of incidence of the beam.

Refraction

Refraction is the change in direction of a beam when it crosses a boundary, at an angle to the perpendicular of the boundary **(i)** and where the speeds of sound in the two media are different **(Fig. 2.15).** **Table 2.3** shows examples of the small deviations that occur at soft tissue boundaries. Refraction is not a severe problem in most tissue imaging. At tissue/bone boundaries, big deviations are caused by large differences in speed of ultrasound between soft tissue and bone.

Lenses and Mirrors

Lenses and mirrors can be constructed for ultrasound as for light by exploiting reflection and refraction **(Fig. 2.16).** Lenses are designed by selecting material in which the speed of ultrasound differs from that of water or tissue.

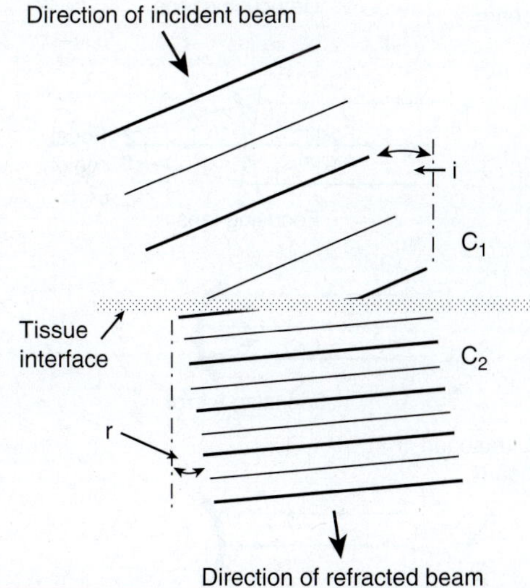

Figure 2.15. Refraction of a beam on passing through an interface at an angle where there is a change in speed of ultrasound.

TABLE 2.3.	Refraction at Tissue Interfaces for Angle of Incidence of 30°	
Bone/soft tissue		19°
Muscle/blood		1°
Muscle/fat		2°

Mirrors of metal or gas layers produce very strong reflection. Lenses are most commonly found on the front face of transducers. Mirrors work well but are rarely used.

Tip:
- An echo is generated at a change in acoustic impedance. The bigger the change, the bigger the echo. It does not matter whether the change is an increase or decrease.
- The acoustic impedance of a tissue is related to the density and compressibility (rigidity) of the tissue.
- Bone and gas have acoustic impedances that are markedly different from those of soft tissue.
- Reflection is said to occur at surfaces of dimensions greater than the ultrasound wavelength, and for smooth surfaces it is analogous to light reflecting from a mirror or glass plate.
- Scattering occurs at small structures of dimensions similar to or smaller than the ultrasound wavelength.
- Very small tissue structures and blood cells are scattering centers of interest.
- Refraction occurs at a tissue interface where the speed of ultrasound changes.

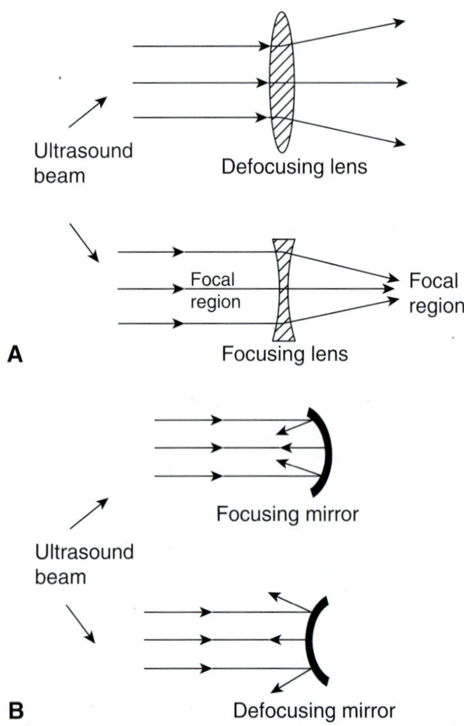

Figure 2.16.   Ultrasound lenses (**A**) and mirrors (**B**).

Absorption and Attenuation

On passing through tissue, the orderly vibrational energy of an ultrasound wave is converted into random vibrational heat energy. The wave pressure amplitude therefore reduces with distance traveled. This process of reduction in wave energy is known as absorption. Absorption rate depends on the tissue involved. Also, the higher the ultrasound frequency, the higher is the absorption rate. In addition to absorption, other effects contribute to the total attenuation of the wave amplitude. These are reflection, scattering, and beam divergence. The last two are also frequency-dependent. Attenuation increases over the diagnostic frequency range. Within a scanner, the electronics can compensate for the reduction of echo amplitude with depth, and the appropriate controls should be set to do this as well as possible. Some machines use adaptive compensation by which the computing system detects the rate of amplitude reduction and compensates automatically. **Table 2.4** presents attenuation commonly encountered. Examination of the attenuation of different tissues shows that many soft tissues have similar attenuation but that of bone is much larger.

Nonlinear Propagation (Harmonics)

The shape of a pulse passing through tissue is altered by a process known as nonlinear propagation. This phenomenon is very evident for high-amplitude waves (e.g., 1 MPa). Pascal (Pa) is the unit of pressure. One Pascal is very low pressure, 0.00001 of atmospheric pressure. Megapascals (MPa) are encountered in clinical beams. The process arises since the speed of ultrasound is higher in regions of the wave of high positive pressure amplitude than in negative pressure regions. The difference in speed is due to the density of the tissue being altered by pressure. As the waveform passes through a tissue, the positive half-cycles catch up on the negative half-cycles and distort the waveform since the speed of sound is higher in the denser compressed tissue (**Fig. 2.17**). The distorted pulses become more spiked and therefore contain more high-frequency components. Nonlinear distortion is widely employed in a technique called harmonic imaging since it can be exploited to produce narrow

TABLE 2.4.	Thickness (mm) of Tissue Required to Attenuate Intensity by Half at 10 MHz	
Blood		20
Water		140
Fat		5
Tendon		1.5
Muscle		1.5
Bone		0.2
Soft tissue (average)		4

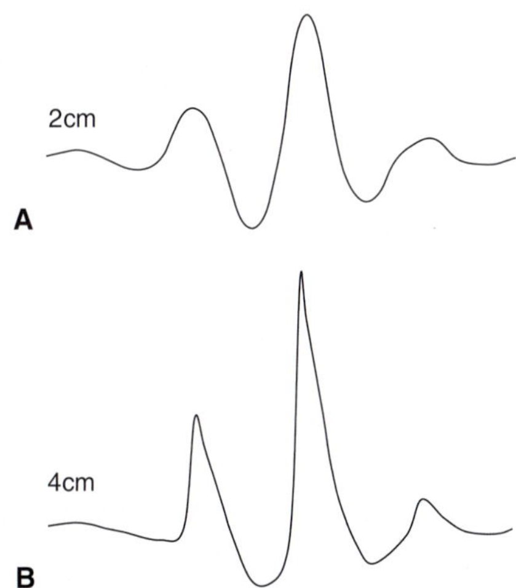

Figure 2.17. Distortion of an ultrasound pulse (**A**) on passing through tissue. The deeper spiked pulse (**B**) contains more frequencies, that is, harmonics.

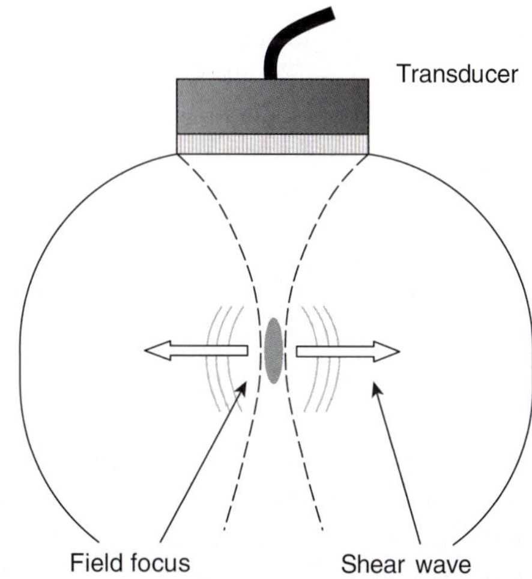

Figure 2.18. Shear wave generation by the radiation force at the focus of an ultrasonic field.

beams and hence greater image detail. The waveform is distorted more in high-pressure regions of the beam than in low-pressure regions. In effect, this means higher frequencies in pulses along the central axis of the beam. Distortion is less at the side of the beam and in the side lobes. After electronic filtering out of low frequencies, only echoes from near the central axis are used. Harmonic imaging is widely employed and is often the default setting when a machine is switched on.

Tissue Characterization

In some applications of medical ultrasound, there is interest in obtaining information on the nature of the tissue that produced the echoes. Measurements of parameters such as speed of sound, attenuation, and scattering coefficient are attempted. Tissue characterization is often made difficult by degradation of the ultrasound beam by fat or muscle between the transducer and the site of interest.

Elastography

There is interest in the measurement of tissue elasticity in the study of, for example, tumors or contracted versus relaxed muscle.[5] By applying a force to a tissue, changes in position of the echo speckle pattern can be used to evaluate the elasticity. The aim is to provide quantitative palpation for tissues deep within the body. But elastography has also been used to investigate superficial tendons such as the tendo Achilles, which lies only a few millimeters deep under the skin. Methods employed to apply force to a tissue range from simply pushing the transducer to exploiting the radiation force of a second sound beam to generate shear waves that spread out around the focus of this second (force) beam. As shown in **Figure 2.18**, a target tissue at the focus of the force beam will experience an impulse when subjected to an ultrasound pulse. This impulse produces a shear wave that travels sideways from the direction of the ultrasound beam. Labels such as "radiation force" or "supersonic" are used for these techniques.

Shear waves of a few hundred hertz travel well through tissue, whereas those in the megahertz range are strongly attenuated. The frequencies of the shear wave in this approach are determined by the rate of pulsing of the force transducer (a few hundred hertz). The speed of a shear wave and its wavelength (speed, 1 m/second; wavelength, 1 mm) are different from those of ultrasound waves as commonly encountered in diagnostic imaging (speed, 1500 m/second; wavelength, 0.5 mm). As the tissue moves under the influence of the shear wave, for example, back and forth over typically 50 μm, the ultrasound scanner operating at a very high frame rate can image these small motions and measure the shear wave speed at each point. The elasticity is calculated from this speed. By using a number of focuses along the beam, the shear wave can be made to spread out over a bigger area, allowing an image of elasticity to be constructed. The elasticity measure is called the shear modulus, the unit of which is pascal. A pascal equals 1 kg/ms^2.

- Nonlinear propagation occurs most near the axis of the beam where the wave amplitude is high relative to the sides of the beam. By only detecting the harmonics, the beam is effectively made narrower, giving better lateral resolution (see later).
- Harmonics frequencies are also generated when ultrasound interacts with contrast microbubbles. Detection of these frequencies is exploited in the location of bubbles in vivo.
- Many operators use harmonic imaging as the method of choice.
- Many attempts have been made to identify tissue types by measuring the acoustic properties of tissue, for example, attenuation, scattering, and speed of sound. Some success has been achieved where there is well-defined anatomy, but difficulties often arise where the ultrasound beam is distorted by overlying layers of fat and muscle.
- Present research into tissue characterization seeks to develop elastography.

DOPPLER TECHNIQUES

Doppler Effect

The Doppler effect is the change (shift) in the observed frequency of a wave due to motion of the source of the wave or the observer. If there is no relative movement, the observed frequency equals the transmitted frequency (**Fig. 2.19A**). If the observer is moving toward a static source, an increase in frequency is observed since more wave cycles per second are encountered (**Fig. 2.19B**). For motion away from the source, fewer wave cycles per second are encountered (**Fig. 2.19C**). The size of the Doppler shift is directly related to the size of the velocity of motion. In another situation, the source may move toward a static observer, the wavelengths are compressed as the source follows the wave, and hence there is an increase in frequency (**Fig. 2.19D**). Motion of the source away from the observer stretches the wavelength and gives a decrease in frequency (**Fig. 2.19E**).

In Doppler technology, a beam from a static transducer is scattered back from tissues to produce echo signals (**Fig. 2.20**). If blood cells are moving toward the transducer, the total Doppler effect is produced by the cells moving through the waves plus the cells following the reflected ultrasound, and hence increasing the frequency further. The motion of the cells toward the transducer produces an increase in ultrasound frequency because of this "double Doppler" effect. Likewise, a reduction in frequency is produced by cells moving away from the transducer. The electronics of the machine can identify these upward and downward frequency shifts; that is, directional information along the ultrasound beam is preserved. Signals are presented above or below a baseline

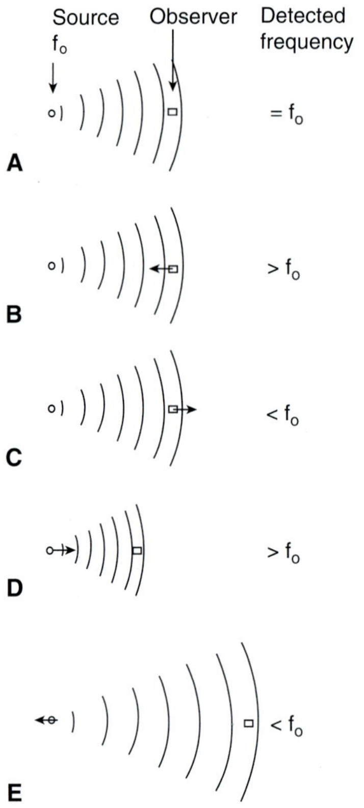

Figure 2.19.   The Doppler effect as observed for different relative motion of the source and observer (**A–E**).

in a spectrogram (see later) or as different colors in an image, depending on the direction of motion.

As shown in **Figure 2.21**, it should be noted that for a beam at an angle to the direction of motion, it is the velocity component along the beam axis (v_1) that is measured when the Doppler effect is used. If blood vessel walls are imaged and flow is assumed to be parallel to the walls, the beam/flow angle may be measured on a B-mode image, allowing the velocity along the vessel to be calculated with the Doppler shift equation. The machine

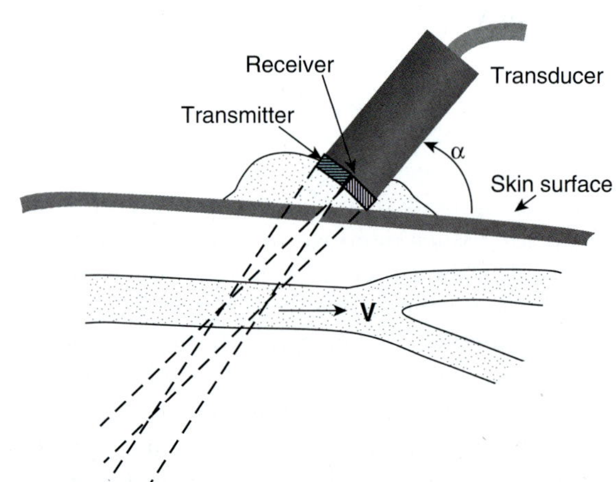

Figure 2.20.   Examination of a blood vessel with a continuous wave Doppler device.

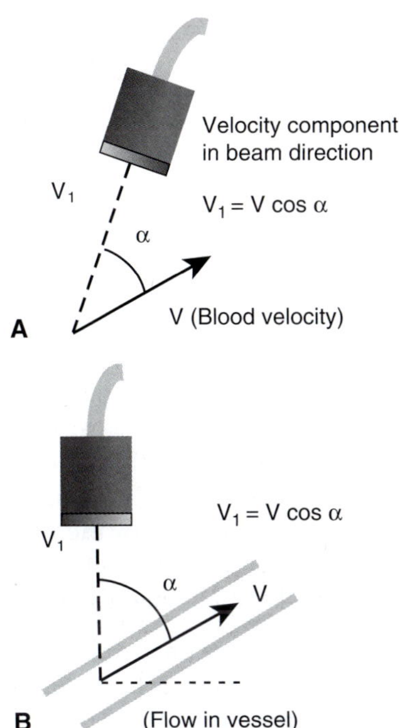

Figure 2.21. **A:** V_1 is the component of the velocity V along the beam axis. **B:** Measurement of a velocity component when an ultrasound beam interrogates blood flow at an angle.

does this automatically after the angle calliper is lined up parallel to the vessel walls.

The Doppler equation links Doppler shift, transmitted frequency, velocity, and ultrasound beam/motion angle:

$$f_d = 2vf_t \cos \alpha /c \quad \text{or} \quad v = f_d c/2f_t \cos \alpha$$

where f_d is the Doppler shift frequency, f_t is the transmitted frequency, v is the velocity, α is the angle, and c is the speed of ultrasound.

In blood flow there can be many moving groups of cells with different velocities. Each group of cells gives rise to an echo signal with a particular Doppler frequency shift, and all of these signals combine to produce the Doppler signal from the blood. This signal can be analyzed into a spectrum of frequencies by Fourier techniques. The frequency components in the spectrum can then be converted to velocities in the blood by using the Doppler equation.

At present, the terms "speed" and "velocity" are used interchangeably in clinical Doppler. Strictly speaking, speed is the rate of change of position, and velocity has two aspects—speed and true direction. Velocity is called a "vector" and speed is "scalar." Vector Doppler techniques are being developed where speed is depicted as color and velocity direction as arrows superimposed on the color image. Alternatively, velocity vectors can be presented with arrow direction for blood flow direction and arrow length for blood speed.

The Doppler effect is exploited in various ways to present information on blood flow and tissue motion. It can provide very detailed information on blood flow.

Continuous Wave Doppler

In very basic, yet sensitive, CW Doppler instruments, the transducer contains two adjacent crystals. One transmits continuously, while the other receives continuously. The transmitted beam and the zone of reception are of the same shape and at a small angle to each other so that they cross at a crude focus in front of the transducer. Since reception is the converse of transmission, the zone of reception has the same shape as the transmission beam. The "focus" is at a depth determined by having the crystal faces at a fixed angle to each other. The focus for a Doppler 2-MHz fetal heart detector could be around 10-cm depth, whereas that for a 10-MHz blood flow device could be at 2 cm. These devices are often small pocket instruments.

Basic Pulsed Wave Doppler

A basic PW Doppler instrument has one crystal and transmits pulses which may be regarded as equally spaced samples of a CW beam. Since pulses are used, echoes from a selected region (sample volume) can be obtained by noting the echo return time. In a manner similar to that of a CW Doppler, the electronics can extract Doppler shift to obtain velocity. At present, the only widely used basic PW Doppler is for transcranial examinations.

Combined B-Mode and Doppler (Duplex Doppler)

Pulse wave Doppler is usually combined with a B-mode imager to aid selection of the site of the sample volume from which Doppler signals are collected and to permit measurement of the beam/motion angle. The size of the sample volume can be varied to suit the application. This combination is often referred to as duplex Doppler.

Color Flow Imaging and B-Mode

Pulse wave Doppler can be expanded to obtain Doppler information from many neighboring sites along the ultrasound beam. Then by scanning the beam, a two-dimensional Doppler image can be constructed. The mean velocity at each site is presented as a color-coded pixel, and the beam/flow angle is taken to be zero when the color coding is related to velocity. This could obviously be a large source of error; therefore, interpretation of images normally involves differences from known patterns at specific sites. Conventionally, flow toward the transducer is coded in shades of red and orange, and flow away as shades of blue and green. This imaging technique is known by several names, such as color flow Doppler, color flow imaging (CFI), and color velocity imaging. Collection of the necessary number of echo signals and signal processing take more time in Doppler

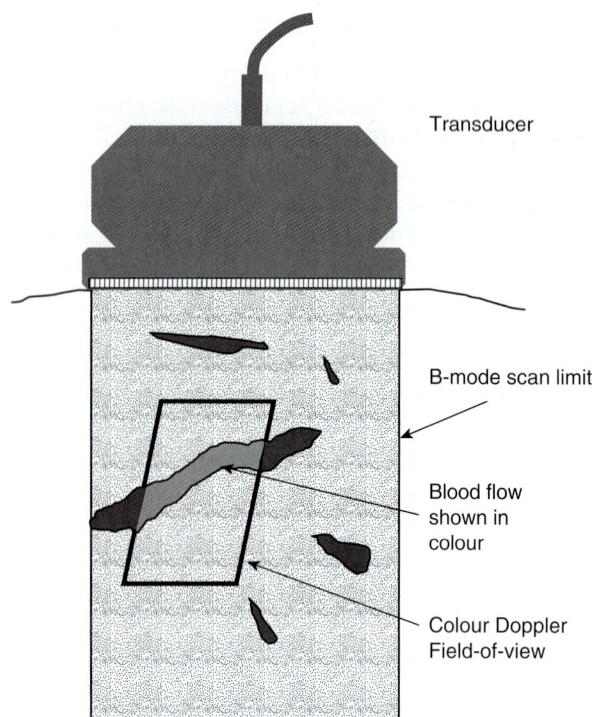

Figure 2.22.   The color flow imaging box located within the B-mode field of view.

imaging than in B-mode imaging. The frame rates are therefore slower in color Doppler than in B-mode, for example, 15 frames per second versus 100. To help speed up the Doppler frame rate, the field of view (image box) is often made smaller for this mode **(Fig. 2.22)**.

Power Doppler

Doppler images can also be created in which the power of Doppler-shifted echoes is presented in each pixel. The power shows the magnitude of the signal from moving blood rather than the velocity. Averaging can be performed over several consecutive frames. This reduces the noise in the image and hence permits weaker blood flow signals from small vessels to be depicted. Velocity images are less suited to averaging since forward and reverse flows cancel out. Power Doppler images are popular for portraying the blood pool rather than the flow.

Doppler Tissue Imaging

Doppler techniques used for imaging tissue motion are similar to those used for imaging blood flow. With tissue the echo signals are stronger and the speeds lower, so the technology is adjusted to suit this situation. Doppler tissue imaging (DTI) is mostly employed to study myocardial action, but it can be used with other muscles and tissues.

Spectral Doppler

When a sample volume is located at a blood site, there will be a range of blood velocities within the sample volume, which typically might be 1 or 2 mm in diameter. There will therefore be a range of Doppler shifts in the composite echo signal received at the transducer. It was noted in the discussion on interference that individual waves combine to produce a complex signal that contains the frequencies of the component waves (Fourier components). This complex signal contains the Doppler shifts of the echoes and hence information on the speeds of the targets that produced the echoes. The complex signal can be broken down into the frequency components, which provide the speeds of the moving targets in the sample volume. The process goes by the name of Fourier or frequency analysis. It is an extremely widely used technique for analyzing all sorts of electronic signals.

If a Doppler shift signal is divided into short time segments, say of 5 or 10 milliseconds, each section can be analyzed into its frequency components; that is, an instantaneous Doppler spectrum is obtained for each segment. Each spectrum can be drawn as a line of gray or coloured spots. When the consecutive lines are placed vertically and adjacent to each other, a "spectrogram" or "sonogram" is constructed. This is a popular way of depicting the changing Doppler frequencies through the cardiac cycle **(Fig. 2.23)**. The operator can alter the scale of presentation of the vertical (frequency/velocity) and horizontal (time) axes for convenience of observation. It is good practice to regard the spectrogram as a type of image in which more detail is seen if it is well presented. If the beam/motion angle is measured by manipulating a calliper at the sample volume site, the machine will convert the vertical axis from frequency to velocity.

Tip:
- The Doppler effect is a very sensitive and accurate detector of motion. It is mostly used to study blood flow, but it can also be employed for tissue motion.
- Users of Doppler techniques should be aware of the large effect of beam/motion angle on velocity measurement.
- Most Doppler devices measure the velocity component along the ultrasound beam axis.
- Most Doppler instruments can provide directional information.
- Processes such as absorption, attenuation, scattering, refraction, and nonlinear propagation discussed for pulse-echo imaging also apply to Doppler methods.
- Doppler images and spectrograms are produced in real time, making them very useful for the study of physiological function.
- Doppler spectra contain a great deal of information on flow at the interrogated site.

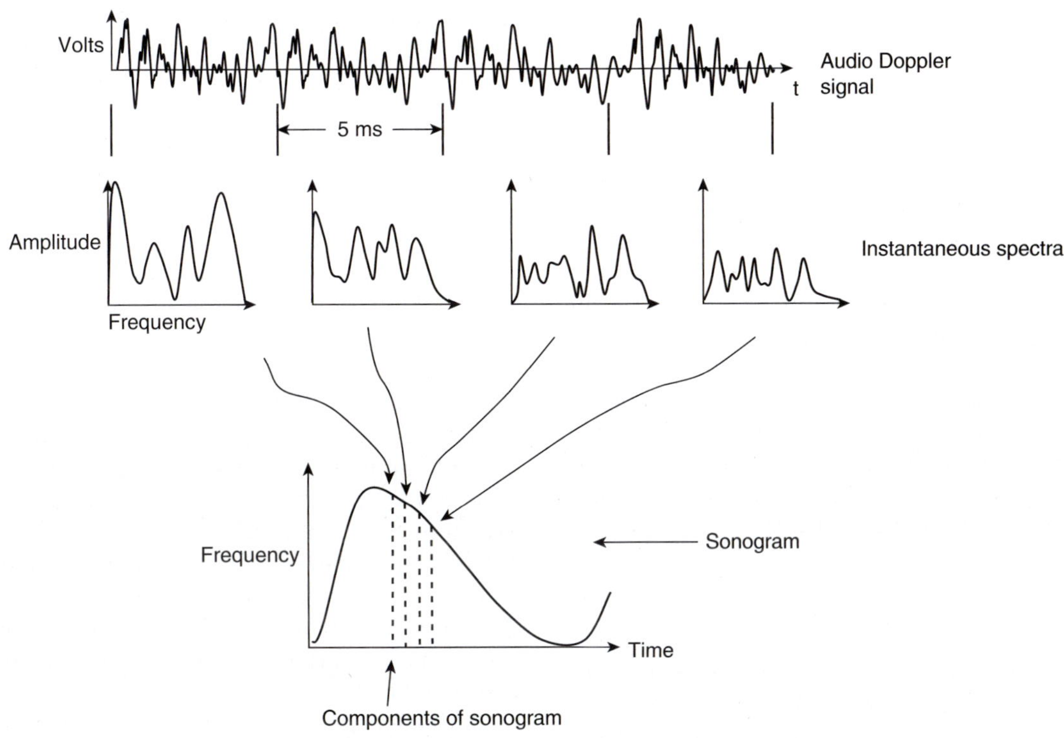

Figure 2.23. Doppler spectra for each section of a Doppler signal combined to produce a sonogram (spectrogram).

RESOLUTION

The detail (resolution) in a particular image, spectrum, or trace depends on a number of factors related to the shape of the ultrasound beam, the rate of data collection, and the signal processing in the ultrasound machine. It is important to have a working knowledge of resolution since it has a direct bearing on the interpretation of the information presented to the clinical operator. The high resolution of ultrasound imaging, particularly along the beam direction, makes it a technique well-suited for measuring length, area, and volume. Calliper packages are a feature of most machines.

Pulse-Echo Mode Resolution (B-Mode, 3D-Mode, M-Mode, and Panoramic)

The spatial resolution in B-mode imaging has three components—axial, lateral, and elevational. Their combined effect determines the detail that can be seen in an image.

The axial resolution is the smallest separation of two targets lying along the beam axis for which individual echoes can be seen. It depends on the length of the transmitted ultrasound pulse. Shorter pulses may be produced at higher frequencies and hence better axial resolution. For a 10-MHz pulse it is typically 0.4 mm.

The lateral resolution is the smallest separation of two discernible targets placed side by side at the same depth in the scan plane. It depends on the beam width.

Narrower beams can be produced at higher frequencies and hence better lateral resolution. For a 10-MHz pulse it is typically 1.0 mm.

The elevational resolution is the smallest separation of two discernible targets placed side by side at the same depth out of the scan plane. It depends on the beam width in the out of scan plane direction. For a 10-MHz pulse it is typically 2.0 mm.

Contrast resolution is the smallest change in echo signal level (shade of gray) that can be detected between regions in an image. It is determined by the variations in size of the neighboring echoes. Averaging can be used to reduce these noise fluctuations and hence improve the contrast resolution. Contrast resolution is quite poor, typically 20%.

Temporal resolution is the smallest separation in time for which two events can be identified separately. High frame rates replenish echo data rapidly and hence improve the temporal resolution. Fifty frames per second give a temporal resolution of 20 milliseconds.

3D imaging and B-mode have similar beam properties. However, since it takes longer to scan a 3D volume than a 2D plane, the line density in the volume scanned or the volume scan rate may be low. These compromises will adversely affect the spatial resolution or the temporal resolution of the 3D image.

M-mode imaging has spatial components similar to those of B-mode, but since the beam has a fixed direction and pulses rapidly, temporal resolution is very high, for example, 1 millisecond for a pulsing rate of 1000 per second.

Doppler Resolution

The spatial resolution for Doppler techniques is similar to that of pulse-echo imaging since it is determined mainly by the transmitted pulse length and the shape of the beam. The temporal resolution is determined by the time it takes to collect echoes and to process the information to produce a spectrogram or color image. The temporal resolution in a spectrogram is typically 5 to 10 milliseconds. In CFI, the frame rate is typically 30 frames per second, but it can be increased by reducing the size of the field of view. Velocity (frequency) resolution is not considered very often; it is typically 5% in a spectrogram and 10% in a color image.

CONTRAST AGENTS

Contrast agents for medical ultrasound imaging take the form of micrometer-sized thin-walled bubbles containing gas.[6] They are injected into blood vessels and can be detected in major and minor blood vessels throughout the body. They greatly enhance the magnitude of the scattered signal from blood. Different manufacturers use different formulations of gas and wall material, for example, large gas molecules to extend the lifetime of the bubbles by restricting diffusion, and lipid walls to give flexibility and hence a good response to the pressure wave. Microbubbles provide much more scattering than any other type of particle of the same size because of the large change in acoustic impedance at the gas/liquid boundary. Further enhancement of the scattered echo is obtained by the coincidence that microbubbles resonate at megahertz frequencies. Four or five agents are commercially available at present. However, these agents have not found much application in the musculoskeletal field to date.

ARTIFACTS

The phenomena that affect the propagation of ultrasound in tissue give rise to not only genuine information but also artifacts. Artifacts are false results in imaging or Doppler data. It may be possible to avoid some artifacts in a particular situation by the scanning technique, but most often they are recognized from experience and either explained or ignored. Occasionally, artifacts provide clinical information on the tissue scanned, for example, reduction in echo amplitudes beyond or within a highly attenuating tumor. Conversely, echo amplitudes are increased (enhanced) in locations beyond a liquid-filled cyst or blood vessel. When a beam intersects the edge of a structure, say a cyst or a tendon, adjacent parts

of the beam can be in different tissues that have different speeds of sound. This defocuses the beam, so weaker echoes are detected beyond intersection and shadowing is evident. Strongly reflecting boundaries such as bone/soft tissue or blood/plaque produce large echoes, but again shadow regions occur beyond them. When there is a lack of a coupling agent between the transducer and the skin, strong shadowing can result. It was noted above that scattering at small structures as in muscle provides images that are a mixture of true boundaries and speckle artifact.

Multiple reflection echo artifacts can be generated when ultrasound bounces around between strongly reflecting boundaries, for example, the transducer face and a fat/muscle boundary. Multiple reflections are depicted as a repeating echo pattern due to later and later arrival of echoes after the instant of transmission. Multiple reflections can occur in thin layers or small structures when the echoes are not resolved and hence extend the pattern rather than register separately. A marked example of this is multiple reflections within the body of a biopsy needle.

Refraction at soft tissue interfaces is weak and not usually appreciated as distinct deviation of the beam but rather as a contribution to beam degradation. At a bone/soft tissue boundary the angle of refraction can be large, and essentially the beam direction is not known beyond it.

Badly set up sensitivity controls result in the overemphasis or underemphasis of regions in the image. It is usually not possible to eliminate this completely. The operator should always strive to produce a well-balanced image.

The artifacts that affect pulse-echo imaging techniques also affect Doppler techniques; however, they are not always noticed since image detail is poorer and is not always scrutinized to the same degree. However, the operator should be aware that attenuation, enhancement, refraction, multiple reflections, and poorly set up controls can affect both Doppler CFI and spectral Doppler. For example, the lack of a Doppler signal may be due the beam being refracted and thereby not interrogating the site of interest.

A common Doppler artifact occurs in PW methods when the ultrasound pulsing rate is too low to handle the high Doppler shifts obtained from rapid flow. In effect, the sampling rate of echoes is too low to permit the electronics to extract Doppler shift frequencies accurately. As a result, high velocities are depicted as going in the wrong direction both in spectra and in color flow images. This artifact is called "aliasing." Recognition of it can be used clinically to identify pathology, for example, high velocities through a stenosis. Switching to a CW mode can remove aliasing, but then the range information on the site interrogated is lost. Adjusting the velocity scale of both Doppler images and spectra to cater for high values can help to remove aliasing since this alters the pulsing rate. However, interrogation of deep sites requires low pulsing rates to allow time for the echoes to return, and it may not be possible to avoid aliasing.

Again Doppler artifacts are coped with by building up experience in normal and pathological cases. Flow can be extremely complex, so careful consideration of likely flow patterns should be the norm.

SAFETY

Hazard in ultrasound scanning of musculoskeletal structures is not a concern since specially sensitive tissues are not insonated. Discussion of the safety of ultrasound usually relates to the eye or the fetus, and even there no harmful effects have been confirmed for clinical techniques. Several national and international organizations have monitored the situation over recent decades. Further information can be found via the British Medical Ultrasound Society website[7] and in review articles.[8] That said, it is good practice to avoid unnecessary exposure of sites such as nerves, bone/soft tissue or gas/soft tissue boundaries. This is easily done by not leaving the transducer resting on one location.

While reading the safety literature, technical aspects of any study need to be compared with those employed in clinical work. For example, check out ultrasound frequency, power, intensity definition, details of a PW or CW beam, and exposure time. If the conditions are not close to those of clinical practice, the results may be of biological interest but have little relevance to patient safety.

Two indices have been developed for user guidance as to the possibility of tissue damage during an examination. These are Mechanical Index (MI) and Thermal Index (TI), related to tissue heating and mechanical damage, respectively. The manufacturer is required to display these indices on the screen of clinical scanners. Acceptable values for these indices should be obtained from the literature describing a particular technique. Typically a machine is set up to keep the index values <1.

REFERENCES

1. Allan PL, McDicken WN, Pozniak MA, et al. *Clinical Doppler Ultrasound.* 2nd ed. Edinburgh, Scotland: Churchill Livingstone; 2006.
2. Duck FA. *Physical Properties of Tissue: A Comprehensive Reference Book.* London, England: Academic Press; 1990.
3. Hoskins PR, Thrush A, Martin K, et al. *Diagnostic Ultrasound: Physics and Equipment.* London, England: Greenwich Medical Media; 2003.
4. McDicken WN. *Diagnostic Ultrasonics: Principles and Use of Instruments.* 3rd ed. Edinburgh, Scotland: Churchill Livingstone; 1991.
5. Shinohara M, Sabra K, Gennisson JL, et al. Real-time visualization of muscle stiffness distribution with ultrasound shear wave imaging during muscle contraction. *Muscle Nerve.* 2010;42(3):438–441.
6. Claudon M, Cosgrove D, Albrecht T, et al. Guidelines and good clinical practice recommendations for contrast enhanced ultrasound (CEUS)—update 2008. *Ultraschall Med.* 2008;29(1):28–44.
7. The British Medical Ultrasound Society (BMUS). http://www.bmus.org.
8. Starritt H, Duck FA. Safety. In: Allan PL, Baxter GM, Weston MJ, eds. *Clinical Ultrasound.* 3rd ed. Edinburgh, Scotland: Churchill Livingstone; 2011.

INTRODUCTION

Ultrasound has become increasingly important in the assessment of the shoulder in recent years. It is as accurate as magnetic resonance imaging (MRI) in diagnosing rotator cuff tears[1] and is also cheap and quick. Patients prefer ultrasound to MRI.[2] The relative ease of access makes ultrasound ideal for a "one-stop shop" approach.[3] Ultrasound-guided interventions are widely used. The objection that ultrasound is operator-dependent applies to other imaging techniques, clinical assessment, and surgical interventions.

ANATOMY AND EXAMINATION TECHNIQUE

The anatomy and examination technique of the shoulder is well illustrated on the website of the European Society of Musculoskeletal Radiology.[4]

The tendons of the four muscles that contribute to the rotator cuff coalesce to insert on the greater and lesser tuberosities of the humerus **(Fig. 3.1)**. Subscapularis

originates from the anterior surface of the scapular blade and inserts on the lesser tuberosity. Supraspinatus originates from the suprascapular fossa and infraspinatus and teres minor from the dorsal surface of the scapula inferior to its spine. They insert in sequence from anterior to posterior on the greater tuberosity: supraspinatus on the superior facet and infraspinatus on the middle facet, although the footprint of the infraspinatus tendon is larger than that of supraspinatus and occupies much more of the tuberosity than previously thought. Teres minor inserts posterior to infraspinatus. Overlapping tendon fibers diffuse the load across the cuff rather than being concentrated in a single tendon.[5,6] The subacromial/subdeltoid bursa is interposed between the rotator cuff tendons and the coracoacromial arch, which comprises the coracoid, acromion, coracoacromial ligament (CAL), and acromioclavicular joint (ACJ) **(Fig. 3.2)**.

The long head of biceps (LHB) tendon is not part of the rotator cuff, but it is an important anatomical landmark. It originates from the superior glenoid labrum at the supraglenoid tubercle and runs through the joint,

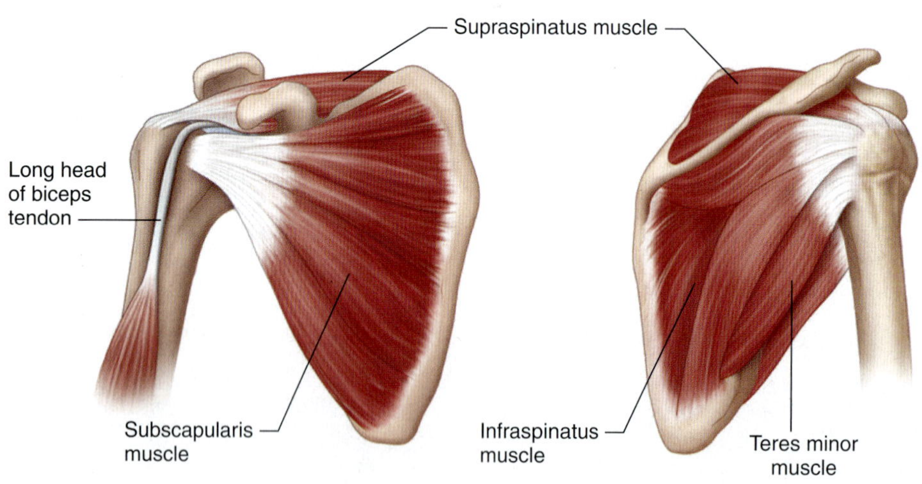

Figure 3.1.   Subscapularis originates from the anterior surface of the scapular blade. Supraspinatus originates from the supraspinatus fossa on the posterior aspect of the scapula. Infraspinatus and teres minor originate below the scapular spine. The long head of biceps tendon lies between subscapularis and supraspinatus and is an important ultrasound landmark.

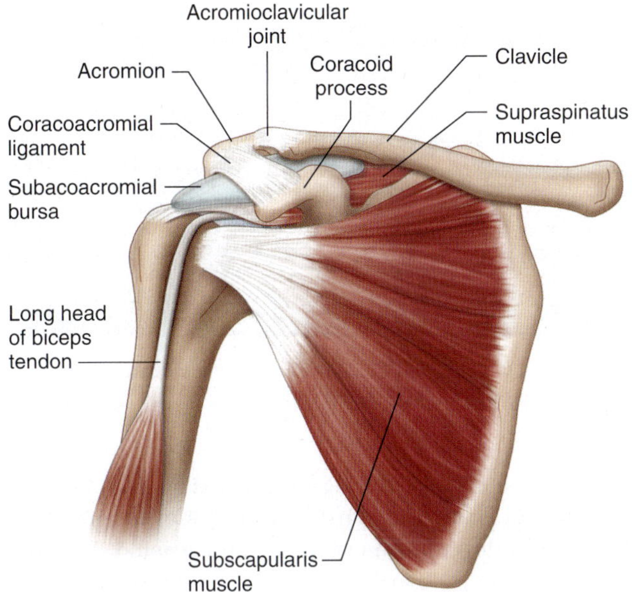

Figure 3.2.   The subacromial bursa lies between the rotator cuff tendons and the coracoacromial arch.

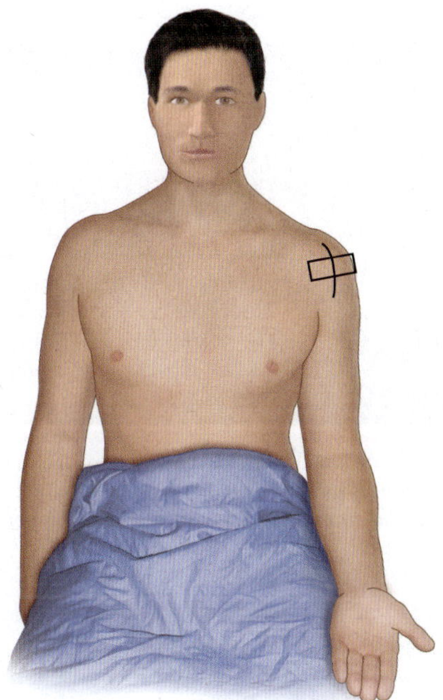

Figure 3.3.   The LHB tendon is examined with the patient's elbow flexed at 90 degrees and the hand palm-up on the lap. Black line, long head of biceps tendon (LHB), black box, position of transducer for transverse scan of LHB.

separating subscapularis from the other rotator cuff tendons at the rotator interval **(Fig. 3.1)**, then enters the bicipital groove and runs distally to its myotendinous junction in the mid-arm.

Supraspinatus and infraspinatus are innervated by the suprascapular nerve, a branch of the brachial plexus that passes through the suprascapular notch to supply supraspinatus and then through the spinoglenoid notch to supply infraspinatus. Subscapularis is supplied by subscapular branches of the brachial plexus and teres minor by the axillary nerve.

The articular cortex of the humeral head is usually smooth, although small pits are common. The greater and lesser tuberosities are usually slightly flat and depressed relative to the articular cortex. Hyaline cartilage covers the articular cortex. Enthesis fibrocartilage covers the tuberosities. Both types of cartilage are anechoic on ultrasound and appear in continuity.

ULTRASOUND EXAMINATION: TECHNIQUE AND APPEARANCES

In contrast to most other joints where the examination is targeted at a particular part of the joint to address a specific problem, ultrasound of the shoulder is usually a "whole joint" examination and is performed in a routine sequence.[7,8]

The patient is seated on a swivel chair and the height adjusted so that the patient's shoulder is at a comfortable level for the examiner who stands in front of or behind the patient. I prefer to stand behind the patient. I can look over the patient at the ultrasound screen, lean forward to adjust the controls, and, importantly, support my hand

on the patient's shoulder. Standing in front of the patient places more stress on the examiner's own shoulder.

The examination starts with the patient's elbow flexed at 90 degrees and the hand supine on the lap **(Fig. 3.3)**. A transverse scan shows the biceps tendon as a round, well-defined, homogeneously echogenic structure in the bicipital groove **(Fig. 3.4)**. A thin echogenic transverse "ligament," probably actually fibers of the subscapularis tendon that continue from the lesser tuberosity to the greater tuberosity, covers the tendon at the entrance to the groove.

If the transducer is positioned slightly proximally, the biceps sling may be identified **(Fig. 3.5)**. Moving the elbow posteriorly and rotating the transducer with the medial end slightly inferiorly may help. The sling is thought to be a more important stabiliser than the

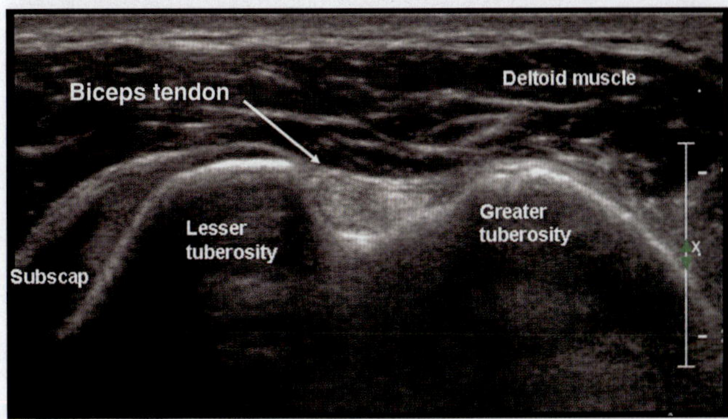

Figure 3.4.   Biceps lies in the bicipital groove and appears round and echogenic on short-axis scans.

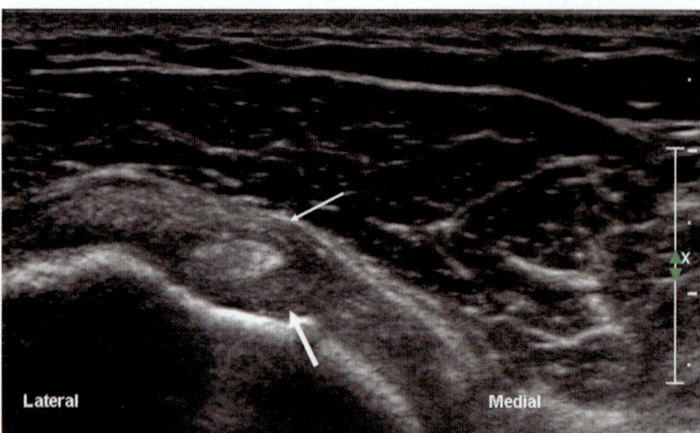

Figure 3.5. Transverse scan of LHB just proximal to bicipital groove. The tendon is stabilised by the biceps sling: the coracohumeral ligament (*thin arrow*) and the superior glenohumeral ligament (*thick arrow*).

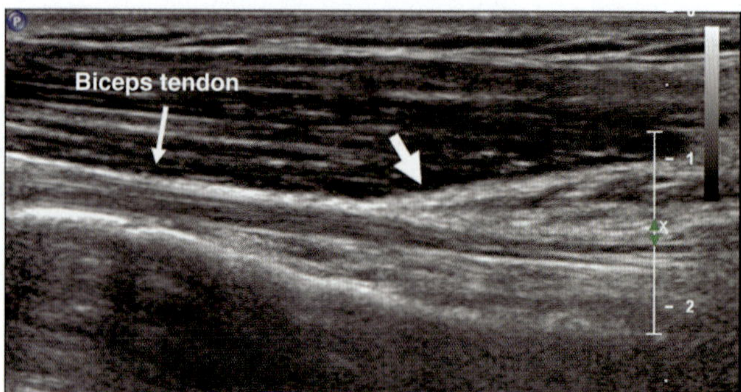

Figure 3.7. Longitudinal scan of LHB (*thin arrow*) and musculotendinous junction (*thick arrow*).

transverse ligament. It is echogenic and has a horizontal U-shape with the base lying medially. The superior limb of the sling is the coracohumeral ligament (CHL), which merges with the anterior fibers of the supraspinatus tendon and also inserts on the greater tuberosity. The inferior limb is the superior glenohumeral ligament, which runs to the lesser tuberosity with some fibers of the CHL.[9,10]

The full length of the extra-articular biceps tendon is easily examined in transverse images by an "elevator" technique, running the transducer proximally and distally between the bicipital groove and the musculotendinous junction of biceps, which lies level with the insertion of the pectoralis major tendon **(Fig. 3.6)**, on the humeral shaft. The normal biceps tendon is well defined and homogeneously echogenic. Small amounts of fluid in the tendon sheath are normal. If the transducer is rotated 90 degrees

biceps can be examined longitudinally **(Fig. 3.7)**, but this is less useful than transverse scanning. On longitudinal scans the tendon appears cord-like and striated. Variable amounts of the intra-articular biceps can be seen, but ultrasound is not an appropriate examination for suspected proximal biceps lesions such as SLAP tears.

Next, to examine the subscapularis, the hand is externally rotated, still palm up with the elbow by the patient's side and flexed at 90 degrees **(Fig. 3.8)**. A long-axis scan of subscapularis **(Fig. 3.9)**, with the transducer lying transversely on the anterior shoulder, shows the hypoechoic muscle emerging from under the coracoid process and running as echogenic tendon to insert on the lesser tuberosity. The distal 1 cm or so of the tendon may appear hypoechoic owing to anisotropy if the transducer is not angled "round the corner" of the tuberosity. On transverse images the tendon is echogenic and has curved superior and inferior margins. Alternating

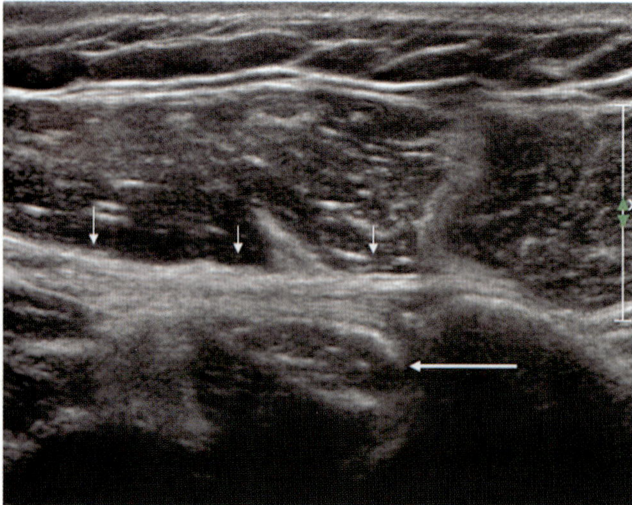

Figure 3.6. Transverse scan of arm at the level of pectoralis major tendon (*short arrows*), which inserts on the anterior humerus alongside the myotendinous junction of LHB (*long arrow*).

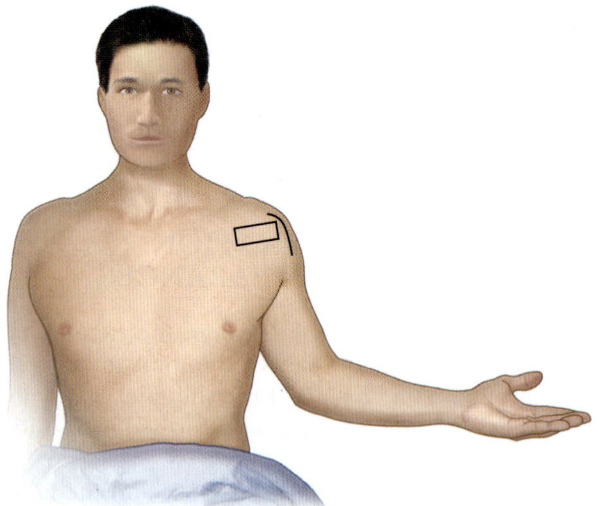

Figure 3.8. Subscapularis is examined with the elbow flexed at 90 degrees and the hand externally rotated. Place the transducer (*black box*) transversely, just medial to biceps (*black line*) to obtain a long-axis scan of subscapularis. Rotate the transducer through 90 degrees for a short-axis scan.

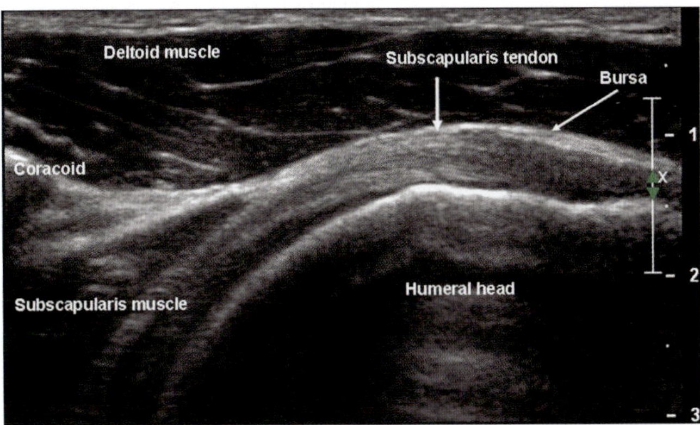

Figure 3.9. Long-axis scan of subscapularis. The muscle runs laterally under the coracoid process and is hypoechoic. The tendon is echogenic except distally where it appears hypoechoic due to anisotropy. The transducer must be angled or beam steering used to compensate.

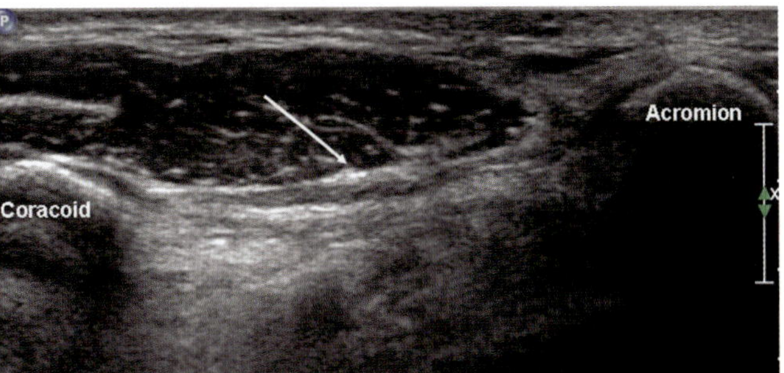

Figure 3.11. Coracoacromial ligament (*arrow*) is thin and broad and runs between the coracoid process and the acromion.

hypoechoic and echogenic areas at the myotendinous junction (**Fig. 3.10**) are due to muscle interspersed between multiple tendon slips.

Placing the transducer on the coracoid process and angling superiorly toward the acromion shows the CAL (**Fig. 3.11**). It is a thin, linear structure, small and oval on cross section.

Supraspinatus is examined with the shoulder internally rotated and extended to pull the tendon out from under the acromion. Three positions may be used. First, the hand is placed behind the lower back with palm facing backward (**Fig. 3.12**). This may be too painful in patients with severe tendinosis or impingement, and in young patients may result in too much internal rotation to show the anterior edge of supraspinatus. The alternatives, which achieve progressively less internal rotation, are to use the "hand-in-back-pocket" position with the hand prone on the lateral buttock, or simply to have the arm hanging by the side with the palm facing backward.

If you can't see the rotator interval and anterior fibers of supraspinatus when the patient's hand is behind his or her back, the shoulder is too internally rotated. Try the "hand-in-back-pocket" or "hand-by-side" positions.

The transducer is placed parallel to the long axis or short axis of the tendon, equivalent to the coronal oblique and sagittal oblique views obtained with MRI. It is important to align the transducer to the axes of the tendon and not to body planes.

On long-axis views (**Fig. 3.13**) the tendon tapers smoothly toward its insertion on the greater tuberosity and has a convex superior surface. The thin, hypoechoic subacromial/subdeltoid bursa is superficial to supraspinatus and the other tendons of the cuff. Thin, parallel echogenic stripes of peribursal fat lie deep and superficial to the bursa. Fluid in the bursa can be an important clue to pathology, but may only be seen by scanning quite far distally, inferior to the tuberosities. Hypoechoic deltoid muscle overlies the bursa. There should therefore be three layers, deltoid, bursa/peribursal fat, and tendon, between the subcutaneous fat and the humeral head.

Always identify three layers when examining supraspinatus: deltoid, bursa, and supraspinatus.

Supraspinatus is echogenic and has a uniformly striated appearance on long-axis images, but may appear hypoechoic if the angle of insonation is not 90 degrees. This occurs particularly distally where the tendon fibers swoop deeply to their insertion, and care must be taken to overcome the effect of anisotropy by altering the angle of the transducer and trying to "fill in" any hypoechoic areas.

Try to "fill in" any hypoechoic areas in the rotator cuff by altering the angle of the transducer.

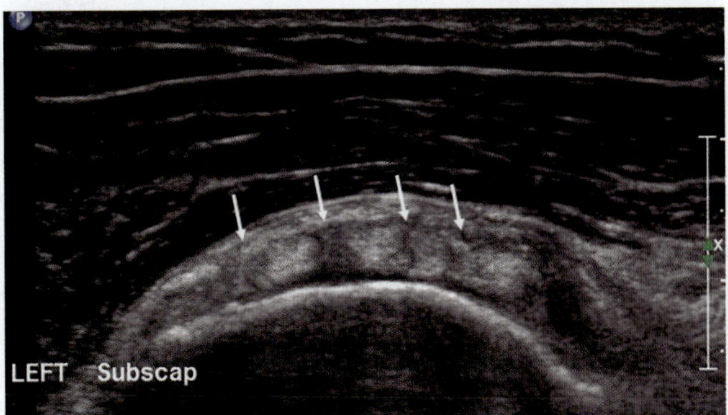

Figure 3.10. Short-axis scan of subscapularis at its musculotendinous junction. The slightly heterogeneous appearance is due to hypoechoic muscle (*arrows*) interposed between the echogenic tendon slips.

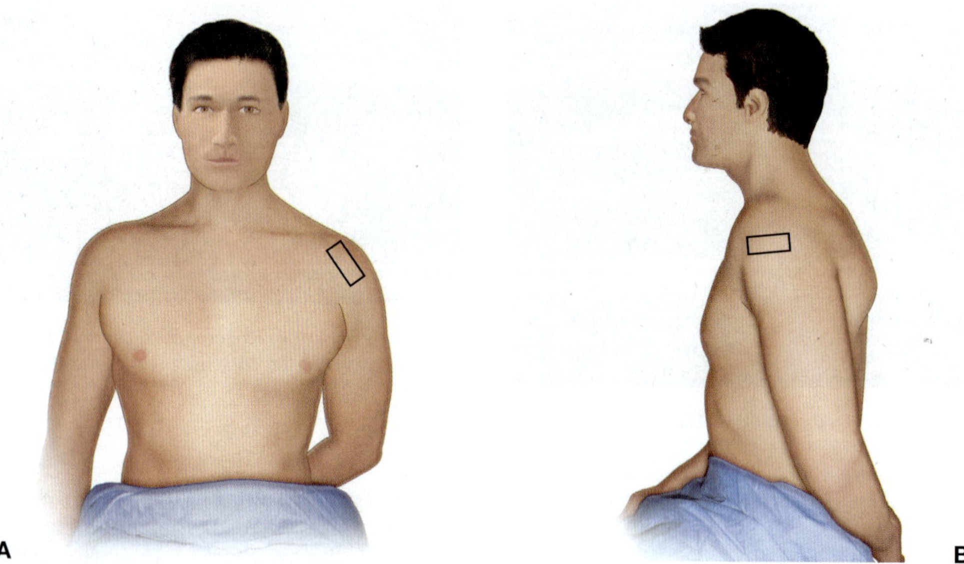

A

B

Figure 3.12.   Supraspinatus is examined with the arm extended, adducted, and internally rotated, with the hand behind the lower back and the palm facing backward to obtain long-axis (**A**) and short-axis (**B**) scans. Black boxes represent transducer positions.

The entheseal fibrocartilage where the tendon inserts on the tuberosity is anechoic and appears virtually continuous with the hyaline cartilage on the articular cortex (**Fig. 3.13**), although a small bare area may be present at the junction between hyaline and entheseal cartilage. On short-axis images, supraspinatus has an echogenic speckled texture and is of uniform caliber, thinning progressively as it runs to its insertion. The anterior edge of supraspinatus normally overlaps the biceps tendon (**Fig. 3.14**).

The distal supraspinatus and infraspinatus tendons, which form the "rotator crescent," are relatively hypovascular[11] and are liable to injury. Occasionally, a small band of echogenic fibers, a few mm thick, runs transversely on the deep aspect of the tendon. This "rotator cable"

appears to protect against tear propagation and reduces the functional disability caused by a rotator cuff tear.[12]

Infraspinatus is examined with the elbow flexed, the forearm across the chest, the patient's hand palm down on the contralateral anterior chest wall, and the transducer placed transversely on the posterior aspect of the shoulder and angled slightly obliquely (**Fig. 3.15**). The hypoechoic infraspinatus muscle runs laterally and slopes gently superiorly. As it does so, the initially narrow intramuscular echogenic tendon widens to merge with the supraspinatus tendon and the hypoechoic muscle thins inversely. Deep to the infraspinatus (**Fig. 3.16**) is the posterior glenohumeral joint margin with the curved humeral head and the echogenic glenoid labrum. This is a good site to detect an effusion (**Fig. 3.17**), which elevates the capsule, or to inject into the joint. The spinoglenoid notch lies medially. A gangion due to internal derangement of the joint may extend to the notch and

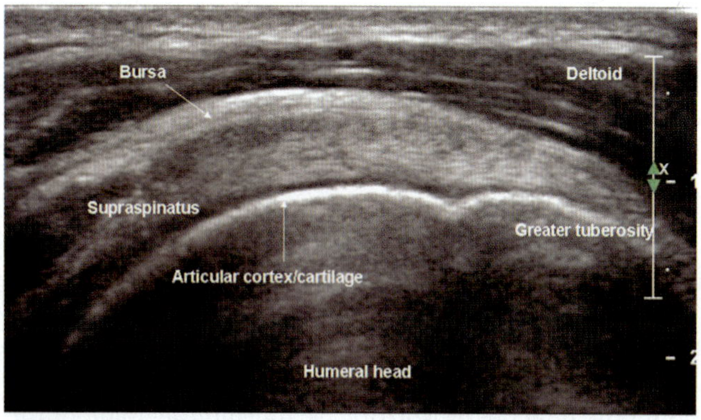

Figure 3.13.   Longitudinal scan of supraspinatus. The tendon is homogeneously echogenic and tapers uniformly to its insertion on the greater tuberosity. There is a dip in the cortex between the tuberosity and the articular cortex. Anechoic cartilage covers the humerus: hyaline cartilage over the articular cortex and fibrocartilage at the tuberosity. The thin hypoechoic bursa and the echogenic peribursal fat lie between the supraspinatus and deltoid.

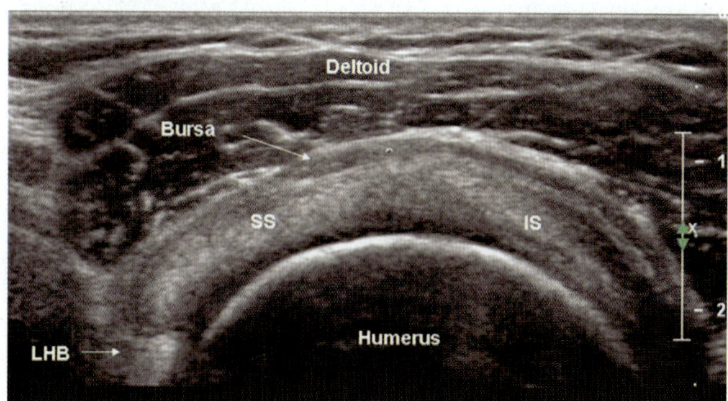

Figure 3.14.   Short-axis scan of supraspinatus (*SS*) and infraspinatus (*IS*). The anterior edge of supraspinatus overlaps biceps (*LHB*). The bursa is thickened.

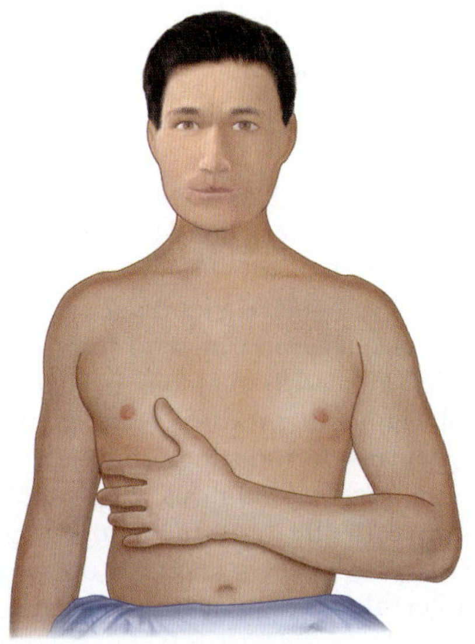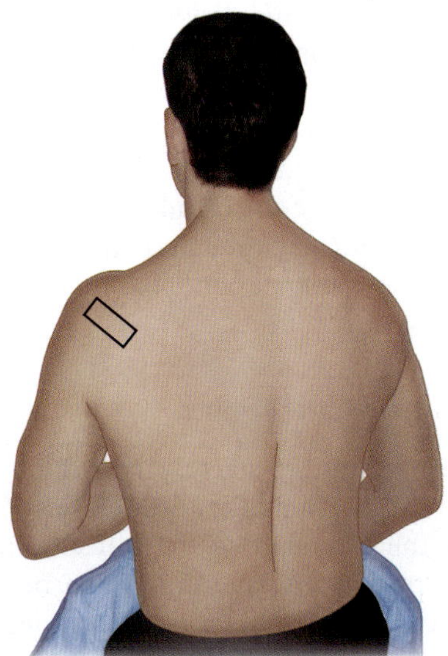

Figure 3.15. Infraspinatus is examined with the hand across the lower chest. The transducer (*black box*) is placed on the posterior glenohumeral joint line and angled obliquely upward to obtain long-axis views of the tendon.

compress the suprascapular nerve. The resulting infraspinatus weakness simulates a cuff tear.

Supraspinatus and infraspinatus form a continuous tendon sheet. Their junction may be recognised because of the slightly different orientations of the two tendons. It may be possible to identify the separate superior and middle facets of the greater tuberosity, the insertion sites of supraspinatus and infraspinatus, respectively. In practice, a distance of 1.5 cm behind the anterior edge of supraspinatus is said to mark the junction between the two tendons, although recent work suggests that infraspinatus may extend more anteriorly than this.[5] If supraspinatus is torn, biceps is a good proxy for its anterior edge.

This concludes the standard examination, although some examiners routinely include the ACJ or dynamic assessment of impingement. Teres minor is not usually examined. Muscle integrity should be assessed if a full-thickness rotator cuff tear is identified.

ROTATOR CUFF TENDINOSIS AND TEARS

Complete thickness tears; partial thickness tears; tendinosis; accuracy; asymptomatic tears; muscle atrophy and fatty infiltration; impingement.

Management of the painful shoulder is based on the concept of rotator cuff impingement. Neer[13] proposed that the interplay between the supraspinatus tendon and the coracoacromial arch, which includes the coracoid, anterior acromion, CAL, and ACJ, damages the tendon.

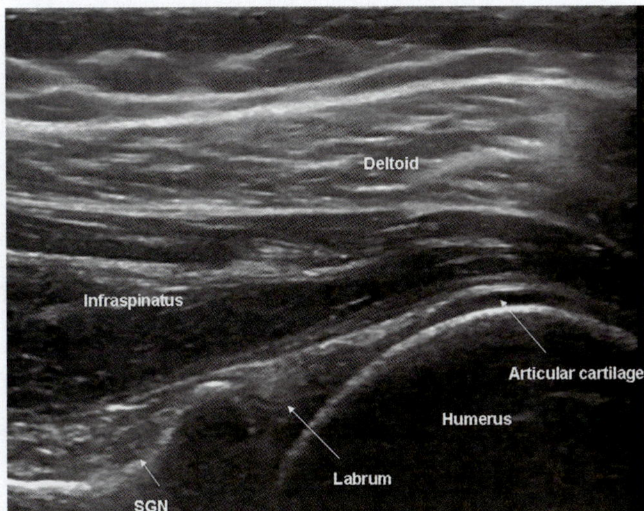

Figure 3.16. Transverse scan of the posterior joint line. The infraspinatus muscle sweeps anteriorly and superiorly toward the rotator cuff across the spinoglenoid notch (*SGN*), posterior labrum, and humeral head. This is a good position to detect small joint effusions and to inject into the glenohumeral joint.

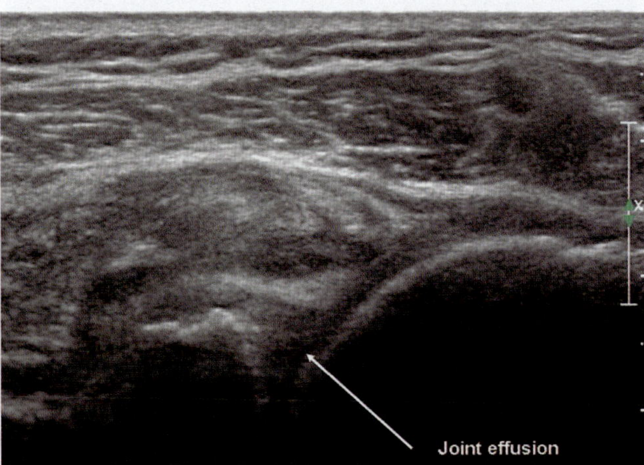

Figure 3.17. Small joint effusion (*arrow*) in a patient with a massive rotator cuff tear.

The distal anterior supraspinatus tendon is especially vulnerable because it is avascular.[11,14] Initially, reversible damage is followed by irreversible tendinosis and fibrosis and finally by rotator cuff tears.

Clinical tests have only moderate sensitivity for rotator cuff tears[15,16] and are subject to considerable interobserver variability.[17] Experienced clinicians can accurately exclude rotator cuff tears, but depend on imaging to confirm if a tear is present.[18]

Full-thickness Rotator Cuff Tears

Most rotator cuff tears are said to start in the vulnerable zone in the anterior supraspinatus tendon close to the greater tuberosity of the humerus, while mid-substance tears that start more posteriorly are thought to be less frequent. However, recent work shows that most degenerate tears start close to the junction of the supraspinatus and infraspinatus tendons, about 15 mm posterior to the biceps tendon.[19] As tears enlarge, they extend proximally and/or in anterior or posterior directions and may eventually involve all the rotator cuff tendons and the biceps tendon.

Full-thickness rotator cuff tears extend all the way from the superficial or bursal surface of the tendon to the deep or articular surface, but not necessarily across the full width from front to back, whereas partial-thickness tears extend only part way between bursal and articular surfaces.

A defect that extends from the bursal surface to the joint surface of the tendon is the primary ultrasound sign of a full-thickness tear, and it should be present on both long-axis and short-axis scans of the tendon **(Fig. 3.18)**. If an apparent defect is identified, the transducer should be angled to try to "fill in" the defect in case the appearance is due to anisotropy, and the defect should be shown on both longitudinal and transverse images. If the tear is very large and the tendon retracted under the acromion, no tendon is visible.

Fluid-filled defects are easy to identify because of the contrast differences between the fluid and the edges of the torn tendon, which may be slightly depressed. Tears are more difficult to identify if the fluid is echogenic or the defect occupied by synovium, debris, or by deltoid muscle **(Fig. 3.19)** that has herniated into the defect. Small tears can produce focal thinning or bursal surface depression indistinguishable from partial-thickness tears or severe tendinosis. Repeatedly pressing on the tendon with the transducer may move fluid or debris and make a small tear more obvious or distinguish a complete-thickness tear from a partial-thickness tear.

Tear margins may be well defined or irregular. Delamination results in hypoechoic clefts that run transversely from the tear edge into the tendon. Rarely such a cleft communicates with a fluid-filled intramuscular cyst.

Tear extension >15 mm posterior to the anterior edge of supraspinatus tendon, which in practice is defined by the biceps tendon, indicates that the infraspinatus tendon is also torn. This measurement technique cannot be used if biceps is also torn, but the combination of biceps and supraspinatus tears usually indicates that the cuff tear is very large.

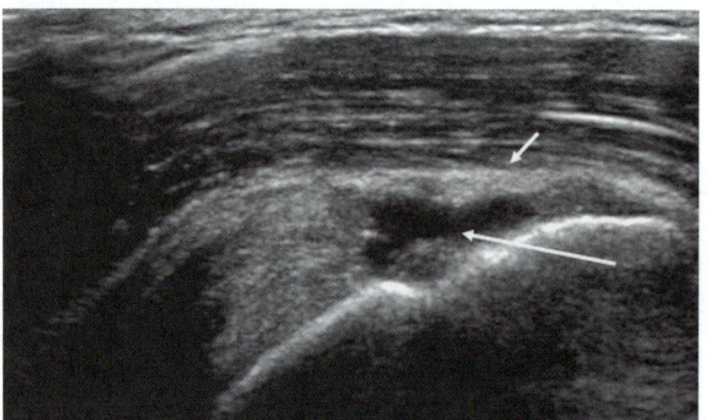
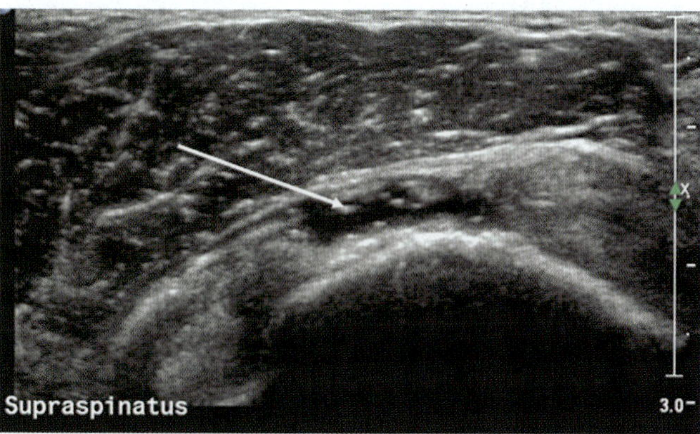

Figure 3.18. Long-axis (**A**) and short-axis (**B**) scans of small full-thickness supraspinatus tear. The defect is occupied by fluid (*long arrows*) and there is slight herniation of peribursal fat (*short arrow* in **A**) into the defect.

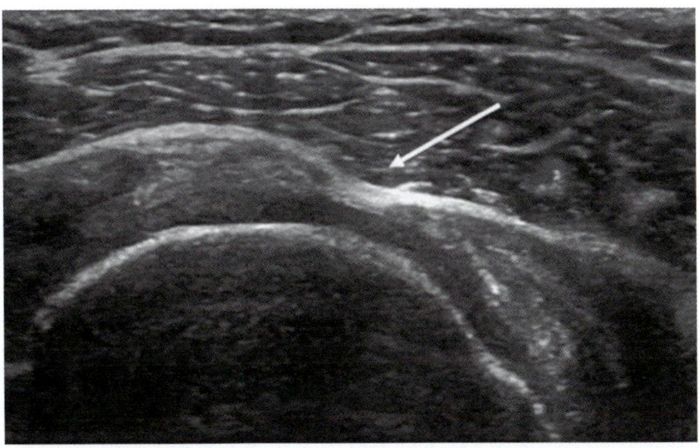

Figure 3.19. Short-axis scan of narrow full-thickness supraspinatus tear (*arrow*) with herniation of deltoid into defect.

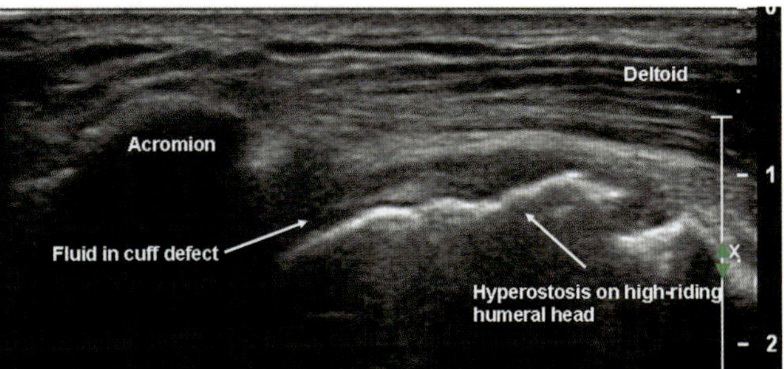

Figure 3.21. Massive rotator cuff tear. The cuff is retracted under the acromion, and the humeral head is high-riding.

Tip:
Bursal surface flattening or depression are sensitive indicators of cuff pathology, but are nonspecific.

Large tears result in tendon retraction under the acromion **(Fig. 3.20)**, when the proximal edge of the tear cannot be seen. The deltoid muscle may herniate into the defect and be in direct contact with the humerus. It is important to recognise that there is a missing layer. Proximal migration of the humeral head to be in direct contact with the acromion **(Fig. 3.21)** occurs with very large chronic tears.

Full-thickness tears are associated with synovial inflammation[20] and abnormal signal is occasionally seen on Doppler ultrasound, but this is not a regular feature.

If a full-thickness tear is identified, the supraspinatus and infraspinatus muscles should be assessed for atrophy and fatty infiltration.

Secondary signs are highly suggestive of full-thickness tears but are not diagnostic. Depression or flattening of the bursal surface **(Fig. 3.22)** is a powerful indicator of pathology. It is nonspecific and occurs in both tears and tendinosis, although the deeper the depression, the more likely a full-thickness tear.

The combination of glenohumeral joint fluid and hyperostosis at the greater tuberosity **(Fig. 3.20)** has a positive predictive value (PPV) and specificity of 100% for full-thickness tears. Fluid in the subdeltoid bursa and joint has a PPV of 95% and specificity of 99%. The bursa extends distal to the greater tuberosity **(Fig. 3.23)**, and sometimes fluid is seen only in the distal segment. My experience is that fluid in the bursa and biceps tendon sheath also strongly suggests a tear, although a PPV of only 54% has been reported. Hyperostosis at the greater tuberosity or fluid in any one of the joint, bursa or biceps tendon sheath are less useful, having PPV value of 60% to 70%. A smooth tuberosity is likely to be associated with an intact tendon.[21–24]

The cartilage interface sign **(Fig. 3.24)** is an echogenic line at the surface of the hyaline cartilage on the humeral head deep to a cuff tear, and is due to reduced attenuation and altered acoustic interface. I do not find this a useful sign. The surface of the articular cartilage is often quite echogenic, especially with modern equipment, and

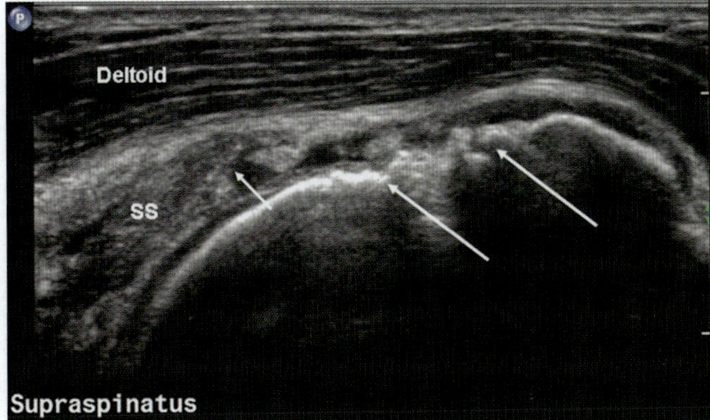

Figure 3.20. Long-axis scan of large full-thickness supraspinatus tear. The tendon is retracted (*short arrow*). Deltoid and fluid occupy the defect, and there is considerable hyperostosis on the humeral head (*long arrow*).

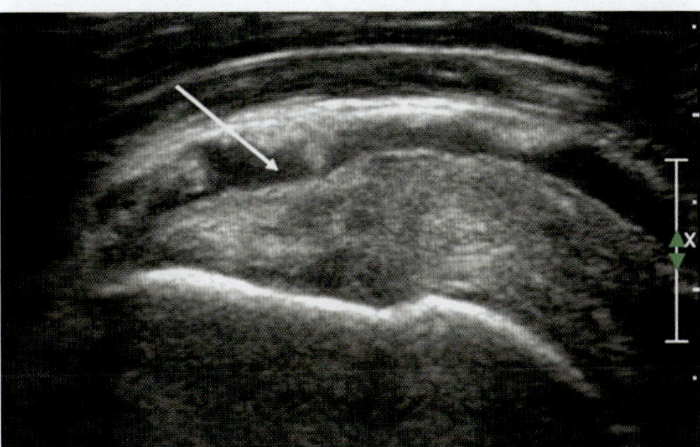

Figure 3.22. The effusion in the subdeltoid bursa shows that the bursal surface of supraspinatus is depressed (*arrow*).

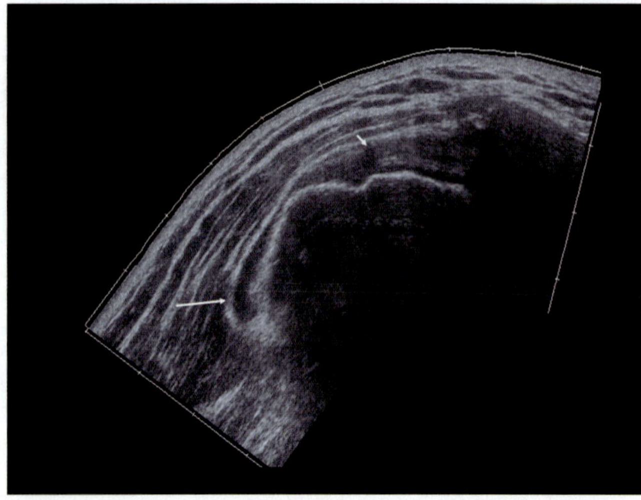

Figure 3.23. It is important to look quite far distally for bursal fluid. The fluid in this patient lies distal (*long arrow*) to the greater tuberosity of the humerus. There is no fluid overlying the rotator cuff (*short arrow*).

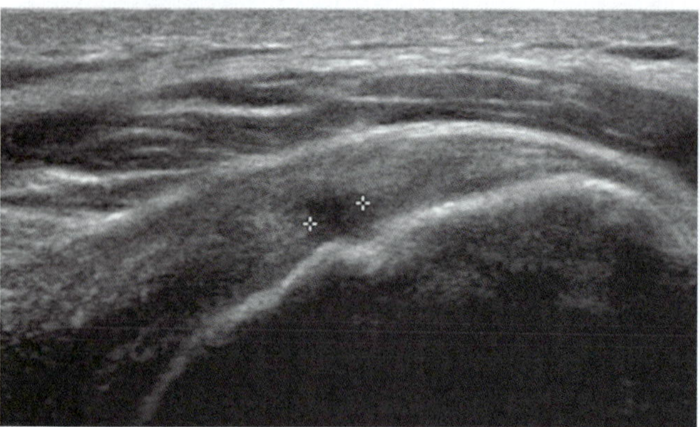

Figure 3.25. Joint side partial-substance tear between caliper marks.

hyperechoity is subjective. In any case, the sign is frequently most conspicuous when there is an obvious tear and fluid is present.

> **Tip:**
> These two combinations have high PPV for full-thickness rotator cuff tears:
> 1. Hyperostosis at the greater tuberosity **and** fluid in the glenohumeral joint.
> 2. Fluid in the glenohumeral joint/biceps tendon sheath **and** subdeltoid bursa.

Partial-Thickness Rotator Cuff Tears

Partial-thickness tears extend part way between the bursal and the articular surfaces of the cuff and may be at the surface or intratendinous. Joint side tears are most common.[25]

Bursal-side tears cause defects or depressions (**Fig. 3.22**) in the bursal surface of the cuff, usually near the greater tuberosity. The bursa may dip into the defect and may be conspicuous because of intrabursal fluid or echogenic peribursal fat. Intrasubstance tears are hypoechoic. A longitudinal split in the tendon may be identified. Articular-side tears (**Fig. 3.25**) are easily identified if the defect is fluid-filled, but are frequently quite difficult to identify and may have a mixed hypoechoic and hyperechoic appearance. Rim-rent tears (**Fig. 3.26**) are partial-substance tears that are minimally retracted from the greater tuberosity and characteristically have a central echogenic "streak" surrounded by hypoechoic fluid.[26,27]

Rotator Cuff Tendinosis or Tendinopathy

Tendinopathy initially results in swelling and altered echogenicity. Swelling can be confirmed by comparing the affected segment with adjacent tendon or with the same position at the opposite shoulder. The difference in measurement is usually <2.5 mm. Thickness of >8 mm is also considered abnormal.[28]

Subsequently, the tendon may become thinned. Alterations in texture (**Figs. 3.27 and 3.28**) include reduced

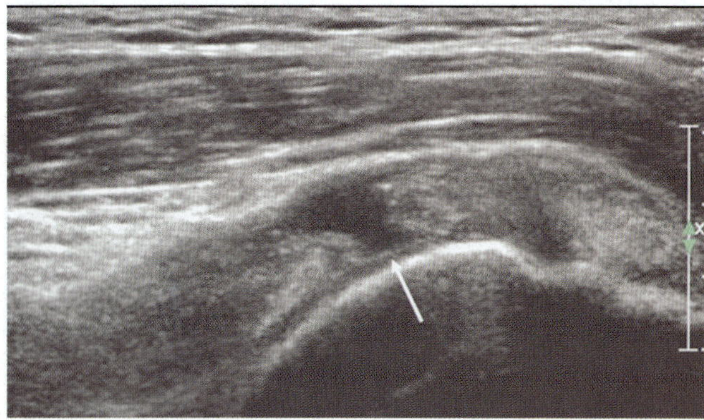

Figure 3.24. Articular cartilage (*arrow*) deep to a tear is brighter than adjacent cartilage.

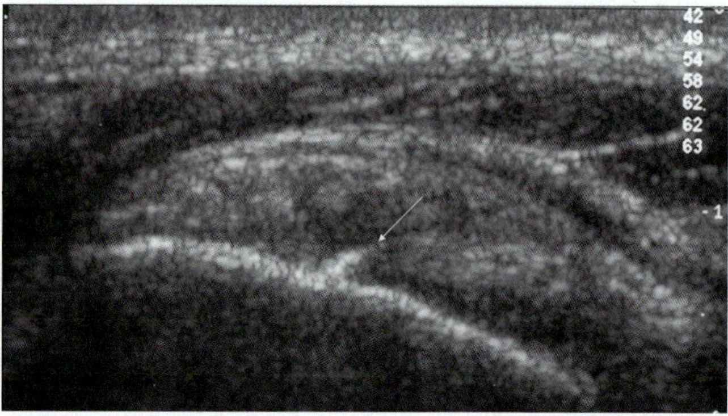

Figure 3.26. Echogenic streak (*arrow*) surrounded by hypoechoic fluid in supraspinatus adjacent to greater tuberosity typical of a "rim rent."

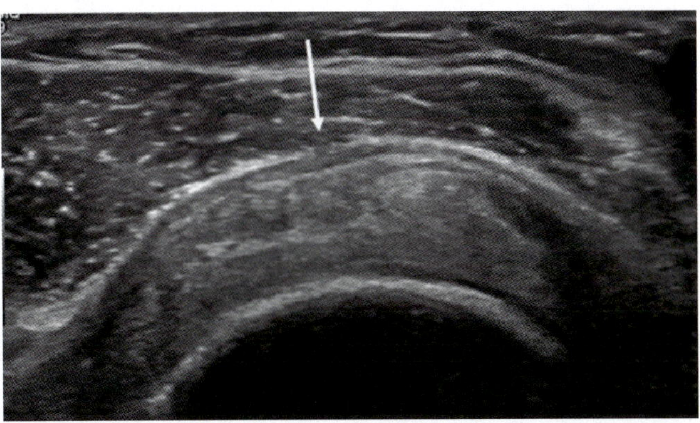

Figure 3.27. Supraspinatus tendinosis: the arrow points to bursal thickening, depression of the bursal surface of the tendon, and heterogeneous tendon texture.

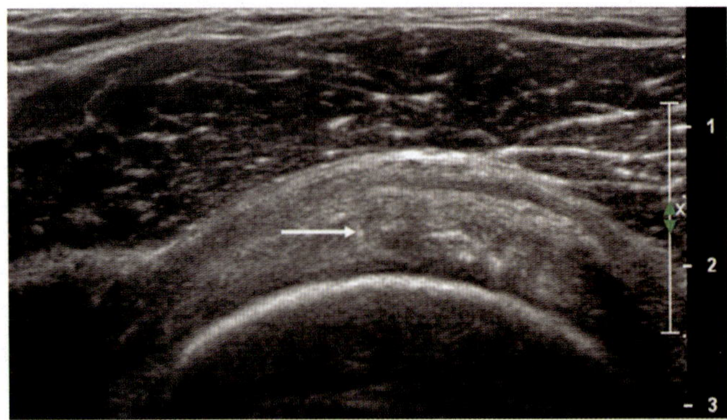

Figure 3.29. Short-axis scan of supraspinatus showing tendinosis. Microcalcification (*arrow*) and heterogeneous tendon texture are present.

echogenicity, mixed hypoechoity and hyperechoity, and foci of microcalcifications (**Fig. 3.29**), although heterogeneity is often seen in older patients without clinical evidence of tendinosis. Thickening of the subdeltoid bursa and small amounts of fluid in the bursa may be present, and there may be subtle loss of definition between tendon and bursa.[24,28–31]

Neer's theory postulates that increasingly severe grades of tendinosis develop into partial-thickness tears and then into full-thickness tears. Just as there are theoretical overlaps, there are overlaps between the ultrasound appearances of tendinosis and partial-thickness tears and between partial-thickness and full-thickness tears.

Accuracy of Ultrasound Detection of Rotator Cuff Tears

Ultrasound of the shoulder has been criticised as inaccurate and operator-dependent. Some initial reports recorded poor results. Subsequent studies have shown that there are no statistically significant differences between ultrasound and MRI in the detection of rotator cuff tears or the assessment of tear size compared with surgical results.[32–34] Performing MRI after normal ultrasound of the rotator cuff confers no benefit.[35]

A series of meta-analyses[1,18,36] has confirmed that ultrasound and MRI are equally accurate in the detection of rotator cuff tears, although results for both modalities are poorer for partial-thickness tears than full-thickness tears, and MR arthrography is a more accurate technique by a very small margin (**Table 3.1**).

Ultrasound errors include simple misses, usually of very small (<5 mm) tears, miscategorisation between full-thickness and partial-thickness tears or between partial-thickness tears and tendinosis, and when patients are too big (heavily muscled or obese) or have such a restricted range of movement that parts of the rotator cuff are inaccessible.[37]

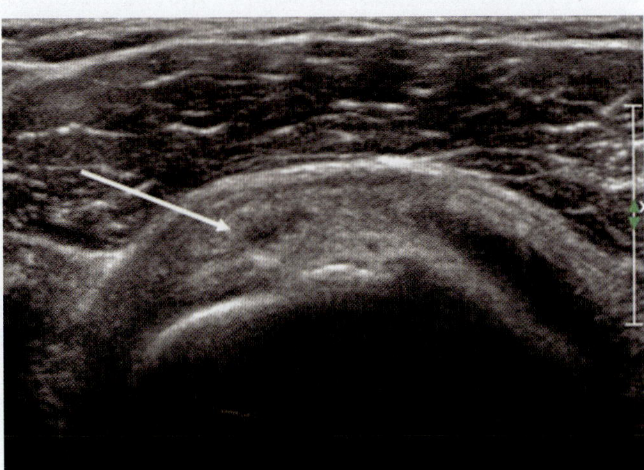

Figure 3.28. Supraspinatus tendinosis: the arrow points to an intrasubstance tear. The adjacent tendon is heterogeneous, and there is bursal surface flattening.

TABLE 3.1.	Accuracy of Imaging in Rotator Cuff Tears	
	Sensitivity (%)	*Specificity (%)*
FULL-THICKNESS TEARS		
MRA	95.4	98.9
US	92.3	94.4
MRI	92.1	92.9
PARTIAL-THICKNESS TEARS		
MRA	85.9	96.0
US	66.7	93.5
MRI	63.6	91.7

MRA, magnetic resonance arthrogram; US, ultrasound; MRI, magnetic resonance imaging.
(Adapted with permission from de Jesus JO, Parker L, Frangos AJ, et al. Accuracy of MRI, MR arthrography, and ultrasound in the diagnosis of rotator cuff tears: a meta-analysis. *AJR Am J Roentgenol.* 2009;192(6):1701–1707; Published with permission from Beggs I. Shoulder ultrasound. *Semin Ultrasound CT MR.* 2011;32(2):101–113.)

There is no doubt that partial-thickness tears are more difficult to diagnose than full-thickness tears.[38] Large bursal-side partial-thickness tears may be indistinguishable from full-thickness tears. When faced with this dilemma, I report frankly that I cannot make the distinction, and the surgeon will usually operate. In some cases, the difficulty is in distinguishing between tendinosis and partial tears, but as the management of both conditions is initially conservative, this is not usually of major practical significance. Subacromial decompression is performed if conservative treatment of impingement fails and debridement of partial tears can be performed at that time.[25,37]

Discrepant results have been found for tear measurement. Teefey et al.[32] found that ultrasound correctly assesses length in 73% and width in 86% of full-thickness tears compared with surgical measurements. Discrepancies are three times as likely to overestimate as underestimate tear length while over- and underestimates are equally likely when measuring width.[32] Curved measurements are more accurate than straight line measurements.[39] Tissue harmonic imaging improves image quality and may also help.[40]

The miscalculation of tear length is partly, not wholly, attributable to non-visualisation due to retraction under the acromion, as similarly poor results occur with MRI. Discrepancies may be due to the position of the shoulder when the tear is measured. Ferri et al.[41] found no differences between ultrasound and surgical measurements in full internal rotation ("hand-behind-the-back position") but lesser degrees of internal rotation ("hand-in-back-pocket position") underestimated tear length.

> **Tip:**
> Measure rotator cuff tear size with the patient in the "hand-behind-the-back" position.

The criticism that shoulder ultrasound is operator-dependent usually comes from surgeons, as if their own work is not operator-dependent. Standard clinical tests for rotator cuff pathology have sensitivities of 23% to 76% and specificities of 47% to 88% and are subject to considerable inter-observer variability, and it would be strange to think that there are not also variations in surgical results.[5,17,42]

In experienced hands, ultrasound has high (>90%) inter-observer agreement. Most significant discrepancies concern the distinction between full-thickness and large partial-thickness tears or whether a supraspinatus tear extends into the infraspinatus.[43–45]

Interobserver agreement improves with experience.[45] The learning curve is usually considered to be quite lengthy. However, Rutten et al.[46] showed excellent agreement between an experienced musculoskeletal sonologist and an experienced abdominal sonologist with no prior musculoskeletal experience.

Several surgeons have reported their experience of performing ultrasound with little or no training, although in many cases they interpreted the ultrasound only after examining the patient and previous imaging studies. Moosmayer,[47] a surgeon, reported excellent results unbiased by any clinical information, but had already performed several hundred shoulder ultrasound examinations by the start of his study.[48] Hedtmann and Fett[48] also reported excellent results after extensive training. Good results have prompted some surgeons to perform their own ultrasound examinations as part of a "one-stop shop" shoulder clinic.[3,34]

Asymptomatic Rotator Cuff Tears

The reported prevalence of asymptomatic rotator cuff tears over the age of 50 ranges from 6% to 40%, and increases with age to 51% at 80 years or older. Although patients are pain-free, objective testing shows reduced shoulder strength, especially when the tear is large.[49–53] About half of the patients become symptomatic within 3 years. About one-third show tear progression, and most of these become symptomatic.[54] Symptomatic rotator cuff tears are associated with rotator cuff tears on the opposite side. These may or may not be asymptomatic; 56% of patient had a tear in the opposite asymptomatic shoulder in one series.[55]

It follows that many patients who present with an injury and are found to have a rotator cuff tear may have a long-standing, previously unrecognised tear, and immediate tendon repair may be inappropriate. A massive tear, paucity of fluid, hypertrophied biceps tendon, high-riding humeral head, and muscle atrophy and fatty infiltration are all features of chronic tears.[56,57]

> **Tip:**
> A massive tear, no fluid, thick biceps, high humerus, and fatty muscle indicate long-standing tear.

Muscle Atrophy and Fatty Infiltration

Atrophy and fatty infiltration of the rotator cuff muscles are frequent consequences of rotator cuff tears and may affect the functional outcome of tendon repair, and hence the decision to operate or the type of surgery performed. Fatty atrophy is not an inevitable consequence of a rotator cuff tear, but the larger the tear the greater is the degree of fatty infiltration likely to be.[58]

Infraspinatus atrophy is commonly seen when the supraspinatus tendon is torn and infraspinatus appears intact. This apparent paradox may be explained by the finding that the infraspinatus footprint is much larger and extends more anteriorly than previously thought. A tear that apparently involves only supraspinatus may therefore also involve infraspinatus.[5]

The "tangent sign" assesses supraspinatus atrophy on sagittal oblique computed tomography (CT) and MRI images of the supraspinatus fossa by drawing a line across the superior margins of the coracoid process and the spine of the scapula. A similar tangent line assessment can be performed on sagittal oblique ultrasound scans. Supraspinatus is considered to be atrophic if it does not reach the tangent line (**Fig. 3.30**). This finding correlates with objective measurements of muscle strength and the occupancy ratio measure of atrophy.[59,60] The occupancy ratio is calculated on sagittal oblique images at the level of the suprascapular notch by drawing separate ellipses around the margins of the muscle and the fossa. Supraspinatus is considered normal if it occupies 0.6 to 1.0 of the fossa, moderately atrophied if 0.4 to 0.6, and severely atrophied if <0.4.[61,62]

CT and MRI grading systems show that muscles that contain no fat or streaks of fat have good functional outcomes after rotator cuff repair, while muscles that contain more fat (Grade 2, "fat less than muscle" or greater) have poor outcomes.[61,63–67]

Scattered deposits of fat result in increased echogenicity of the muscle and loss of definition of its contour, pennate pattern, and central tendon (**Fig. 3.30**). Increased echogenicity is easily recognised by comparing supraspinatus or infraspinatus with the overlying deltoid or trapezius muscles (**Fig. 3.31**), which also helps to distinguish between normal age-related atrophy and atrophy from a rotator cuff tear. The ultrasound grading of fatty infiltration is subjective, but a muscle that is clearly

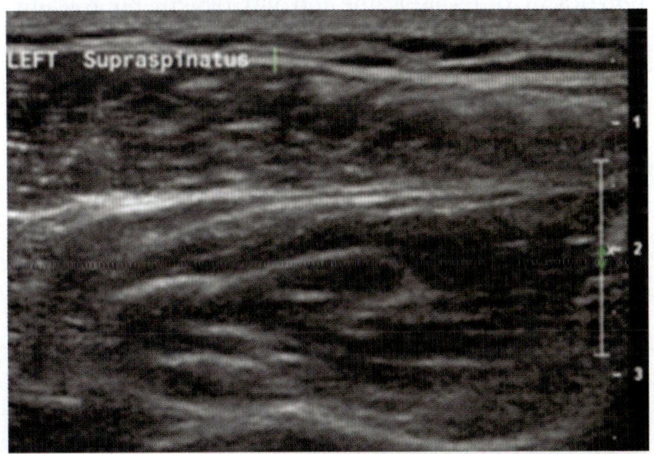

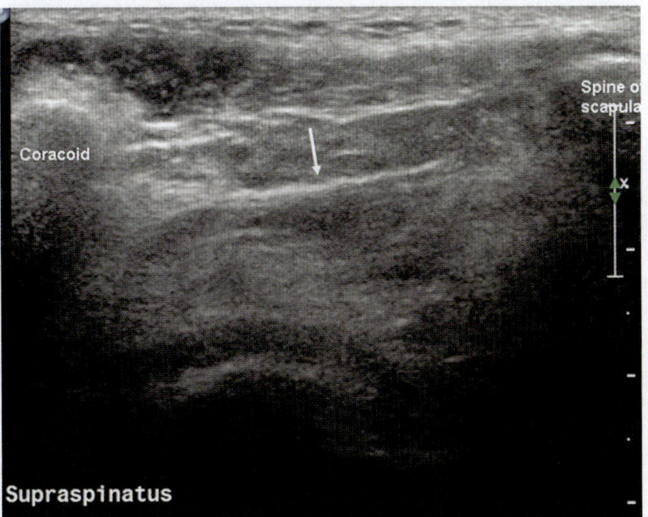

Figure 3.30. **A:** Sagittal scan of supraspinatus fossa showing normal architecture and bulk of supraspinatus muscle. **B:** Sagittal scan of supraspinatus fossa showing atrophy and fatty infiltration of supraspinatus muscle. The superficial surface of supraspinatus normally reaches a line between the coracoid process and the spine of the scapula. In this case the superficial margin of the muscle (*arrow*) lies deep to the line, indicating that the muscle is atrophic. The muscle is diffusely echogenic and has lost its internal architecture in keeping with fatty infiltration.

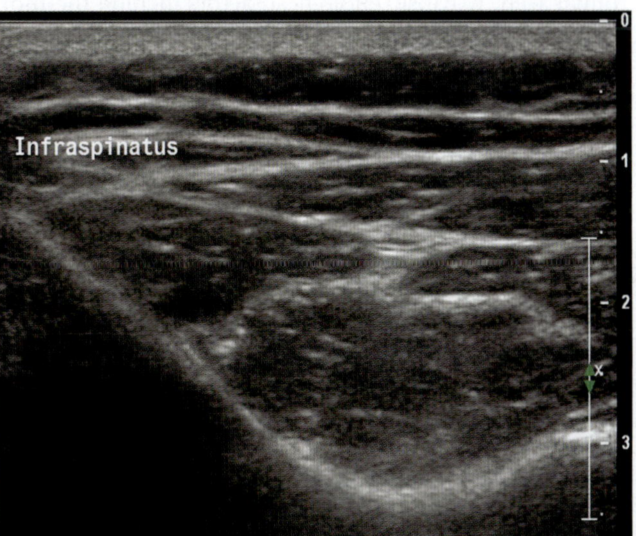

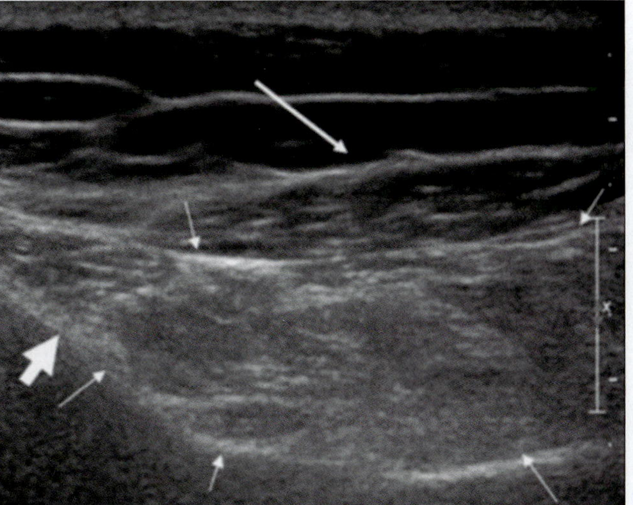

Figure 3.31. Sagittal scans of infraspinatus muscle (*short arrows* in **B**). The scapula (*broad arrow* in **B**) is deep and trapezius (*long arrow*) is superficial. **A:** Normal infraspinatus muscle that is isoechoic to trapezius and has well-defined internal architecture. **B:** Fatty atrophy. The muscle is diffusely more echogenic than trapezius, is reduced in size, and has lost its internal architecture.

more echogenic than the overlying deltoid has a substantial degree of fatty infiltration, equivalent to at least Grade 2 on MRI or CT. Assessment of infraspinatus is easier than supraspinatus and can be aided by extended-field-of-view imaging.[62,68,69]

> **Tip:**
> Fatty infiltration is easily identified by comparing the echogenicity of infraspinatus and the overlying deltoid or trapezius muscles.

Impingement

Most cases of rotator cuff impingement are anterosuperior and involve the supraspinatus tendon and the coracoacromial arch. Extrinsic etiological factors include the morphology of the arch, repetitive and tensile overload, and biomechanical factors, while intrinsic factors include tendon vascularity. It is now accepted that changes at the coracoacromial arch are also consequences of impingement.[6,70]

Neer described three progressive stages of tendon abnormality as a result of impingement. Stage I, characterised by subacromial bursitis and minor or no tendon changes, is reversible. Stage II additionally shows evidence of irreversible tendinosis and may require decompression of the coracoacromial arch to halt progression and relieve symptoms. Stage III damage includes partial-thickness and full-thickness tears and may need decompression and tendon repair.[13]

Clinical features of impingement include pain, particularly on overhead movement, stretching, or internal rotation, painful arc, pain that disturbs sleep and localised tenderness over the greater tuberosity. Radiographs may show hyperostosis at the greater tuberosity and spurs on the acromion.

Clinical tests of impingement are widely used but are, at least in some cases, of doubtful validity.[16]

A widely used clinical test is to inject local anesthetic into the subacromial bursa to try to abolish pain and a painful arc. Long-acting steroids may be added for therapeutic purposes. Blind injections into the bursa may be accurate in experienced hands,[71] but most studies show that "blind" injections frequently miss the bursa and may result in a false negative "impingement test."[72–76]

Ultrasound-guided bursal injections (Fig 3.23) are widely used for both diagnostic and therapeutic purposes. In addition to the evidence that ultrasound-guidance ensures accurate needle placement, it seems intuitively reasonable to assume that intrabursal injections will improve therapeutic response and there is evidence to support this.[77] However, a double blind study failed to show any benefit for ultrasound-guided bursal injections over blind gluteal injections of steroid.[78]

Ultrasound evidence of impingement includes bursal thickening and rotator cuff damage (**Fig. 3.27**). Dynamic scanning is performed during active or passive abduction. Passive abduction is easily achieved if the examiner grasps the patient's flexed elbow and abducts the arm. Alternatively, the patient is asked to abduct the arm. Abduction in internal rotation and 60° forward flexion may help. The transducer is placed on the edge of the acromion and CAL, parallel to the long axis of supraspinatus. Ultrasound shows pooling of bursal fluid or buckling of the bursa or bursal surface of the cuff against the acromion or CAL (**Fig. 3.32**). In more severe cases, the greater tuberosity of the humerus may block against the acromion. However, these findings have not been objectively verified, and pooling of bursal fluid or buckling of the bursa may be seen in asymptomatic patients.[28,29,30,79]

My own preference in assessing impingement is to perform ultrasound-guided bursal injections. I use a combination of 1mL of 1% lidocaine and 5mL of 0.5% bupivacaine, which are short-acting and long-acting local anesthetics, respectively and monitor response by asking the patient to subsequently complete a VAS (visual analogue pain score) at hourly intervals, although in most patients a positive response (or its absence) is obvious almost immediately. I also inject 40 mg of methylprednisolone, a long-acting steroid, for possible longer-term benefit. I prefer methylprednisolone because of its reduced risk of skin depigmentation but others prefer triamcinolone because of its reduced risk of causing synovitis.

I perform the injection with the patient supine to avoid a vasovagal reaction. The patient's hand is usually in a neutral position by the patient's side but sometimes a degree of internal or external rotation is needed to visualise the bursa optimally. I scan along the long-axis of supraspinatus to identify the bursa and mark the skin so that the needle will run (from inferolateral to superomedial) as close to parallel to the transducer as possible. After cleaning the skin and injecting subcutaneous local anaesthetic I insert a green needle attached to a 5mL syringe loaded with local anaesthetic. The bevel of the needle should point down. The needle is then inserted into the bursa and a small test dose of local anaesthetic is injected. If the needle is in the bursa, the sensation when injecting is like a "knife through

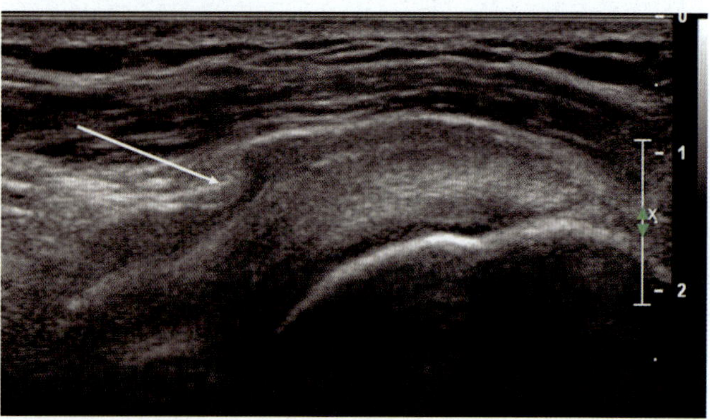

Figure 3.32.   Rotator cuff impingement: the bursa is thickened and the CAL (*arrow*) protrudes into the bursa.

butter" and there is very little to see as the injected fluid runs away from the needle tip into the bursa. Pooling of fluid around the needle tip indicates that the needle is outside the bursa and the needle should be repositioned. Occasionally intrabursal adhesions are present and the bursa has to be 'forced' to distend by pushing harder on the syringe but care must be taken to ensure that the injection is truly intra-bursal. After distending the bursa with local anaesthetic, the steroid is injected. I tell patients that they might experience 2 to 3 days of modest discomfort after the injection but warn them that severe pain due to a steroid 'flare' is a possibility. I ask them to avoid strenuous activities and to refrain from physiotherapy for 2 to 3 weeks after the injection. My experience is that about 60% of patients still benefit 6 months after injection.

Frozen Shoulder

Frozen shoulder or adhesive capsulitis results in stiffness, globally restricted range of active and passive movement, and severe pain that disturbs sleep. Patients are middle-aged, often diabetic. The cause of frozen shoulder is unknown. Arthroscopy shows fibrous soft tissue thickening in the rotator interval, particularly around the CHL.[80,81] Inflammation is not a feature of established disease, but synovial inflammation may be present initially.[82] Frozen shoulder is usually a clinical diagnosis that does not require imaging.

Ultrasound shows increased soft tissue density in the rotator interval, thickening of the CHL, and vascularity in the rotator interval on Doppler imaging. Restricted abduction is seen during dynamic examination, but this is obvious clinically. Magnetic resonance arthrography shows changes in the rotator interval including thickening of the capsule, synovium, and CHL.[83–85]

Frozen shoulder is a self-limiting condition that has a protracted course and may last several years. Complete functional recovery may never be achieved. Image-guided intra-articular steroid injections may help, although severe or recalcitrant cases may require operative intervention.[81,86] I use fluoroscopy to perform image-guided injections for frozen shoulder but ultrasound - guidance can be employed. An identical ultrasound technique can be used to inject contrast for MR arthrography or to aspirate the joint for organisms or crystals. The patient either sits on the examination couch or lies semiprone, facing away from the operator, with the hand on the opposite shoulder. The infraspinatus muscle/tendon and underlying posterior gleno-humeral joint line are identified by placing the transducer obliquely on the posterior shoulder with the outer end of the transducer rotated superiorly and the skin is marked for either an inferomedial to superolateral needle trajectory or the reverse trajectory. After skin preparation, including infiltration with local anaesthetic, a 22G spinal needle is advanced under ultrasound guidance towards the posterior glenohumeral

joint line and the posterior aspect of the humeral head. When it touches bone a small test injection of anaesthetic is made to show if the needle is in joint or has to be repositioned. If the needle is intra-articular, I then inject 40 mg of triamcinolone, 5mL of 0.5% bupivacaine and 15 mL of air or normal saline to distend the joint. The purpose of the injection is to alleviate pain and to restore the range of joint movement and all of my patients receive physiotherapy within a few days of the injection, although the evidence for the efficacy of post-injection physiotherapy is mixed. Audit shows that 70 to 80% of patients benefit from the procedure. As with all intra-articular steroid injections, I warn patients to expect mild discomfort or pain and the possibility of severe pain due to a "steroid flare" in the next 2 to 3 days.

CALCIFICATION

Deposits of calcium hydroxyapatite in the rotator cuff include foci of microcalcification that are radiographically occult, and larger "hard" or "soft" deposits that are visible on radiographs. Supraspinatus is the most frequent site, but any of the tendons may be involved. The cause remains unknown although hypoxia and metaplasia have been suggested. Large foci of calcification are initially hard and often clinically occult, although chronic pain may subsequently develop. After a latent period, which is often prolonged, an inflammatory resorptive phase follows and the calcium softens or fragments. This phrase often causes severe pain and lasts for several weeks. As the overlying skin may be hot and erythematous and inflammatory markers are elevated, patients are often thought to have septic arthritis and are referred for urgent ultrasound and aspiration. Rupture of calcium into the subdeltoid bursa may result in bursitis and exacerbation of pain or more frequently relieve pain, presumably by reducing the pressure and inflammation in the tendon. Rarely, calcium may extend into the humerus or rupture between the tendon and the bursa.[87]

Microcalcification produces small echogenic foci (**Fig. 3.29**) in the rotator cuff that are usually seen in the context of tendinosis. Acoustic shadows are infrequent. Distinguishing microcalcification in the tendon from hyperostosis on the cortex may be impossible if the echogenic focus is adjacent to the bone.

Most large calcifications are hard and have a densely echogenic convex superficial surface (**Fig. 3.33**). Multiple foci may be present. Distal acoustic shadowing is typical unless the calcification is too close to the humerus for shadowing to be seen. Rotator cuff tears and abnormal signal on Doppler ultrasound are rare. Deposits occasionally elevate the bursal surface of the tendon, causing pain on abduction when the bursa impinges on the acromion.

Soft calcification is often exquisitely painful and tender. Even gentle transducer pressure may be very uncomfortable. Soft calcification (**Fig. 3.34**) is less echogenic

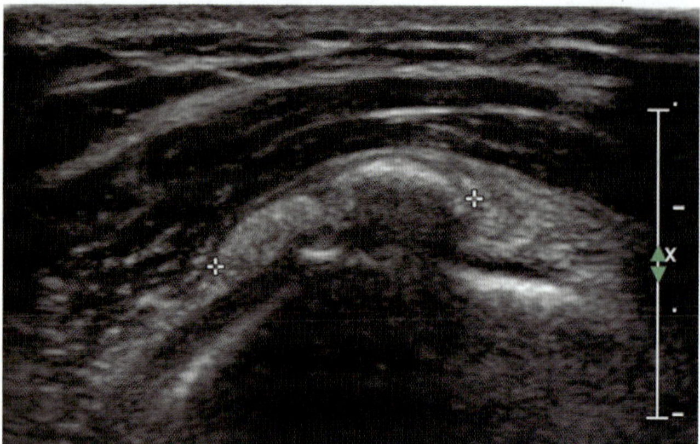

Figure 3.33. Large dense focus of "hard" calcification (between caliper marks) in supraspinatus. The calcium has a convex superficial surface, casts an acoustic shadow, and elevates the bursal surface.

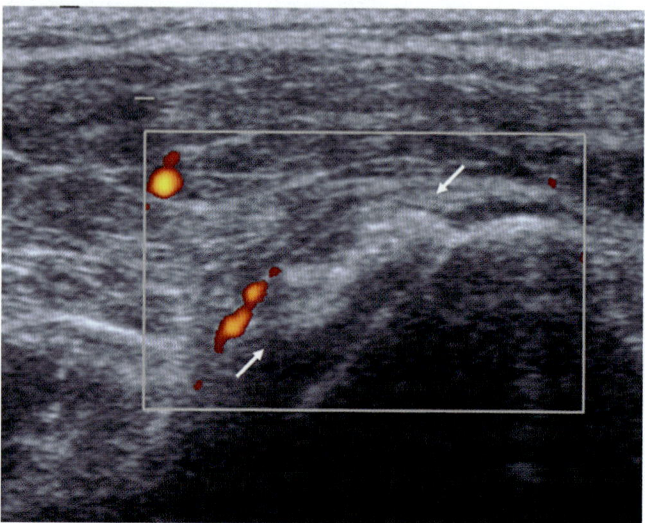

Figure 3.35. Large, acutely painful calcific deposit (*arrows*) in subscapularis. There is a small effusion in the bursa. Power Doppler shows neovascularity. Ultrasound-guided needle aspiration provides immediate and lasting pain relief.

than hard calcification and may be difficult to see if it is almost isoechoic with the tendon. Acoustic shadowing is uncommon. Hyperaemia **(Fig. 3.35)** in and around the calcification on Doppler ultrasound is associated with pain and a good response to needling. If the patient can tolerate it, increased transducer pressure may show fluid movement within the calcium deposit. Rupture into the subdeltoid bursa leaves echogenic streaks of calcium in the tendon and fluid and increased echogenicity in the bursa.

> **Tip:**
> Soft calcification responds well to aspiration, particularly if Doppler signal is present.

Several ultrasound-guided needle techniques have been advocated to treat rotator cuff calcification,[88–92] and the procedure is discussed in more detail in the interventional chapter (see Chapter 14).

I use a similar approach for both hard and soft calcifications. The patient is supine so as to avoid a vasovagal reaction. I use a 19G green needle to inject a mixture of long- and short-acting local anaesthetic and methylpredisolone into the bursa as described previously then advance the needle into the calcium. Hard calcium feels firm and may "crunch" when the needle enters. It does not usually yield an aspirate. I perform multiple needle perforations while trying to inject long-acting local anesthetic to disrupt the calcium. Soft calcium often spurts from the end of the needle when the syringe is detached. Even if it does, I try to aspirate as much calcium as possible by alternately injecting local anesthetic and aspirating. Sometimes the needle becomes blocked by calcium and has to be replaced. I do not inject steroid into the tendon. My experience is that this technique almost invariably relieves the pain of acute calcific tendonitis even if no aspirate is obtained. A similar technique also shows good short- and long-term results, although a proportion of patients suffer a recurrence of pain several weeks after the procedure and a minority requires a repeat procedure.[90]

Alternative techniques using needle sizes from 16G to 20G and one or two needles have been described.[89–93] The double needle technique flushes the calcium with saline using one needle to inject and the other to aspirate. Some authors advocate injecting steroid into the bursa or the calcium or not injecting steroid. All report good results.[91–95]

Postoperative Shoulder

Assessment of the postoperative shoulder requires detailed information about the previous surgery. Recurrent tears are common and often asymptomatic, and there is frequently poor correlation between the clinical and imaging findings; but ultrasound assessment is accurate. Large tears, older patients, and multiple procedures are risk factors for recurrent tears.[93–95]

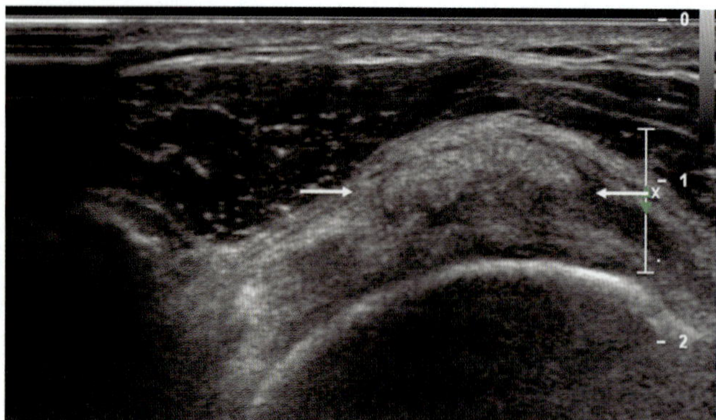

Figure 3.34. Large acute/soft calcific deposit (*arrows*) in subscapularis. The calcium is isoechoic to the tendon and elevates the bursal surface.

Most surgeons use arthroscopy whenever possible rather than open arthrotomy. Subacromial decompression for impingement involves resection of the subdeltoid bursa and inferior acromion and release or resection of the CAL. Rotator cuff tears are treated by subacromial decompression and tendon repair. Partial-thickness tears may be debrided. Small full-thickness tears can be repaired by side-to-side sutures. Larger tears require the tendon to be reattached to bone, usually by bioabsorbable anchors placed in drill holes. Double row repair using distal and proximal anchors is said to promote healing and is currently popular. The distal anchors lie beyond the edge of the tendon.

Both the bursa and the CAL re-form after decompression and appear normal or thickened (**Figs. 3.36 and 3.37**). If the rotator cuff was intact at the time of surgery, the same criteria to diagnose a rotator cuff tear apply postoperatively as in a non-operated shoulder (**Figs. 3.38 and 3.39**).

A repaired tendon is often heterogeneously echogenic and has a flattened or depressed bursal surface. Thinning of the tendon is normal postoperatively. Anchors result in small defects in the humeral cortex. The tendon should be identified running to the defects (**Fig. 3.40**) or to a wider surgical trough in older repairs, but not to the distal anchor holes in double row repairs. If the tear is large and cannot be pulled fully back to the tuberosity, the anchor defects lie proximally, and the tuberosity is bare. Partial-thickness tears result in hypoechoic or mixed hypoechoic and hyperechoic defects on the articular side of the tendon.[93]

> **Tip:**
> Rotator cuff repair often results in heterogeneously increased echogenicity and bursal surface flattening.

Large recurrent tears that retract under the acromion result in non-visualisation of the tendon, usually with deltoid in direct contact with the humeral head and often with proximal migration of the humerus. Smaller tears result in discrete defects in the tendon. A gap between the tendon and the surgical defects in the humerus is

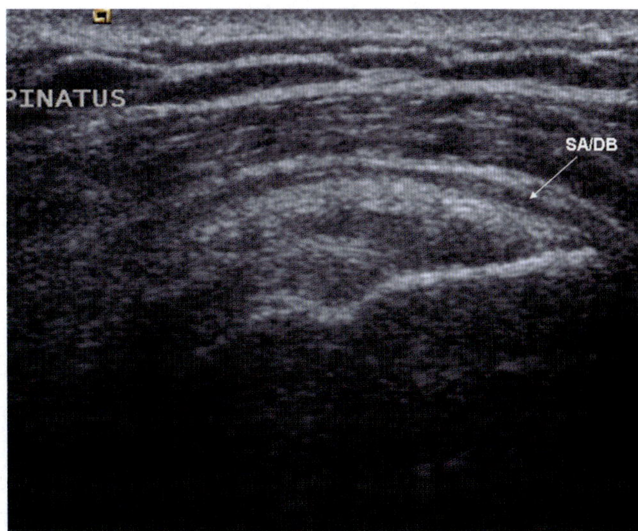

Figure 3.37.   Subacromial decompression and excision of bursa 5 years previously. Good results but left with thickened bursa. SA/SB, subacromial/deltoid bursa.

convincing evidence of a tear. Occasionally in the immediate postoperative period, an anchor can be seen loose in the joint.[93,96,97]

Poor functional results following rotator cuff repair may be due to fatty atrophy of the muscles. Atrophy generally does not improve after cuff repair and may deteriorate. The same criteria apply as in the unoperated shoulder for the assessment of muscle atrophy.

Appearances vary after removal of calcium from the cuff. Complete resorption may be seen several years later. Other patients have residual streaks of calcium.

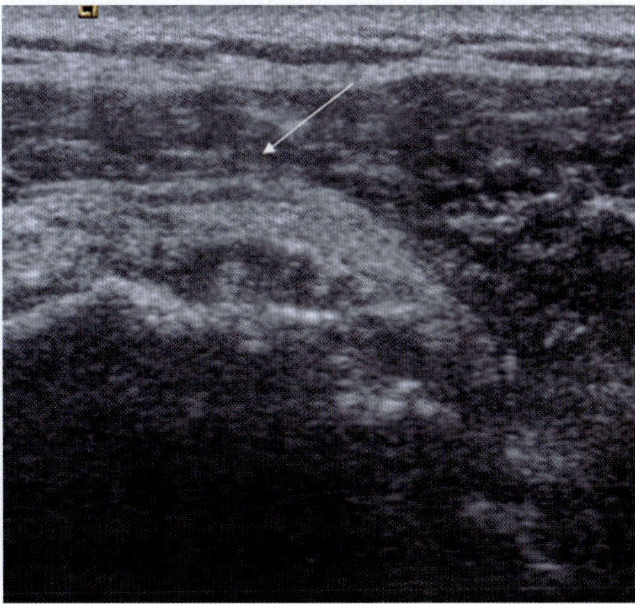

Figure 3.38.   Previous subacromial decompression. Cuff intact at time of surgery. Now has thick bursa that is within normal limits, but there is bursal surface depression of supraspinatus, (*arrow*) indicating that there is a partial tear.

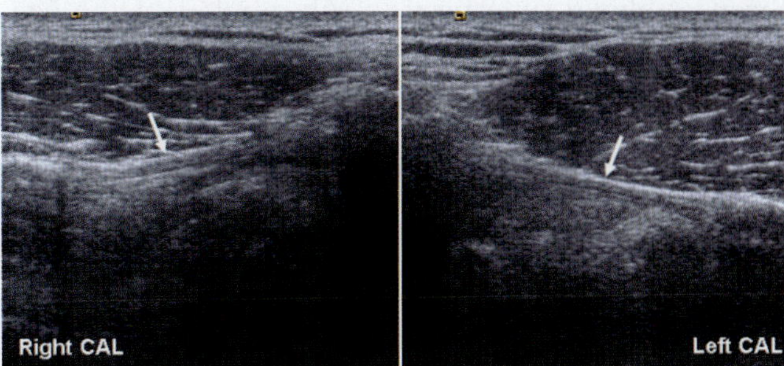

Figure 3.36.   Previous subacromial decompression on right with release of the CAL. No surgery on left. The CALs appear identical.

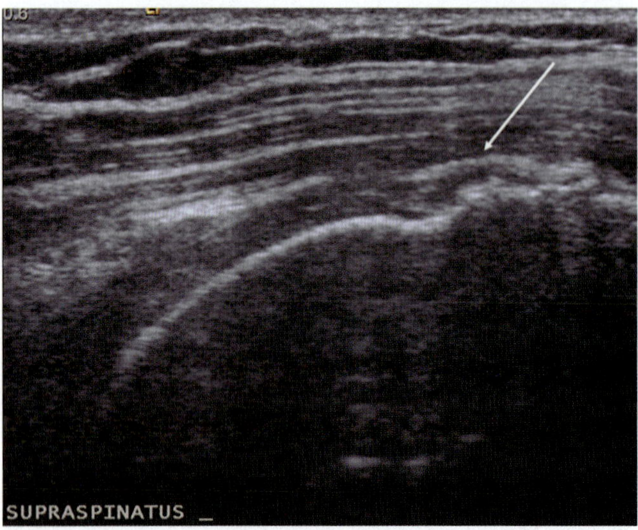

Figure 3.39.   Previous decompression and debridement of partial thickness tear 7 years previously. Recent recurrence of pain. There is now a full-thickness tear, and the deltoid (*arrow*) is in direct contact with the humeral head.

Tenodesis of the LHB is performed for biceps tears and severe tendinosis. The tendon is detached from its origin at the superior rim of the glenoid and reattached to the humerus. If reattached proximally, the tendon may appear subluxed (**Fig. 3.41**) or dislocated from the bicipital groove. Distal reattachment results in an empty groove. Biceps tenotomy is sometimes performed in association with rotator cuff repairs in older or less active patients. The tendon is cut close to its origin and allowed to slip distally, resulting in an empty bicipital groove.

Conventional shoulder arthroplasty or hemiarthroplasty is performed for severe arthropathy when the rotator cuff is substantially intact; small tears can be repaired at the time of surgery. Reverse shoulder arthroplasty is performed in patients who have severe arthropathy and irreparable rotator cuff damage; the construction of the reverse prosthesis allows the deltoid to abduct the shoulder. The rotator cuff should be present following

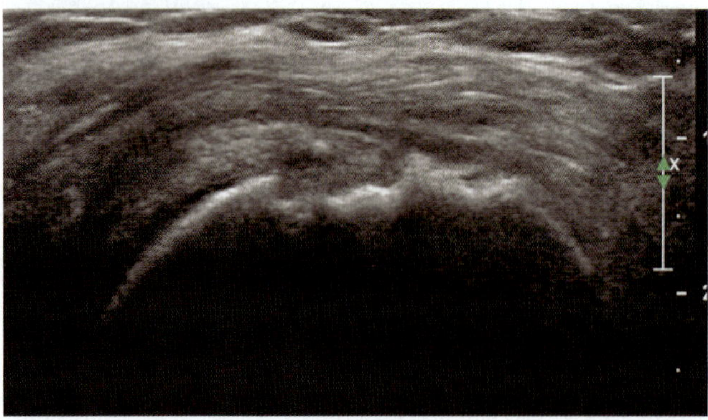

Figure 3.40.   Intact supraspinatus following previous repair. The tendon runs into the surgical defect where it has been reattached.

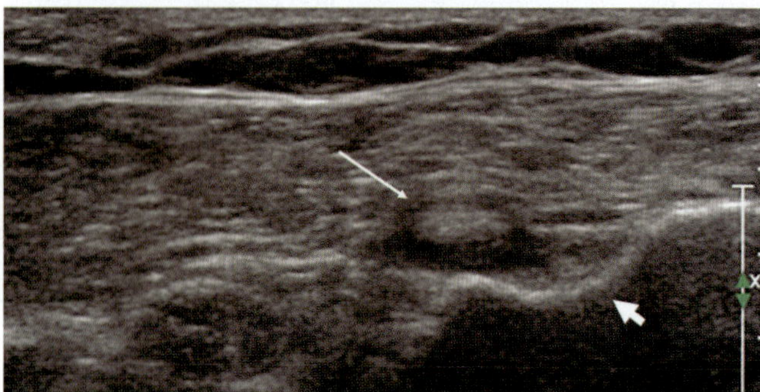

Figure 3.41.   Following biceps tenodesis, the LHB tendon (*long arrow*) lies outside the bicipital groove (*wide arrow*).

conventional arthroplasty, although postoperative tears are common. No cuff is visible after reverse arthroplasty.

Long head of Biceps Tendon

Biceps tendinopathy results from impingement against the coracoacromial arch and bicipital groove, and is often seen in patients with rotator cuff tears. Osteophytes and hyperostosis are frequently present at the entrance to the groove.[98]

Tendinopathy is best identified on transverse scans (**Fig. 3.42A**), which show an irregular contour, heterogeneous texture, and thickening or thinning of the tendon. Thinning occurs typically at the entrance to the bicipital groove, where osteophytes and hyperostosis may be identified. Longitudinal splits can be difficult to distinguish from congenitally bifid tendons, but other features of tendinopathy help, and the presence of a mesotendon for each moiety indicates a bifid tendon.

Fluid is frequently identified in the biceps tendon sheath. There is no definition of the difference between small normal, and large abnormal amounts of fluid, although it has been suggested that only a tiny amount of fluid posterior to the tendon is normal. A large effusion may be the result of intra-articular rather than biceps pathology, but it is always worth trying to identify tenosynovitis (**Fig. 3.42B**) using Doppler.[8]

Biceps instability (**Fig. 3.43**) results from rupture of its ligamentous stabilisers, particularly the CHL, either alone or in association with rupture of subscapularis. Biceps subluxes superficial to subscapularis if the ligaments are ruptured, and subscapularis is intact or only partly torn, and deep to subscapularis if the latter is completely torn.

The most obvious sign of a dislocated biceps is an empty groove. Biceps dislocation is distinguished from rupture by identifying the tendon lying medially, possibly as far medially as the coracoid process when subscapularis is ruptured and retracted. If biceps is not identified or cannot be distinguished from the short head of biceps tendon that arises from the coracoid process, it helps to place the transducer on the insertion of

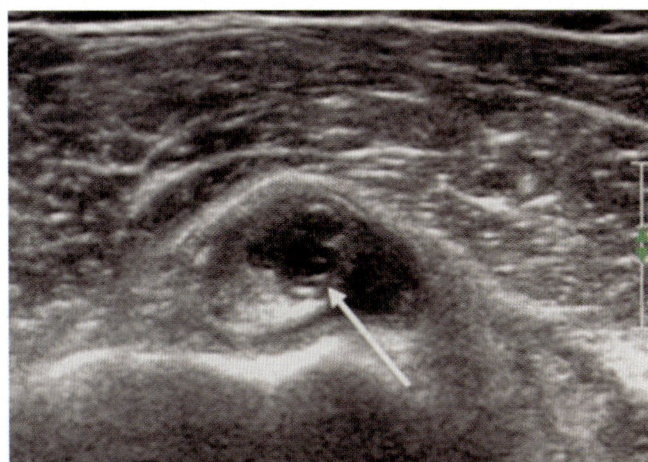

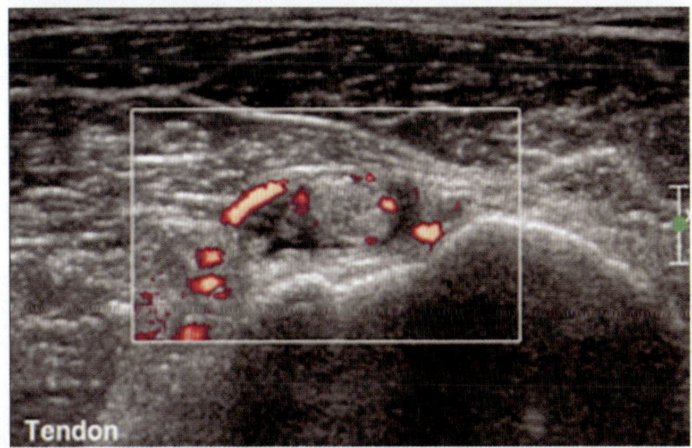

Figure 3.42. **A:** Short-axis scan of LHB, which is swollen and contains an intrasubstance tear (*arrow*). **B:** Power Doppler shows neo-vascularity in the LHB and its tendon sheath in keeping with tendinosis and associated tenosynovitis.

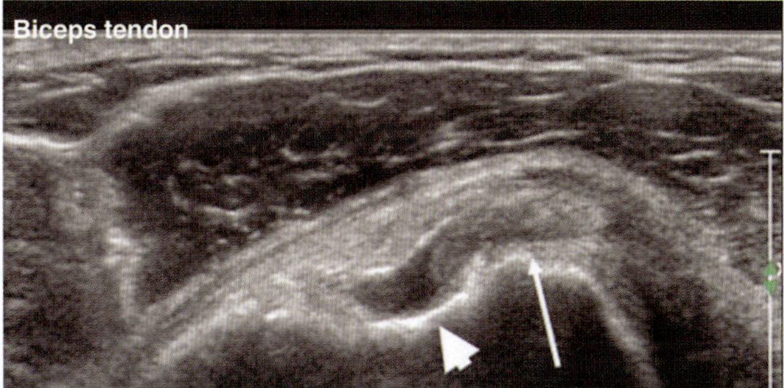

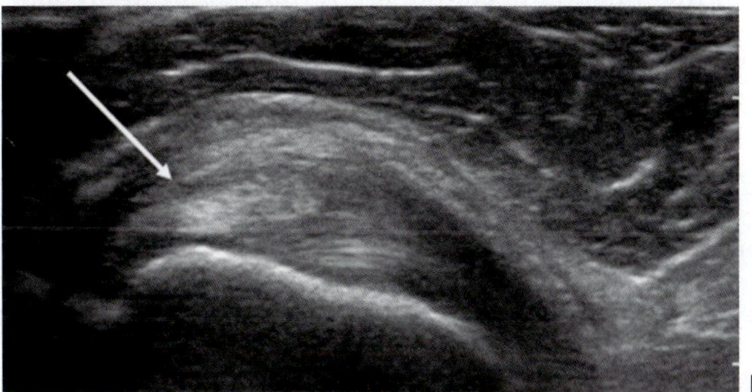

Figure 3.43. **A:** Transverse scan showing subluxed LHB (*thin arrow*) slipping out of bicipital groove (*short arrow*). **B:** Longitudinal scan showing subscapularis fibers superficial and deep to LHB (*arrow*), indicating a delaminating tear of subscapularis.

pectoralis major tendon on the humerus. This is at the level of the musculotendinous junction of the LHB, and it should be possible to follow the tendon proximally from there if it is present.[99,101]

> **Tip:**
> If the biceps tendon is not visible, use transverse images to identify the pectoralis major insertion, which is at the level of the myotendinous junction of the biceps. Run the transducer proximally from the myotendinous junction to pick up the LHB tendon.

Particularly when the subscapularis is intact, the subluxed biceps usually remains close to the groove or partly subluxed and lying at the edge of the groove. Intermittent subluxation can be demonstrated by dynamic examination with the elbow flexed at 90°. The biceps slips medially out of the groove on external rotation and back in again on internal rotation.[101,102]

Tenodesis of biceps may move the tendon outside the bicipital groove, but it remains fixed in position during dynamic scanning.

Complete rupture of the biceps tendon often occurs in association with large rotator cuff tears that extend across the rotator interval. Isolated tears are often clinically obvious as retraction of the muscle belly results in the "Popeye" sign. The fluid-filled tendon sheath lies in the bicipital groove and may contain debris or remnants of the tendon.

SLAP tears of the biceps origin cannot be identified on ultrasound. Magnetic resonance arthrography is the appropriate investigation for suspected SLAP tears.

Infection

Risk factors for infection include diabetes, renal failure, and immune suppression. Patients present with acute severe pain, pyrexia, and elevated inflammatory markers. The differential diagnosis is acute calcific tendonitis.

Fluid is the ultrasound hallmark of infection at the glenohumeral joint, subdeltoid bursa, or ACJ. The fluid may be thick and echogenic, but the ultrasound characteristics are nonspecific. Aspiration is essential if fluid is identified when infection is suspected. Ultrasound demonstrates even small-volume effusions that elevate the joint capsule at the posterior glenohumeral joint margin, best demonstrated with the hand across the chest **(Fig. 3.17)**. This is a good site for aspiration. The biceps tendon sheath is the other reliable site to detect fluid.[103] In addition to distension with fluid, an infected bursa may be thick-walled and hyperaemic; and erosions may be present at an infected ACJ.[104,105]

Tip:
The posterior margin of the glenohumeral joint is the best place to identify and aspirate a joint effusion.

Instability

US may show a Hill-Sachs or reverse Hill-Sachs defect in the humeral head due to previous dislocation, damage to the glenoid or labrum or apparent joint laxity, but has no role in the assessment of glenohumeral instability.

Pectoralis Major

Injury to the pectoralis major is uncommon and due to forced extreme external rotation. Tears may involve muscle, musculotendinous junction, or tendon. Ultrasound shows a large hypoechoic haematoma, and muscle or tendon retraction.[106,107] The musculotendinous junction of the biceps is a good landmark for the pectoralis major insertion (**Fig. 3.6**).

Fractures

Ultrasound has no formal role in the assessment of fractures, but may show a depression in the posterolateral cortex of the humeral head due to the Hill-Sachs defect of anterior dislocation, or deep to subscapularis due to a reverse Hill-Sachs defect from posterior dislocation. Radiographically, occult tuberosity fractures can be associated with prolonged pain, restricted range of movement, and an intact but clinically weak supraspinatus following trauma. The cortex is undisplaced or minimally depressed or elevated, and the fracture line is seen as a tiny defect in the cortex. Overlying callus develops after several weeks.[102] With larger, displaced fragments, the tendon can usually be identified attached to the displaced bone.

Acromioclavicular Joint

Soft tissue hypertrophy and osteophytes occur with osteoarthritis (OA). Soft tissue swelling and erosions may be seen with rheumatoid arthritis (RA). Infection results in an effusion and possibly erosions.

Post-traumatic osteolysis of the clavicle results in irregular erosions at the outer end of the clavicle and widening, soft tissue swelling, and an effusion at the ACJ. Joint widening is also a feature of ACJ sprains. The "geyser sign" is a large cystic swelling filled with synovial fluid and extending superficially from the ACJ. It is due to direct communication between the glenohumeral joint and the ACJ through a large rotator cuff tear. Transducer pressure may

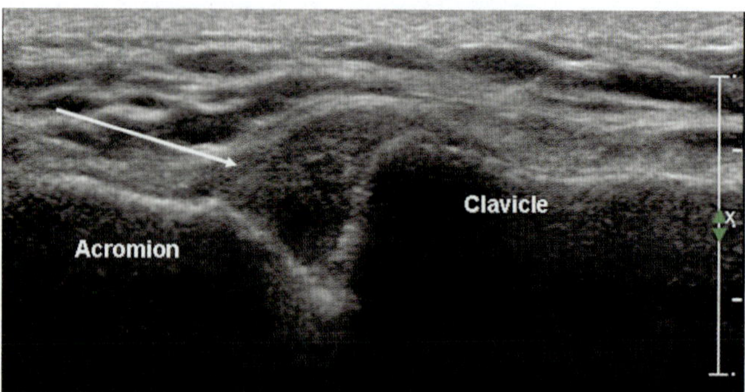

Figure 3.44.   Long-axis scan of the ACJ (*arrow*).

demonstrate fluid moving through the ACJ, although not all ACJ cysts are associated with rotator cuff tears.[102,108]

Blind injection of the ACJ is difficult, particularly if there is much overlying soft tissue, because the joint is so narrow (**Fig. 3.44**). Ultrasound-guided injection is easy. The transducer is placed on the clavicle, oriented sagittally, and moved laterally to the acromion and back again. The bony structures are flat and densely echogenic. The ACJ is hypoechoic and disc-shaped (**Fig. 3.45**). After skin preparation, I use a green needle attached to a 5mL syringe. The needle is inserted into the joint either superior or inferior to the transducer. As the joint is often thick-walled, the needle position may have to be adjusted to ensure that the needle tip is in the joint space. This is confirmed by injecting a small volume of local anaesthetic. The ACJ has a small capacity and usually accepts <1 mL. If the injection is purely diagnostic (ie to see if it abolishes pain), I inject about 1mL of a mixture of lidocaine and bupivacaine. If steroid is to be injected for therapeutic benefit, the volume of anaesthetic injected should be just sufficient to show that the needle is intraarticular. I use methylprednisolone because it has a lower risk of causing skin depigmentation than triamcinolone. Most ACJ's injected in this way will accept 20 to 30 mg of methylpredisolone. Pain relief as a result of the injection is a good prognostic test for surgical intervention but the effect of the steroid injection is usually short-lived.[109]

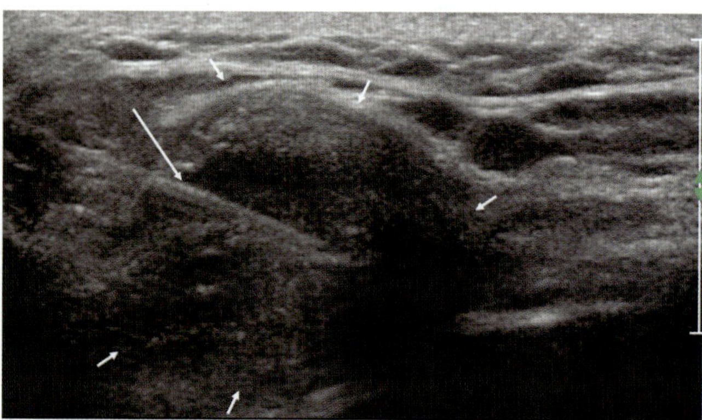

Figure 3.45.   Sagittal scan showing needle insertion (*long arrow*) into hypoechoic, disc-like ACJ (*short arrows*).

Masses

Lipomas are by far the most common tumours at the shoulder. If a mass cannot confidently be diagnosed as a lipoma or cyst on ultrasound, MRI and possibly biopsy will be needed.[110]

The other mass with a predilection for the shoulder region is elastofibroma dorsi, which almost always occurs deep to the inferior scapula. It is a pseudotumour composed of fat and fibroelastic tissue, probably due to friction between the scapula and chest wall, and is bilateral in about 50% of cases. The patient should be examined with the arm positioned to throw the scapula off the mass. Ultrasound shows multiple linear hypoechoic streaks against an echogenic background due to alternating tissue layers. Magnetic resonance imaging shows a poorly defined mass with alternating layers of fat and muscle signal intensity. The location, particularly if bilateral masses are present, and the ultrasound and MRI appearances, are characteristic. Biopsy and resection are unnecessary unless the lesion is symptomatic.[111–113]

Arthropathy: Osteoarthritis, Rheumatoid Arthritis, Crystal Deposition Disease, and Loose Bodies

Osteoarthritis causes osteophytes at the margins of the glenoid and humeral articular surfaces, joint space narrowing, and an effusion that may contain debris, loose bodies, and synovial hypertrophy.

Crystal deposition disease produces multiple small echogenic foci in cartilage, synovium, and joint fluid. Calcium pyrophosphate crystals are deposited within the hyaline cartilage, whereas monosodium urate crystals are deposited on the surface.[114,115]

Rapidly progressive joint destruction associated with a massive rotator cuff tear and deposition of hydroxyapatite and pyrophosphate crystals occurs in "cuff tear arthropathy" or "Milwaukee shoulder." The humerus is high-riding. Large and painful haemorrhagic joint effusions may contain debris, loose bodies, and hyperplastic synovium. Clinically, the effusion may simulate a large mass.[116]

Rheumatoid arthritis may affect the glenohumeral joint, ACJ, biceps tendon sheath, or, most frequently, the subdeltoid bursa. Ultrasound shows effusions, synovial proliferation, and hyperemia. It may be difficult to distinguish pannus from fluid even using sonopalpation. Early bone erosions may be present. Contrast-enhanced MRI is slightly superior to ultrasound in the detection of early inflammatory arthropathy at the shoulder.[117,118] Ultrasound can locate the inflammation and be used to guide steroid injections.

Multiple small echogenic filling defects in the glenohumeral joint or subdeltoid bursa may be due to synovial chondromatosis or to rice bodies in association with RA or tuberculosis.[108]

CONCLUSION

Ultrasound is an important diagnostic tool in the management of many shoulder conditions. A good understanding of the anatomy and pathologic processes and meticulous technique are essential for good results. Ultrasound-guided interventions are widely employed, although their efficacy remains unproven.

REFERENCES

1. de Jesus JO, Parker L, Frangos AJ, et al. Accuracy of MRI, MR arthrography, and ultrasound in the diagnosis of rotator cuff tears: a meta-analysis. *AJR Am J Roentgenol.* 2009;92(6):1701–1707.
2. Middleton WD, Payne WT, Teefey SA, et al. Sonography and MRI of the shoulder: comparison of patient satisfaction. *AJR Am J Roentgenol.* 2004;183(5):1449–1452.
3. Miller D, Frost A, Hall A. A 'one-stop clinic' for the diagnosis and management of rotator cuff pathology: getting the right diagnosis first time. *Int J Clin Pract.* 2008;62(5):750–753.
4. Beggs I, Bianchi S, Buero A, et al. Musculoskeletal ultrasound technical guidelines. I shoulder. http://essr.org/html/img/pool/shoulder.pdf.
5. Mochizuki T, Sugaya H, Uomizu M, et al. Humeral insertion of the supraspinatus and infraspinatus. New anatomical findings regarding the footprint of the rotator cuff. *J Bone Joint Surg Am.* 2008;90(5):962–969.
6. Soslowsky LJ, Carpenter JE, Bucchieri JS, et al. Biomechanics of the rotator cuff. *Orthop Clin North Am.* 1997;28(1):17–30.
7. Jamadar DA, Jacobson JA, Caoili EM, et al. Musculoskeletal sonography technique: focused versus comprehensive examination. *AJR Am J Roentgenol.* 2008;190(1):5–9.
8. Jacobson JA. Shoulder US: anatomy, technique, and scanning pitfalls. *Radiology.* 2011;260(1):6–16.
9. Krief OP. MRI of the rotator interval capsule. *AJR Am J Roentgenol.* 2005;184(5):1490–1494.
10. Petchprapa CN, Beltran LS, Jazrawi LM, et al. The rotator interval: a review of anatomy, function, and normal and abnormal MRI appearances. *AJR Am J Roentgenol.* 2010;195(3):567–576.
11. Adler RS, Fealy S, Rudzki JR, et al. Rotator cuff in asymptomatic volunteers: contrast-enhanced US depiction of intratendinous and peritendinous vascularity. *Radiology.* 2008;248(3):954–961.
12. Morag Y, Jacobson JA, Lucas D, et al. US appearance of the rotator cable with histologic correlation: preliminary results. *Radiology.* 2006;241(2):485–491.
13. Neer CS 2nd. Anterior acromioplasty for the chronic impingement syndrome in the shoulder: a preliminary report. *J Bone Joint Surg Am.* 1972;54(1):41–50.
14. Biberthaler P, Wiedemann E, Nerlich A, et al. Microcirculation associated with degenerative rotator cuff lesions. In vivo assessment with orthogonal polarization spectral imaging during arthroscopy of the shoulder. *J Bone Joint Surg Am.* 2003;85-A(3):475–480.
15. Park HB, Yokota A, Gill HS, et al. Diagnostic accuracy of clinical tests for the different degrees of subacromial impingement syndrome. *J Bone Joint Surg Am.* 2005;87(7):1446–1455.
16. Kelly SM, Brittle N, Allen GM. The value of physical tests for subacromial impingement syndrome: a study of diagnostic accuracy. *Clin Rehabil.* 2010;24(2):149–158.
17. Beaudreuil J, Nizard R, Thomas T, et al. Contribution of clinical tests to the diagnosis of rotator cuff disease: a systematic literature review. *Joint Bone Spine.* 2009;76(1):15–19.
18. Dinnes J, Loveman E, McIntyre L, et al. The effectiveness of diagnostic tests for the assessment of shoulder pain due to

soft tissue disorders: a systematic review. *Health Technol Assess.* 2003;7(29):iii,1–166.

19. Kim HM, Dahiya N, Teefey SA, et al. Location and initiation of degenerative rotator cuff tears: an analysis of three hundred and sixty shoulders. *J Bone Joint Surg Am.* 2010;92(5):1088–1096.

20. Shindle MK, Chen CC, Robertson C, et al. Full-thickness supraspinatus tears are associated with more synovial inflammation and tissue degeneration than partial-thickness tears. *J Shoulder Elbow Surg.* 2011;20(6):917–927.

21. Hollister MS, Mack LA, Patten RM, et al. Association of sonographically detected subacromial/subdeltoid bursal effusion and intraarticular fluid with rotator cuff tear. *AJR Am J Roentgenol.* 1995;165(3):605–608.

22. Wohlwend JR, van Holsbeeck M, Craig J, et al. The association between irregular greater tuberosities and rotator cuff tears: a sonographic study. *AJR Am J Roentgenol.* 1998;171(1):229–233.

23. Arslan G, Apaydin A, Kabaalioglu A, et al. Sonographically detected subacromial/subdeltoid bursal effusion and biceps tendon sheath fluid: reliable signs of rotator cuff tear? *J Clin Ultrasound.* 1999;27(6):335–339.

24. Jacobson JA, Lancaster S, Prasad A, et al. Full-thickness and partial-thickness supraspinatus tendon tears: value of US signs in diagnosis. *Radiology.* 2004;230(1):234–242.

25. Fukuda H. The management of partial-thickness tears of the rotator cuff. *J Bone Joint Surg Br.* 2003;85(1):3–11.

26. Vinson EN, Helms CA, Higgins LD. Rim-rent tear of the rotator cuff: a common and easily overlooked partial tear. *AJR Am J Roentgenol.* 2007;189(4):943–946.

27. Bouffard JA, Lee SM, Dhanju J. Ultrasonography of the shoulder. *Semin Ultrasound CT MR.* 2000;21(3):164–191.

28. Crass JR, Craig EV, Feinberg SB. Clinical significance of sonographic findings in the abnormal but intact rotator cuff: a preliminary report. *J Clin Ultrasound.* 1988;16(9):625–634.

29. Farin PU, Jaroma H, Harju A, et al. Shoulder impingement syndrome: sonographic evaluation. *Radiology.* 1990;176(3):845–849.

30. Read JW, Perko M. Shoulder ultrasound: diagnostic accuracy for impingement syndrome, rotator cuff tear, and biceps tendon pathology. *J Shoulder Elbow Surg.* 1998;7(3):264–271.

31. Lewis JS, Raza SA, Pilcher J, et al. The prevalence of neovascularity in patients clinically diagnosed with rotator cuff tendinopathy. *BMC Musculoskelet Disord.* 2009;10:163.

32. Teefey SA, Rubin DA, Middleton WD, et al. Detection and quantification of rotator cuff tears. Comparison of ultrasonographic, magnetic resonance imaging, and arthroscopic findings in seventy-one consecutive cases. *J Bone Joint Surg Am.* 2004;86-A(4):708–716.

33. Fotiadou AN, Vlychou M, Papadopoulos P, et al. Ultrasonography of symptomatic rotator cuff tears compared with MR imaging and surgery. *Eur J Radiol.* 2008;68(1):174–179.

34. Al-Shawi A, Badge R, Bunker T. The detection of full-thickness rotator cuff tears using ultrasound. *J Bone Joint Surg Br.* 2008; 90(7):889–892.

35. Rutten MJ, Spaargaren GJ, van Loon T, et al. Detection of rotator cuff tears: the value of MRI following ultrasound. *Eur Radiol.* 2010;20(2):450–457.

36. Smith TO, Back T, Toms AP, et al. Diagnostic accuracy of ultrasound for rotator cuff tears in adults: a systematic review and meta-analysis. *Clin Radiol.* 2011;66(11):1036–1048.

37. Teefey SA, Middleton WD, Payne WT, et al. Detection and measurement of rotator cuff tears with sonography: analysis of diagnostic errors. *AJR Am J Roentgenol.* 2005;184(6):1768–1773.

38. Teefey SA, Hasan SA, Middleton WD, et al. Ultrasonography of the rotator cuff: A comparison of ultrasonographic and arthroscopic findings in one hundred consecutive cases. *J Bone Joint Surg Am.* 2000;82(4):498–504.

39. Kluger R, Mayrhofer R, Kröner A, et al. Sonographic versus magnetic resonance arthrographic evaluation of full-thickness rotator cuff tears in millimeters. *J Shoulder Elbow Surg.* 2003;12(2): 110–116.

40. Strobel K, Zanetti M, Nagy L, et al. Suspected rotator cuff lesions: tissue harmonic imaging versus conventional US of the shoulder. *Radiology.* 2004;230(1):243–249.

41. Ferri M, Finlay K, Popowich T, et al. Sonography of full-thickness supraspinatus tears: comparison of patient positioning technique with surgical correlation. *AJR Am J Roengenol.* 2005;184(1):180–184.

42. Sasyniuk TM, Mohtadi NG, Hollinshead RM, et al. The interrater reliability of shoulder arthroscopy. *Arthroscopy.* 2007;23(9): 971–977.

43. Middleton WD, Teefey SA, Yamagichi K. Sonography of the rotator cuff: analysis of interobserver variability. *AJR Am J Roentgenol.* 2004;183(5):1465–1468.

44. O'Connor PJ, Rankine J, Gibbon WW, et al. Interobserver variation in sonography of the painful shoulder. *J Clin Ultrasound.* 2005;33(2):53–56.

45. Le Corroller T, Cohen M, Aswad R, et al. Sonography of the painful shoulder: role of the operator's experience. *Skeletal Radiol.* 2008;37(11):979–986.

46. Rutten MJ, Jager GJ, Kiemeney LA. Ultrasound detection of rotator cuff tears: observer agreement related to increasing experience. *AJR Am J Roentgenol.* 2010;195(6):W440–W446.

47. Moosmayer S, Heir S, Smith HJ. Sonography of the rotator cuff in painful shoulders performed without knowledge of clinical information: results from 58 sonographic examinations with surgical correlation. *J Clin Ultrasound.* 2007;35(1):20–26.

48. Hedtmann A, Fett H. Ultrasonography of the shoulder in subacromial syndromes with disorders and injuries of the rotator cuff [in German]. *Orthopade.* 1995;24(6):498–508.

49. Schibany N, Zehetgruber H, Kainberger F, et al. Rotator cuff tears in asymptomatic individuals: a clinical and ultrasonographic screening study. *Eur J Radiol.* 2004;51(3):263–268.

50. Worland RL, Lee D, Orozco CG, et al. Correlation of age, acromial morphology, and rotator cuff tear pathology diagnosed by ultrasound in asymptomatic patients. *J South Orthop Assoc.* 2003; 12(1):23–26.

51. Moosmayer S, Smith HJ, Tariq R, et al. Prevalence and characteristics of asymptomatic tears of the rotator cuff: an ultrasonographic and clinical study. *J Bone Joint Surg Br.* 2009;91(2):196–200.

52. Tempelhof S, Rupp S, Seil R. Age-related prevalence of rotator cuff tears in asymptomatic shoulders. *J Shoulder Elbow Surg.* 1999;8(4):296–299.

53. Kim HM, Teefey SA, Zelig A, et al. Shoulder strength in asymptomatic individuals with intact compared with torn rotator cuffs. *J Bone Joint Surg Am.* 2009;91(2):289–296.

54. Yamaguchi K, Tetro AM, Blam O, et al. Natural history of asymptomatic rotator cuff tears: a longitudinal analysis of asymptomatic tears detected sonographically. *J Shoulder Elbow Surg.* 2001;10(3):199–203.

55. Yamaguchi K, Ditsios K, Middleton WD, et al. The demographic and morphological features of rotator cuff disease. A comparison of asymptomatic and symptomatic shoulders. *J Bone Joint Surg Am.* 2006;88(8):1699–1704.

56. Wallny T, Wagner UA, Prange S, et al. Evaluation of chronic tears of the rotator cuff by ultrasound. A new index. *J Bone Joint Surg Br.* 1999;81(4):675–678.

57. Teefey SA, Middleton WD, Bauer GS, et al. Sonographic differences in the appearance of acute and chronic full-thickness rotator cuff tears. *J Ultrasound Med.* 2000;19(6):377–378.

58. Kim HM, Dahiya N, Teefey SA, et al. Relationship of tear size and location to fatty degeneration of the rotator cuff. *J Bone Joint Surg Am.* 2010;92(4):829–839.

59. Schaefer O, Winterer J, Lohrmann C, et al. Magnetic resonance imaging for supraspinatus muscle atrophy after cuff repair. *Clin Orthop Relat Res.* 2002;(403):93–99.

60. Morag Y, Jacobson JA, Miller B, et al. MR imaging of rotator cuff injury: what the clinician needs to know. *Radiographics.* 2006;26(4):1045–1065.

61. Thomazeau H, Rolland Y, Lucas C, et al. Atrophy of the supraspinatus belly. Assessment by MRI in 55 patients with rotator cuff pathology. *Acta Orthop Scand.* 1996;67(3):264–268.

62. Khoury V, Cardinal E, Brassard P. Atrophy and fatty infiltration of the supraspinatus muscle: sonography versus MRI. *AJR Am J Roentgenol.* 2008;190(4):1105–1111.

63. Goutallier D, Postel JM, Lavau L, et al. Impact of fatty degeneration of the suparspinatus and infraspinatus muscles on the prognosis of surgical repair of the rotator cuff [in French]. *Rev Chir Orthop Reparatrice Appar Mot.* 1999;85(7):668–676.

64. Goutallier D, Postel JM, Bernageau J, et al. Fatty muscle degeneration in cuff ruptures. Pre- and postoperative evaluation by CT scan. *Clin Orthop Relat Res.* 1994;(304):78–83.

65. Goutallier D, Postel JM, Gleyze P, et al. Influence of cuff muscle fatty degeneration on anatomic and functional outcomes after simple suture of full-thickness tears. *J Shoulder Elbow Surg.* 2003;12(6):550–554.

66. Zanetti M, Gerber C, Hodler J. Quantitative assessment of the muscles of the rotator cuff with magnetic resonance imaging. *Invest Radiol.* 1998;33(3):163–170.

67. Mellado JM, Calmet J, Olona M, et al. Surgically repaired massive rotator cuff tears: MRI of tendon integrity, muscle fatty degeneration, and muscle atrophy correlated with intraoperative and clinical findings. *AJR Am J Roentgenol.* 2005;184(5):1456–1463.

68. Strobel K, Hodler J, Meyer DC, et al. Fatty atrophy of supraspinatus and infraspinatus muscles: accuracy of US. *Radiology.* 2005;237(2):584–589.

69. Kavanagh EC, Koulouris G, Parker L, et al. Does extended-field-of-view sonography improve interrater reliability for the detection of rotator cuff muscle atrophy? *AJR Am J Roentgenol.* 2008;190(1):27–31.

70. DeFranco MJ, Cole BJ. Current perspectives on rotator cuff anatomy. *Arthroscopy.* 2009;25(3):305–320.

71. Rutten MJ, Maresch BJ, Jager GJ, et al. Injection of the subacromial-subdeltoid bursa: blind or ultrasound-guided? *Acta Orthop.* 2007;78(2):254–257.

72. Henkus HE, Cobben LP, Coerkamp EG, et al. The accuracy of subacromial injections: a prospective randomized magnetic resonance imaging study. *Arthroscopy.* 2006;22(3):277–282.

73. Yamakado K. The targeting accuracy of subacromial injection to the shoulder: an arthrographic evaluation. *Arthroscopy.* 2002;18(8):887–891.

74. Kang MN, Rizio L, Prybicien M, et al. The accuracy of subacromial corticosteroid injections: a comparison of multiple methods. *J Shoulder Elbow Surg.* 2008;17(suppl 1):61–66.

75. Partington PF, Broome GH. Diagnostic injection around the shoulder: hit and miss? A cadaveric study of injection accuracy. *J Shoulder Elbow Surg.* 1998;7(2):147–150.

76. Ucuncu F, Capkin E, Karkucak M, et al. A comparison of the effectiveness of landmark-guided injections and ultrasonography guided injections for shoulder pain. *Clin J Pain.* 2009;25(9):786–789.

77. Naredo E, Cabero F, Beneyto P, et al. A randomized comparative study of short term response to injection versus sonographic-guided injection of local corticosteroids in patients with painful shoulder. *J Rheumatol.* 2004;31:308–314.

78. Ekeberg OM, Bautz-Holter E, Tveitå EK, et al. Subacromial ultrasound guided or systemic steroid injection for rotator cuff disease: randomised double blind study. *BMJ.* 2009;338:A3112.

79. Bureau NJ, Beauchamp M, Cardinal E, et al. Dynamic sonography evaluation of shoulder impingement syndrome. *AJR Am J Roentgenol.* 2006;187(1):216–220.

80. Bunker TD, Anthony PP. The pathology of frozen shoulder. A Dupuytren-like disease. *J Bone Joint Surg Br.* 1995;77:677–683.

81. Dias R, Cutts S, Massoud S. Frozen shoulder. *BMJ.* 2005;331(7530):1453–1456.

82. Rodeo SA, Hannafin JA, Tom J, et al. Immunolocalization of cytokines and their receptors in adhesive capsulitis of the shoulder. *J Orthop Res.* 1997;15(3):427–436.

83. Lee JC, Sykes C, Saifuddin A, et al. Adhesive capsulitis: sonographic changes in the rotator cuff interval with arthroscopic correlation. *Skeletal Radiol.* 2005;34(9):522–527.

84. Homsi C, Bordalo-Rodrigues M, da Silva JJ, et al. Ultrasound in adhesive capsulitis of the shoulder: is assessment of the coracohumeral ligament a valuable diagnostic tool? *Skeletal Radiol.* 2006;35(9):673–678.

85. Mengiardi B, Pfirrmann CW, Gerber C, et al. Frozen shoulder: MR arthrographic findings. *Radiology.* 2004;233(2):486–492.

86. Carette S, Moffet H, Tardif J, et al. Intraarticular corticosteroids, supervised physiotherapy, or a combination of the two in the treatment of adhesive capsulitis of the shoulder: a placebo-controlled trial. *Arthritis Rheum.* 2003;48(3):829–838.

87. Uhthoff HK, Loehr JW. Calcific tendinopathy of the rotator cuff: pathogenesis, diagnosis and management. *J Am Acad Orthop Surg.* 1997;5(4):183–191.

88. Farin PU, Jaroma H, Soimakallio S. Rotator cuff calcifications: treatment with US-guided technique. *Radiology.* 1995;195(3):841–843.

89. Aina R, Cardinal E, Bureau NJ, et al. Calcific shoulder tendinitis: treatment with modified US-guided fine-needle technique. *Radiology.* 2001;221(2):455–461.

90. del Cura JL, Torre I, Zabala R, et al. Sonographically guided percutaneous needle lavage in calcific tendinitis of the shoulder: short- and long-term results. *AJR Am J Roentgenol.* 2007;189(3):W128–W134.

91. Lin JT, Adler RS, Bracilovic A, et al. Clinical outcomes of ultrasound-guided aspiration and lavage in calcific tendinosis of the shoulder. *HSS J.* 2007;3(1):99–105.

92. Serafini G, Sconfienza LM, Lacelli F, et al. Rotator cuff calcific tendonitis: short-term and 10-year outcomes after two-needle us-guided percutaneous treatment—nonrandomized controlled trial. *Radiology.* 2009;252(1):157–164.

93. Prickett WD, Teefey SA, Galatz LM, et al. Accuracy of ultrasound imaging of the rotator cuff in shoulders that are painful postoperatively. *J Bone Joint Surg Am.* 2003;85-A(6):1084–1089.

94. Galatz LM, Ball CM, Teefey SA, et al. The outcome and repair integrity of completely arthroscopically repaired large and massive rotator cuff tears. *J Bone Joint Surg Am.* 2004;86-A(2):219–224.

95. Gulotta LV, Nho SJ, Dodson CC, et al. Prospective evaluation of arthroscopic rotator cuff repairs at 5 years: part II—prognostic factors for clinical and radiographic outcomes. *J Shoulder Elbow Surg.* 2011;20(6):941–946.

96. Crass JR, Craig EV, Feinberg SB. Sonography of the postoperative rotator cuff. *AJR Am J Roentgenol.* 1986;146(3):561–564.

97. Mack LA, Nyberg DA, Matsen FR 3rd, et al. Sonography of the postoperative shoulder. *AJR Am J Roentgenol.* 1998;150(5):1089–1093.

98. Pfahler M, Branner S, Refior HJ. The role of the bicipital groove in tendinopathy of the long biceps tendon. *J Shoulder Elbow Surg.* 1999;8(5):419–424.

99. Bennett WF. Subscapularis, medial, and lateral head coracohumeral ligament insertion anatomy. Arthroscopic appearance and incidence of "hidden" rotator interval lesions. *Arthroscopy.* 2001;17(2):173–180.

100. Patton WC, McCluskey GM 3rd. Biceps tendinitis and subluxation. *Clin Sports Med.* 2001;20(3):505–529.

101. Farin PU, Jaroma H, Harju A, et al. Medial displacement of the biceps brachii tendon: evaluation with dynamic sonography during maximal external shoulder rotation. *Radiology.* 1995;195(3):845–848.

102. Martinoli C, Bianchi S, Prato N, et al. US of the shoulder: non-rotator cuff disorders. *Radiographics.* 2003;23(2):381–401.

103. Zubler V, Mamisch-Saupe N, Pfirrmann CW, et al. Detection and quantification of glenohumeral joint effusion: reliability of ultrasound. *Eur Radiol.* 2011;21(9):1858–1864.

104. Cardinal E, Bureau NJ, Aubin B, et al. Role of ultrasound in musculoskeletal infections. *Radiol Clin North Am.* 2001;39(2):191–201.

105. Widman DS, Craig JG, van Holsbeeck M. Sonographic detection, evaluation, and aspiration of infected acromioclavicular joints. *Skeletal Radiol.* 2001;30(7):388–392.

106. Beloosesky Y, Grinblat J, Katz M, et al. Pectoralis major rupture in the elderly: clinical and sonographic findings. *Clin Imaging.* 2003;27(4):261–264.

107. Weaver JS, Jacobson JA, Jamadar DA, et al. Sonographic findings of pectoralis major tears with surgical, clinical, and magnetic resonance imaging correlation in 6 patients. *J Ultrasound Med.* 2005;24(1):25–31.

108. Mellado JM, Salvadó E, Camins A, et al. Fluid collections and juxta-articular cystic lesions of the shoulder: spectrum of MRI findings. *Eur Radiol.* 2002;12(3):650–659.

109. Bain GI, Van Riet RP, Gooi C, et al. The long-term efficacy of corticosteroid injection into the acromioclavicular joint using a dynamic fluoroscopic method. *Int J Shoulder Surg.* 2007;1:104–107.

110. Kransdorf MJ, Murphey MD. Soft tissue tumors in a large referral population: prevalence and distribution of diagnoses by age, sex and location. In: *Imaging of Soft Tissue Tumors.* Philadelphia, PA: WB Saunders,1997:3–35.

111. Naylor MF, Nascimento AG, Sherrick AD, et al. Elastofibroma dorsi: radiologic findings in 12 patients. *AJR Am J Roentgenol.* 1996;167(3):683–687.

112. Bianchi S, Martinoli C, Abdelwahab IF, et al. Elastofibroma dorsi: sonographic findings. *AJR Am J Roentgenol.* 1997;169(4):1113–1115.

113. Dalal A, Miller TT, Kenan S. Sonographic detection of elastofibroma dorsi. *J Clin Ultrasound.* 2003;31(7):375–378.

114. Ciapetti A, Filippucci E, Gutierrez M, et al. Calcium pyrophosphate dihydrate crystal deposition disease: sonographic findings. *Clin Rheumatol.* 2009;28(3):271–276.

115. Dalbeth N, McQueen FM. Use of imaging to evaluate gout and other crystal deposition disorders. *Curr Opin Rhuematol.* 2009;21(2):124–131.

116. Llauger J, Palmer J, Rosón N, et al. Nonseptic monoarthritis: imaging features with clinical and histopathologic correlation. *RadioGraphics.* 2000;20 Spec No:S263–S278.

117. Alasaarela E, Leppilahti J, Hakala M. Ultrasound and operative evaluation of arthritic shoulder joints. *Ann Rheum Dis.* 1998;57(6):357–360.

118. Hermann K-GA, Backhaus M, Schneider O, et al. Rheumatoid arthritis of the shoulder joint: comparison of conventional radiography, ultrasound, and dynamic contrast-enhanced magnetic resonance imaging. *Arthritis and Rheum.* 2003;48(12):3338–3349.

Elbow

Theodore T. Miller

INTRODUCTION

The elbow is commonly injured in sports and occupational activities. Elbow injuries account for approximately 20% of upper extremity sports injuries[1] and the elbow is the second most commonly dislocated joint after the shoulder.[2] The elbow is well suited to sonographic evaluation: it is small and easily manipulated by the examiner, enabling dynamic assessment; it is accessible around its entire circumference, allowing long and short axis scanning of every segment of the joint; and the structures of interest are superficial and linear and thus easily examined.

ANATOMY AND TECHNIQUE

Linear high-frequency transducers should be used since the ligaments, tendons, and nerves about the elbow are superficial and linear. Unlike the shoulder, which has a standard scanning protocol, the elbow is scanned by placing the transducer over the site of clinical concern. Nonetheless, for the purpose of the description of anatomy, the elbow can be divided into four quadrants: anterior, lateral, posterior, and medial.[3]

Anterior Quadrant

The anterior quadrant contains the biceps muscle and tendon, the radial and median nerves, and the anterior aspects of the radiocapitellar and humeroulnar joints. Scanning is performed with the elbow extended and supinated (**Fig. 4.1**). The transducer is placed transversely across the distal arm. The pulsating brachial artery is midline and is a major landmark. Lateral to the brachial artery is the distal biceps tendon, and medial to the brachial artery is the median nerve. The biceps aponeurosis (also called the lacertus fibrosus) is a fascial layer that extends from the flexor pronator muscle group to the biceps tendon (**Figs. 4.2 and 4.3**).

Tip:
You may have to rock the transducer cranially to make the tendons and nerves echogenic.

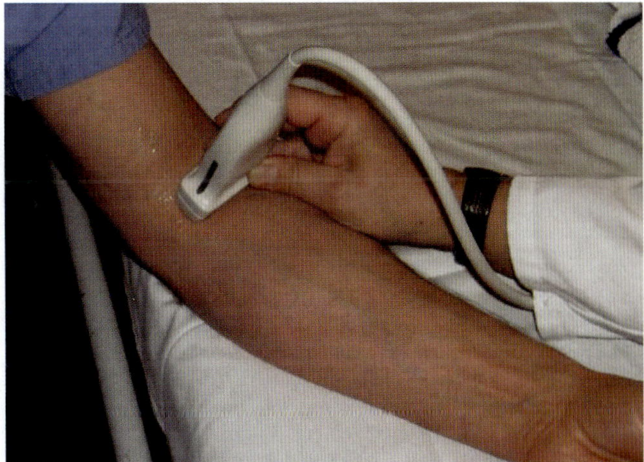

Figure 4.1. Scanning of the anterior quadrant. The transducer is placed transversely across the antecubital fossa.

As the transducer slides distally, the anterior aspects of the radiocapitellar and humeroulnar joints come into view. The curvilinear bony surfaces are covered by anechoic articular cartilage. The radial nerve is visible deep to the brachioradialis muscle at this level (**Fig. 4.3**). As the transducer moves distally, the deep branch of the radial nerve can be identified as it enters the supinator muscle between the superficial and deep muscle heads (**Fig. 4.4**). Rotating the transducer 90 degrees over either the radial or median nerves demonstrates the hypoechoic fibrillar appearance of the nerve in long axis (**Fig. 4.5**).

The radial nerve is the terminal branch of the posterior cord of the brachial plexus (C5–8, T1). In the arm it courses posterior to the humerus in the spiral groove, and pierces the intermuscular septum in the distal arm to lie anterior to the lateral condyle of the humerus. The radial nerve supplies the triceps, anconeus, brachioradialis, and the lateral half of the brachialis.

At the level of the elbow joint, the radial nerve divides into a superficial sensory branch, which courses in the forearm along the deep surface of the brachioradialis, and a deep motor branch, which enters the radial tunnel. The radial tunnel extends from the level of the radiocapitellar joint to the proximal aspect of the supinator,[4] and is bounded by the joint capsule posteriorly, the

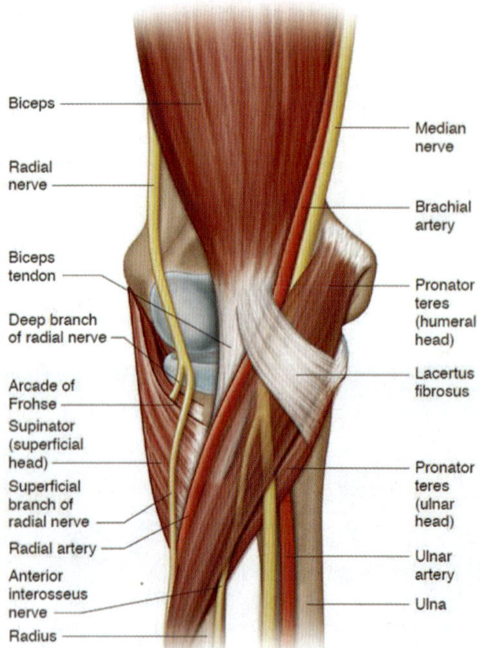

Figure 4.2.   Anatomy of the anterior aspect of the elbow. In the distal arm, the biceps tendon is lateral to the brachial artery and the median nerve is medial to the brachial artery. The lacertus fibrosus (the biceps aponeurosis) extends from the common flexor mass to the distal biceps tendon. The median nerve and its anterior interosseous branch pass between the two heads of the pronator muscle. The deep branch of the radial nerve courses between the superficial and deep heads of the supinator muscle.

brachialis muscle and biceps tendon medially, and the brachioradialis muscle and the extensor carpi radialis brevis and longus muscles laterally.[5]

At the distal aspect of the radial tunnel, the deep branch pierces the supinator muscle anteriorly between

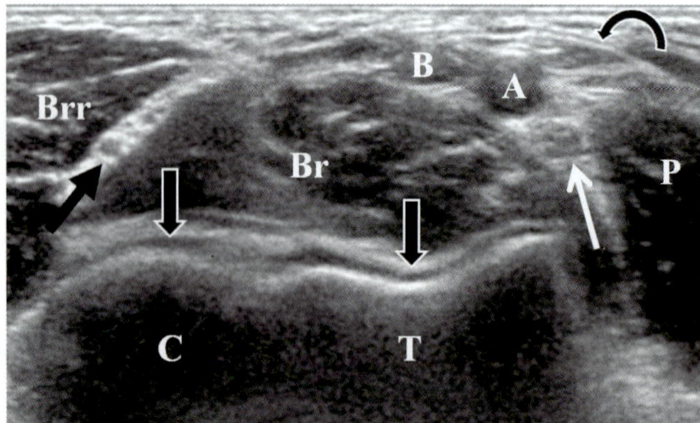

Figure 4.3.   Transverse sonographic image of the antecubital fossa. The biceps tendon (*B*) is lateral to the brachial artery (*A*), and the median nerve (*white arrow*) is medial and deep to the brachial artery. The thin biceps aponeurosis (*curved black arrow*) extends from the pronator muscle (*P*) to the biceps tendon. The brachialis (*Br*) is a large muscle directly anterior to the humerus. Deep to the brachialis is the thin hypoechoic articular cartilage (*straight block arrows*) of the capitellum (*C*) and trochlea (*T*). The radial nerve (*straight black arrow*) lies between the brachialis and brachioradialis (*Brr*) muscles.

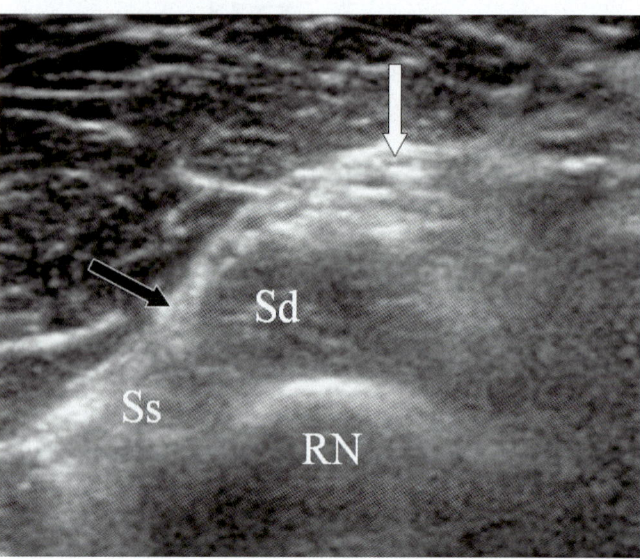

Figure 4.4.   Short-axis image at the radial neck (*RN*) shows the superficial branch of the radial nerve (*white arrow*) and the deep branch (*black arrow*) in the proximal plane between the superficial (*Ss*) and deeps heads (*Sd*) of the supinator.

the superficial and deep heads of the supinator **(Figs. 4.2 and 4.5).** The proximal edge of the superficial head of the supinator is called the Arcade of Frohse and is the most common site of radial nerve entrapment **(Fig. 4.2).** The deep branch of the radial nerve exits the posterior aspect of the supinator as the posterior interosseous nerve (PIN) and enters the posterior compartment of the forearm. At the elbow, the deep branch supplies the extensor carpi radialis brevis and the supinator. In the posterior compartment of the forearm, the deep branch, now called the PIN, supplies the extensor carpi ulnaris, the extensor digitorum communis, the extensor digiti minimi, the abductor pollicis longus, the extensor pollicis longus and brevis, and the extensor indicis proprius.[4]

The median nerve arises from the medial and lateral cords of the brachial plexus (C6–8, T1) and courses

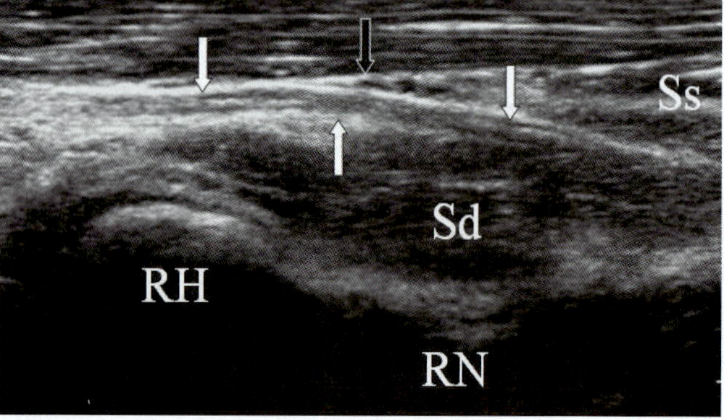

Figure 4.5.   Long-axis image shows the echogenic fibrillar appearance of the deep branch of the radial nerve (*white arrows*) as it enters between the superficial (*Ss*) and deep (*Sd*) heads of the supinator. The proximal edge of the superficial head is the Arcade of Frohse (*black arrow*). RH, radial head; RN, radial neck.

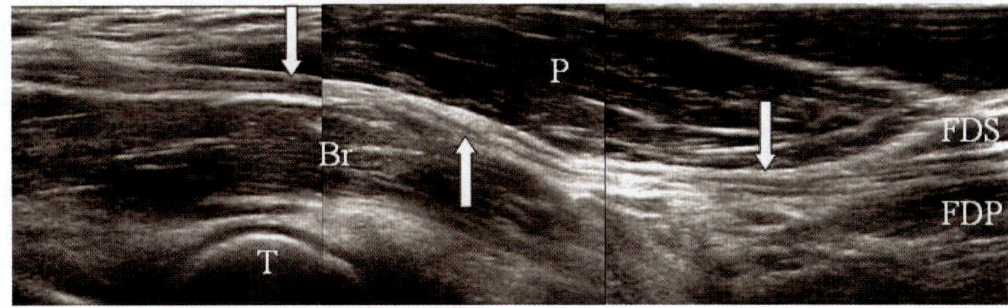

Figure 4.6. Composite long-axis image shows the median nerve (*arrows*) passing between the humeral head of the pronator teres (*P*) and the brachialis (*Br*) at the level of the elbow joint (*T* is the trochlea), and entering the forearm between the flexor digitorum superficialis (*FDS*) and flexor digitorum profundus (*FDP*). The ulnar head of the pronator teres is not visualized well in this image.

alongside the brachial artery in the anterior compartment of the arm and at the elbow, passing through the antecubital fossa deep to the biceps aponeurosis (see below) and anterior to the brachialis muscle. The nerve lies between the humeral (superficial) and ulnar (deep) heads of the pronator teres muscle at the level of the elbow joint **(Fig. 4.2)**, and enters the anterior compartment of the forearm by passing beneath the fibrous arch of the heads of the flexor digitorum superficialis (FDS)[6] **(Fig. 4.6)**. At the elbow and proximal aspect of the forearm the median nerve supplies the pronator teres, flexor carpi radialis, palmaris longus, and FDS.[7] Within the forearm, the nerve courses between the FDS and FDP.

The anterior interosseous nerve (AIN) arises from the median nerve at the level of the humeral head of the pronator teres, and travels along the anterior aspect of the interosseous membrane of the forearm between the flexor pollicis longus and the flexor digitorum profundus **(Fig. 4.7)**. The AIN is purely motor and supplies the pronator quadratus muscle, the flexor pollicis longus muscle, and the FDP muscle for the index and the middle fingers.[4,8]

Longitudinal scanning over the radiocapitellar joint shows the joint space and the thin stripe of anechoic articular cartilage of the capitellum **(Fig. 4.8)**. Sliding the transducer medially demonstrates the coronoid fossa of the distal humerus. This is a good place to look for joint fluid and intra-articular loose bodies.

The distal biceps tendon can be challenging to image because it dives deep in the antecubital fossa to insert on the radial tuberosity and because it does not have a straight sagittal orientation. There are several techniques for scanning the distal biceps:

1. Anterior approach[3,9]—With the arm extended and maximally supinated, find the tendon in short axis in the distal arm, just proximal to the elbow crease, and then rotate the transducer 90 degrees **(Fig. 4.9)**. Alternatively, place the transducer longitudinally on the antecubital fossa, find the brachial artery, and then slide the transducer just lateral to the artery **(Fig. 4.10)**.

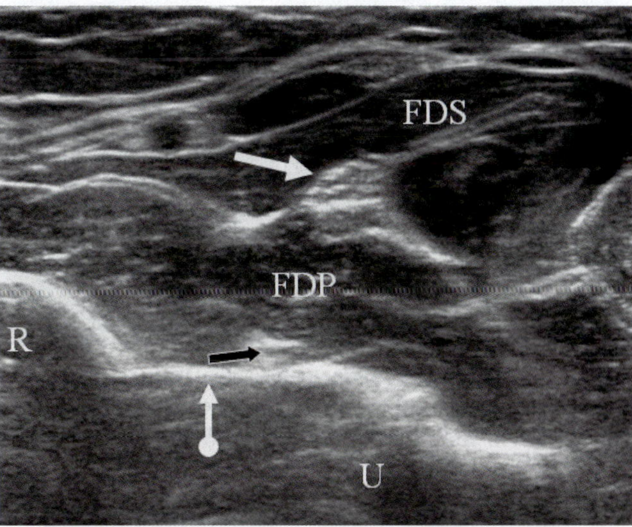

Figure 4.7. Transverse image of the proximal forearm shows the hypoechoic anterior interosseous nerve (*black arrow*) along the anterior surface of the echogenic interosseous membrane (*round tail white arrow*). The median nerve (*straight white arrow*) lies between the flexor digitorum superficialis (*FDS*) muscle and the flexor digitorum profundus (*FDP*) muscle. R, radius; U, ulna.

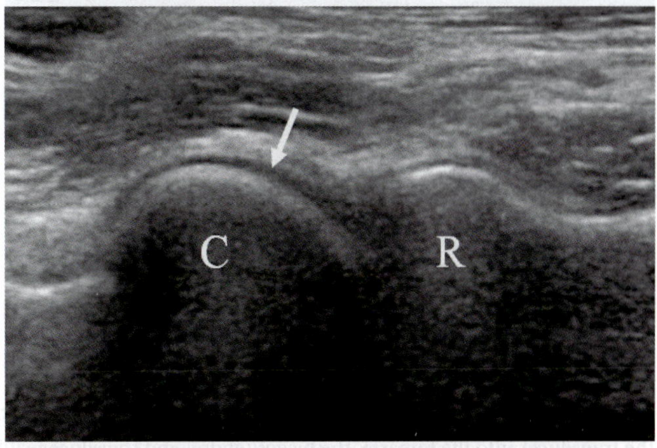

Figure 4.8. Long-axis image shows the capitellum (*C*), thin hypoechoic cartilage (*arrow*), and the radial head (*R*).

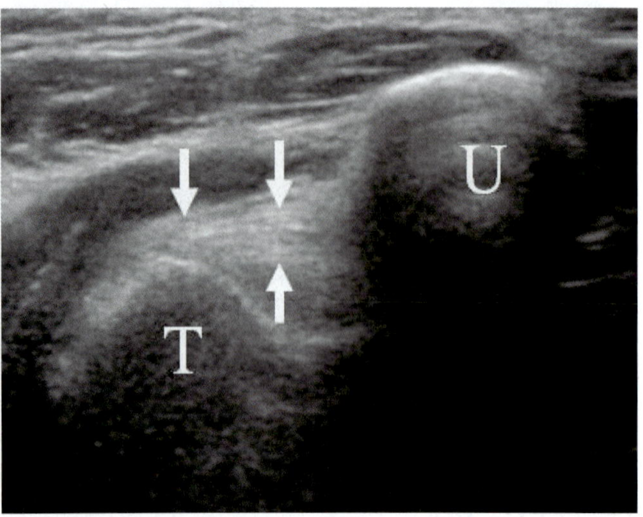

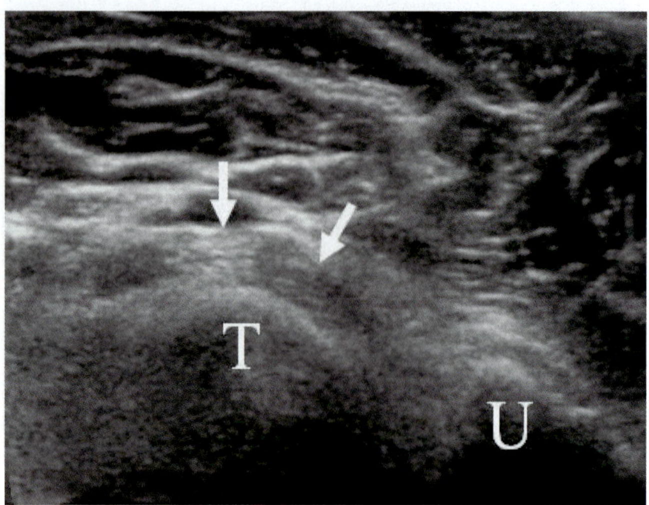

Figure 4.18.   Short-axis biceps tendon insertion. **A:** Using the short-axis posterior approach, the distal biceps tendon (*arrows*) is well seen between the radial tuberosity (*T*) and the ulna (*U*). **B:** Using the short-axis conventional anterior approach, the distal biceps tendon (*arrows*) is not as well seen attaching to the radial tuberosity (*T*) due to anisotropy. Ulna (*U*).

distal biceps tendon to protect it from osseous friction during pronation of the forearm.[14] It is not normally distended.

Lateral Quadrant

The lateral quadrant contains the lateral aspect of the radiocapitellar joint, the common extensor tendon, and the lateral collateral ligament complex that consists of the radial collateral ligament, lateral ulnar collateral ligament, and the annular ligament.[15–17] With the patient's elbow flexed 80 to 90 degrees and the forearm on the examination table, the transducer is placed longitudinally on the lateral elbow at the level of the radiocapitellar joint using the bony landmarks of the radial head and lateral epicondyle (**Fig. 4.19**). The common extensor tendon originates from the lateral epicondyle of the humerus and is comprised of the extensor carpi radialis brevis, extensor carpi ulnaris, extensor digitorum communis, and extensor digiti minimi (**Fig. 4.20**). The common tendon has a long thin echogenic fibrillar appearance (**Fig. 4.21**).

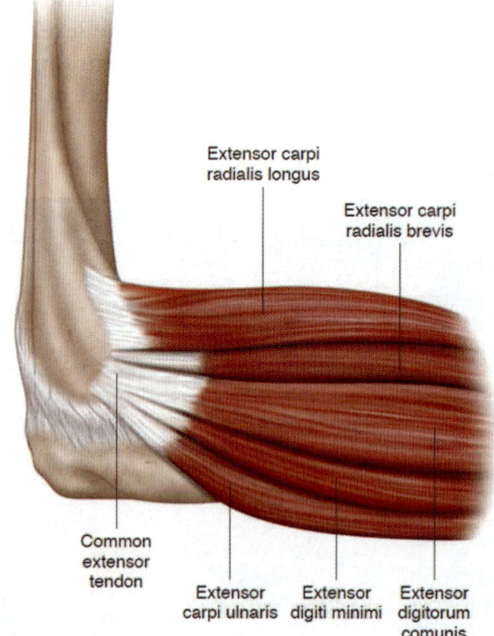

Figure 4.20.   Diagram of the common extensor tendon. The extensor carpi radialis brevis component is the deep portion of the tendon and is the most commonly involved component in lateral epicondylitis. The extensor carpi radialis longus inserts more proximally, on the supracondylar ridge, and is not part of the common extensor tendon.

Figure 4.19.   Scanning the lateral quadrant. The elbow is flexed, the thumb is up, and the transducer is placed long axis over the radial head.

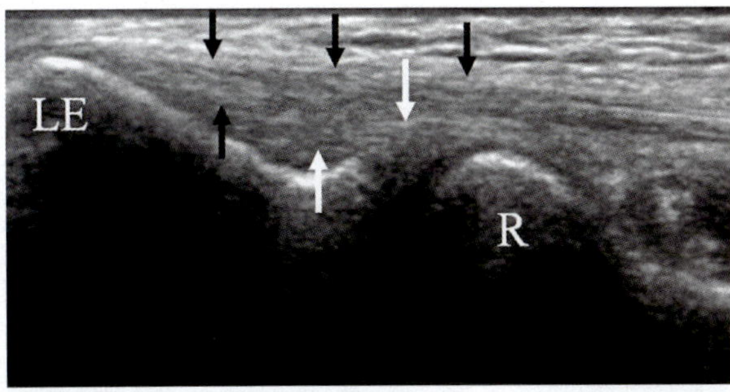

Figure 4.21.   Long-axis image of the lateral quadrant shows the thin long common extensor tendon (*black arrows*) inserting on the lateral epicondyle (*LE*). The echogenic fibrillar radial collateral ligament (*white arrows*) extends from the radial head (*R*) to the LE, and is often difficult to distinguish from the overlying common extensor tendon.

The radial collateral ligament complex is composed of the radial collateral ligament, the lateral ulnar collateral ligament, and the annular ligament[15–17] **(Fig. 4.22).** The radial collateral ligament lies deep to the common extensor tendon, extending from the undersurface of the lateral epicondyle to blend with the fibers of the annular ligament. It is often difficult to distinguish the radial collateral ligament as a distinct structure from the overlying common extensor tendon **(Fig. 4.21).**

Short axis scanning over the radial head demonstrates the thin annular ligament. Oblique scanning is necessary to visualize the lateral ulnar collateral ligament, which extends from the undersurface of the lateral epicondyle, passes posterior to the radial head and neck, thus acting as a supporting sling, and inserts on the supinator crest of the ulna.[15,16]

Posterior Quadrant

The posterior quadrant contains the triceps tendon, olecranon fossa, and ulnar nerve, and it can be scanned in several ways:

1. The "crawling crab" position, in which the patient's hand is placed on the examination table with the elbow up and rotated toward the examiner **(Fig. 4.23).** The disadvantage of this position is that it is static.
2. The elbow is flexed 90 degrees with the forearm resting on the examination couch in front of the patient **(Fig. 4.24).** This position is good for the triceps but is difficult for the ulnar nerve since the medial aspect of the elbow is lying against the table.
3. The patient's arm is elevated by the examiner who holds the patient's forearm with one hand and places the transducer against the posterior aspect of the elbow with the other hand. The patient's elbow rests against the palm of the examiner **(Fig. 4.25).** The advantage of this technique is that it allows dynamic scanning as the examiner flexes and extends the elbow by moving the patient's forearm. This is particularly helpful for the evaluation of a clinically suspected

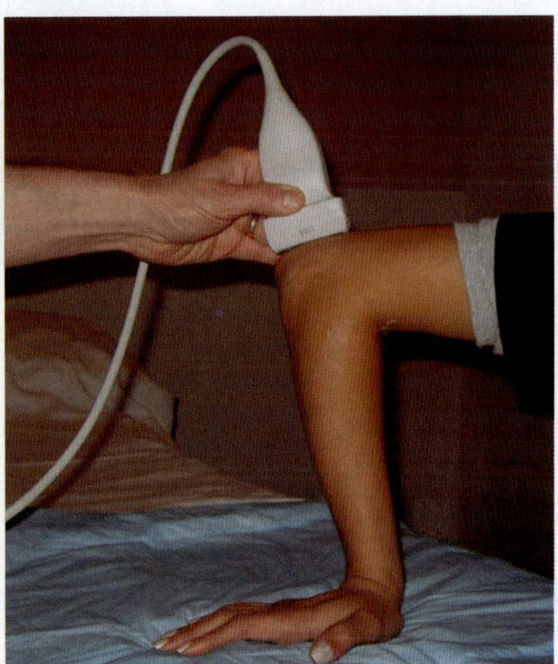

Figure 4.22.   Diagram of the radial collateral ligament complex. The radial collateral ligament blends with the annular ligament. The lateral ulnar collateral ligament passes from the posterior aspect of the lateral condyle to the supinator crest of ulna, and supports the posterior aspect of the radial head.

Figure 4.23.   Crawling crab position. The posterior quadrant is well accessible but the elbow is static.

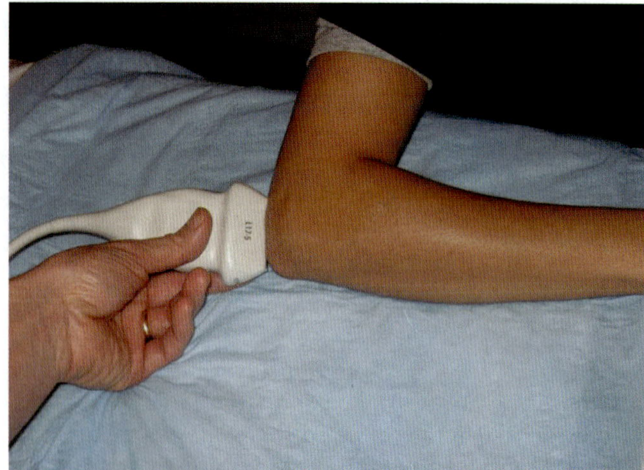

Figure 4.24. The elbow is flexed 90 degrees with the forearm resting on the examination table. The ulnar nerve is difficult to assess in this position.

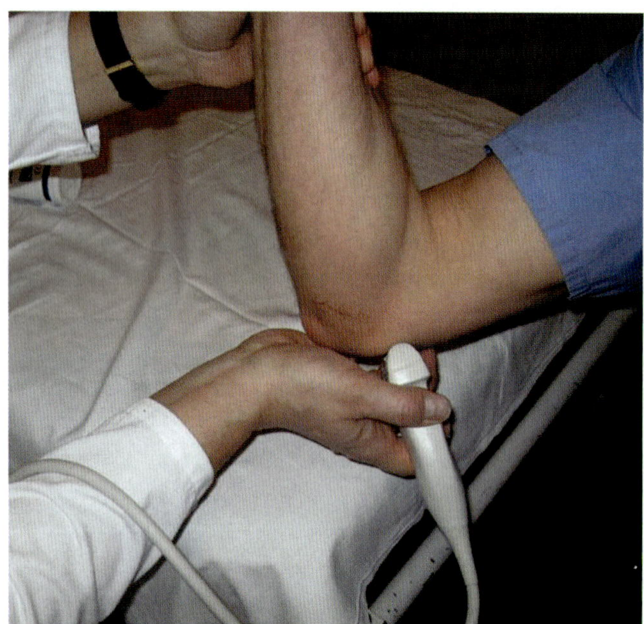

Figure 4.25. Posterior approach for dynamic scanning. This technique is good for assessment of a snapping ulnar nerve or triceps muscle.

snapping ulnar nerve. The disadvantage is that it requires a steady and experienced hand since both the patient's elbow and the examiner's hand are free-floating in the air.

The triceps tendon is a short broad structure with an echogenic fibrillar appearance composed of contributions of the long and lateral heads,[18] and inserts on the superficial aspect of the olecranon process The medial head of the triceps muscle has a separate insertion on the olecranon process, deep to the tendon **(Fig. 4.26).**

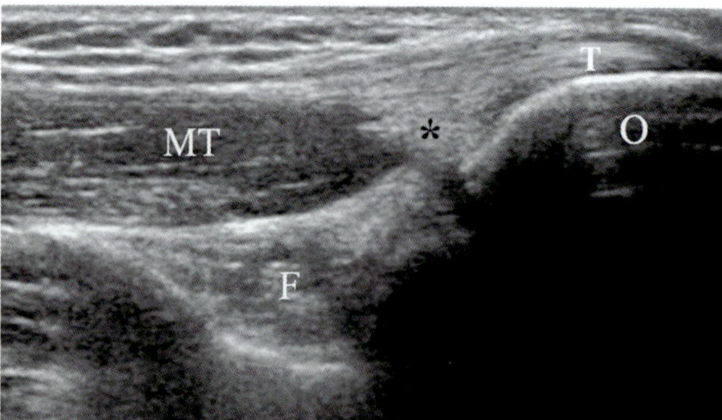

Figure 4.26. Long-axis view of the posterior quadrant. The triceps tendon (*T*) inserts on the olecranon process (*O*). The medial head of the triceps (*MT*) has a separate, short insertion (*asterisk*) deep to the tendon. By flexing the elbow, the olecranon moves distally, exposing the fossa (*F*).

With the elbow flexed, the olecranon fossa of the humerus is exposed and can be viewed both in short and long axis **(Fig. 4.27).**

> **Tip:**
> The olecranon fossa is a good place to look for synovitis, joint effusion, and loose bodies, and is a good target for elbow aspiration.

In short axis, slide the transducer medially, posterior to the medial epicondyle to visualize the ulnar nerve. The ulnar nerve arises from the medial cord of the brachial plexus (C8, T1) and courses along the medial side of the brachial artery in the anterior compartment of the proximal arm. It then passes posterior to the medial epicondyle of the humerus in the cubital tunnel, a fibro-osseous channel formed by the olecranon process

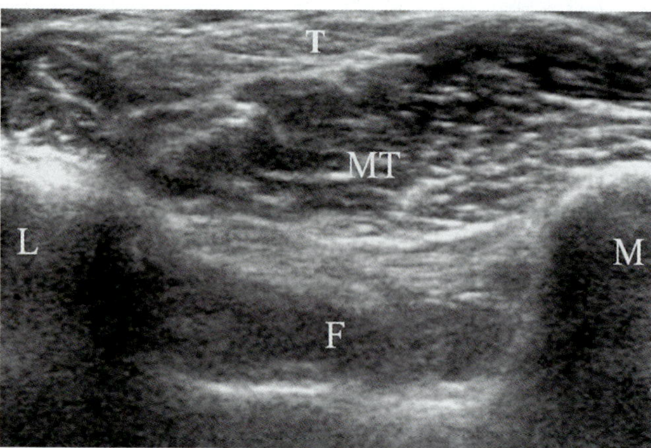

Figure 4.27. Short axis of the posterior quadrant shows the olecranon fossa (*F*) between the medial (*M*) and lateral (*L*) condyles of the humerus. The medial head of the triceps (*MT*) and the triceps tendon (*T*) overlie the fossa.

laterally, the posterior cortex of the medial epicondyle medially, the elbow joint capsule and posterior bundle of the medial collateral ligament (MCL) anteriorly, and the Ligament of Osborne (the cubital retinaculum) posteriorly (**Fig. 4.28**). The nerve exits the cubital tunnel to enter the medial aspect of the forearm between the superficial and deep heads of the flexor carpi ulnaris muscle. At the elbow, the ulnar nerve supplies the flexor carpi ulnaris and the medial half of the FDP.

In the cubital tunnel, the ulnar nerve appears round and hypoechoic, surrounded by echogenic fat in transverse scans, and narrow, linear, and hypoechoic in longitudinal scans. Nerve stability is assessed while scanning transversely during flexion and extension of the elbow.

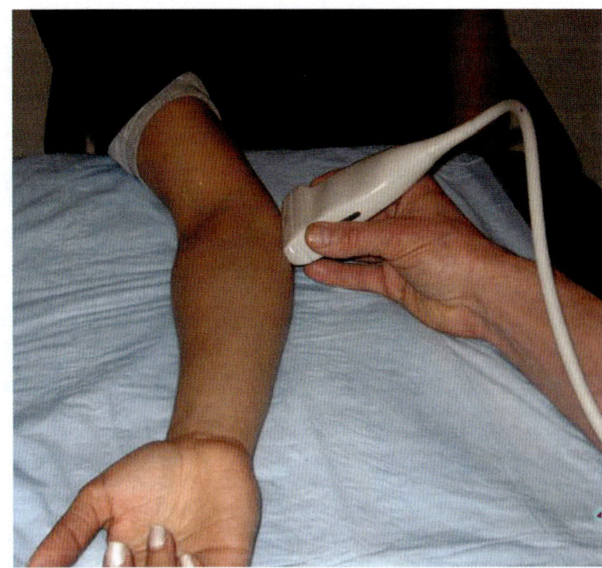

Figure 4.29. Scanning the medial quadrant. The elbow is extended, the forearm is supinated, and the patient may have to lean away from the examiner.

Medial Quadrant

The medial quadrant contains the common flexor tendon and MCL and is scanned with the elbow extended and the forearm supinated (**Fig. 4.29**). The common flexor tendon originates from the medial epicondyle of the humerus. It is composed of the flexor–pronator group of muscles: pronator teres, flexor carpi radialis, palmaris longus, and flexor carpi ulnaris (**Fig. 4.30**).

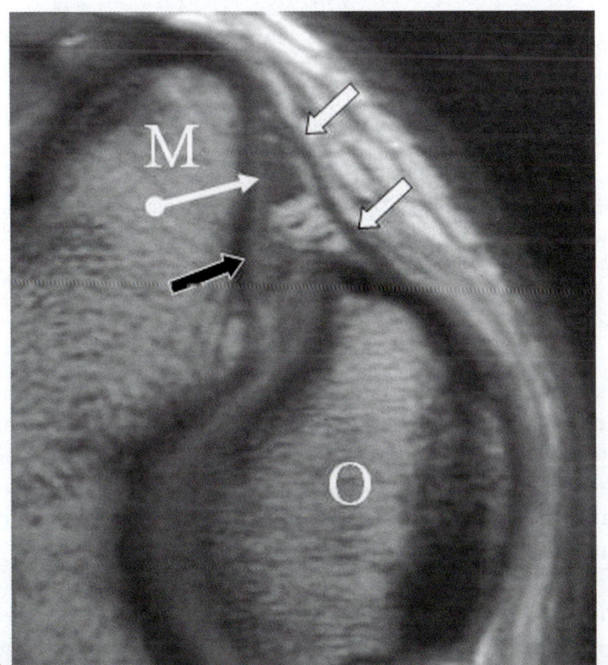

A

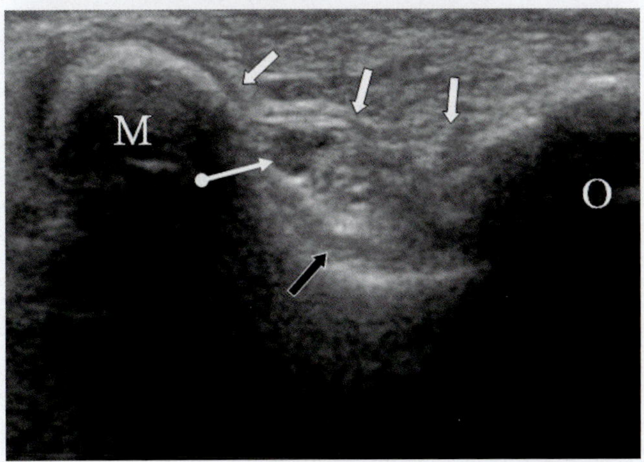

B

Figure 4.28. Cubital tunnel and ulnar nerve. Axial proton density MR image (**A**), oriented to match the sonographic image (**B**). The ulnar nerve (*round tail arrow*) is bounded by the posterior bundle of the medial collateral ligament (*black arrow*), the medial condyle (*M*), the cubital retinaculum (*white arrows*), and the olecranon process (*O*).

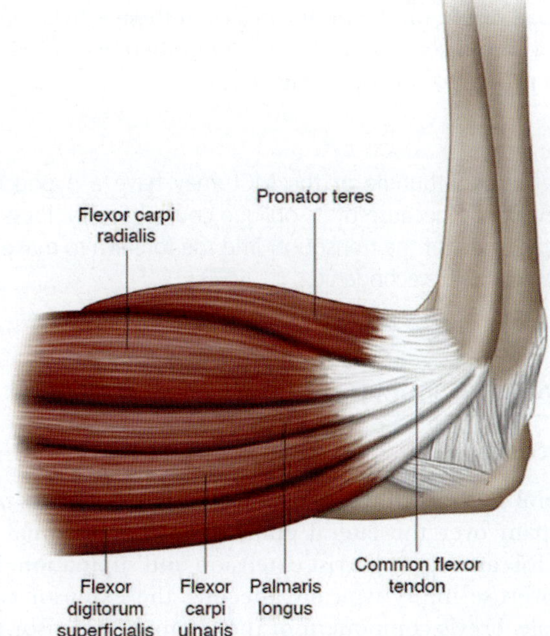

Figure 4.30. Diagram of the flexor pronator group, forming the common flexor tendon. The pronator teres and flexor carpi radialis components are most commonly involved in medial epicondylitis.

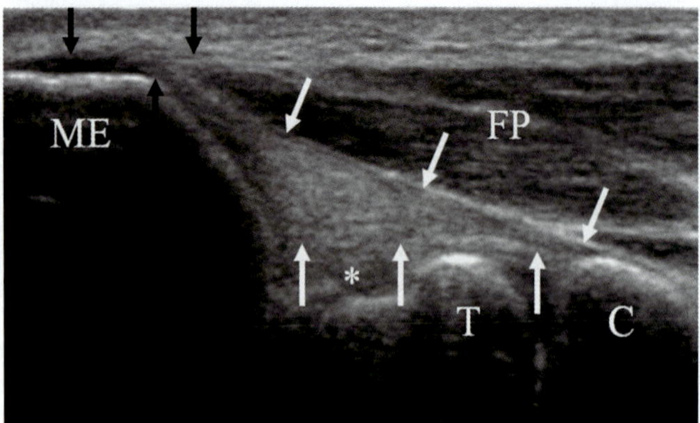

Figure 4.31. Long-axis image of the medial side of the elbow shows the short common flexor tendon (*black arrows*) of the flexor–pronator (*FP*) muscle group, with hypoechoic anisotropy at its attachment on the medial epicondyle (*ME*). The anterior bundle of the MCL (*white arrows*) has a fan shape, with a broad origin on the medial condyle and a tapered insertion on the sublime tubercle of the coronoid process (*C*) of the ulna. The ligament crosses the joint space between the coronoid process and trochlea (*T*) of the humerus, and has echogenic fibrofatty material (*asterisk*) between it and the humerus.

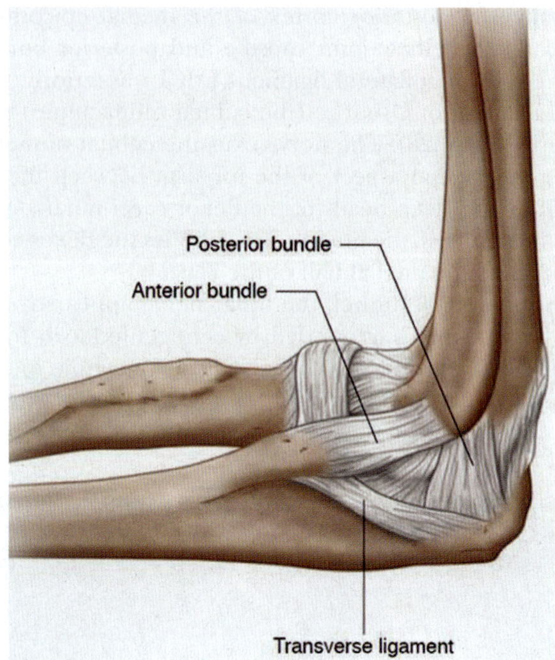

Figure 4.32. Diagram of the medial collateral ligament, showing the anterior and posterior bundles and the transverse ligament component.

The common flexor tendon is shorter and broader than the common extensor tendon, and has an echogenic fibrillar appearance as it attaches on the medial epicondyle **(Fig. 4.31)**. It is well demonstrated by placing the transducer longitudinally over the medial joint line.

Deep to the common flexor tendon is the anterior bundle of the MCL. The MCL is also composed of a posterior bundle and a transverse bundle, but the anterior bundle is the primary restraint to valgus stress, is the bundle that is usually of clinical concern, and is most visible at imaging **(Fig. 4.32)**. The anterior bundle has a fan shape, with a broad origin on the undersurface of the medial condyle and a thin insertion on the sublime tubercle of the coronoid process of the ulna **(Fig. 4.31)**.

> **Tip:**
> The anterior bundle of the MCL may have a hypoechoic appearance because of its oblique course distally. Press the distal aspect of the transducer into the forearm to make the ligament more echogenic.

TENDON PATHOLOGY

Epicondylitis

Lateral epicondylitis ("tennis elbow") is the term used for pain over the lateral epicondyle and proximal lateral forearm during wrist extension and supination. It is an overuse injury typically affecting the extensor carpi radialis brevis component of the common extensor tendon,[19] and got the name "tennis elbow" because of its association with poor backhand technique in amateur players,[20] but most cases are not due to tennis, and it

may be encountered in the lead elbow of professional golfers[21] and activities that require repetitive extension and supination of the wrist.[19] Lateral epicondylitis and radial nerve neuropathy may have similar clinical presentations, and imaging plays an important role in distinguishing the two conditions.[22]

Medial epicondylitis is the term used for pain over the medial epicondyle with wrist and finger flexion and wrist pronation. It is less common than lateral epicondylitis. Medial epicondylitis is also called "golfer's elbow", affecting the trail arm as a result of poor swing technique in amateur golfers,[21] but most cases are not due to golf. Weight lifting, bowling, and throwing are all associated with medial epicondylitis due to the valgus stress that accompanies these activities.[23] The pronator teres and flexor carpi radialis components are predominantly affected.[24] Patients with medial epicondylitis may also have ulnar neuritis due to tensile and valgus compressive loads that produce medial epicondylitis.

The term "epicondylitis" is a misnomer, since histologically there is no acute inflammatory process.[25–27] Rather, it is a degenerative process due to repetitive microtrauma of the common extensor or flexor tendons, with micro tearing of the fibers leading to mucoid degeneration, angiofibroblastic proliferation, and eventual macro tearing if the offending activity continues.

Sonographically, the process looks similar regardless of the side affected. In the early stages the tendon may be hypoechoic and/or thickened **(Fig. 4.33)**.

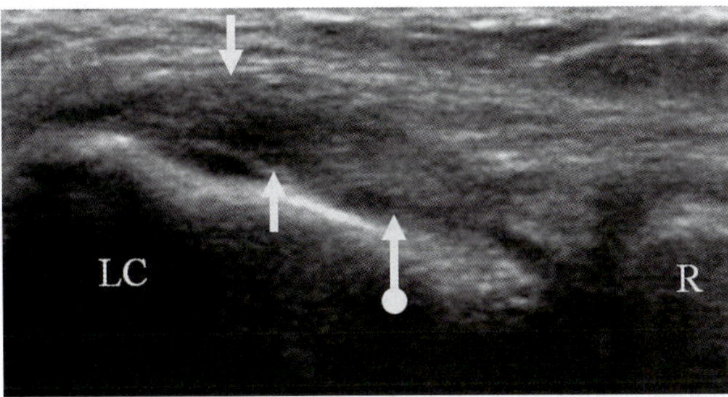

Figure 4.33. Long-axis image shows a thickened and hypoechoic common extensor tendon (*straight white arrows*). The radial collateral ligament, deep to the tendon, is also degenerated hypoechoic (*round tail arrow*). LC, lateral condyle; R, radial head.

Tip:
Rock the transducer to eliminate anisotropy as an artifactual cause of decreased echogenicity.

Occasionally, calcium hydroxyapatite is deposited in the degenerated tendon, giving a patchy echogenic appearance (**Fig. 4.34**). More severe disease may show linear hypoechoic clefts in the tendon or partial tearing of the deep surface at its condylar attachment, and scanning in the short axis helps to confirm a partial tear (**Fig. 4.35**). Hyperemia due to angiofibroblastic proliferation may be demonstrated using color or power Doppler[24,28,29] (**Fig. 4.36**) but is not always present. Enthesophytes may be present at the apex of the epicondyle in long-standing cases. Sonoelastography may demonstrate softening of the tendon.[30] The underlying radial collateral and medial collateral ligaments may also be degenerated or torn as a result of the overlying tendon abnormality and should be examined when scanning for epicondylitis.

Sonography has variable sensitivity and specificity for detecting epicondylitis. Miller et al. reported sensitivities ranging from 64% to 82% and specificities of 67% to 100%,[29] whereas Levin reported sensitivities of 80% to 92% but specificities of only 41% to 59%.[31] Struijs reported positive predictive values of 78% to 82%.[32] Lee et al. found that more than 4.2 mm of thickening of the common extensor tendon had 78% sensitivity and 95% specificity for lateral epicondylitis,[33] but their overall

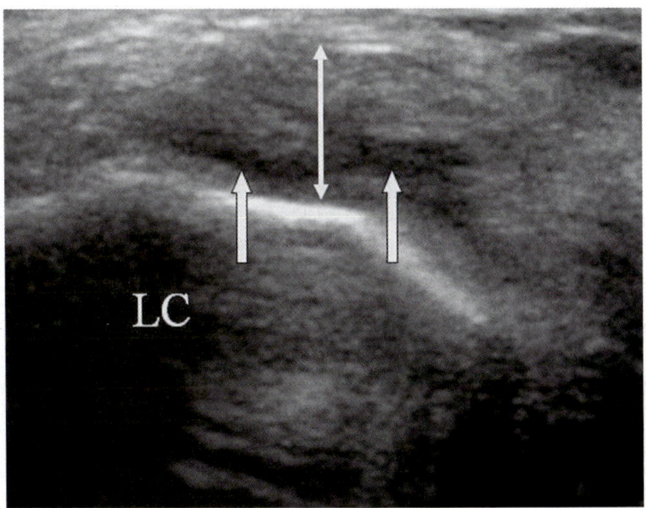

Figure 4.35. Short-axis image shows a tear (*arrows*) of the common extensor tendon. Note the thickening of the tendon (*double-headed arrow*). LC, lateral condyle.

sensitivity and specificity were only 76.5% and 76%, respectively. On the other hand, Park et al. reported 95% sensitivity and 92% specificity for the sonographic diagnosis of medial epicondylitis.[34]

Epicondylitis may be treated with ultrasound-guided needle techniques such as fenestration,[35] steroid injection,[36] lavage of hydroxyapatite, and platelet-rich plasma (PRP) or autologous blood injections.[37] Regardless of the procedure, the needle technique is the same, using a long- or short-axis approach, whichever gives better access to the abnormal tissue. As with other ultrasound-guided techniques, success depends on keeping the transducer in plane with the needle. There is no scientific evidence regarding the most effective needle size for fenestration, nor how many fenestrations are needed to stimulate healing. Typically, the needle sizes range from 20G to 25G. Similarly, there is no evidence regarding efficacy of any particular corticosteroid. A typical injectate consists of 0.5 mL of 1% lidocaine, 0.5 mL of 0.25% bupivacaine, and 1 mL of betamethasone (Celestone

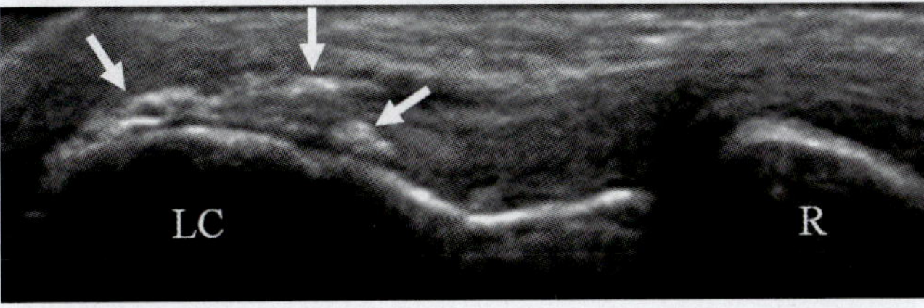

Figure 4.34. Long-axis image of common extensor origin shows focal areas of speckled echogenic calcification (*arrows*). LC, lateral condyle; R, radial head.

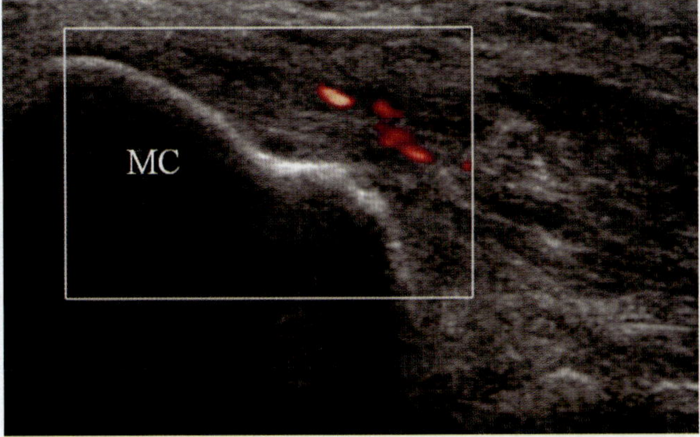

Figure 4.36. Power Doppler long-axis image shows hyperemia within a degenerated common flexor tendon. MC, medial condyle.

Soluspan 6 mg/mL). Betamethasone is less likely to cause skin depigmentation and atrophy of subcutaneous fat than long-acting depot preparations, which is a particular issue in such a visible joint as the elbow. Fenestration is always performed as part of a steroid injection. Fenestration of the tendon is performed first, followed by injection of the anesthetic–steroid mixture around the tendon. Steroid is not directly injected into the tendon so as to minimize the risk of tendon rupture. On the other hand, autologous blood or PRP are injected directly into the tendon after fenestration, and will occasionally demonstrate intrasubstance tears that were not otherwise visible. Various commercially available kits are used to produce PRP from the patient's autologous blood. Typically, 3 mL of PRP are obtained after spinning 20 mL of the patient's blood, and all 3 mL are injected into the degenerated or torn tendon after fenestration.

Distal Biceps Tendon

Degeneration of the distal biceps is the result of repetitive microtrauma from exercise or manual labor, but large partial tears or complete rupture are usually the result of a single episode affecting a degenerated tendon. The mechanism of injury is an eccentric contraction of the tendon (i.e., the elbow is forcibly extended during active flexion) such as grabbing a banister while falling down steps, jerking an object that is too heavy to lift, or doing "negatives" as part of a biceps curl exercise. Weight lifting and anabolic steroid abuse are risk factors.[38]

The patient may experience sudden pain in the antecubital fossa, and may demonstrate the "Popeye" sign of the retracted muscle and tendon on physical examination. Retraction of the tendon is limited if the biceps aponeurosis (the lacertus fibrosus) remains intact and this may make the diagnosis more difficult. The aponeurosis is a thin fascial layer that extends from the superficial surface of the common flexor muscle mass of the medial side of the forearm to blend with the fibers of the distal biceps tendon. If it remains intact, the biceps does not usually retract beyond the radiocapitellar joint. Clinically, the patient with a ruptured biceps tendon has weak but not absent flexion and supination, since other supinators and flexors remain intact (e.g., the supinator and brachialis muscles, respectively). The examiner may be able to palpate a defect in the antecubital fossa.

Sonographically, biceps tendinosis or low-grade partial tearing demonstrates thickening or thinning, irregular contour, and hypoechogenicity of the tendon, and there may be distension of the adjacent bicipitoradial bursa[9,39] (**Fig. 4.37**).

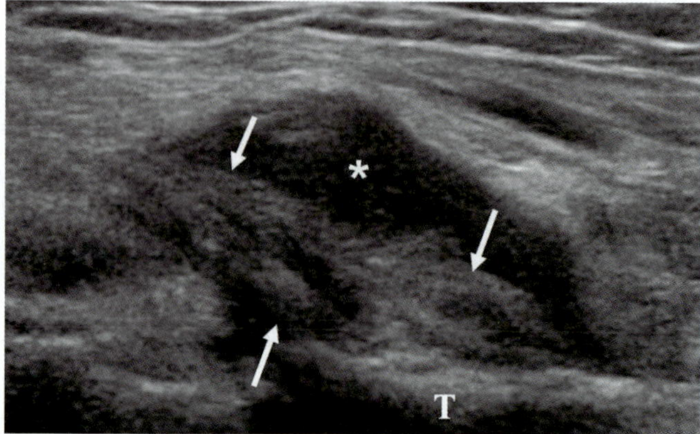

Figure 4.37.   Long-axis image of distal biceps tendinosis and partial tearing shows a thickened tendon (*arrows*) with intrasubstance hypoechoic clefts, and distension of the bicipitoradial bursa (*asterisk*). Radial tuberosity (*T*).

Complete rupture results in discontinuity and variable retraction of the tendon (**Fig. 4.38**). The extent of retraction is important as it will assist the surgeon in planning the surgical repair and the level of incisions. It is also important to evaluate the torn tendon ends to determine the tissue quality: A frayed end suggests poor tissue quality. Heterogeneous hypoechoic edema/hematoma may be present in the tendon gap or in the bicipitoradial bursa.

Da Gama Lobo et al. reported 95% sensitivity, 71% specificity, and 91% accuracy for the diagnosis of complete versus partial tears of the distal biceps tendon, and found that posterior acoustic shadowing emanating from the ruptured tendon edge had 98% accuracy for distinguishing a ruptured tendon from normal, and 91%

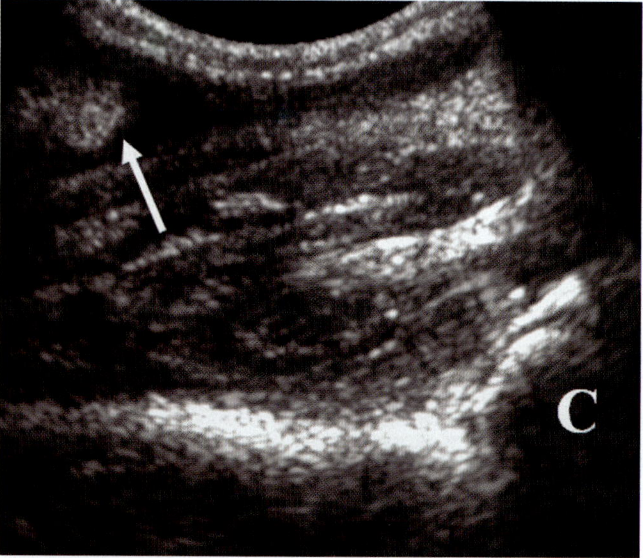

Figure 4.38.   Long-axis image shows a ruptured biceps tendon, with its torn edge (*arrow*) retracted several centimeters proximal to the capitellum (*C*).

Tip:
Scanning from the extensor surface of the forearm while the patient supinates and pronates can be helpful.

accuracy for distinguishing a ruptured tendon from a partially torn tendon.[40]

Distal Triceps Tendon

Distal triceps tendon injuries occur as a result of repetitive extension, such as in bench press exercises, or a fall on an outstretched arm with resultant concentric contraction, but triceps tendon injuries in general are rare.[18] Chronic systemic diseases, such as rheumatoid arthritis, diabetes, renal failure, and steroid use may weaken the tendon and predispose to injury.[18] The patient usually complains of pain during resisted elbow extension, with or without weakness depending on the severity of tendon injury. Degeneration results in a thickened hypoechoic tendon, and partial tears produce clefts or gaps in the tendon[41,42] (**Fig. 4.39**). Rupture of the tendon can occur but actually represents a delamination type of injury since the medial head insertion on the olecranon remains intact[41,42] (**Fig. 4.40**).

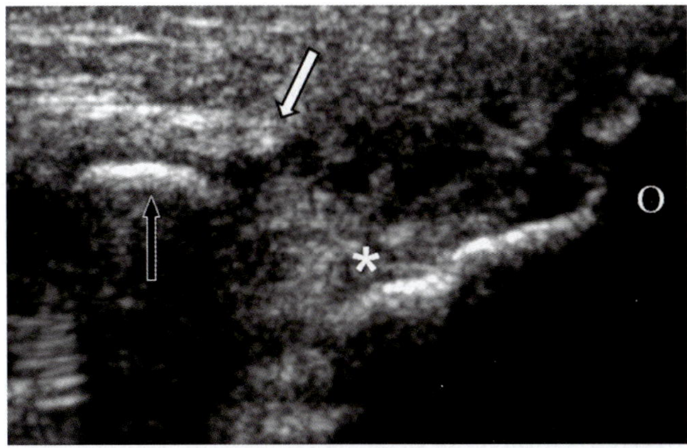

Figure 4.40.   Long-axis image shows a torn and retracted triceps tendon (*white arrow*) with heterogeneous blood between it and the olecranon (*O*). The attachment of the medial head of the triceps is degenerated but intact (*asterisk*). A large focus of dystrophic ossification with posterior shadowing is present in the retracted tendon (*black arrow*), indicating chronic degeneration of the tendon.

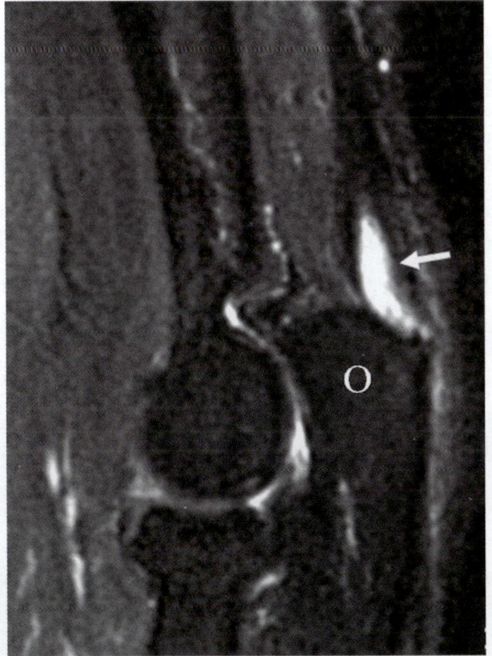

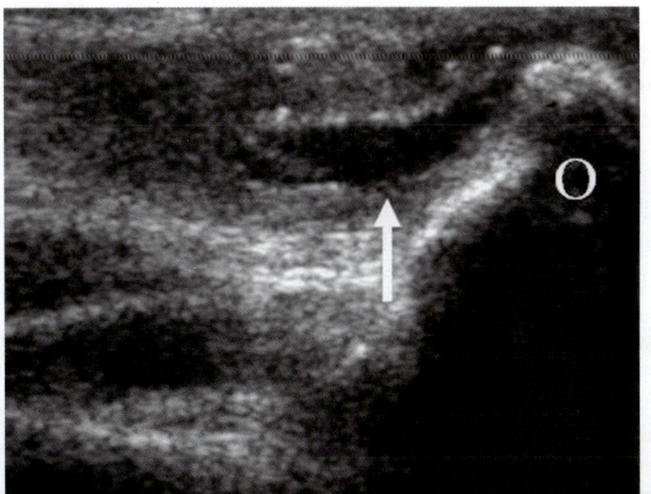

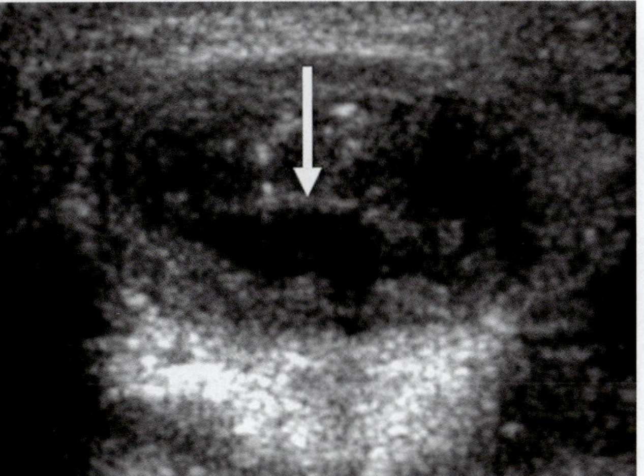

Figure 4.39.   Partial tear of triceps tendon. **A:** Sagittal fat-suppressed T2-weighted MR image shows a large high-signal intensity tear (*arrow*) within a thickened distal triceps tendon. Olecranon (*O*). **B:** Long-axis sonographic image shows the hypoechoic tear (*arrow*) in the thickened tendon, inserting on the olecranon (*O*). **C:** Short-axis sonographic image shows the intrasubstance tear (*arrow*).

Another triceps abnormality is the snapping medial head during elbow flexion, usually associated with a snapping ulnar nerve. During elbow flexion, both the ulnar nerve and medial head of the triceps can be seen to dislocate anteriorly, snapping over the medial epicondyle. Usually the nerve and triceps dislocate simultaneously, producing a single snapping sensation, but occasionally they are temporally separated and the patient reports a double snap sensation.[43]

LIGAMENT PATHOLOGY

Medial Collateral Ligament

The anterior bundle of the MCL, the primary restraint against valgus stress, is composed of anterior and posterior bands that are reciprocally taut as the elbow flexes.[44,45] Consequently, the anterior bundle is usually injured by repetitive valgus loads in throwing activities such as baseball, javelin, and volleyball spiking.[46] In the late cocking–early acceleration phase of baseball throwing, the tensile force across the flexed elbow is as much as 120 N-m,[47] with an angular velocity of over 3,000 degrees/second.[48] Less commonly, injury to the MCL is the result of a fall or posterior dislocation of the elbow. The posterior bundle of the MCL, which forms the floor of the cubital tunnel, is a secondary restraint to valgus load of the flexed elbow, and the transverse bundle has no known mechanical function.[44,49]

The normal MCL adapts to repetitive stress. Studies on asymptomatic baseball and handball players have shown that the MCL of the dominant (throwing) arm is thicker than the nondominant arm **(Fig. 4.41)**, and that the medial joint line may gap by 1 to 2 mm more in the dominant than nondominant arm with valgus stress[50–52] **(Fig. 4.42)**. Valgus stress can be achieved in the sonography suite by having the patient lie supine and hang the flexed elbow over the edge of the couch, or, with the patient sitting or

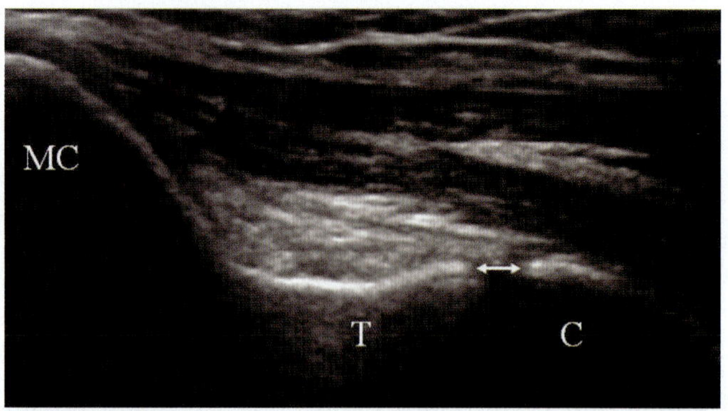

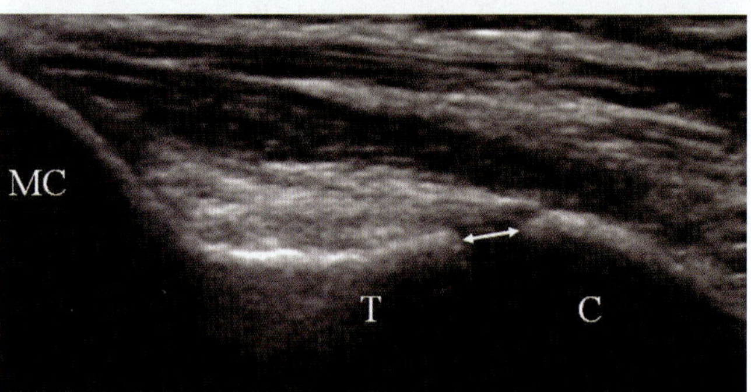

Figure 4.42. Widening of the medial joint line. **A:** Long-axis image at rest shows the joint line (*double headed arrow*) between the coronoid process of the ulna (*C*) and the trochlea (*T*). **B:** Long-axis image with valgus stress shows widening of the joint line (*double headed arrow*) between the coronoid process of the ulna (*C*) and the trochlea (*T*). MC, medial condyle.

standing with the elbow flexed, by placing the supinated forearm against the examiner's side while the examiner pushes against the lateral side of the elbow **(Fig. 4.43)**.

Tip:
The elbow must be flexed at least 30 degrees when testing valgus stress so as to unlock the osseous stability provided by the olecranon process within the olecranon fossa.

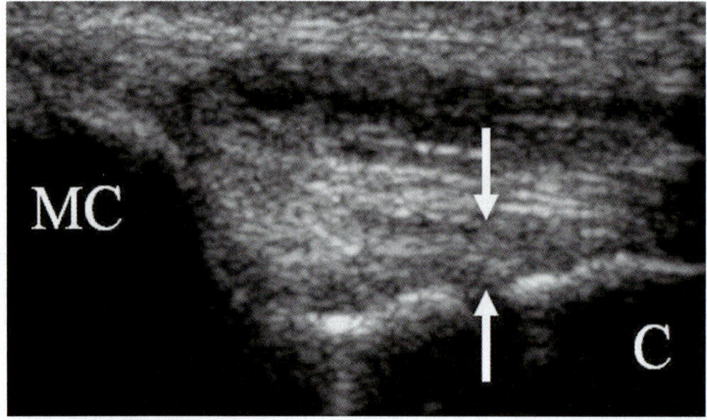

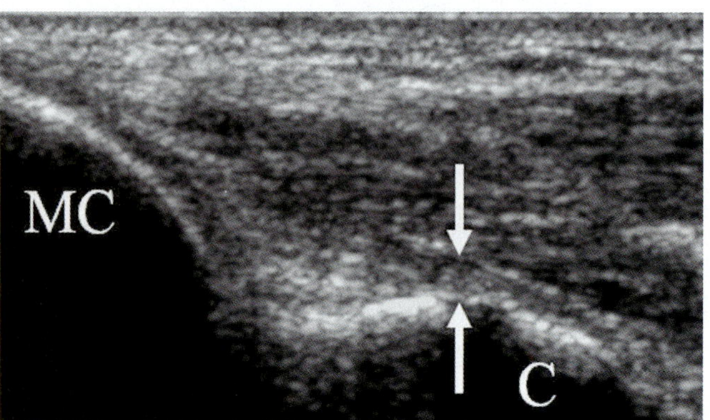

Figure 4.41. Thick MCL. **A:** Long-axis image of the dominant elbow shows a thickened distal aspect of the MCL (*arrows*). **B:** Long-axis image of the patient's nondominant arm shows normal thickness of the MCL (*arrows*). C, coronoid process of the ulna; MC, medial condyle.

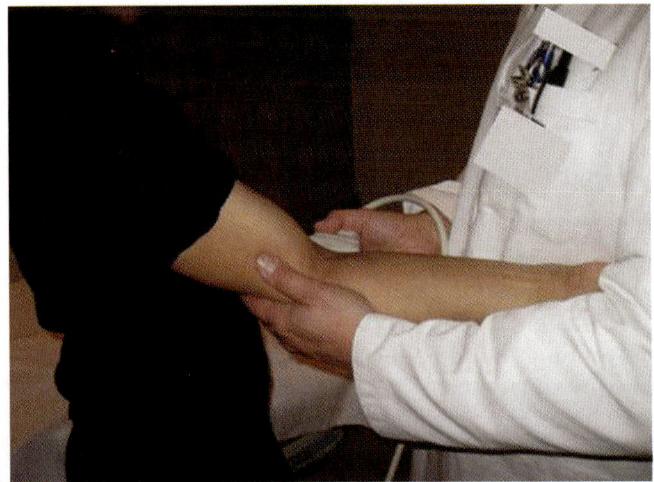

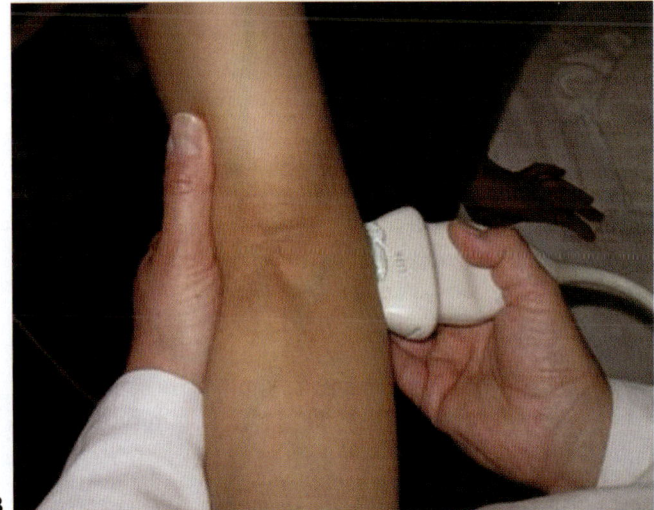

Figure 4.43. Valgus stress testing. **A:** Side view shows the patient's forearm supinated and tucked under the examiner's arm. The patient's elbow is flexed at least 30 degrees. **B:** Frontal view shows the transducer against the medial side of the elbow while the examiner pushes the elbow toward the transducer with his/her other hand.

In throwers, MCL injury may be an isolated event or part of the larger spectrum of the "valgus extension overload" syndrome. This syndrome represents a constellation of findings that results from valgus stress on the medial side of the elbow and resultant compressive forces on the radiocapitellar joint[53,54,55]:

1. MCL injury.
2. Medial epicondylitis or strain of the common flexor mass.
3. Ulnar neuritis
4. Osteochondral injury of the capitellum.
5. Stress reactions or fracture of the olecranon process.
6. Osteophytes along the medial margins of the olecranon and olecranon fossa.

When the MCL is injured, the patient complains of medial elbow pain during valgus loads. Throwers will also complain of decreased velocity of the throw and inability to control the pitch. Mild sprains may be difficult to detect sonographically as the only clue may be subtle hypoechoic edema around the ligament.[56] High-grade partial tears demonstrate thickening, thinning, or contour irregularity, and ruptures can be diagnosed by discontinuity or non-visualization of the ligament[56] **(Fig. 4.44).**

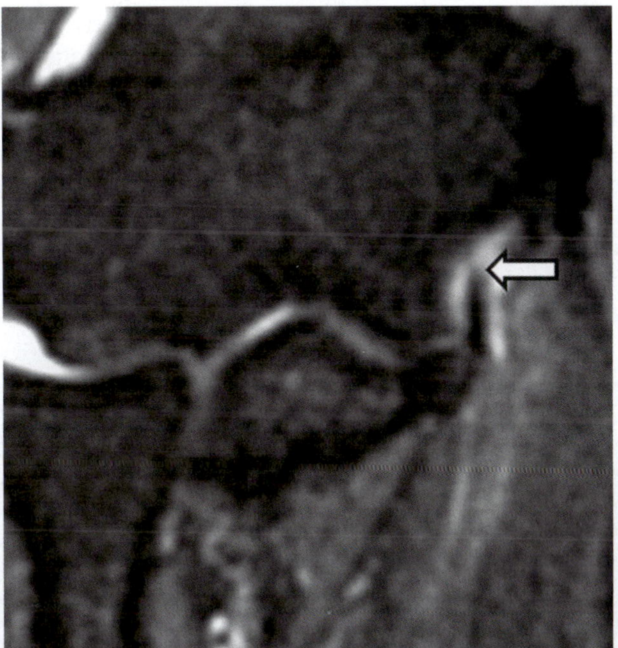

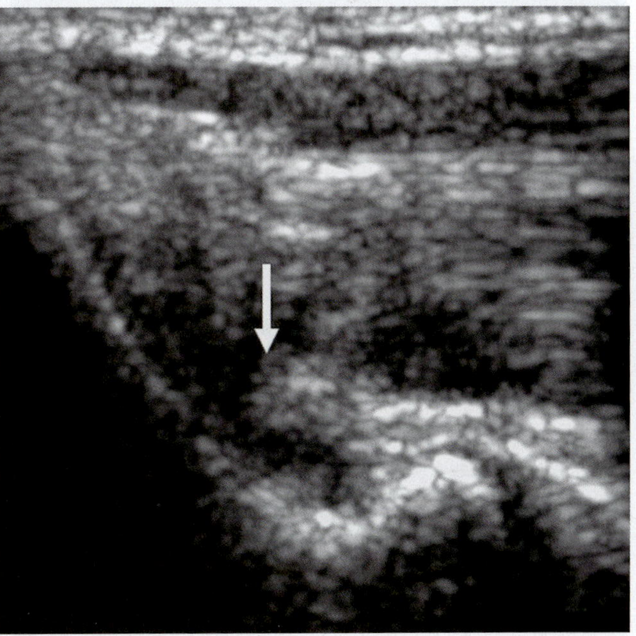

Figure 4.44. Ruptured MCL. **A:** Coronal fat-suppressed T2-weighted image of the elbow in a collegiate baseball player shows a ruptured MCL proximally (*arrow*). **B:** Corresponding long-axis sonographic image of the same patient shows the discontinuity of the ruptured ligament (*arrow*).

A particular type of partial tear occurs at the deep surface of the distal aspect of the ligament due to focal stripping of the deep fibers. On MR-arthrography and CT-arthrography, contrast insinuates into the space between the MCL and sublime tubercle of the coronoid process, producing the "T-sign" on coronal images.[57] Such a deep surface distal tear can also be visualized on sonography, although the sensitivity and specificity of ultrasound is currently unknown.

In the skeletally immature thrower, the growth plate of the medial epicondylar apophysis is the weakest portion of the ligament–bone and tendon–bone units, and the tensile load placed on the apophysis by the MCL and common flexor tendon can occasionally avulse the apophysis ("little leaguer's elbow") instead of tearing the ligament or common flexor tendon.[58,59] Thus, little leaguer's elbow is a Salter I injury, and is treated conservatively if the apophysis is displaced less than 5 mm. Sonographically, the hypoechoic apophysis will be displaced **(Fig. 4.45)**.

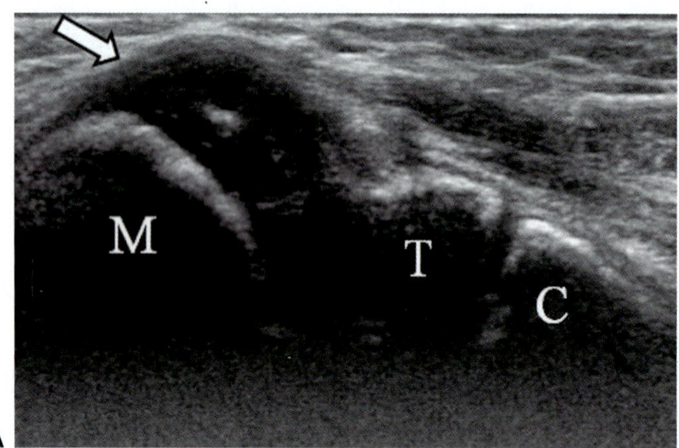

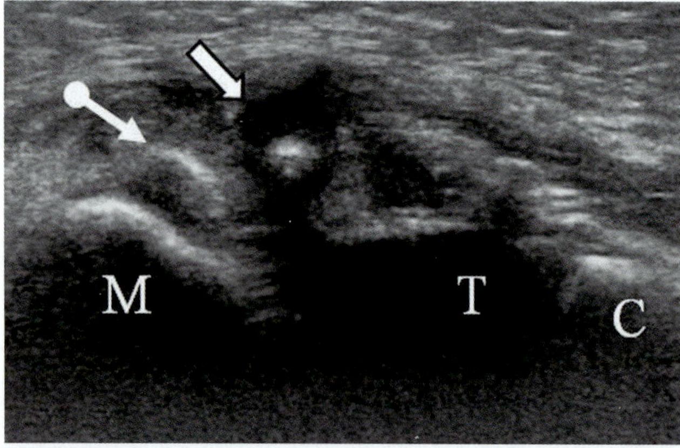

Figure 4.45. Little leaguer's elbow. **A:** Long-axis image of the patient's contralateral normal elbow shows the hypoechoic medial epicondylar apophysis (*arrow*) with an early echogenic ossification center, located immediately adjacent to the medial condyle (*M*). T, trochlea; C, coronoid process of ulna. **B:** Long-axis image of the injured elbow in the same patient shows the displaced apophysis (*straight arrow*) and a separate fragment of growth plate (*round tail arrow*). M, medial condyle; T, trochlea; C, coronoid process of ulna.

Tip:
Comparison with the patient's normal contralateral side can be helpful.

Radial Collateral Ligament Complex

The radial collateral ligament is the primary restraint to varus stress, and the lateral ulnar collateral ligament is the primary restraint to posterolateral stress. The annular ligament maintains the proximal radioulnar joint by restraining the radial head against the sigmoid notch of the proximal ulna.

The radial collateral and lateral ulnar collateral ligaments are usually injured as a result of a fall, either leading to a varus load or a posterior dislocation. Ligament injury as a result of elbow dislocation occurs in a predictable fashion dependent on the force of injury, beginning with the radial collateral and lateral ulnar collateral ligaments, followed by the joint capsule with continued injury, and lastly by the MCL.[60] The annular ligament remains intact. Rupture of the lateral ulnar collateral ligament leads to posterolateral instability of the elbow.[17,60,61] Although the lateral ulnar collateral ligament can be visualized sonographically, patients with instability after dislocation are best assessed with MRI.

The radial collateral ligament and lateral ulnar collateral ligament may also be affected in cases of lateral epicondylitis, and it is important to look at these ligaments when scanning for abnormalities of the common extensor tendon[62] **(Figs. 4.33 and 4.46)**. In addition, the lateral ulnar collateral ligament may be iatrogenically injured during surgical debridement of lateral epicondylitis.

The annular ligament is not often injured. In young children, the radial head may be pulled out of the annular ligament by a forceful yank on the forearm, usually by

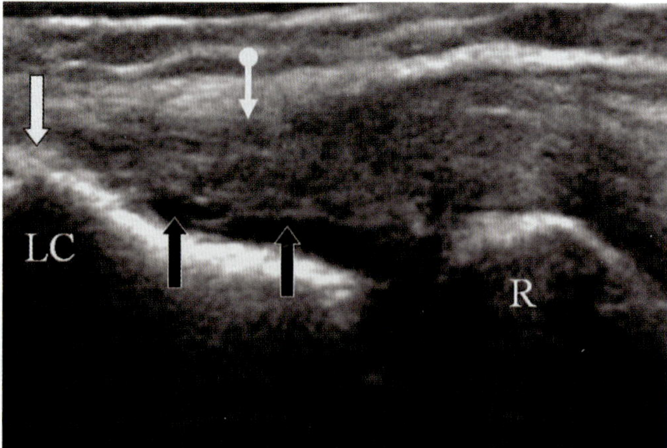

Figure 4.46. Long-axis image shows a high-grade partial tear of the radial collateral ligament (*black arrows*), associated with lateral epicondylitis, seen as a thickened and hypoechoic common extensor tendon (*round tail arrow*) with an epicondylar enthesophyte (*straight white arrow*). LC, lateral epicondyle; R, radial head.

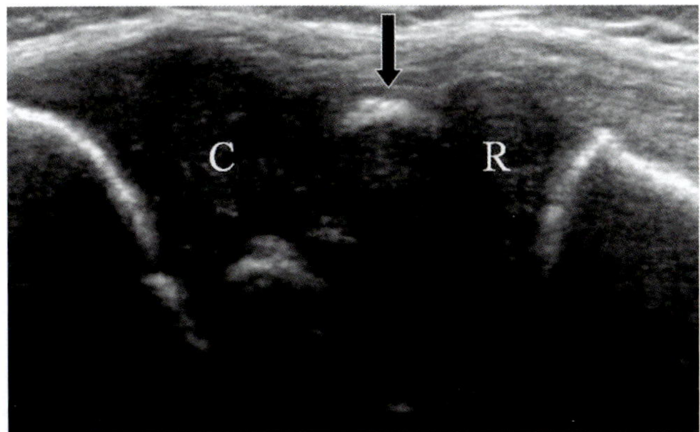

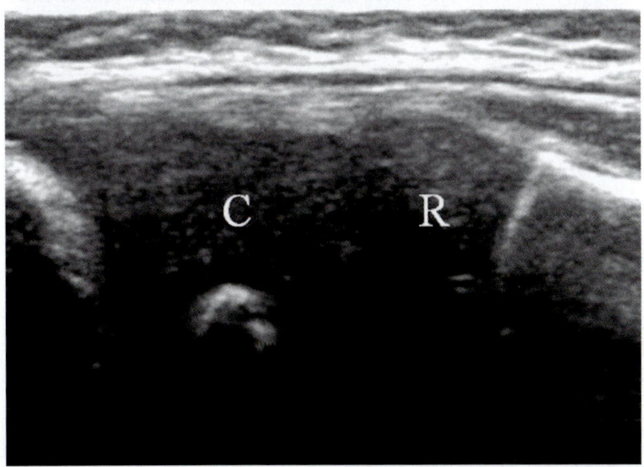

Figure 4.47. Nursemaid's elbow. **A:** Long-axis image over the radiocapitellar joint shows interposition of the displaced annular ligament (*arrow*) between the hypoechoic cartilaginous capitellum (*C*) and radial head (*R*). **B:** Long-axis image of the patient's contralateral elbow shows the capitellum (*C*) directly against the radial head (*R*).

an aggravated adult ("nursemaid's elbow"), and can be diagnosed sonographically by a widened radiocapitellar space compared to the contralateral side[63,64] **(Fig. 4.47)**.

> **Tip:**
> Scan the radiocapitellar joint longitudinally along the lateral joint line to detect widening of the radiocapitellar joint in "nursemaid's elbow". Comparison with the contralateral elbow can be helpful.

The echogenic annular ligament can sometimes be seen interposed between the hypoechoic cartilaginous epiphyses of the capitellum and radial head.

NERVES

The nerves of interest at the elbow are the ulnar nerve, the radial nerve and its deep branch that becomes the posterior interosseous nerve, and the median nerve and its branch, the AIN.

Ulnar Nerve

Ulnar nerve compression at the elbow is the second most common nerve entrapment of the upper extremity after carpal tunnel syndrome, with an estimated annual incidence of 21 to 25 cases per 100,000.[65,66] There is no agreement on risk factors, although physical labor is commonly reported.[65,66] Flexion of the elbow causes increased tensile load on the ulnar nerve and increases the pressure in the cubital tunnel up to 20 times the pressure at rest.[67,68] Populations at risk for flexion-induced ulnar neuropathy include truck drivers who lean the flexed elbow against the open window of the truck[69] and constant cell phone users.[68] Baseball pitchers are also at risk due to the valgus stress that is induced in the late cocking and early acceleration phases of throwing.[70]

Patients with ulnar neuropathy complain of pain, paresthesia, and weakness in the little finger and ulnar side of the ring finger, and numbness in the dorsal ulnar aspect of the hand and fingers.[67] Chronic compression may lead to claw deformities of the ring and little fingers and loss of grip.[68]

Compression of the ulnar nerve may occur at four different locations at the elbow from proximal to distal[67]:

1. At the intermuscular septum in the medial aspect of the mid arm.
2. Posterior to the medial epicondyle at the entrance to the cubital tunnel.
3. Within the cubital tunnel.
4. At the flexor–pronator aponeurosis between the heads of the flexor carpi ulnaris as the nerve enters the forearm.

The cubital tunnel is the most common location of ulnar nerve compression, and the most common structural abnormality in the cubital tunnel is the anconeus epitrochlearis muscle. This is an anomalous muscle reported in 23% of asymptomatic elbows on MR imaging and in up to 34% of the population in anatomic dissections.[71] Located along the posterior aspect of the cubital tunnel, the anconeus epitrochlearis muscle may compress the ulnar nerve against the medial epicondyle or olecranon. Osteophytes may also compress the ulnar nerve in the cubital tunnel.[72]

Ulnar neuritis is demonstrated sonographically by nerve enlargement[73,74] **(Fig. 4.48)**. Comparison of the nerve with the contralateral asymptomatic nerve[73] or comparison of the cross-sectional area at the site of maximal nerve swelling with the cross-sectional area at a non-swollen location[74] can be helpful.

> **Tip:**
> When scanning the contralateral elbow or other locations in the ipsilateral elbow, make sure that images are obtained in same degree of elbow flexion as the cross-sectional area of the nerve decreases with increased flexion.[67]

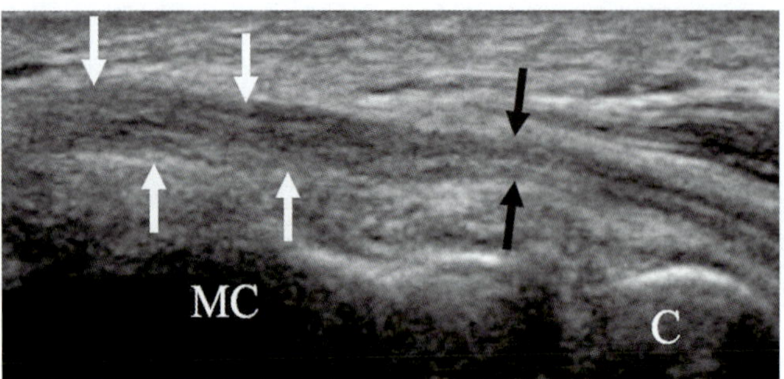

Figure 4.48.   Long-axis image of the ulnar nerve shows proximal enlargement (*white arrows*) compared to more distal fibers (*black arrows*). MC, medial condyle; C, coronoid process.

If the nerve is bifid or trifid, the separate moieties must be evaluated additively[75] **(Fig. 4.49)**.

Another group at risk for ulnar neuropathy are people with recurrent anterior dislocation of the ulnar nerve that occurs asymptomatically in 16% to 20% of the population.[76,77] Risk factors for ulnar nerve dislocation include cubitus varus deformity, absent or lax ligament of Osborne (the fascia that forms the roof of the cubital tunnel), hypertrophic medial head of triceps, or an accessory head of triceps.[43,78–80] The dislocation may be associated with activities that involve resisted elbow extension such as the early acceleration phase of throwing and bench press.[78] The abnormal movement of the nerve may be felt as a snap by the patient during elbow flexion, but the snapping may also include the medial head of the triceps or an accessory triceps muscle; in these instances the patient may report a double-snap sensation.[78,79] The repetitive translation of the nerve over the bony prominence of the epicondyle as it dislocates in flexion and reduces in extension can cause frictional neuritis,[76] and patients can present with a spectrum of clinical abnormalities such as medial elbow pain, snapping, ulnar neuropathy, or combinations thereof.[78,79]

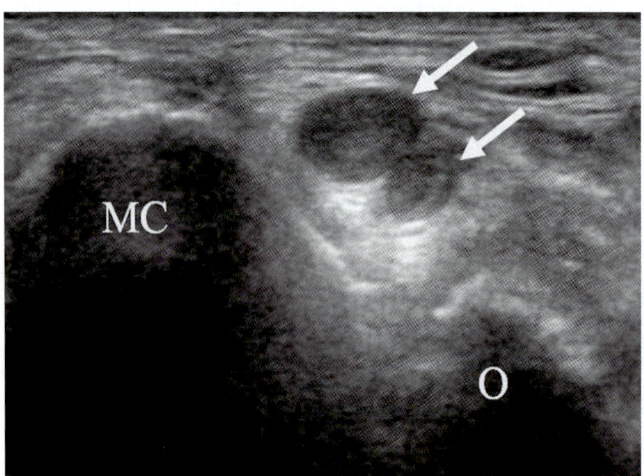

Figure 4.49.   Short-axis image through the cubital tunnel shows enlargement of both portions of a bifid ulnar nerve (*arrows*). MC, medial condyle; O, olecranon process.

Sonographic imaging during flexion and extension is a real-time method of evaluating ulnar nerve dislocation. Transverse scans over the cubital tunnel demonstrate both the nerve and medial head of the triceps[43] **(Fig. 4.50)**. Scanning during resisted extension and flexion may be needed to demonstrate the abnormal movement.[79] Recognition of concomitant triceps dislocation is crucial to correct treatment, since surgical anterior transposition of the nerve without correction of the snapping triceps will lead to persistent symptoms.[78,79,81]

Radial Nerve

Compression of the deep branch of the radial nerve may occur at five different locations at the elbow from proximal to distal[4]:

1. At the level of the radial head by fibrous bands between the brachioradialis muscle and joint capsule.
2. Distal to the radial head by the "Leash of Henry," an arcade of anastomosing branches of the radial recurrent artery.
3. At the level of the tendinous edge of the overlying extensor carpi radialis brevis muscle.
4. At the "arcade of Frohse" along the proximal aspect of the supinator muscle.
5. At the distal aspect of the supinator muscle.

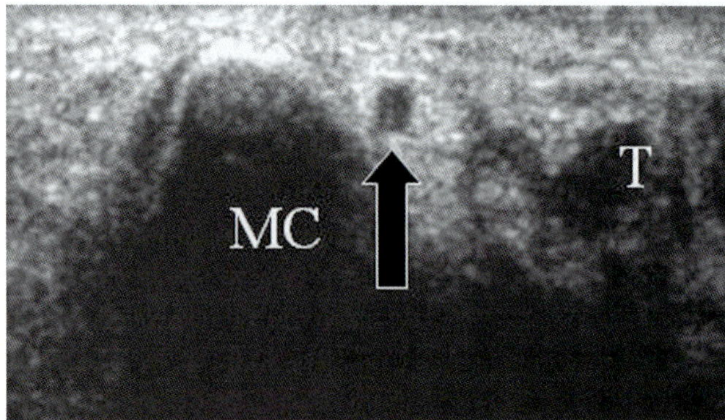

A

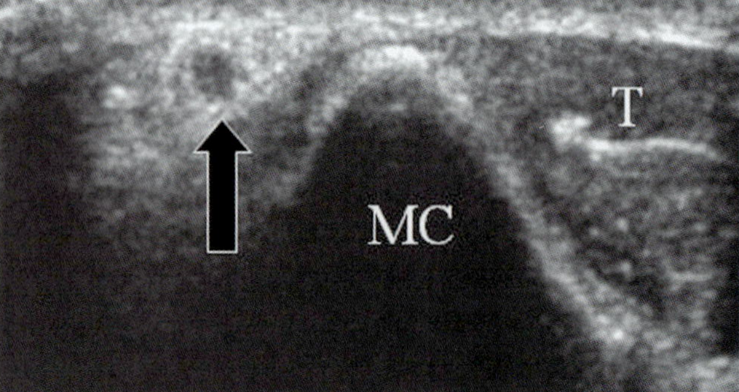

B

Figure 4.50.   Snapping ulnar nerve. **A:** Short-axis image through the cubital tunnel in elbow extension shows normal location of the nerve (*arrow*), posterior to the medial condyle (*MC*). T, medial head of triceps. **B:** Short-axis image in elbow flexion shows dislocation of the nerve (*arrow*) anterior to the medial condyle (*MC*), with the medial head of the triceps muscle (*T*) now filling the cubital tunnel.

The arcade of Frohse is the most common site of compression and represents a thickened tendinous proximal edge of the superficial head of the supinator. The normal edge is thin and membranous. The tendinous thickening is most likely due to repetitive pronation/supination.[82] Deep branch radial nerve compression can lead to either "radial tunnel syndrome" or "posterior interosseous nerve syndrome" (also called "supinator syndrome"), although it is not known why in any individual one syndrome occurs and not the other.[4] Radial tunnel syndrome leads to a burning sensation along the lateral aspect of the forearm mimicking lateral epicondylitis, whereas posterior interosseous nerve syndrome presents with weakness of the extensor muscles of the forearm.

Lateral epicondylitis and deep branch radial nerve compression may coexist, often due to irritation or compression of the nerve by the degenerated or torn extensor carpi radialis brevis tendon. The two clinical entities are also difficult to distinguish on physical examination,[4] and electrodiagnostic tests are usually normal in radial tunnel syndrome.[82] Compression of the lateral antebrachial cutaneous nerve can also cause burning pain in the lateral aspect of the forearm, mimicking both lateral epicondylitis and radial tunnel syndrome, but compression of this nerve is rare.[4]

Caution must be exercised in interpreting structural changes in patients without symptoms of nerve compression; for example, a hypertrophic leash of Henry, arbitrarily defined as more than six vessels, was present in 9 of 60 asymptomatic elbows.[71]

Patients with PIN syndrome may have a hypoechoic swollen deep branch, with a mean diameter of 4.2 mm, as well as hyperemia of the nerve on color Doppler imaging.[83]

The sonographic appearances of radial nerve abnormalities include compression within the radial tunnel, as described above **(Fig. 4.51)**, compression by masses such as ganglion cysts, or intrinsic abnormalities of the nerve such as a nerve sheath tumor **(Fig. 4.52)**.

> **Tip:**
> The deep branch of the radial nerve may normally have an angulated course at the arcade of Frohse if scanned with the forearm pronated,[84] and this should not be misinterpreted as entrapment.

Median Nerve

The median nerve can be trapped at four locations around the elbow:

1. In the distal humerus by the ligament of Struthers, a fibrous vestigial remnant, present in up to 2.7% of the population that extends from the anteromedial aspect

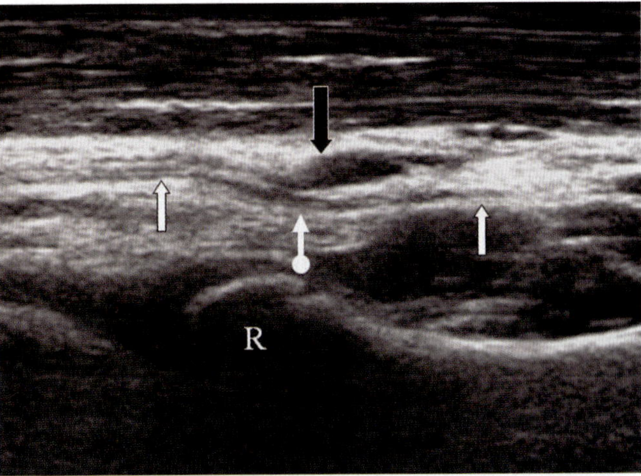

Figure 4.51. Long-axis image shows focal deviation (*round tail arrow*) of the radial nerve (*white arrows*) by a prominent vessel (*black arrow*) at the Leash of Henry. R, radial head.

of the distal humerus to the medial epicondyle.[6,7,85] It is the rarest cause of median nerve compression.[6] The ligament takes its origin from a supracondylar spur on the distal humerus that is present in approximately 1% of the population.[86]

2. At the proximal elbow by a thickened biceps aponeurosis.
3. At the elbow joint between the superficial and deep heads of the pronator teres, which is the most common cause of median nerve compression.
4. At the proximal forearm by a thickened proximal edge of the FDS.[4,6,7,87]

The AIN may be compressed by the pronator teres and by the proximal edge of the FDS,[4,7] and can be dynamically compressed by repetitive elbow flexion or forearm pronation.[4,88]

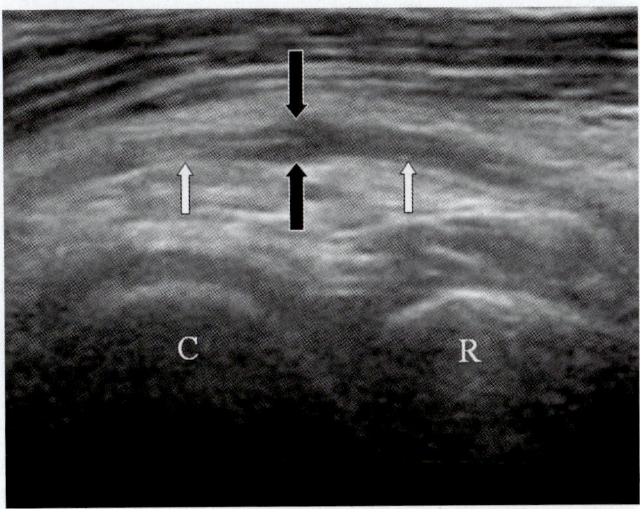

Figure 4.52. Long-axis image of the radial nerve (*white arrows*) at the level of the radio (*R*)-capitellar (*C*) joint shows a focal neurofibroma (*black arrows*).

Similar to radial nerve compression, compression of the median nerve has two presentations: "pronator syndrome" and "AIN syndrome".

Patients with pronator syndrome have pain and paresthesia in the volar aspects of the elbow and forearm and in the hand affecting the thumb, the index and long fingers, and the lateral half of the ring finger.[4,7] The hand symptoms are similar to those of carpal tunnel syndrome. Both syndromes may be aggravated by overuse, but pronator syndrome may also have associated numbness of the palm due to compression of the palmar cutaneous nerve, whereas symptoms that wake the patient at night are more common with carpal tunnel syndrome.[4,88] Tinel's sign should be positive over the wrist in patients with carpal tunnel syndrome and is positive over the elbow and proximal forearm in pronator syndrome.[4,88] Symptom reproduction during resisted forearm pronation suggests median nerve compression by the pronator teres, and symptom reproduction during resisted elbow flexion and supination suggests the biceps aponeurosis as the cause of compression.[4]

Patients with AIN syndrome, also called the "Kiloh-Nevin syndrome",[89] have motor weakness typically manifested by weakened ability to pinch the thumb and index finger together, tested by asking the patient to make an "ok" sign, reflecting the palsy of the flexor pollicis longus muscle and FDP muscle to the index finger.[4,7,88] A nonmechanical cause of AIN syndrome is Parsonage-Turner syndrome (acute brachial neuritis), which can affect the AIN and cause symptoms of AIN syndrome following a transient period of shoulder pain.[4,90]

MR imaging of patients with AIN syndrome shows denervation edema in the muscles supplied by the nerve, or fatty atrophy in chronic cases. The pronator quadratus muscle is always involved, followed by the FDP muscle, and flexor pollicis longus.[8,91] Ultrasound shows increased echogenicity and decreased bulk of the three muscles, suggesting atrophy.[92]

Perineural injection of the ulnar, radial, or median nerves or their branches can be performed as either diagnostic (anesthetic only) or therapeutic (anesthetic and cortisone) procedures. The technique is the same regardless of which nerve is injected: The nerve is identified sonographically in short axis, and a 25G hypodermic needle is placed in-plane with the transducer adjacent to the nerve **(Fig. 4.53)**. For a diagnostic injection, use 0.5 mL of 1% lidocaine and 0.5 mL of 0.25% marcaine, and for therapeutic injections add 1 mL of either triamcinolone (40 mg/mL) or betamethasone (6 mg/mL) to the anesthetics.

BURSAE

The two bursae of clinical concern are the olecranon bursa posteriorly, and the bicipitoradial bursa in the antecubital fossa. The olecranon bursa is subcutaneous

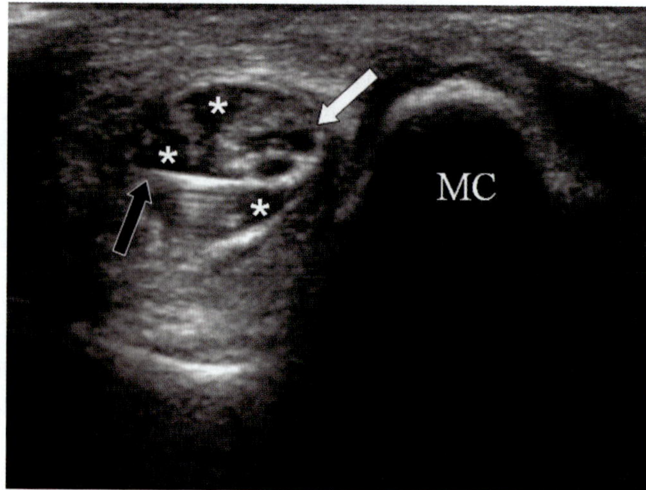

Figure 4.53.   Short-axis image during a sonographically guided ulnar nerve injection shows the needle (*black arrow*), with reverberation artifact, adjacent to the ulnar nerve, which has a fascicular appearance (*white arrow*). The hypoechoic injectate (*asterisks*) surrounds the nerve. MC, medial condyle.

and overlies the posterior aspect of the olecranon. It is usually distended as a result of systemic diseases such as rheumatoid arthritis and gout, but can be inflamed due to mechanical irritation. Sonography shows a distended bursa with irregular synovial thickening and hypoechoic or anechoic fluid **(Fig. 4.54)**. Power Doppler may demonstrate hyperemia.[93]

The bicipitoradial bursa is adjacent to the distal biceps tendon insertion, and acts to cushion the tendon during forearm pronation as the tendon is pulled into the interosseous space.[14] It can be inflamed due to mechanical irritation or inflammatory arthritis and is often distended

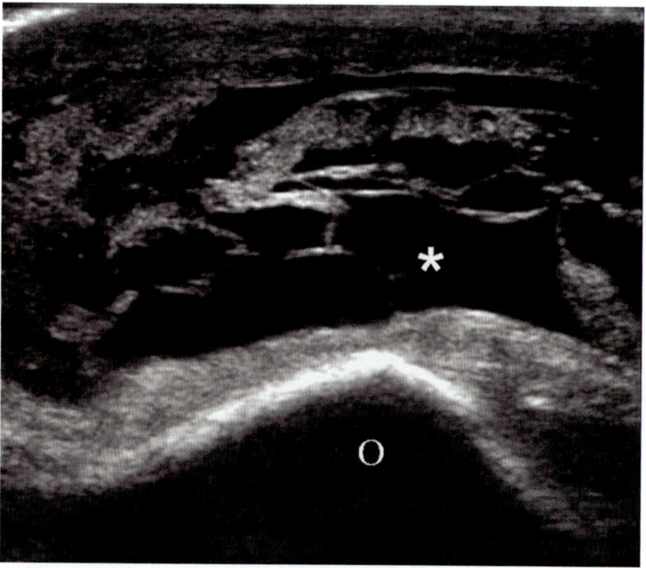

Figure 4.54.   Long-axis sonographic image shows a distended olecranon bursa (*asterisk*) with irregular walls adjacent to the olecranon process (*O*).

when the distal biceps tendon is torn. The distended bursa is usually wrapped around the distal biceps tendon simulating tenosynovitis, but the distal biceps tendon does not have a sheath. The appearance of the distended bursa is variable; it can have a thin or thick and irregular wall **(Fig. 4.37)**, may be complex, and may be hyperemic on Doppler.[94,95]

JOINT SPACE

Joint fluid tends to pool in the recesses of the joint, and the most useful places to look for an effusion are the olecranon fossa, the coronoid fossa, and the annular recess of the radiocapitellar joint.

Tip:
Flex the elbow to move the olecranon process out of the olecranon fossa to show joint fluid **(Fig. 4.55)**.

Effusions are usually hypoechoic or anechoic. In infection or active inflammatory arthritis, the synovium is thickened and irregular, and power Doppler may show hyperemia **(Fig. 4.55)**. In chronic cases, the synovium may be thickened without hyperemia. Aspiration of joint fluid may be required in suspected infection or to look for crystals, and is easily accomplished under ultrasound guidance using a short-axis approach to the olecranon fossa with an 18G or 20G hypodermic needle and the elbow flexed 90 degrees. Alternatively, the needle can be placed short axis to the radiocapitellar joint if fluid is visualized in this location with the elbow bent. Both the olecranon fossa and radiocapitellar joint are also easily accessible sites for injecting anesthetics and steroids into the joint, using a 25G hypodermic needle.

Loose bodies can be detected sonographically as hypoechoic or echogenic, depending on their mineralization, and they tend to collect in areas of capsular laxity, such as the olecranon and coronoid fossae and the annular recess, but the donor site of the loose body is not always visible sonographically.[96,97] The presence of an effusion may make intra-articular bodies more conspicuous.[98] Purely cartilaginous bodies are hypoechoic and visualized only if they cause a contour deformity of the adjacent joint capsule. In the presence of an effusion they may be masked by the low echogenicity of the surrounding fluid. Calcified or ossified bodies have an echogenic surface and posterior shadowing **(Fig. 4.56)**.

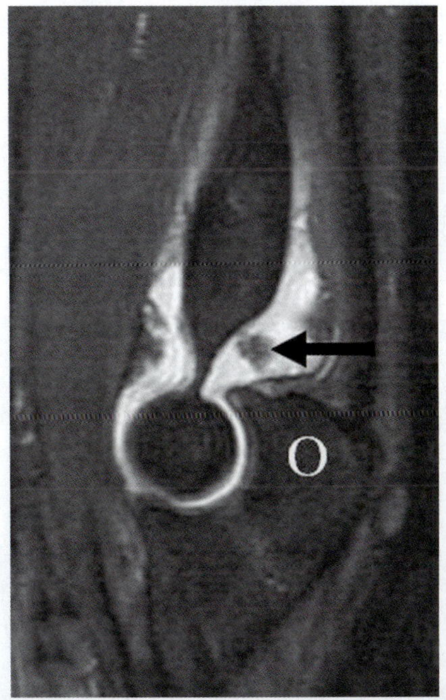

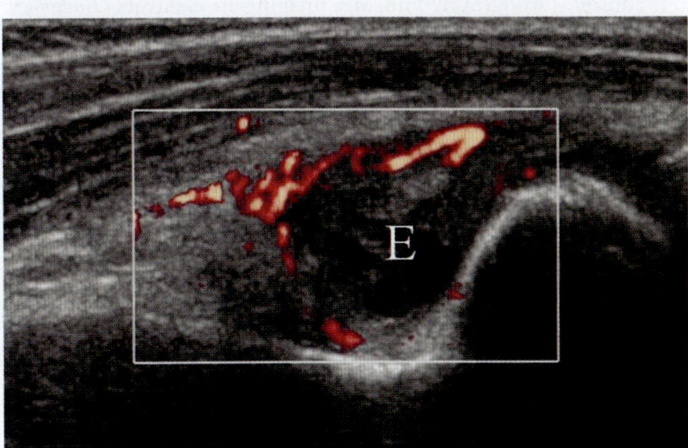

Figure 4.55. Power Doppler long-axis image shows a large effusion (*E*) in the olecranon fossa with marked surrounding hyperemia. The elbow has been flexed to move the olecranon process out of the way.

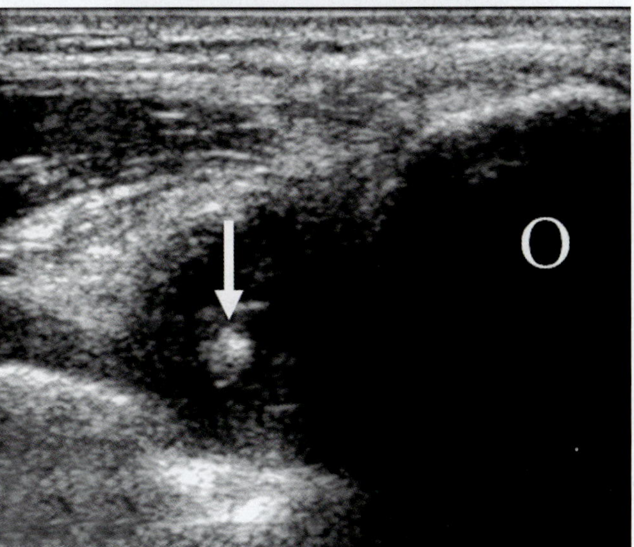

Figure 4.56. Loose body. **A:** Sagittal fat-suppressed T2-weighted MR image shows a low signal intensity loose body (*arrow*) in the olecranon fossa with a large effusion. **B:** Corresponding long-axis sonographic image in the same patient shows the echogenic body (*arrow*) in the large hypoechoic effusion. O, olecranon.

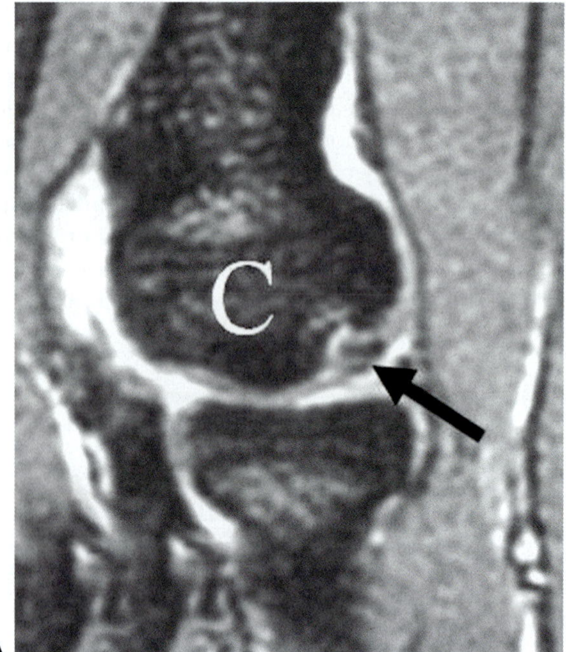

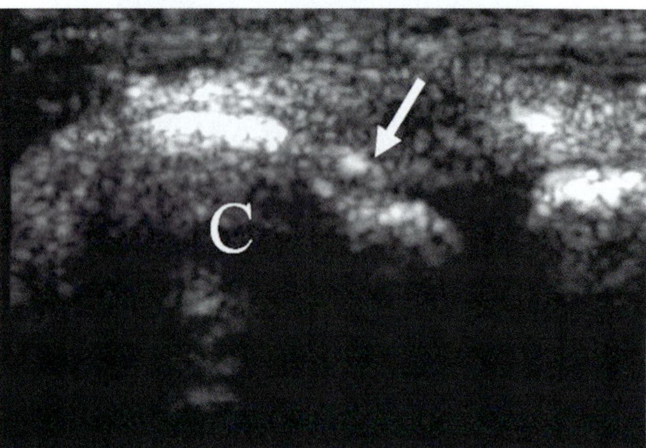

Figure 4.57.   Osteochondral injury. **A:** Sagittal gradient-echo MR image shows an in situ osteochondral fracture (*arrow*) of the capitellum (*C*). **B:** Corresponding long-axis sonographic image in the same patient shows the in situ fragment (*arrow*) of the capitellum (*C*).

Osteochondral injuries of the elbow usually occur at the anterior aspect of the capitellum, due to radiocapitellar impaction of the flexed elbow, often caused by throwing or gymnastics. Longitudinal sonography over the radiocapitellar joint of the extended elbow may demonstrate irregularity of the subchondral plate, fragmentation of the subchondral plate and overlying cartilage, or an osteochondral defect[99,100] **(Fig. 4.57).**

CONCLUSION

Sonography is excellent for the focused assessment of abnormalities of ligaments, tendons, nerves, and bursae around the elbow, and for assessing the joint itself.

Additional advantages are its ability to perform dynamic scanning and guide percutaneous treatments.

REFERENCES

1. Conn JM, Annest JL, Gilchrist J. Sports and recreation related injury episodes in the US population, 1997-99. *Inj Prev.* 2003;9(2):117–123.
2. Yang NP, Chen HC, Phan DV, et al. Epidemiological survey of orthopedic joint dislocations based on nationwide insurance data in Taiwan, 2000–2005. *BMC Musculoskelet Disord.* 2011;12:253.
3. Reijneirse M, Miller TT. Sonography of the elbow: scanning technique and normal anatomy. *AJR:*200, June 2013, In Press.
4. Tsai P, Steinberg DR. Median and radial nerve compression about the elbow. *Instr Course Lect.* 2008;57:177–185.
5. Ferdinand BD, Rosenberg ZS, Schweitzer ME, et al. MR imaging features of radial tunnel syndrome: initial experience. *Radiology.* 2006;240(1):161–168.
6. Lee MJ, LaStayo PC. Pronator syndrome and other nerve compressions that mimic carpal tunnel syndrome. *J Orthop Sports Phys Ther.* 2004;34(10):601–609.
7. Andreisek G, Crook DW, Burg D, et al. Peripheral neuropathies of the median, radial, and ulnar nerves: MR imaging features. *Radiographics.* 2006;26(5):1267–1287.
8. Dunn AJ, Salonen DC, Anastakis DJ. MR imaging findings of anterior interosseous nerve lesions. *Skeletal Radiol.* 2007;36(12):1155–1162.
9. Miller TT, Adler RS. Sonography of tears of the distal biceps tendon. *AJR Am J Roentgenol.* 2000;175(4):1081–1086.
10. Kalume Brigido M, De Maeseneer M, Jacobson JA, et al. Improved visualization of the radial insertion of the biceps tendon at ultrasound with a lateral approach. *Eur Radiol.* 2009;19(7):1817–1821.
11. Smith J, Finnoff JT, O'Driscoll SW, et al. Sonographic evaluation of the distal biceps tendon using a medial approach: the pronator window. *J Ultrasound Med.* 2010;29(5):861–865.
12. Giuffre BM, Lisle DA. Tear of the distal biceps branchii tendon: a new method of ultrasound evaluation. *Australas Radiol.* 2005;49(5):404–406.
13. Tagliafico A, Michaud J, Capaccio E, et al. Ultrasound demonstration of distal biceps tendon bifurcation: normal and abnormal findings. *Eur Radiol.* 2010;20(1):202–208.
14. Skaf AY, Boutin RD, Dantas RW, et al. Bicipitoradial bursitis: MR imaging findings in eight patients and anatomic data from contrast material opacification of bursae followed by routine radiography and MR imaging in cadavers. *Radiology.* 1999;212(1):111–116.
15. Teixeira PA, Omoumi P, Trudell DJ, et al. Ultrasound assessment of the lateral collateral ligamentous complex of the elbow: imaging aspects in cadavers and normal volunteers. *Eur Radiol.* 2011;21(7):1492–1498.
16. Stewart B, Harish S, Oomen G, et al. Sonography of the lateral ulnar collateral ligament of the elbow: study of cadavers and healthy volunteers. *AJR Am J Roentgenol.* 2009;193(6):1615–1619.
17. Reichel LM, Milam GS, Sitton SE, et al. Elbow lateral collateral ligament injuries. *J Hand Surg Am.* 2013;38(1):184–201.
18. Yeh PC, Dodds SD, Smart LR, et al. Distal triceps rupture. *J Am Acad Orthop Surg.* 2010;18(1):31–40.
19. Calfee RP, Patel A, DaSilva MF, et al. Management of lateral epicondylitis: current concepts. *J Am Acad Orthop Surg.* 2008;16(1):19–29.
20. Abrams GD, Renstrom PA, Safran MR. Epidemiology of musculoskeletal injury in the tennis player. *Br J Sports Med.* 2012;46(7):492–498.
21. Bayes MC, Wadsworth LT. Upper extremity injuries in golf. *Phys Sportsmed.* 2009;37(1):92–96.

22. Miller TT, Reinus WR. Nerve entrapment syndromes of the elbow, forearm, and wrist. *AJR Am J Roentgenol.* 2010;195(3):585–594.

23. Plancher KD, Halbrecht J, Lourie GM. Medial and lateral epicondylitis in the athlete. *Clin Sports Med.* 1996;15(2):283–305.

24. Walz DM, Newman JS, Konin GP, et al. Epicondylitis: pathogenesis, imaging, and treatment. *Radiographics.* 2010;30(1):167–184.

25. Nirschl RP. Elbow tendinosis/tennis elbow. *Clin Sports Med.* 1992;11(4):851–870.

26. Potter HG, Hannafin JA, Morwessel RM, et al. Lateral epicondylitis: correlation of MR imaging, surgical, and histopathologic findings. *Radiology.* 1995;196(1):43–46.

27. Regan W, Wold LE, Coonrad R, et al. Microscopic histopathology of chronic refractory lateral epicondylitis. *Am J Sports Med.* 1992;20(6):746–749.

28. Connell D, Burke F, Coombes P, et al. Sonographic examination of lateral epicondylitis. *AJR Am J Roentgenol.* 2001;176(3):777–782.

29. Miller TT, Shapiro MA, Schultz E, et al. Comparison of sonography and MRI for diagnosing epicondylitis. *J Clin Ultrasound.* 2002;30(4):193–202.

30. De Zordo T, Lill SR, Fink C, et al. Real-time sonoelastography of lateral epicondylitis: comparison of findings between patients and healthy volunteers. *AJR Am J Roentgenol.* 2009;193(1):180–185.

31. Levin D, Nazarian LN, Miller TT, et al. Lateral epicondylitis of the elbow: US findings. *Radiology.* 2005;237(1):230–234.

32. Struijs PA, Spruyt M, Assendelft WJ, et al. The predictive value of diagnostic sonography for the effectiveness of conservative treatment of tennis elbow. *AJR Am J Roentgenol.* 2005;185(5):1113–1118.

33. Lee MH, Cha JG, Jin W, et al. Utility of sonographic measurement of the common tensor tendon in patients with lateral epicondylitis. *AJR Am J Roentgenol.* 2011;196(6):1363–1367.

34. Park GY, Lee SM, Lee MY. Diagnostic value of ultrasonography for clinical medial epicondylitis. *Arch Phys Med Rehabil.* 2008;89(4):738–742.

35. McShane JM, Shah VN, Nazarian LN. Sonographically guided percutaneous needle tenotomy for treatment of common extensor tendinosis in the elbow: is a corticosteroid necessary? *J Ultrasound Med.* 2008;27(8):1137–1144.

36. McShane JM, Nazarian LN, Harwood MI. Sonographically guided percutaneous needle tenotomy for treatment of common extensor tendinosis in the elbow. *J Ultrasound Med.* 2006;25(10):1281–1289.

37. Suresh SP, Ali KE, Jones H, et al. Medial epicondylitis: is ultrasound guided autologous blood injection an effective treatment? *Br J Sports Med.* 2006;40(11):935–939.

38. Rantanen J, Orava S. Rupture of the distal biceps tendon. A report of 19 patients treated with anatomic reinsertion, and a meta-analysis of 147 cases found in the literature. *Am J Sports Med.* 1999;27(2):128–132.

39. Belli P, Costantini M, Mirk P, et al. Sonographic diagnosis of distal biceps tendon rupture: a prospective study of 25 cases. *J Ultrasound Med.* 2001;20(6):587–595.

40. Lobo Lda G, Fessell DP, Miller BS, et al. The role of sonography in differentiating full versus partial distal biceps tendon tears: correlation with surgical findings. *AJR Am J Roentgenol.* 2013;200(1):158–162.

41. Tagliafico A, Gandolfo N, Michaud J, et al. Ultrasound demonstration of distal triceps tendon tears. *Eur J Radiol.* 2012;81(6):1207–1210.

42. Downey R, Jacobson JA, Fessell DP, et al. Sonography of partial-thickness tears of the distal triceps brachii tendon. *J Ultrasound Med.* 2011;30(10):1351–1356.

43. Jacobson JA, Jebson PJ, Jeffers AW, et al. Ulnar nerve dislocation and snapping triceps syndrome: diagnosis with dynamic sonography—report of three cases. *Radiology.* 2001;220(3):601–605.

44. Callaway GH, Field LD, Deng XH, et al. Biomechanical evaluation of the medial collateral ligament of the elbow. *J Bone Joint Surg Am.* 1997;79(8):1223–1231.

45. Floris S, Olsen BS, Dalstra M, et al. The medial collateral ligament of the elbow joint: anatomy and kinematics. *J Shoulder Elbow Surg.* 1998;7(4):345–351.

46. Magra M, Caine D, Maffulli N. A review of epidemiology of paediatric elbow injuries in sports. *Sports Med.* 2007;37(8):717–735.

47. Paletta GA Jr, Klepps SJ, Difelice GS, et al. Biomechanical evaluation of 2 techniques for ulnar collateral ligament reconstruction of the elbow. *Am J Sports Med.* 2006;34(10):1599–1603.

48. Dodson CC, Thomas A, Dines JS, et al. Medial ulnar collateral ligament reconstruction of the elbow in throwing athletes. *Am J Sports Med.* 2006;34(12):1926–1932.

49. Pollock JW, Brownhill J, Ferreira LM, et al. Effect of the posterior bundle of the medial collateral ligament on elbow stability. *J Hand Surg Am.* 2009;34(1):116–123.

50. Nazarian LN, McShane JM, Ciccotti MG, et al. Dynamic US of the anterior band of the ulnar collateral ligament of the elbow in asymptomatic major league baseball pitchers. *Radiology.* 2003;227(1):149–154.

51. Sasaki J, Takahara M, Ogino T, et al. Ultrasonographic assessment of the ulnar collateral ligament and medial elbow laxity in college baseball players. *J Bone Joint Surg Am.* 2002;84-A(4):525–531.

52. Popovic N, Ferrara MA, Daenen B, et al. Imaging overuse injury of the elbow in professional team handball players: a bilateral comparison using plain films, stress radiography, ultrasound, and magnetic resonance imaging. *Int J Sports Med.* 2001;22(1):60–67.

53. Cain EL Jr, Dugas JR, Wolf RS, et al. Elbow injuries in throwing athletes: a current concepts review. *Am J Sports Med.* 2003;31(4):621–635.

54. O'Holleran JD, Altchek DW. The thrower's elbow: arthroscopic treatment of valgus extension overload syndrome. *HSS J.* 2006;2(1):83–93.

55. Ahmad CS, ElAttrache NS. Valgus extension overload syndrome and stress injury of the olecranon. *Clin Sports Med.* 2004;23(4):665–676.

56. Miller TT, Adler RS, Friedman L. Sonography of injury of the ulnar collateral ligament of the elbow-initial experience. *Skeletal Radiol.* 2004;33(7):386–391.

57. Timmerman LA, Schwartz ML, Andrews JR. Preoperative evaluation of the ulnar collateral ligament by magnetic resonance imaging and computed tomography arthrography. Evaluation in 25 baseball players with surgical confirmation. *Am J Sports Med.* 1994;22(1):26–31.

58. Brogdon BG, Crow NE. Little leaguer's elbow. *Am J Roentgenol Radium Ther Nucl Med.* 1960;83:671–675.

59. Klingele KE, Kocher MS. Little league elbow: valgus overload injury in thepaediatric athlete. *Sports Med.* 2002;32(15):1005–1015.

60. O'Driscoll SW. Classification and evaluation of recurrent instability of the elbow. *Clin Orthop Relat Res.* 2000;(370):34–43.

61. McKee MD, Schemitsch EH, Sala MJ, et al. The pathoanatomy of lateral ligamentous disruption in complex elbow instability. *J Shoulder Elbow Surg.* 2003;12(4):391–396.

62. Bredella MA, Tirman PF, Fritz RC, et al. MR imaging findings of lateral ulnar collateral ligament abnormalities in patients with lateral epicondylitis. *AJR Am J Roentgenol.* 1999;173(5):1379–1382.

63. Kosuwon W, Mahaisavariya B, Saengnipanthkul S, et al. Ultrasonography of pulled elbow. *J Bone Joint Surg Br.* 1993;75(3):421–422.

64. Kim MC, Eckhardt BP, Craig C, et al. Ultrasonography of the annular ligament partial tear and recurrent "pulled elbow". *Pediatr Radiol.* 2004;34(12):999–1004.

65. Bartels RH, Verbeek AL. Risk factors for ulnar nerve compression at the elbow: a case control study. *Acta Neurochir (Wien)*. 2007;149(7):669–674.

66. van Rijn RM, Huisstede BM, Koes BW, et al. Associations between work-related factors and specific disorders at the elbow: a systematic literature review. *Rheumatology (Oxford)*. 2009;48(5):528–536.

67. Gellman H. Compression of the ulnar nerve at the elbow: cubital tunnel syndrome. *Instr Course Lect*. 2008;57:187–197.

68. Darowish M, Lawton JN, Evans PJ. Q: What is cell phone elbow, and what should we tell our patients? *Cleve Clin J Med*. 2009;76(5):306–308.

69. Jensen A, Kaerlev L, Tüchsen F, et al. Locomotor diseases among male long-haul truck drivers and other professional drivers. *Int Arch Occup Environ Health*. 2008;81(7):821–827.

70. Cummins CA, Schneider DS. Peripheral nerve injuries in baseball players. *Neurol Clin*. 2008;26(1):195–215.

71. Husarik DB, Saupe N, Pfirrmann CW, et al. Elbow nerves: MR findings in 60 asymptomatic subjects—normal anatomy, variants, and pitfalls. *Radiology*. 2009;252(1):148–156.

72. Martinoli C, Bianchi S, Gandolfo N, et al. US of nerve entrapments in osteofibrous tunnels of the upper and lower limbs. *Radiographics*. 2000;20 Spec No:S199–S213.

73. Thoirs K, Williams MA, Phillips M. Ultrasonographic measurements of the ulnar nerve at the elbow: role of confounders. *J Ultrasound Med*. 2008;27(5):737–743.

74. Yoon JS, Walker FO, Cartwright MS. Ultrasonographic swelling ratio in the diagnosis of ulnar neuropathy at the elbow. *Muscle Nerve*. 2008;38(4):1231–1235.

75. Jacob D, Creteur V, Courthaliac C, et al. Sonoanatomy of the ulnar nerve in the cubital tunnel: a multicentre study by the GEL. *Eur Radiol*. 2004;14(10):1770–1773.

76. Childress HM. Recurrent ulnar-nerve dislocation at the elbow. *Clin Orthop Relat Res*. 1975;(108):168–173.

77. Okamoto M, Abe M, Shirai H, et al. Morphology and dynamics of the ulnar nerve in the cubital tunnel. Observation by ultrasonography. *J Hand Surg Br*. 2000;25(1):85–89.

78. Spinner RJ, Goldner RD. Snapping of the medial head of the triceps and recurrent dislocation of the ulnar nerve. Anatomical and dynamic factors. *J Bone Joint Surg Am*. 1998;80(2):239–247.

79. Spinner RJ, Goldner RD, Lee RA. Diagnosis of snapping triceps with US. *Radiology*. 2002;224(3):933–934.

80. Clavert P, Lutz JC, Adam P, et al. Frohse's arcade is not the exclusive compression site of the radial nerve in its tunnel. *Orthop Traumatol Surg Res*. 2009;95(2):114–118.

81. Xarchas KC, Psillakis I, Koukou O, et al. Ulnar nerve dislocation at the elbow: review of the literature and report of three cases. *Open Orthop J*. 2007;24:1–3.

82. Dang AC, Rodner CM. Unusual compression neuropathies of the forearm, Part I: radial nerve. *J Hand Surg Am*. 2009;34(10):1906–1914.

83. Bodner G, Harpf C, Meirer R, et al. Ultrasonographic appearance of supinator syndrome. *J Ultrasound Med*. 2002; 21(11):1289–1293.

84. Martinoli C, Bianchi S, Pugliese F, et al. Sonography of entrapment neuropathies in the upper limb (wrist excluded). *J Clin Ultrasound*. 2004;32(9):438–450.

85. Suranyi L. Median nerve compression by Struthers ligament. *J Neurol Neurosurg Psychiatry*. 1983;46(11):1047–1049.

86. Lordan J, Rauh P, Spinner RJ. The clinical anatomy of the supracondylar spur and the ligament of Struthers. *Clin Anat*. 2005;18(7):548–551.

87. Bilecenoglu B, Uz A, Karalezli N. Possible anatomic structures causing entrapment neuropathies of the median nerve: an anatomic study. *Acta Orthop Belg*. 2005;71(2):169–176.

88. Dang AC, Rodner CM. Unusual compression neuropathies of the forearm, part II: median nerve. *J Hand Surg Am*. 2009;34(10):1915–1920.

89. Kiloh LG, Nevin S. Isolated neuritis of the anterior interosseous nerve. *Br Med J*. 1952;1(4763):850–851.

90. Wong L, Dellon AL. Brachial neuritis presenting as anterior interosseous nerve compression—implications for diagnosis and treatment: a case report. *J Hand Surg Am*. 1997;22(3): 536–539.

91. Grainger AJ, Campbell RS, Stothard J. Anterior interosseous nerve syndrome: appearance at MR imaging in three cases. *Radiology*. 1998;208(2):381–384.

92. Hide IG, Grainger AJ, Naisby GP, et al. Sonographic findings in the anterior interosseous nerve syndrome. *J Clin Ultrasound*. 1999;27(8):459–464.

93. Blankstein A, Ganel A, Givon U, et al. Ultrasonographic findings in patients with olecranon bursitis. *Ultraschall Med*. 2006;27(6):568–571.

94. Liessi G, Cesari S, Spaliviero B, et al. The US, CT, and MR findings of cubital bursitis: a report of five cases. *Skeletal Radiol*. 1996;25(5):471–475.

95. Sofka CM, Adler RS. Sonography of cubital bursitis. *AJR Am J Roentgenol*. 2004;183(1):51–53.

96. Bianchi S, Martinoli C. Detection of loose bodies in joints. *Radiol Clin North Am*. 1999;37(4):679–690.

97. Frankel DA, Bargiela A, Bouffard JA, et al. Synovial joints: evaluation of intraarticular bodies with US. *Radiology*. 1998;206(1):41–44.

98. Miller JH, Beggs I. Detection of intraarticular bodies of the elbow with saline arthrosonography. *Clin Radiol*. 2001;56(3):231–234.

99. Harada M, Takahara M, Sasaki J, et al. Using sonography for the early detection of elbow injuries among young baseball players. *AJR Am J Roentgenol*. 2006;187(6):1436–1441.

100. Takahara M, Ogino T, Tsuchida H, et al. Sonographic assessment of osteochondritis dissecans of the humeral capitellum. *AJR Am J Roentgenol*. 2000;174(2):411–415.

Hand and Wrist

Monique Reijnierse
Nicole C. Fernandes

INTRODUCTION

The complex soft tissue structures of the hand and wrist are ideally suited for ultrasound examination. They are superficial and accessible. Dynamic examination can be performed in real-time and vascularity assessed by color or power Doppler. Standard linear array transducers are adequate for most purposes, but small footprint transducers operating at high frequency (>10MHz) may be valuable.

ANATOMY OF THE WRIST

Bones and Ligaments

Two carpal rows with eight carpal bones form the wrist. From radial to ulnar, the proximal carpal row is formed by scaphoid, lunate, triquetrum, and pisiform, and the distal carpal row by trapezium, trapezoid, capitate, and hamate **(Fig. 5.1)**. Stability is maintained by extrinsic (radiocarpal and ulnocarpal) and intrinsic (intercarpal) ligaments. Palmar and dorsal ligaments are differentiated and are named for the bones from which they originate and into which they insert, starting from proximal to distal and from radial to ulnar.[1,2]

The scapholunate (SLL) and lunotriquetral ligaments (LTL) are the most important intrinsic ligaments. They have thick palmar and dorsal components and thinner central portions.[3]

The triangular fibrocartilage is a biconcave disk between the ulnar styloid and the radius, with a variable thickness. Together with the meniscus homologue,

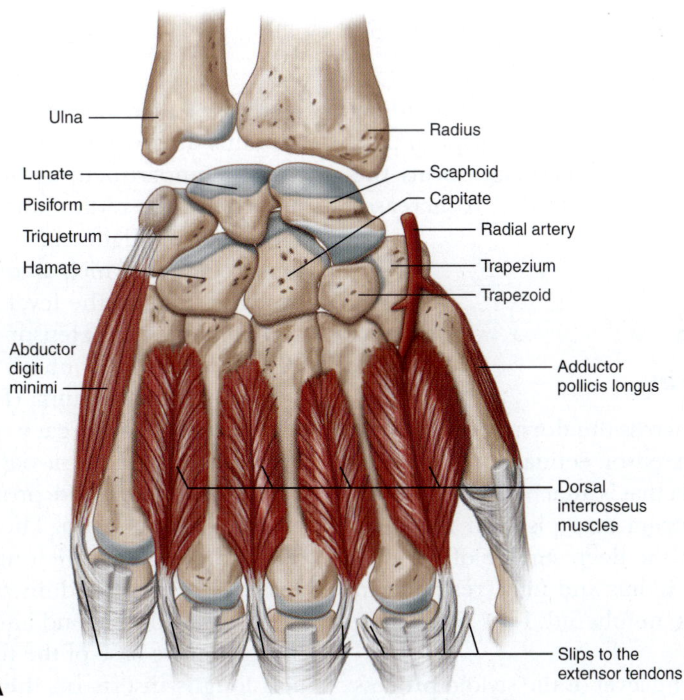

Figure 5.1. Bony anatomy. **A, B**: The anatomy of the proximal and distal carpal rows, as seen from the dorsal (**A**) and palmar (**B**) sides is shown. The landmarks for the carpal tunnel proximally—scaphoid and pisiform—and distally—trapezium and hamate—are clearly visible in **B**. The carpal bones are connected by intrinsic ligaments. The interosseous and lumbrical muscles contribute lateral and central slips to stabilize the extensor tendons.

(Adapted from Netter FH, Woodburne RT, Crelin ES, et al. Upper limb, wrist and hand. In: *Musculoskeletal System, Part 1: Anatomy, Physiology and Metabolic Disorders.* NJ: Ciba-Geigy; 1987:55–73, with permission.)

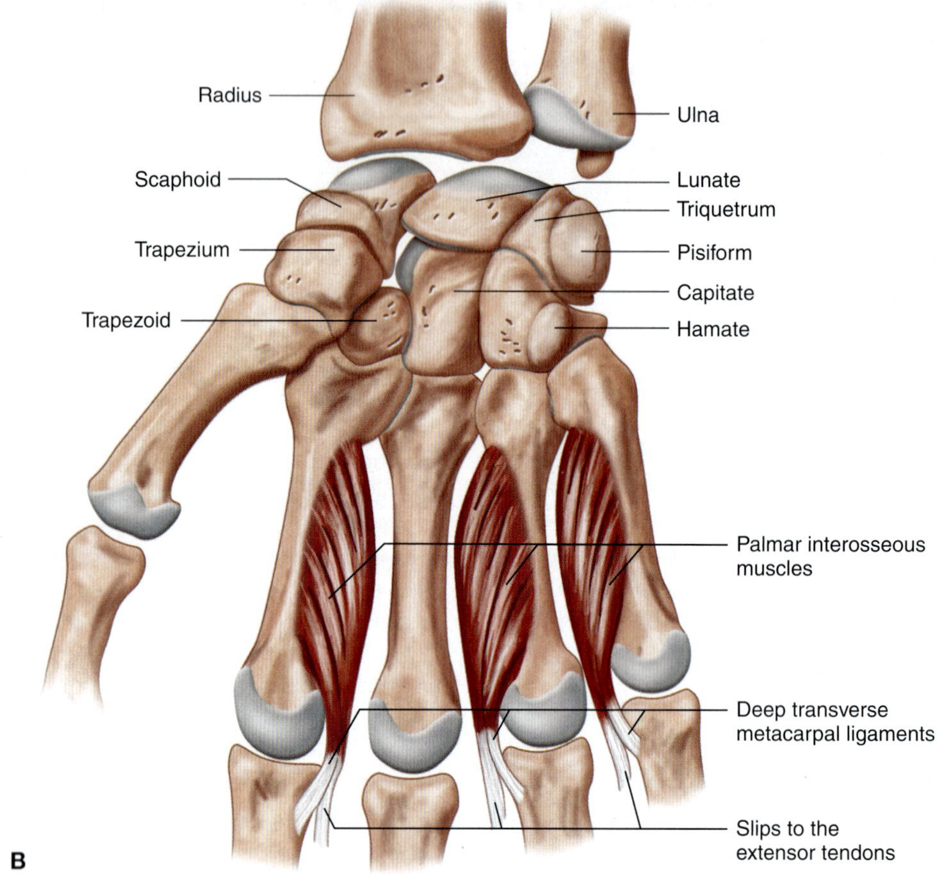

Figure 5.1.   (*Continued*)

the ulnar collateral ligament (UCL), the radioulnar ligament, and the sheath of the extensor carpi ulnaris (ECU) tendon, the triangular fibrocartilage forms the triangular fibrocartilage complex (TFCC).[3] It increases stability of the ulnar side of the wrist.

Tendons and Synovium

Extensor Tendons at the Wrist

The extensor tendons run across the dorsum of the wrist held in position by the extensor retinaculum, a focal thickening of the deep fascia that is attached to the radius laterally and to the triquetrum and pisiform medially. Fibrous bands extend from the deep surface of the retinaculum and attach to the radius and ulna, resulting in six separate compartments numbered 1 to 6, starting from the radial side.

Compartment one is at the level of the styloid process of the radius and contains the tendons of abductor pollicis longus (APL) and extensor pollicis brevis (EPB).

Compartment two lies on the radial side of Lister's tubercle, a bony prominence on the dorsal aspect of the distal radius, and contains the extensor carpi radialis longus (ECRL) and extensor carpi radialis brevis (ECRB)

tendons. Ulnar to Lister's tubercle, compartment three contains the extensor pollicis longus (EPL) tendon. The fourth compartment is the last compartment on the ulnar side of the radius, and contains the four tendons of the extensor digitorum muscle and the tendon of extensor indicis, which is deeper. Compartment five lies over the ulna, at the level of the distal radioulnar joint, and contains the extensor digiti minimi (EDM) tendon. Compartment six contains the tendon of the ECU in the groove of the distal ulna (**Fig. 5.2**).

The tendons of each compartment are enveloped by double-layered synovial sheaths to prevent friction.[4] These sheaths extend proximally and distally from the extensor retinaculum. The sheaths surrounding the tendons to the fingers are longer than those of ECU, ECRB, and ECRL. The tendons of ECRB and ECRL insert on the bases of the second and third metacarpals, and ECU inserts on the base of the fifth metacarpal. Abductor pollicis longus inserts on the base of the first metacarpal. The extensor tendons are vulnerable at the dorsum of the hand, since they are located superficially. The extensor digitorum tendons show intertendinous connections that limit separate movement. Since the tendon of the extensor indicis is extra, separate extension of the index finger is possible.

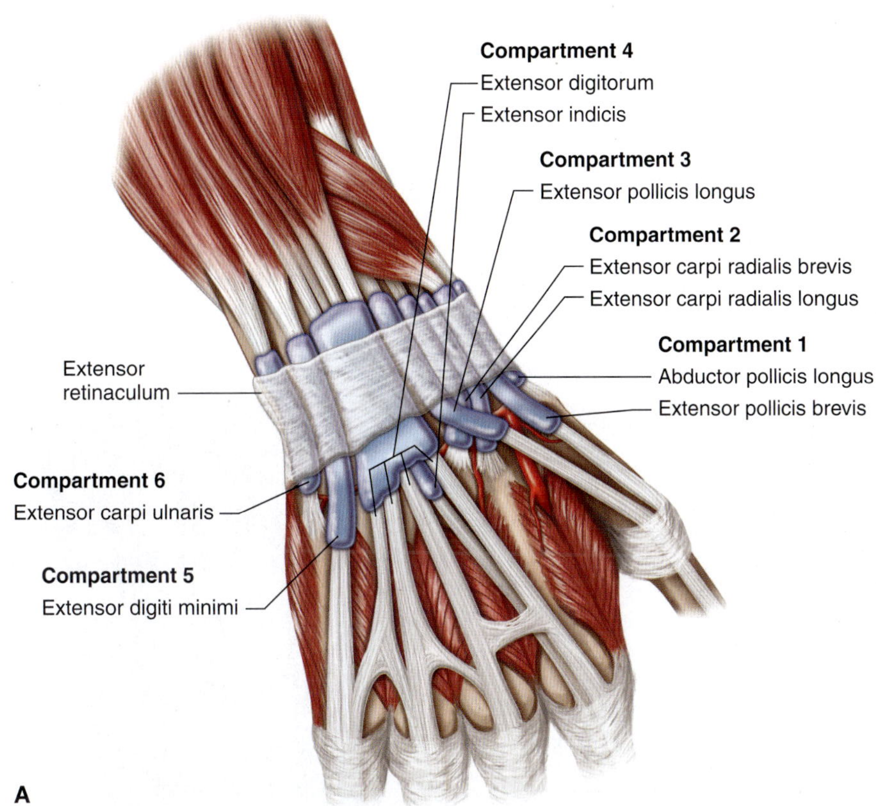

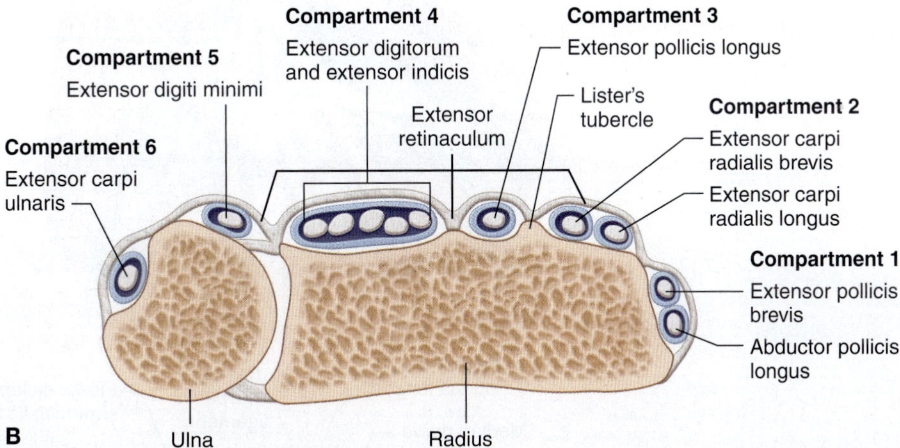

Figure 5.2.   Extensor tendon anatomy at the wrist. **A:** Dorsal view. The extensor tendons lie in six compartments. Each compartment contains a synovial sheath for the tendon(s) it contains. The sheaths extend proximal and distal to the extensor retinaculum. The tendons of compartments two and six insert on the bases of the second/third and fifth metacarpals, respectively. Intertendinous connections are visible on the dorsum of the hand. **B:** Axial view. The extensor compartments are numbered from the radial to the ulnar side. Lister's tubercle is the bony landmark that separates compartments two and three.

(Adapted from Netter FH, Woodburne RT, Crelin ES, et al. Upper limb, wrist and hand. In: *Musculoskeletal System, Part 1: Anatomy, Physiology and Metabolic Disorders.* NJ: Ciba-Geigy; 1987:55–73, with permission.)

Proximal to the extensor retinaculum the tendons of compartment one cross superficial to the tendons of compartment two. Distal to Lister's tubercle, EPL crosses over extensor compartment two.

Flexor Tendons at the Wrist

There are nine flexor tendons in the carpal tunnel. The flexor tendons of the fingers, the flexor digitorum superficialis (FDS) and flexor digitorum profundus (FDP), are arranged in the carpal tunnel, superficial and deep, respectively, and continue distally in pairs to each finger except the thumb **(Fig. 5.3)**. They are invested by a common tendon sheath that starts proximal to the carpal tunnel and extends to within 5 mm of the insertion of the profundus tendon on the distal phalanx. A separate ulnar bursa envelops the flexor tendons of the little finger. There is a gap between ulnar bursa and the synovial sheaths of the index, long, and ring fingers in the distal palm of the hand. The other tendon in the carpal

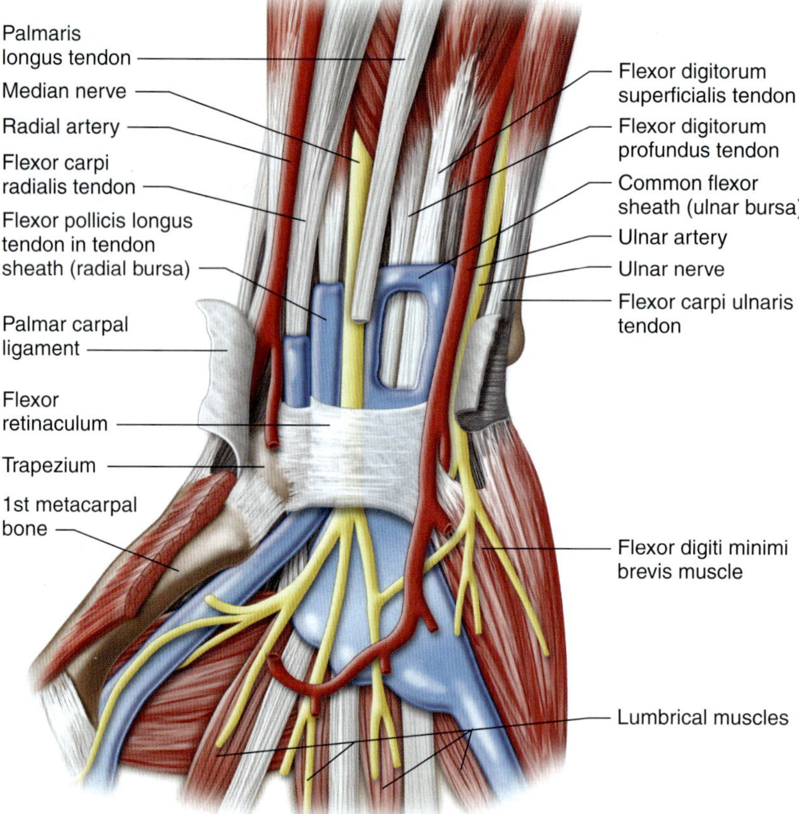

Figure 5.3.   Flexor tendon anatomy at the wrist. **A:** Volar view. The palmar ligament is proximal and superficial to the flexor retinaculum. The tendons of FPL, FDP, and FDS (nine in total) run through the carpal tunnel, accompanied by the median nerve. Flexor carpi radialis runs in a separate compartment and inserts on the bases of the second and third metacarpals and the tuberosity of the trapezium. Flexor carpi ulnaris inserts on the pisiform and has no synovial sheath. The palmaris longus is the only other flexor tendon without a sheath. **B:** Axial view, proximal to the carpal tunnel. Appreciate the typical position of the tendons surrounded by the ulnar bursa.

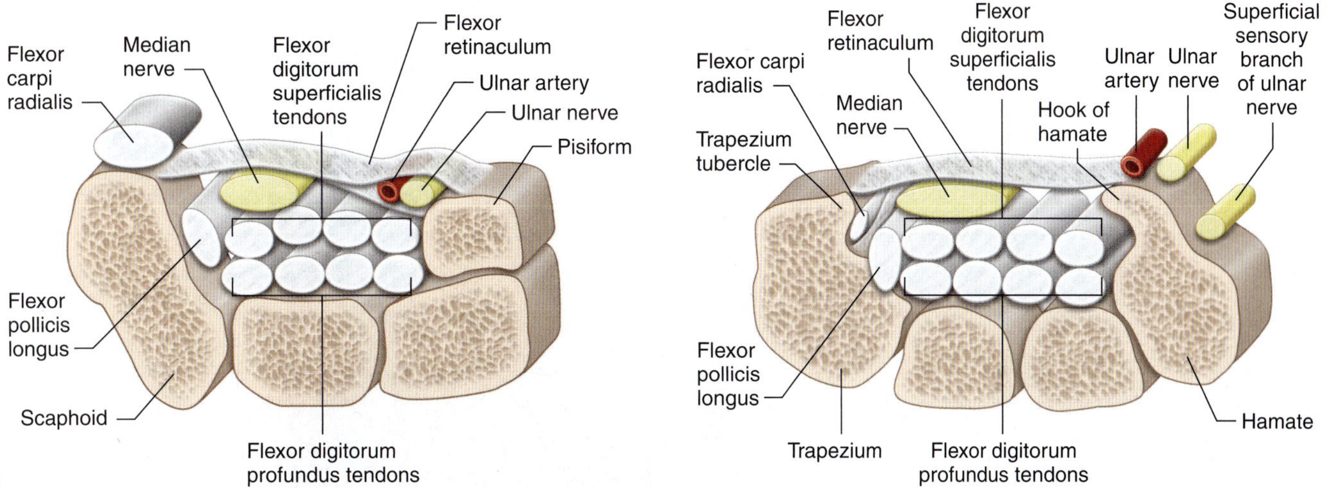

Figure 5.3. (*Continued*) **C:** At proximal carpal tunnel. The bony landmarks are the scaphoid tubercle and the pisiform. The flexor retinaculum forms the roof of the carpal tunnel and the floor of Guyon's canal that contains the ulnar artery and nerve. **D:** Distal carpal tunnel. The bony landmarks are the trapezium tubercle and the hook of the hamate. The FCR tendon sits in a groove in the trapezium separated from the other tendons by a split in the attachment of the retinaculum.

(Adapted from Netter FH, Woodburne RT, Crelin ES, et al. Upper limb, wrist and hand. In: *Musculoskeletal System, Part 1: Anatomy, Physiology and Metabolic Disorders.* NJ: Ciba-Geigy; 1987:55–73, with permission.)

tunnel is the flexor tendon of the thumb, flexor pollicis longus, which has a separate synovial covering, the radial bursa **(Fig. 5.4)**.

There are two primary wrist flexors. They are superficial to the carpal tunnel. The flexor carpi radialis (FCR) tendon inserts on the base of the second metacarpal. It has a separate synovial sheath. Flexor carpi ulnaris (FCU) contains the pisiform, a sesamoid bone, and inserts on the hook of the hamate and the base of the fifth metacarpal. The FCU does not have a tendon sheath. The palmaris longus tendon is a thin, variable tendon that inserts on the transverse carpal ligament and the palmar aponeurosis and is absent in 20% of cases.[4]

Nerves at the Wrist

The median nerve (MN) enters the carpal tunnel with the FDP and FDS tendons of the fingers. The MN is located superficial to the flexor pollicis longus tendon and the FDS tendon of the index finger. Distal to the carpal tunnel, it divides into recurrent motor and common palmar digital nerves.[5] It provides the motor supply for the muscles of the thenar eminence and the sensory supply to the palmar aspect of the thumb, index, and middle fingers and the radial half of the ring finger.[3] Anatomic variants include a persistent median artery of the forearm and bifid MN.

The ulnar nerve and artery run through Guyon's canal. The floor of this small tunnel is formed by the transverse carpal ligament, its ulnar wall by the pisiform, and its roof by the palmar carpal ligament, which is an extension of the flexor retinaculum. The tunnel is demarcated by the pisiform proximally and the hook of hamate distally. The ulnar nerve divides in the distal canal into a superficial sensory branch and a deep motor branch, located on either side of the flexor digiti minimi brevis muscle.[5,6] The sensory branch supplies the palmar aspect of the ulnar portion of the ring finger and the little finger, and the motor branch supplies the muscles of the hypothenar eminence, ulnar lumbrical, and interosseous muscles and the adductor pollicis.[4]

The radial nerve at the wrist is a small superficial branch in the subcutis and pierces the deep fascia proximal to the extensor retinaculum. It crosses the first extensor compartment, subdivides into two branches, which usually split into four or five dorsal digital nerves, and provides sensation to the dorsum of the wrist, hand, thumb, and proximal fingers.[6,4]

ANATOMY OF THE FINGERS

The five metacarpal bones and their phalanges form the metacarpophalangeal (MCP) and proximal (PIP) and distal interphalangeal (DIP) joints, except for the thumb, which has a metacarpal joint and a single interphalangeal joint. In each joint, the bones are united by a loose articular capsule, radial and ulnar collateral ligaments, and a palmar ligament. Dorsally the joints are reinforced by the expansion of the digital extensor tendon.[4]

The collateral ligaments are strong, fan-shaped, cord-like bands that stabilize the joint.

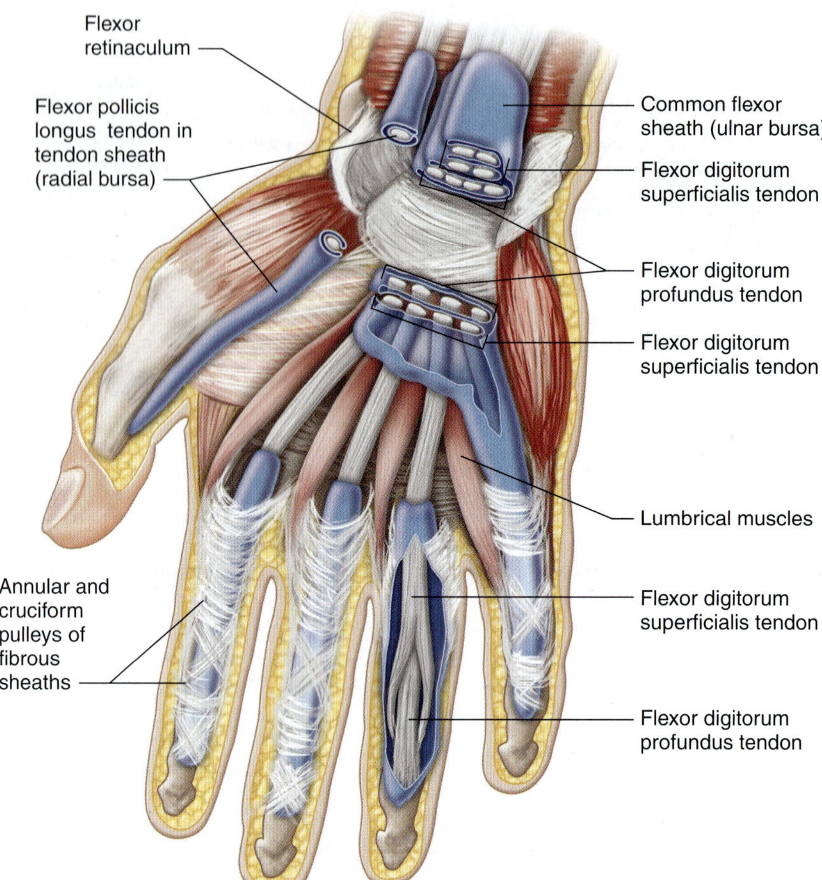

Figure 5.4.   Volar wrist and hand synovial anatomy. The flexor pollicis longus tendon is surrounded by the radial bursa, which extends distally. The other flexor tendons are surrounded by the ulnar bursa, which extends to the little finger. Note the gap between this bursa and the synovial sheaths of the second, third, and fourth digits.

(Adapted from Netter FH, Woodburne RT, Crelin ES, et al. Upper limb, wrist and hand. In: *Musculoskeletal System, Part 1: Anatomy, Physiology and Metabolic Disorders.* NJ: Ciba-Geigy; 1987:55–73, with permission.)

The palmar ligament, also called the palmar or volar plate, consists of thick fibrocartilage, extending from the neck of the proximal bone to the base of the distal bone. Proximally it is loosely attached, distally firmly. At the sides, it is continuous with the collateral ligaments, and at the level of the MCP joints it is also continuous with the deep transverse metacarpal ligament. On the volar side of the palmar plate, a groove holds the flexor digitorum tendons. Fibrous sheaths cover the synovial sheaths and extend from the head of the metacarpals distally. The fibrous sheaths have thick, transversely running fibers, pulleys, which insert on the palmar plate **(Fig. 5.5)**. The pulley system refers to a number of ligaments, including annular pulleys (A1–A5) and cruciform pulleys (C1–3). Their task is to keep the tendons close to the bone in flexion and to prevent "bowstringing." The A2 and A4 pulleys are broader than the others and are functionally more important. **(Fig. 5.5)**

The tendon of FDP inserts on the base of the distal phalanx. The tendon of FDS splits at the level of the proximal phalanx and inserts on the shaft of the middle phalanx **(Fig. 5.5B).**

The four tendons of extensor digitorum longus flatten distally from the MCP joints and divide into three slips: the central slip inserts on the base of the middle phalanx, and the two lateral slips insert on the base of the distal phalanx **(Fig. 5.5C)**. The extensor tendons are closely related to the joint capsule, and an extensor expansion for the MCP, PIP, and DIP joints is formed by the tendons of the lumbrical and interosseous muscles of the hand.[4] At the level of the MCP joint this dorsal expansion is called a hood. A triangular aponeurosis is formed over the distal end of the middle phalanx, with the apex inserting on the distal phalanx. The thumb has two separate extensor tendons: the EPL inserting on the base of the distal phalanx and the EPB inserting on the base of the proximal phalanx. Thus the extensor tendons are attached to the bone by a complex ligamentous structure and do not have a synovial sheath.

ULTRASOUND TECHNIQUE

The patient is seated opposite the examiner, with the hand placed on the examination couch. The height of the couch is adjusted such that it is comfortable for both the patient and the examiner. Abundant ultrasound gel is required to ensure that the ultrasound probe is in good contact with the underlying skin, without the need to exert excessive pressure. The hand is placed on an absorbent pad.

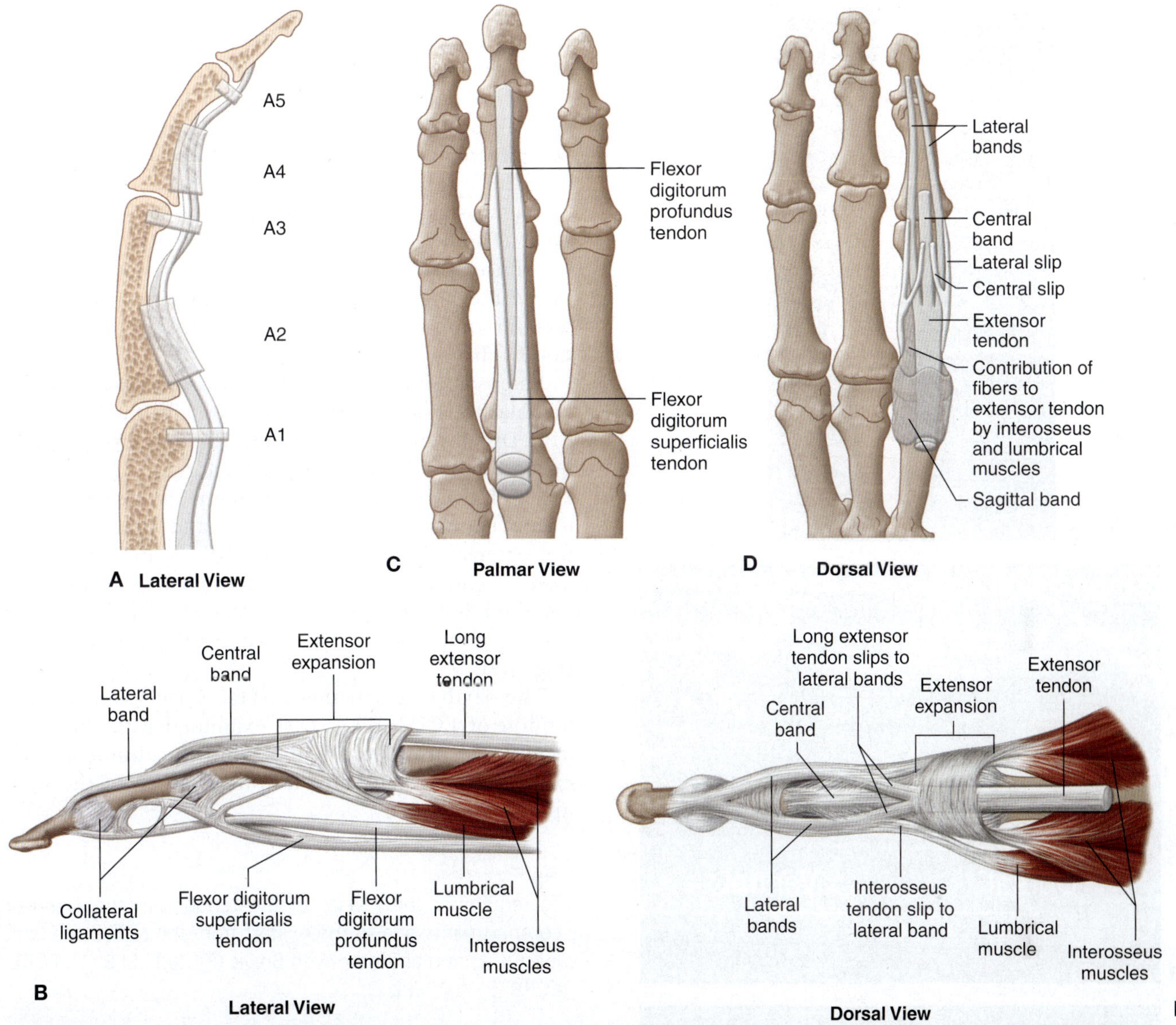

Figure 5.5.   Tendon anatomy of the fingers. **A:** Lateral view of annular pulley system that stops the flexor tendons from bowstringing. **B:** Lateral view: insertion of the extensor and flexor tendons. The extensor tendon has three slips and flattens distally. Flexor tendons are thicker than extensor tendons and have superficial and deep components. The stabilizers of the extensor tendon include the interosseous and lumbrical insertions and a dorsal expansion at the level of the MCP joints. **C:** Palmar view: flexor tendon insertion. The FDP tendon inserts on the base of the distal phalanx, the FDS tendon divides into two at the level of the proximal phalanx and inserts on the shaft of the middle phalanx. **D,E:** Dorsal views: extensor tendon insertion. The extensor tendon with three slips, the lateral ones inserting distally and the central one inserting on the middle phalanx, is stabilized by slips of the interosseous and lumbrical muscles and a dorsal expansion at the level of the MCP joints.

(Adapted from Netter FH, Woodburne RT, Crelin ES, et al. Upper limb, wrist and hand. In: *Musculoskeletal System, Part 1: Anatomy, Physiology and Metabolic Disorders.* NJ: Ciba-Geigy; 1987:55–73, with permission.)

In general, anatomy is identified using a standardized protocol[3,5,7] and important landmarks. Be aware of normal variations.

Dorsal Wrist

Start the examination of the wrist in a transverse plane. Identification of the different tendons is achieved by using the important landmark of Lister's tubercle, a bony prominence on the distal radius that separates the second and third compartments. The six extensor compartments are identified. Compartment one contains the tendons of the APL (palmar) and the EPB (dorsal), which are best shown with the hand placed on its ulnar side, thumb upward (**Fig. 5.6**). A septum may divide this compartment into two. This is important in the case of therapeutic injections as the two sub-compartments may have to be injected separately.

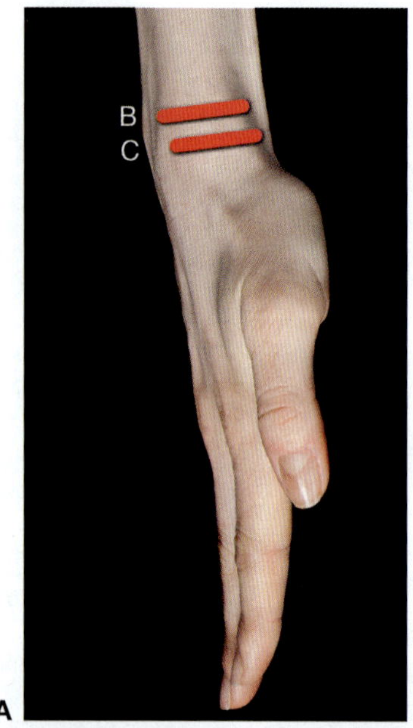

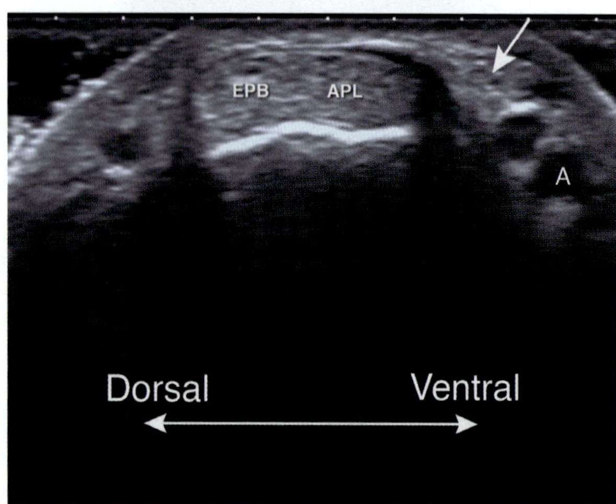

Dorsal ⟷ Ventral

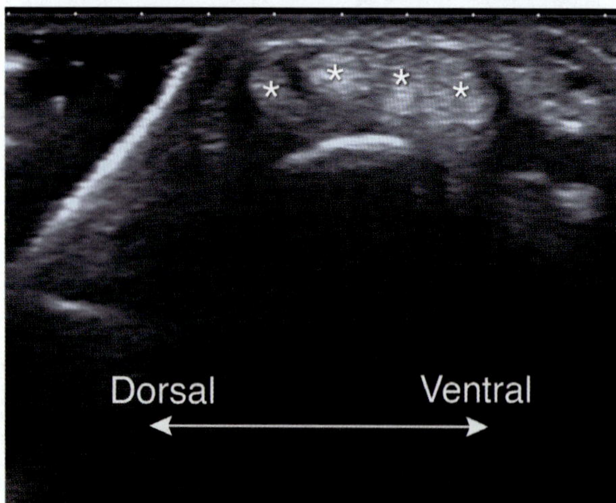

Dorsal ⟷ Ventral

Figure 5.6.   Compartment one. **A:** The right hand is examined on its side, thumb upward. **B:** Extensor pollicis brevis (*EPB*) is dorsal, and abductor pollicis longus (*APL*) lies ventral. The radial artery (*A*) crosses deep to the tendons more distally, and the superficial branch of the radial nerve (*arrow*) crosses superficially. **C:** Distal image demonstrates the multiple tendon slips (*asterisks*) of APL.

The APL may have multiple tendinous slips, a normal finding. The radial artery and the sensory branch of the radial nerve lie palmar to the APL. The artery crosses deep to the tendons, and the nerve crosses superficial. To exclude accessory tendons at the first compartment, the APL should be followed distally over the scaphoid.

The wrist is then turned prone. The second compartment **(Fig. 5.7)** contains ECRL and ECRB. Moving the transducer proximally from Lister's tubercle, the point where the first compartment crosses superficial to the second compartment is identified, the site of intersection syndrome.

Extensor compartment three lies immediately medial or ulnar to Lister's tubercle and contains the tendon of EPL. Distally, the tendon of EPL **(Fig. 5.8)** crosses superficial to the tendons of compartment two.

The fourth compartment contains the extensor digitorum communis (EDC) tendon and the tendon of the extensor indicis proprius (EIP), which is located deeper. The compartment has a thick, hypoechoic retinaculum that should not be mistaken for fluid. The fifth compartment is small and contains the tendon of EDM **(Fig. 5.9)**.

The sixth compartment **(Fig. 5.10)** contains the tendon of ECU, and is best examined with the hand in extreme pronation, that is, with the thumb on the examination couch and the ulnar surface of the wrist upward.

Tip:
To remember the names of the tendons in the extensor compartments one to three, start from the radial side with longus (L) and alternate with Brevis (B): APL, EP**B** (1), ECRL, ECR**B** (2), and EPL (3).

The TFCC is located in the space between the distal ulna and the proximal carpal row, but is not well demonstrated by ultrasound. Suspected TFCC tears should be investigated by magnetic resonance imaging (MRI) or MR arthrography.

To identify the SLL **(Fig. 5.11)**, the transducer is moved distally from Lister's tubercle. Only the dorsal part of the SLL can be seen as a thin band running between the scaphoid and the lunate, but this is a useful screening tool in suspected SLL tears. The LTL may be seen ulnar to the SLL.

Tip:
Use Lister's tubercle as a landmark to identify the second and third compartments. By moving distally from Lister's tubercle, you will find the scapholunate ligament.

Longitudinal imaging is used to image the radiocarpal joint and screen for synovial hypertrophy or joint

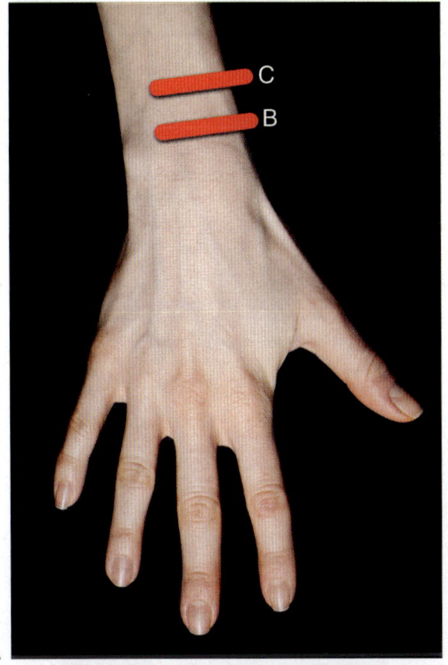

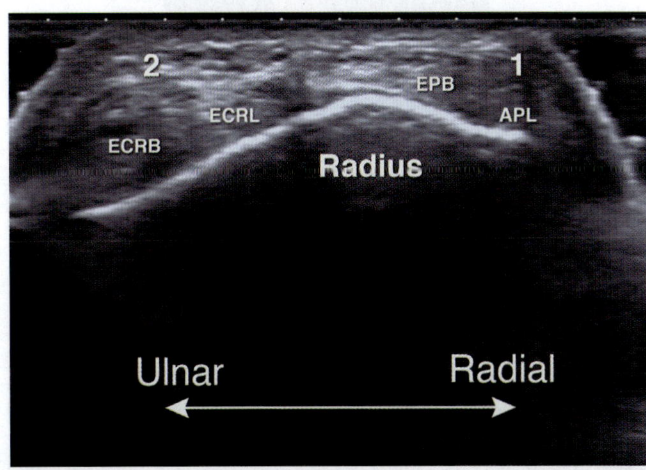

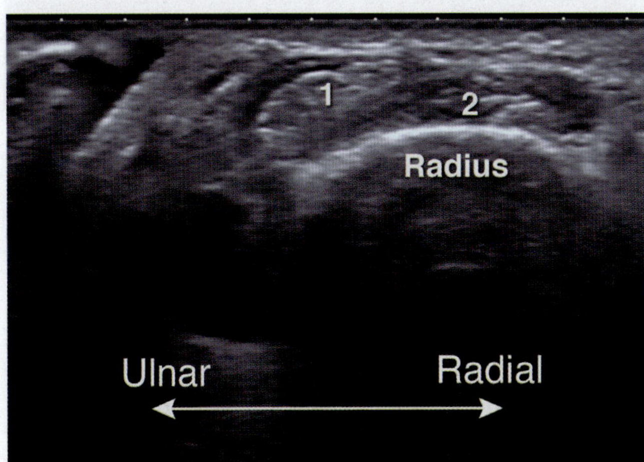

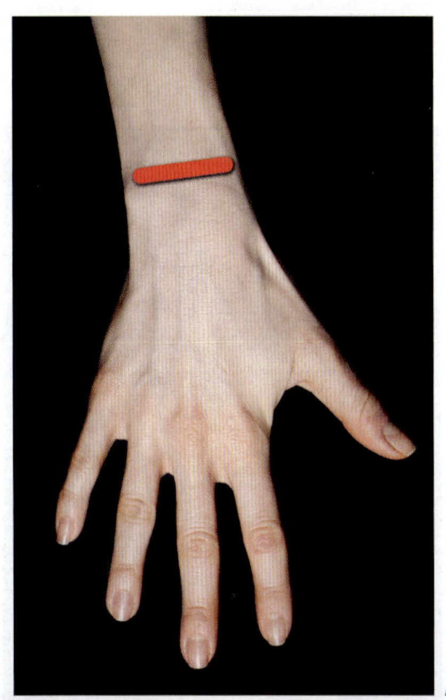

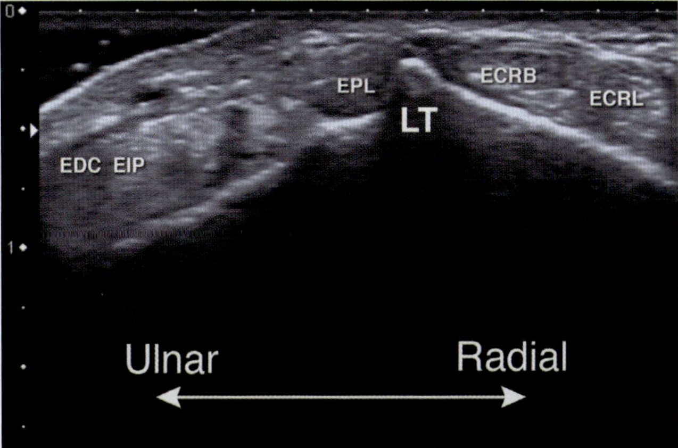

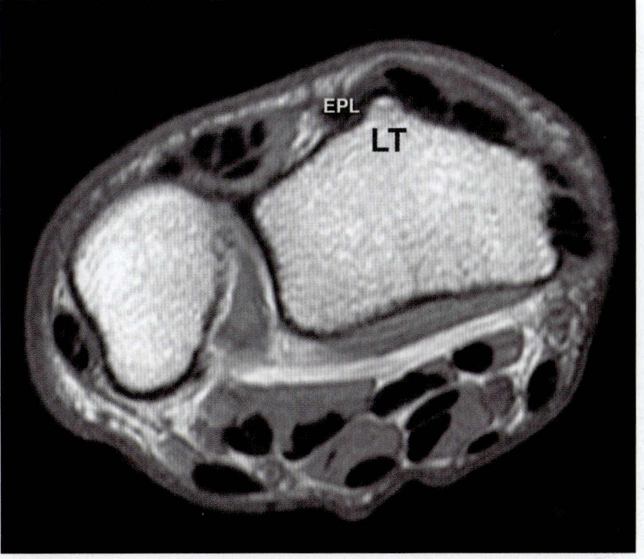

Figure 5.7. Compartment two. **A:** Hand pronated. **B:** Axial image of the second extensor compartment illustrating the extensor carpi radialis longus (*ECRL*) and extensor carpi radialis brevis (*ECRB*). EPB, extensor pollicis brevis; APL, abductor pollicis longus. **C:** Moving the transducer proximally shows the first compartment crossing superficial to the second compartment.

Figure 5.8. Compartments two, three, and four. **A:** Hand pronated. **B:** Axial ultrasound: Lister's tubercle (*LT*) is the bony landmark that separates compartments two (*ECRB, ECRL*) and three (*EPL*). ECRL, extensor carpi radialis longus; ECRB, extensor carpi radialis brevis; EPL, extensor pollicis longus; EDC, extensor digitorum communis; EIP, extensor indicis proprius. **C:** Axial T1 weighted image. EPL lies immediately medial to Lister's tubercle. EPL, extensor pollicis longus.

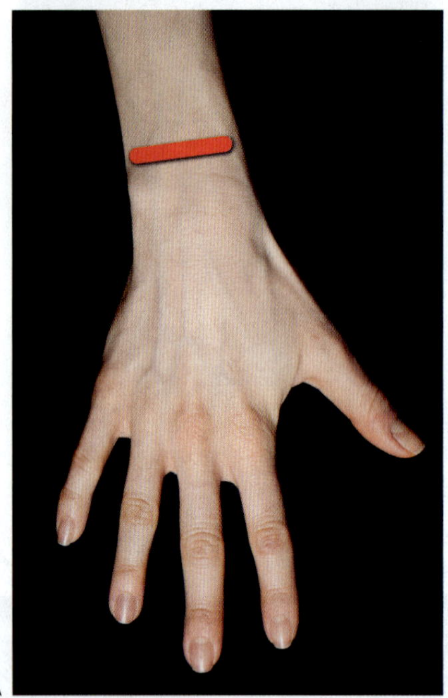

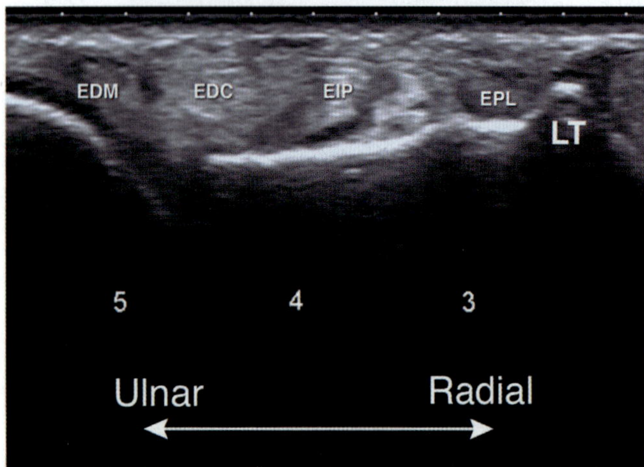

Figure 5.9.   Compartment three, four, and five. **A:** Hand pronated. **B:** Axial ultrasound image. Moving the transducer ulnar from Lister's tubercle and EPL demonstrates the fourth compartment with the extensor indicis proprius (*EIP*) and extensor digitorum communis (*EDC*), and the fifth compartment with extensor digiti minimi (*EDM*). Moving the fingers can be used to identify individual tendons. EPL, extensor pollicis longus; LT, Lister's tubercle.

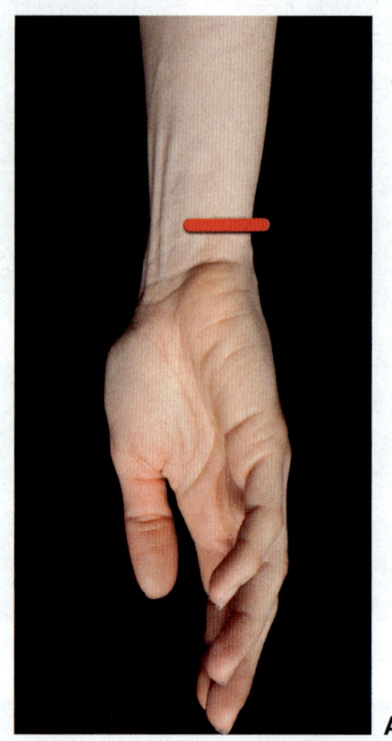

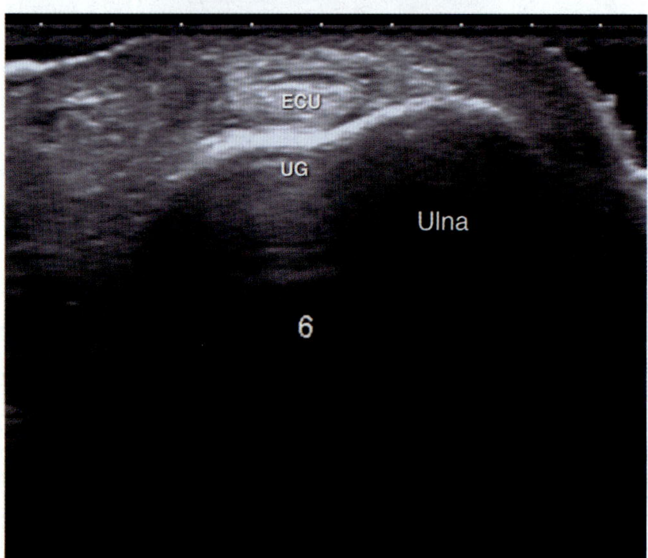

Figure 5.10.   Compartment six. **A:** Extreme pronation of the hand is the ideal position for examining the sixth compartment. **B:** Extensor carpi ulnaris (*ECU*) is situated in the ulnar groove (*UG*).

effusion. The distal radio ulnar (DRU) joint is imaged transversely and lies just proximal to the radiocarpal joint.

Volar Wrist

Carpal Tunnel

The volar wrist is examined with the wrist supinated and slightly extended. The transverse plane is most valuable in identifying the anatomic landmarks. The bony landmarks for the proximal carpal tunnel are the scaphoid tubercle (radial) and pisiform (ulnar). By placing the transducer on these marks, the flexor retinaculum, nine flexor tendons, and MN are demonstrated. **(Fig. 5.12)** Attention should be paid to possible anomalous muscles in the carpal tunnel. The landmarks for the distal carpal tunnel are the trapezium tubercle (radial) and hamate hook (ulnar) **(Fig. 5.13)**. Adjustment of the orientation of the probe or slight flexion of the wrist can help to optimize imaging.

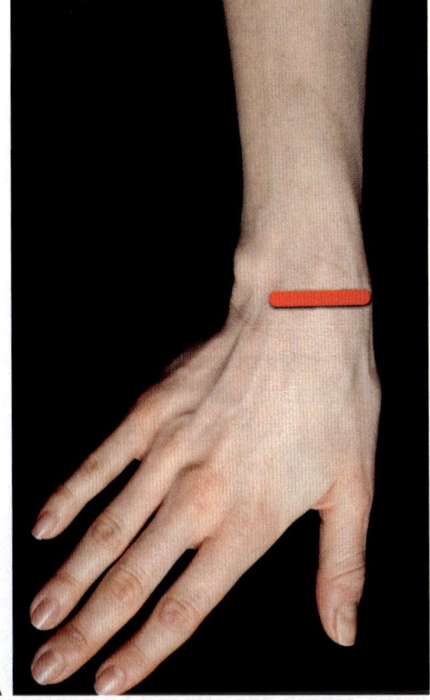

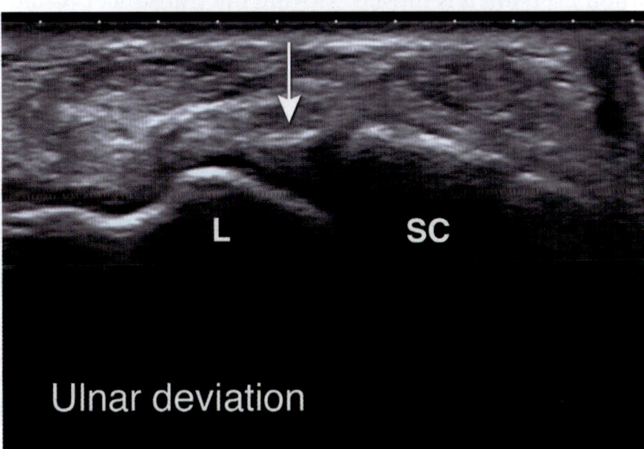

Figure 5.11. Scapholunate Ligament. **A:** Hand pronated and in ulnar deviation. **B:** Moving the transducer distally from Lister's tubercle shows the scapholunate ligament as a thin hyperechoic structure (*arrow*) running between the scaphoid (*SC*) and the lunate (*L*).

The MN is identified in the carpal tunnel in the transverse plane by rocking the transducer back and forward. As transducer angulation alters, the tendons change between hypoechoic and hyperechoic due to anisotropy, whereas the MN does not, or at least not to the same degree. On longitudinal scans, the flexor tendons show quite long excursions on finger flexion/extension, whereas the MN has a shorter excursion. Another way to identify the MN is to scan transversely in the mid-forearm and demonstrate the nerve between the muscle bellies of FDS and FDP, then trace the nerve distally to the carpal tunnel. The cross-sectional area (CSA) of the MN can be calculated proximal to and in the carpal tunnel (see section on carpal tunnel syndrome).[5] As it runs distally through

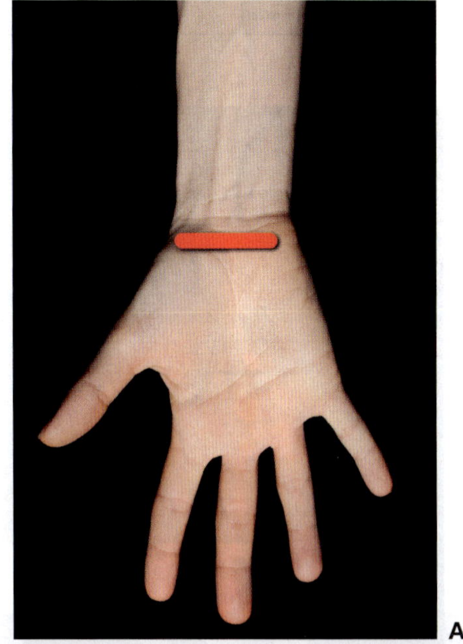

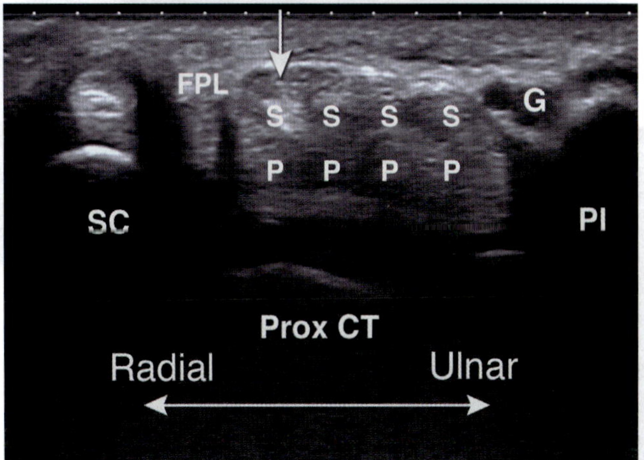

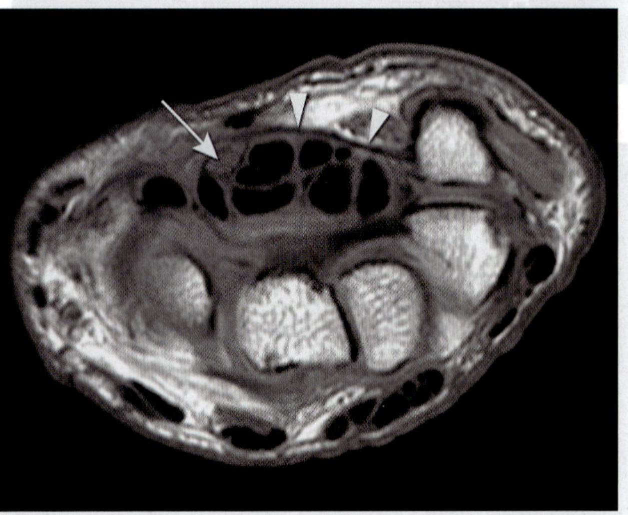

Figure 5.12. Proximal carpal tunnel. **A:** Hand supinated. **B:** Axial ultrasound of the proximal carpal tunnel (*CT*): the bony landmarks are the scaphoid (*SC*) and pisiform (*PI*). Arrow, median nerve and nine tendons run in the carpal tunnel: four tendons of flexor digitorum superficialis (*S*), four tendons of flexor digitorum profundus (*P*), and the flexor pollicis longus (*FPL*) radially. Note Guyon's canal (*G*). **C:** Axial T1-weighted image of the proximal carpal tunnel. The retinaculum (*arrowheads*) is the roof of the carpal tunnel. The median nerve (*arrow*) lies immediately deep to the flexor retinaculum.

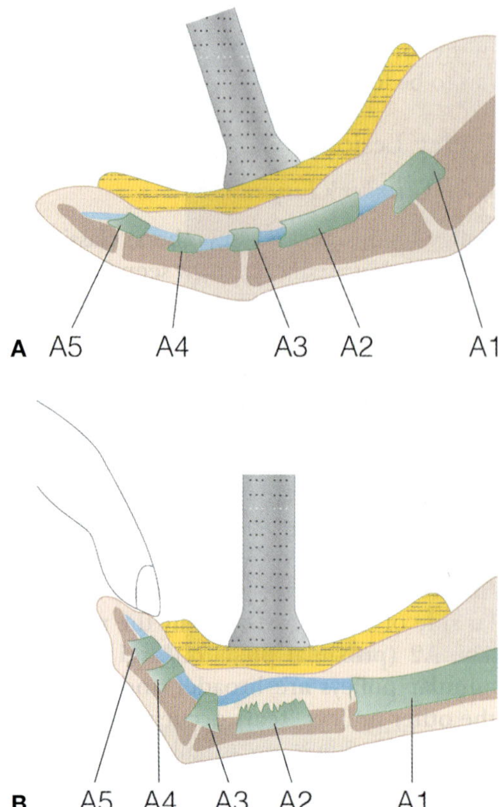

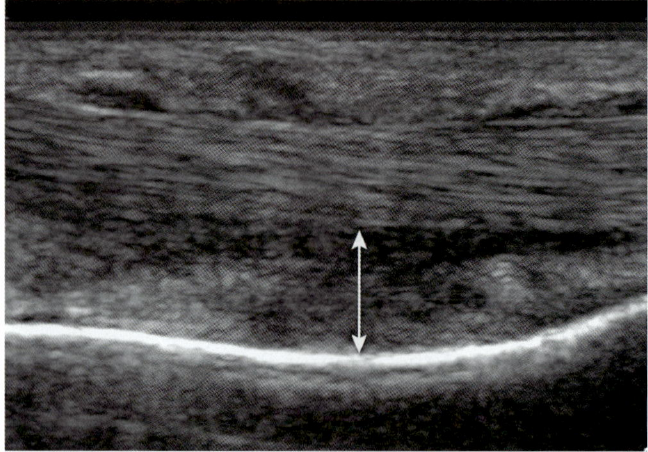

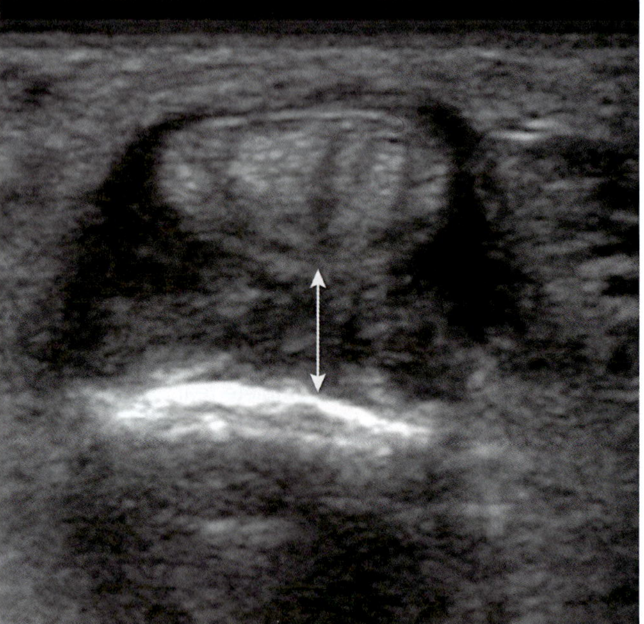

Figure 5.29.   A2 pulley tear. **A, B:** Drawing of dynamic imaging of the annular pulleys. The transducer is placed longitudinally on the finger at rest (**A**) and with forced flexion against the tip of the examiner's finger (**B**). The A2 pulley demonstrates bowstringing, consistent with a complete tear. (**A, B:** Adapted with permission from Klauser A, Frauscher F, Bodner G, et al. Finger pulley injuries in extreme rock climbers: depiction with dynamic US. *Radiology*. 2002;222(3): 755–761.) Acute A2 pulley tear longitudinal (**C**) and axial (**D**) images show the increased distance between the flexor tendon and the proximal phalanx. (**C, D:** Courtesy: Dr **Carlo Martinoli**. Associate Professor of Radiology. University of **Genoa, Italy**.)

without surgery,[43] although reconstruction of isolated A2 or A4 pulley tears is performed in selected cases.[3,44] Other patients are treated conservatively.

Trigger Finger

Trigger finger is transient locking of the finger in flexion, followed by a painful snapping sensation during extension. It is a clinical diagnosis. Most cases are idiopathic, but activities requiring repetitive flexion and extension may lead to chronic, stenosing tenosynovitis with secondary thickening of the A1 pulley. The incidence of triggering is increased in patients with diabetes mellitus, RA, gout, amyloid, and acromegaly.[45] Ultrasound shows a thick, hypoechoic A1 pulley constricting the tendon sheath and may show hypervascularization. Tendinosis and tenosynovitis may be observed.[46] Dynamic ultrasound performed in the long axis at the level of the metacarpal

joint during flexion and extension of the finger may show the tendon "blocking" at the A1 pulley, followed by sudden release. Comparison with adjacent fingers can help. Treatment is often corticosteroid injection near the level of the A1 pulley or in the tendon sheath[46,47] (**Fig. 5.30**) and can be performed under ultrasound guidance. Failed conservative management may require surgical release.[48] Ultrasound-guided release using a bent 19 or 25 G hypodermic needle has been described.[49]

LIGAMENTS

Ligaments of the wrist can be divided into extrinsic, that is, radiocarpal and ulnocarpal, and intrinsic, that is, intercarpal and involved in carpal stability.

The SLL and LTL are important stabilizers of the wrist. They have volar and dorsal segments and a central segment, which is also known as the proximal or

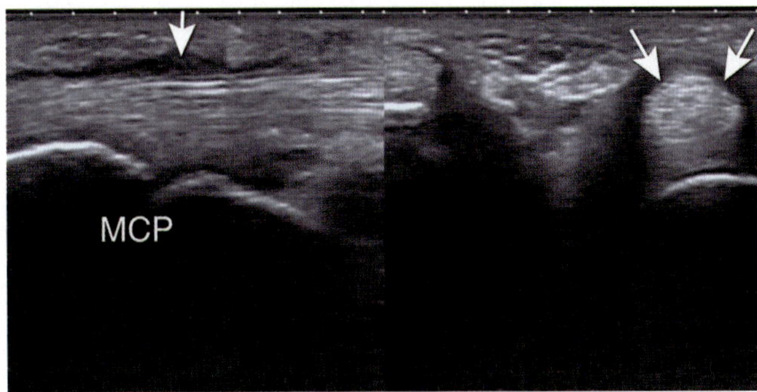

Figure 5.30. Trigger finger. Longitudinal and axial scans showing thickening (*arrows*) of the A1 pulley, resulting in triggering.

membranous component. The site and extent of a tear may be used to differentiate between traumatic (peripheral) and degenerate (central) tears.[50] Tears of the dorsal segment of the SLL alter the normal relationship between the scaphoid and the lunate and may result in dynamic scapholunate instability, causing wrist pain and instability with a normal radiograph.[1]

Diagnostic modalities advocated in the diagnosis of ligament tears include radiography in ulnar and radial deviation, arthrography, scintigraphy, and CT and MRI with and without arthrography.[51,52] In cadaver wrists, CT arthrography and MR imaging are almost equally accurate in depicting palmar and central segment tears, whereas CT arthrography is superior to MR imaging in detecting dorsal segment tears.[53] The diagnostic performance of MR varies considerably, and the sensitivity for SLL tears is consistently better than that for LTL tears.[54]

Ultrasound studies focus on the SLL. The dorsal aspect of the SLL can be depicted as a thin hyperechoic structure **(Fig. 5.11)**,[55,56] completely or partially visible in 78% of normal wrists. Its detection following injury excludes scapholunate dissociation **(Fig. 5.31)**, but the

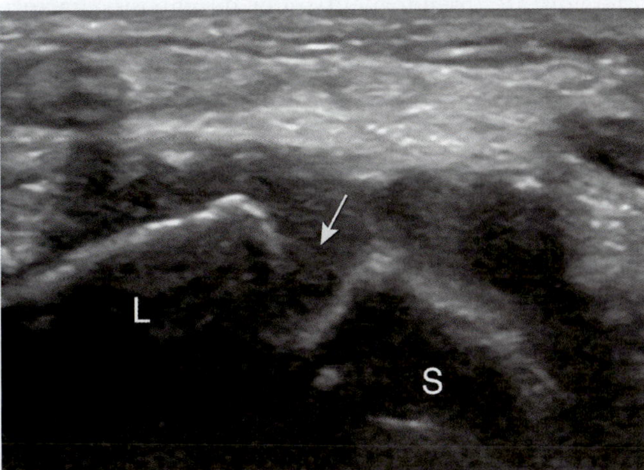

Figure 5.31. Scapholunate ligament tear. Axial ultrasound image shows an SL ligament tear with hematoma. (Courtesy: Dr. Eugene McNally, Consultant Musculoskeletal Radiologist at the Nuffield Orthopaedic Centre & University of Oxford.)

absence of a visible SLL does not necessarily indicate injury.[55] There is considerable variation in scapholunate interval widths on sonography and an unpredictable response with stress testing.

In spite of this, ultrasound distinguishes between normal and abnormal or possibly abnormal wrists.[57] Comparison with tricompartmental arthrography shows that ultrasound accurately detects SLL tears, but misses many LTL and TFCC tears.[58]

The introduction of a new generation of ultrasound machines with advanced probes and software and increased spatial resolution has improved visualization of the extrinsic and intrinsic carpal ligaments[59,60] as thin fibrillar hyperechoic structures. Dynamic examination in flexion and extension may be useful,[60] but the radioscapholunate and UCL of the wrist are not usually seen. A standardized protocol has been proposed for evaluating the intrinsic and extrinsic wrist ligament and the TFC as a screening tool,[2] but as the imaging of chronic wrist pain wrist includes assessment of the TFCC, hyaline cartilage, ligaments, tendons, and bones, ultrasound can only be used as part of the diagnostic work-up and the role of ultrasound remains to be determined.

Triangular Fibrocartilage Complex

The TFC is a triangular structure of homogeneous hyperechogenicity on transverse and oblique sagittal scans at the level of the distal radioulnar joint, and is normally thicker than 2.5 mm on both transverse and oblique sagittal sections. A tear appears as a hypoechoic region or as thinning of the TFC (<2.5 mm) on either transverse or oblique sagittal sections.[61]

Ultrasound[62] shows a degree of correlation with MRI and arthroscopy for TFCC tears, but is not sufficiently accurate for clinical practice.[63,64]

MR arthrography with injection of contrast into the distal radioulnar joint is recommended for evaluation of the TFCC. Clinically meaningful ulnar-sided peripheral tears are otherwise hard to diagnose.[54] Multi Detector Computed Tomography (MDCT) arthrography may also be used.[65]

Ulnar wrist pain has a large differential diagnosis including ECU tendinitis **(Fig. 5.32)**, FCU tendinitis, pisotriquetral arthritis, TFCC lesions, ulnar impaction, LT instability, and distal radioulnar joint instability.[66]

Ulnar Collateral Ligament Tears of the Thumb and Stener Lesion

Acute injury of the UCL of the MCP joint of the thumb, "gamekeeper's thumb," or "skier's thumb" is due to valgus stress (hyperabduction) and hyperextension. Acute thumb pain after trauma requires prompt evaluation of structural integrity to avoid long-term morbidity from instability, chronic pain, and osteoarthritis.[67]Clinical examination is limited by pain and swelling. Imaging of the

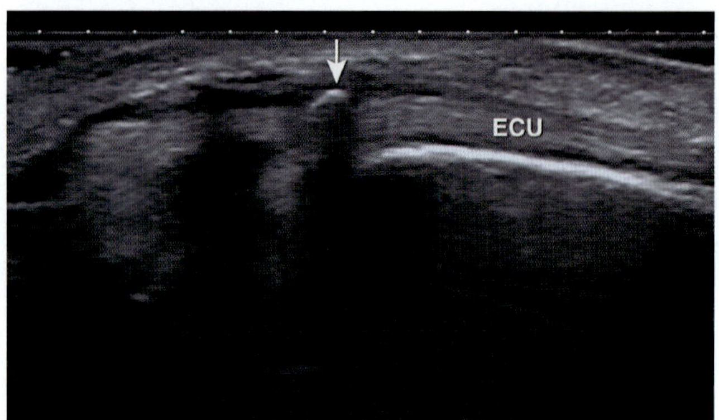

Figure 5.32. Extensor carpi ulnaris calcific tendinitis. Longitudinal image of the ECU tendon at the level of the distal ulna. The patient presented with acute wrist pain. A small calcific deposit (*arrow*) is present.

thumb is indicated to identify injuries that require surgery, that is, a displaced bone fragment or a Stener lesion.[67,68]

A tear of the UCL usually occurs at its distal insertion at the base of the proximal phalanx. An avulsed bone fragment may be identified on radiographs. "Stress radiographs" are sometimes requested, but are often difficult to interpret and may increase damage. Both ultrasound and MRI offer detailed anatomic information. Ultrasound is easy to perform and is quick **(Fig. 5.18)**.[67]

Ulnar collateral ligament injury is graded into sprain, partial tear, and full thickness tear **(Fig. 5.33A)**. Sprained ligaments appear thickened and hypoechoic owing to edema and hemorrhage. Tears usually occur at the distal insertion and remain deep to the adductor aponeurosis. Ultrasound shows obvious discontinuity in the ligament. Additional findings may include bone avulsion, joint effusion, and volar plate injury.[67] Full-thickness UCL tears are divided[68] into intra-aponeurosis tears, when the ligament remains deep to the adductor aponeurosis, and extra-aponeurosis tears, when the displaced proximal fragment of the torn ligament is retracted and trapped superficial to the aponeurosis, the so-called Stener lesion **(Figs. 5.33B, and 5.34)**. Ultrasound of a Stener lesion shows the hypoechoic mass of torn and retracted proximal ligament superficial to the adductor aponeurosis at the level of the metacarpal head. The torn ligament cannot return to its normal position and the two torn ends of the ligament are not in contact; therefore, healing is impossible. Surgery is indicated to prevent chronic instability of the joint.[67,69] The diagnosis is more difficult if the injury is more than 1 week old because of reactive changes.

NERVES

Carpal Tunnel Syndrome

Compression of the MN in the carpal tunnel is a clinical diagnosis and confirmed by electrodiagnostic testing

(EDX). Ultrasound is not routinely performed in CTS. A recent meta-analysis confirms that ultrasound-derived CSA measurement of the MN is not an alternative to EDX, but gives complementary results **(Fig. 5.35)**.[70] The diagnostic accuracy of ultrasound is increased by comparing CSA measurements of the MN at the levels of the carpal tunnel and the pronator quadratus muscle.[71]

Color Doppler ultrasound may confirm the severity of CTS by showing intraneural hypervascularity.[72,73]

Ultrasound can identify normal variants such as a persistent median artery (incidence 2% to 4%) and a bifid MN (incidence 3%)[74] and mass lesions including anomalous muscles **(Fig. 5.19)**, ganglion cysts, and tenosynovitis.[75]

Steroid injections into the carpal tunnel can be performed under ultrasound guidance and produce short-term benefits compared with placebo, oral steroids, anti-inflammatories, and splinting.[76]

Surgical decompression results in decreased MN caliber within 2 weeks of surgery,[77] although EDX studies take much longer to normalize. Surgery is associated with a greater decrease in MN CSA than nonsurgical treatment. Smaller postoperative CSAs may be associated with better clinical outcomes.[78]

Guyon's Canal

There is a high prevalence of anomalous muscles in Guyon's canal (see Normal anatomy: anomalous muscles), and if the AADM muscle is not significantly thicker than 1.7 mm,[6] alternative causes of ulnar nerve compression should be sought. A ganglion cyst is the most frequent cause. Ultrasound shows a well-defined anechoic/hypoechoic mass.[79] The pedicle, which is often difficult to identify, originates from the joints between the hamate and triquetrum or between the pisiform and triquetrum. Other causes of compression are neuritis, ulnar artery disease (pseudoaneurysm or thrombosis), fracture (hook of hamate), or nerve sheath tumor. At the level of the hook of the hamate, the deep branch of the ulnar nerve and the ulnar artery may be injured by compression against the hook owing to single or repeated episodes of trauma, often occupational, causing hypothenar hammer syndrome. Intimal damage causes ulnar artery thrombosis or pseudoaneurysm. In thrombosis, the artery is increased in size, filled with echogenic thrombus, and shows no flow on Doppler. With pseudoaneurysm, the artery is dilated and shows swirling, abnormal flow on Doppler.[80]

Radial Nerve

The radial nerve at the wrist can become inflamed, for example, by a tight watch strap or wrist band, as it crosses the first extensor compartment to reach the dorsal aspect of the wrist. This Wartenberg syndrome has to be differentiated from de Quervain tenosynovitis and

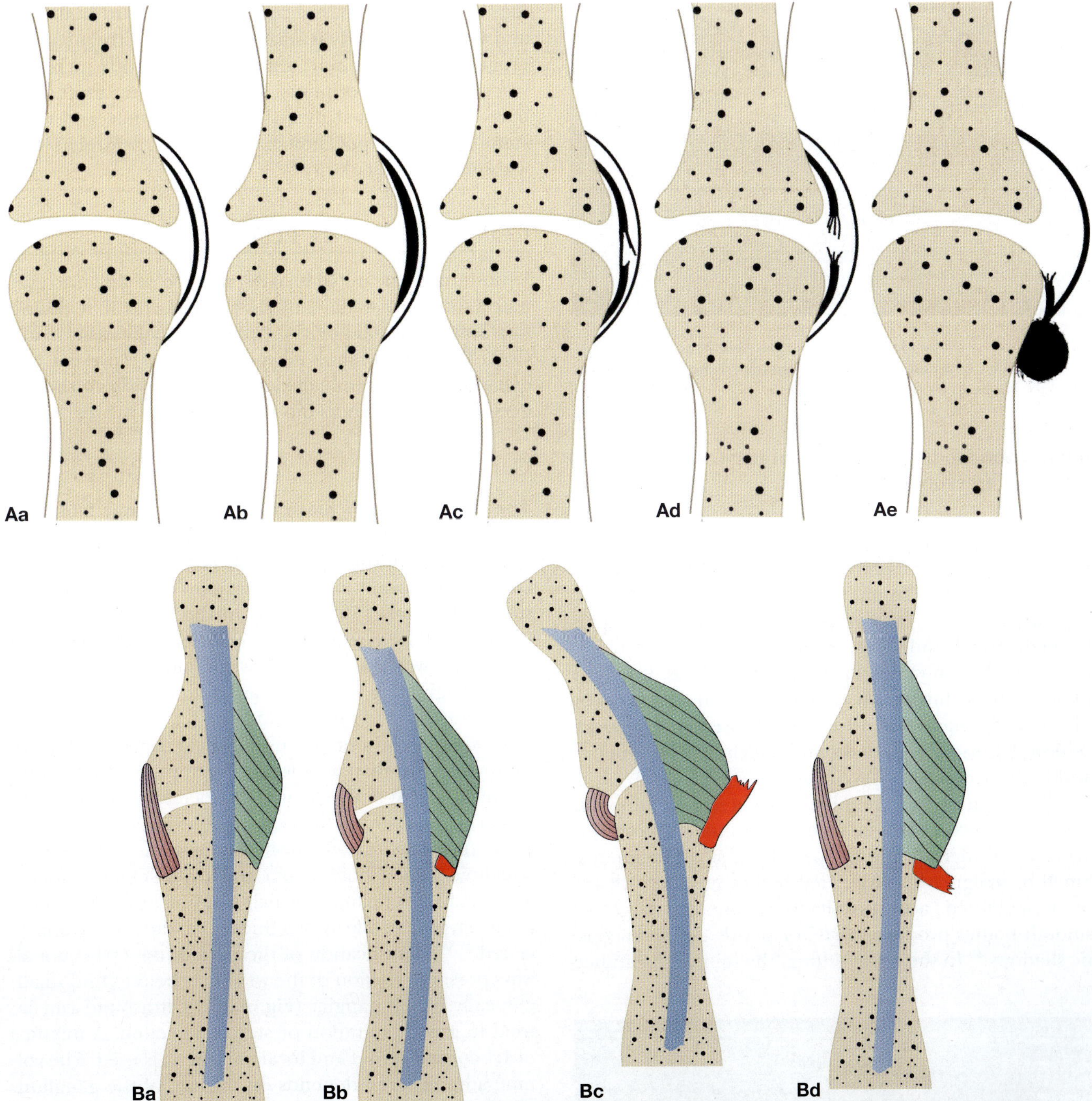

Figure 5.33. Tears of the UCL of the thumb. **A:** Drawing showing UCL pathology of the thumb. **a.** normal appearance, **b.** sprain, **c.** partial-thickness tear, **d.** full-thickness tear, and **e.** Stener lesion. The adductor aponeurosis remains intact in all grades of UCL injury. In a Stener lesion, the aponeurosis becomes interposed between the proximally retracted UCL and its distal insertion. (Drawings adapted with permission from Ebrahim FS, De Maeseneer M, Jager T, et al. ultrasound diagnosis of UCL tears of the thumb and Stener lesions: technique, pattern-based approach, and differential diagnosis. *Radiographics.* 2006;26(4):1007–1020.). **B:** Mechanism of a Stener lesion. **a.** The normal UCL is covered by the adductor aponeurosis (*green*). **b.** In abduction, the ligament (*red*) is torn distally, deep to the aponeurosis. **c.** In extreme abduction, the torn ligament slips superficial to the aponeurosis. **d.** With the joint back in the neutral position, the torn ligament remains trapped superficial to the adductor aponeurosis. (Adapted with permission from Shinohara T, Horii E, Majima M, et al. Sonographic diagnosis of acute injuries of the ulnar collateral ligament of the metacarpophalangeal joint of the thumb. *J Clin Ultrasound.* 2007;35(2):73–77.)

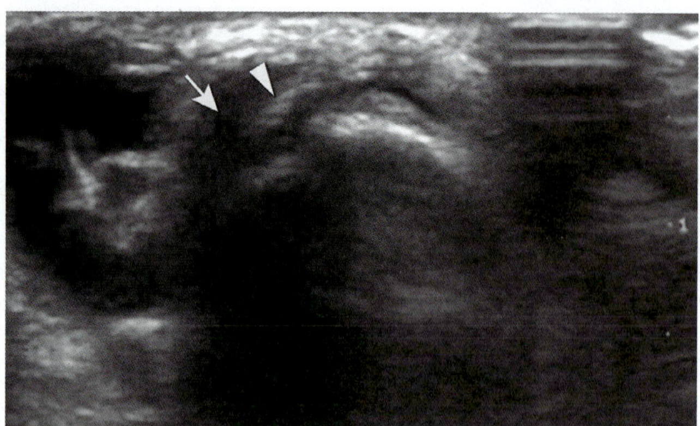

Figure 5.34. Stener lesion. A hypoechoic soft tissue mass (*arrow*) of retracted UCL lies superficial to the thin hyperechoic band of the adductor aponeurosis (*arrowhead*).

intersection syndrome. The radial nerve can also be injured by intravenous cannulation.

FOREIGN BODIES

Foreign bodies are frequently encountered in the hand and wrist. Initial radiographs should always be performed. Metal and glass, even lead-free glass, are radiopaque.[81] Non-radiopaque bodies such as wood or plastic can be missed on radiographs, but detected by ultrasound, which also provides exact preoperative localization. Ultrasound-guided removal can be performed,[82] and high success rates have been reported.[83]

All foreign bodies are initially hyperechoic, although wood may become less echogenic over time.[84] Posterior artifacts aid identification, especially of small fragments. Small or irregularly marginated bodies produce "clean" or well-defined acoustic shadows, whereas large or smooth bodies produce "dirty" or poorly defined acoustic shadows.[85] In the acute setting, the initial appearance

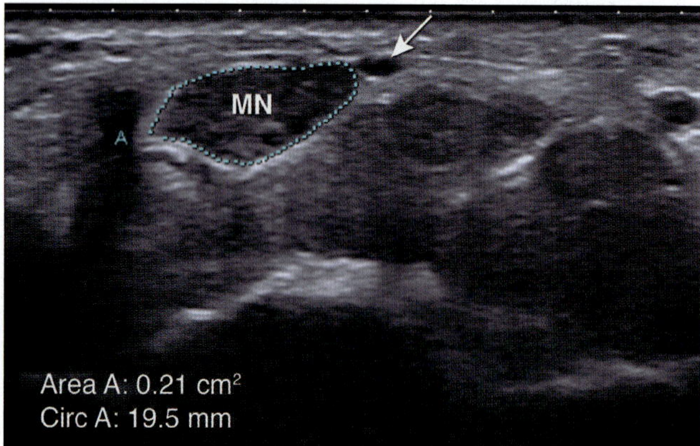

Figure 5.35. Swollen median nerve (*MN*). Swollen MN in a patient with CTS. The cross-sectional area of the MN is 21 mm², which is greater than the upper limit of the normal (10 mm²). There is a persistent median artery (*arrow*).

may be a localized mass secondary to infection or abscess, and the foreign body is surrounded by an irregular, heterogenous, hypoechoic fluid collection with increased vascularity at the periphery. In chronic cases, a soft tissue mass may be caused by a sterile granuloma, and ultrasound shows a hypoechoic halo around the foreign body without hypervascularity.[24,86]

COMMON HAND TUMORS

Ultrasound is the initial imaging method of choice to evaluate a soft tissue swelling of the hand or wrist. The distinction between a solid or cystic mass is usually easily made. Color Doppler will show if hypervascularity is present, and dynamic imaging with flexion and extension of the fingers shows the relationship of the lesion to the tendon.

Ganglia

The most common masses of the wrist and hand are ganglia. The cyst is filled with thick viscous fluid and surrounded by a fibrous capsule. There is no synovial lining. Ganglia are usually attached to a joint capsule or tendon sheath.[24,87] Most (70%) occur in the dorsal wrist[87] and are attached by a pedicle of variable length to a damaged SLL. Volar wrist ganglia are less common and located radially, originating from the scaphoradial or scaphotrapezial joints, close to the radial artery.

Cysts at flexor tendons, usually near the A1 pulley, are more common than at extensor tendons.[24,86] Ultrasound often shows well-demarcated hypoechoic masses, with posterior acoustic enhancement, but appearances vary depending on size and chronicity. Larger cysts tend to be anechoic/hypoechoic. Septa and hyperechoic contents are seen in older ganglia, which may not appear obviously cystic. Hypervascularity of a thickened wall may be appreciated.[87,88] Identification of the neck of the cyst is not always possible. Flexion of the wrist may help to find small, clinically occult ganglia (**Fig. 5.36**). Ultrasound can be used to guide aspiration or steroid injection. A mixture of 1:1 corticosteroid and local anesthetic is used. The volume administered depends on the size of the ganglion. The long-term results of aspiration/injection are identical to those of nonintervention.[89]

> **Tip:**
> In assessing the vascularity of a soft tissue mass, do not push too hard or the vessels may be effaced. A large amount of gel is helpful.

Giant Cell Tumor of Tendon Sheath

Also called nodular tenosynovitis, it is histologically identical to pigmented villonodular synovitis (PVNS). Giant cell tumor of tendon sheath (GCTTS) is the most

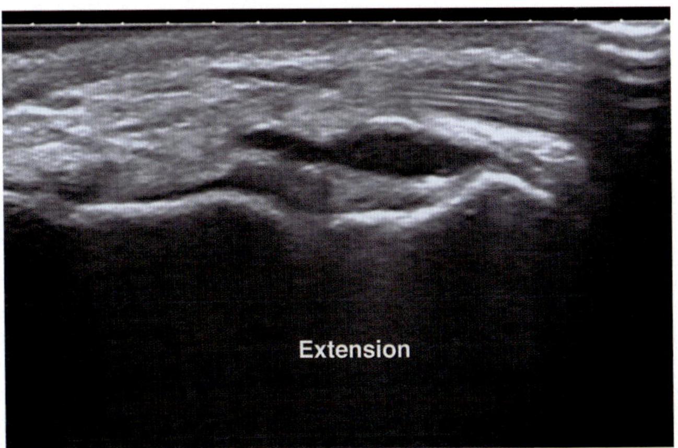

Figure 5.36. Ganglion cyst. Longitudinal image of the dorsal wrist in extension shows a ganglion deep to the extensor tendon. Dynamic imaging can help to identify a clinically occult ganglion cyst.

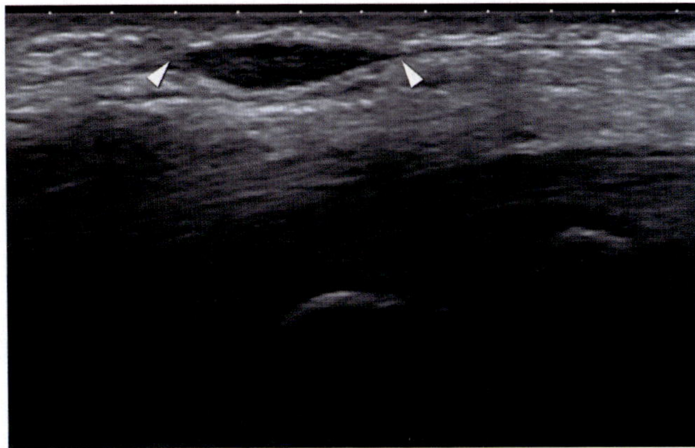

Figure 5.37. Peripheral nerve sheath tumor. Longitudinal image of the volar wrist shows an oval hypoechoic mass in direct continuity with the cutaneous branch (*arrowheads*) of the MN.

common soft tissue tumor of the hand and wrist, and is usually seen on the volar aspect of the distal fingers.[90] Synovial proliferation with dense collagen and hemosiderin deposition is characteristic. Giant cell tumor of tendon sheath arises from the tendon sheath in close contact with the tendon and may even encase the tendon. Uncommonly, satellite lesions are seen adjacent to the primary lesion, and there may be diffuse involvement of the tendon sheath. The origin of the mass on the tendon sheath can be confirmed by flexing and extending the finger, showing that the tumor is not moving with the tendon.

Ultrasound shows a well-defined, hypoechoic mass, predominantly homogeneous, although heterogeneous lesions are described.[91] Color or power Doppler imaging shows internal vascularity, peripheral or central, or a combination of the two. The ultrasound appearance is not diagnostic, but the proximity to the tendon sheath is highly suggestive of GCTTS.[24] Progressive enlargement can cause bone erosions, predominantly at or distal to the MCP joints, or even present as an intrinsic osseous lesion.[92] MRI[92,93] shows low to intermediate signal intensity on both T1- and T2-weighted images, with a variable degree of heterogeneity, an unusual appearance in other extra-articular soft tissue masses and suggestive of the diagnosis, especially in the hand or foot. Enhancement is seen after intravenous gadolinium. Gradient echo images characteristically show variable "blooming" or susceptibility artifact due to hemosiderin GCTTS.[93]

Nerve and Nerve Sheath Tumors

Tumors of peripheral nerves are rare in the hand and are usually benign and subcutaneous. Benign lesions include schwannoma and neurofibromas, which can originate from any nerve. Most peripheral nerve sheath tumors are homogeneous, hypoechoic, and show posterior acoustic enhancement. Continuity of a mass with a peripheral nerve suggests the diagnosis **(Fig. 5.37)**.

Careful scanning may be needed to identify the nerve proximally and/or distally as it may be displaced.[17] Internal blood flow on Doppler ultrasound helps to differentiate nerve sheath tumors from avascular ganglion cysts. Ultrasound cannot reliably distinguish neurofibromas from schwannomas.[94,95] A rare neurogenic mass with a predilection for the MN is fibrolipohamartoma, also known as neural fibrolipoma or intraneural lipoma. Its presentation is a sausage-like, fusiform mass at the volar wrist usually before 20 years of age. Histology shows fatty and fibrous components surrounding the nerve fascicles.[96] Ultrasound shows fusiform enlargement of the nerve at the level of the distal radius and carpal tunnel. The hypoechoic, enlarged nerve fascicles are separated by echogenic fat.

Vascular Tumors

Glomus tumors are rare, benign hamartomas that develop from the neuromyoarterial glomus bodies that regulate blood flow in the skin. Up to 75% of all glomus tumors occur in the hand, and approximately 65% of these are in the fingertips, particularly the subungual space. They account for 1% to 4.5% of all hand tumors.[97] Patients present with pain, evoked by pressure or cold exposure. Ultrasound shows a hypoechoic mass, which is highly vascularized, with arteriovenous shunting. Comparison with another finger may be valuable as the subungual area is normally highly vascularized. Erosion of the underlying bone may be present **(Fig. 5.38)**. On MR, most glomus tumors are of intermediate signal intensity on T1-weighted images, hyperintense on T2-weighted images, and show inhomogeneous contrast enhancement. The differential diagnosis includes mucoid cyst and angioma.[98]

Hemangioma can involve any soft tissue, and may be intramuscular, but in the finger is usually located

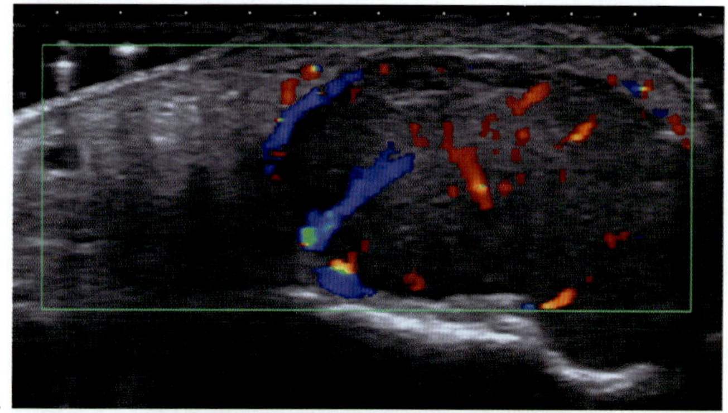

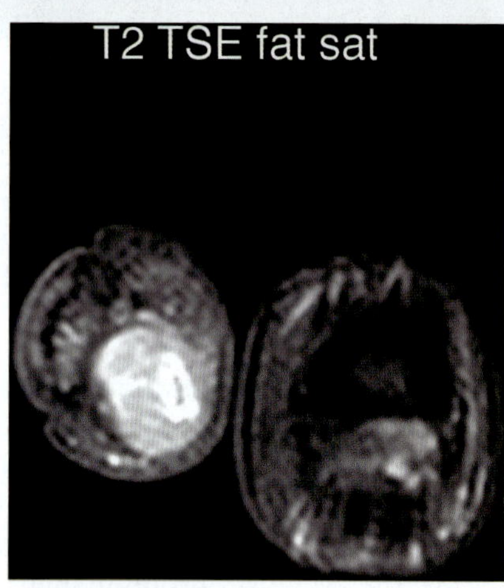

Figure 5.38. Glomus tumor. **A:** Longitudinal color Doppler image showing a hypervascular hypoechoic well-defined soft tissue mass volar to the distal phalanx of the thumb. **B:** Axial fat-suppressed T2-weighted TSE image showing a hyperintense mass. Post-contrast images showed enhancement. The location and appearances are consistent with a glomus tumor, although a subungual position is more common.

in the superficial dermis.[97] Ultrasound usually shows a hypoechoic mass that is inhomogeneous due to hypoechoic vascular channels and hyperechoic fat. Slow flow is typical.[99]

Lipoma

A superficial lipoma presents as a soft, painless, well-delineated, and mobile mass. Its echogenicity is variable and ranges from hypoechoic to anechoic, related to cellular variability.[100,101] Lipomas have an elongated shape, and most are oriented parallel to the skin. In 66% of cases,[100] superficial lipomas are well marginated, and occasionally a distinct echogenic capsule can be defined. The absence of internal vascularization helps to exclude malignancy. Larger and deeper masses are better evaluated with MRI.[24]

Miscellaneous

Accessory muscles **(Fig. 5.19)** and tenosynovitis can present as masses and mimic tumors or compress nerves.

If ultrasound fails to provide an answer, MRI is an accurate problem solver for evaluating mass lesions, but is relatively infrequently needed.[96]

ACKNOWLEDGMENT

The authors acknowledge the help of Maria Kelemouridou, MD, Radiology Department, A.H.E.P.A. University Hospital, Thessaloniki, Greece and Gerrit Kracht, Radiology Department, Leiden University Medical Center, The Netherlands.

REFERENCES

1. Taleisnik J. Post-traumatic carpal instability. *Clin Orthop Relat Res.* 1980;(149):73–82.
2. Taljanovic MS, Goldberg MR, Sheppard JE, et al. US of the intrinsic and extrinsic wrist ligaments and triangular fibrocartilage complex—normal anatomy and imaging technique. *Radiographics.* 2011;31(1):E44.
3. Bianchi S, Martolini C. Wrist and hand. In: *Ultrasound of the Musculoskeletal System.* Berlin Heidelberg, NY: Springer; 2007:425–548.
4. Netter FH, Woodburne RT, Crelin ES, et al. Upper limb, wrist and hand. In: *Musculoskeletal System, Part 1: Anatomy, Physiology and Metabolic Disorders.* NJ: Ciba-Geigy; 1987:55–73.
5. McNally EG. Upper limb: Anatomy and technique. In: *Practical Musculoskeletal Ultrasound.* Philadelphia, PA: Elsevier Churchill Livingstone; 2005:1–21.
6. Martinoli C, Serafini G, Bianchi S, et al. Ultrasonography of peripheral nerves. *J Peripher Nerv Syst.* 1996;1(3):169–178.
7. Beggs I, Bianchi S, Bueno A, et al. *Musculoskeletal Ultrasound Technical Guidelines: III. Wrist.* Vienna, Austria: European Society of MusculoSkeletal Radiology. Available at http://www.essr.org/html/img/pool/wrist.pdf
8. Timins ME. Muscular anatomic variants of the wrist and hand: findings on MR imaging. *AJR Am J Roentgenol.* 1999;172(5):1397–1401.
9. Harvie P, Patel N, Ostlere SJ. Prevalence and epidemiological variation of anomalous muscles at Guyon's canal. *J Hand Surg Br.* 2004;29(1):26–29.
10. Zeiss J, Guilliam-Haidet L. MR demonstration of anomalous muscles about the volar aspect of the wrist and forearm. *Clin Imaging.* 1996;20(3):219–221.
11. Anderson MW, Benedetti P, Walter J, et al. MR appearance of the extensor digitorum manus brevis muscle: a pseudotumor of the hand. *AJR Am J Roentgenol.* 1995;164(6):1477–1479.
12. Gama C. Extensor digitorum brevis manus: a report on 38 cases and a review of the literature. *J Hand Surg Am.* 1983;8(5, pt 1):578–582.
13. Ogura T, Inoue H, Tanabe G. Anatomic and clinical studies of the extensor digitorum brevis manus. *J Hand Surg Am.* 1987;12(1):100–107.
14. Sanger JR, Krasniak CL, Matloub HS, et al. Diagnosis of an anomalous superficialis muscle in the palm by magnetic resonance imaging. *J Hand Surg Am.* 1991;16(1):98–101.
15. Smith RJ. Anomalous muscle belly of the flexor digitorum superficialis causing carpal-tunnel syndrome. Report of a case. *J Bone Joint Surg Am.* 1971;53(6):1215–1216.
16. Touborg-Jensen A. Carpal-tunnel syndrome caused by an abnormal distribution of the lumbrical muscles. Case report. *Scand J Plast Reconstr Surg.* 1970;4(1):72–74.
17. Roberts PH. An anomalous accessory palmaris longus muscle. *Hand.* 1972;4(1):40–41.

18. Polesuk BS, Helms CA. Hypertrophied palmaris longus muscle, a pseudomass of the forearm: MR appearance—case report and review of the literature. *Radiology.* 1998;207(2):361–362.

19. Genc H, Cakit BD, Tuncbilek I, et al. Ultrasonographic evaluation of tendons and enthesal sites in rheumatoid arthritis: comparison with ankylosing spondylitis and healthy subjects. *Clin Rheumatol.* 2005;24(3):272–277.

20. Backhaus M. Ultrasound and structural changes in inflammatory arthritis: synovitis and tenosynovitis. *Ann N Y Acad Sci.* 2009;1154:139–151.

21. Boutry N, Morel M, Flipo RM, et al. Early rheumatoid arthritis: a review of MRI and sonographic findings. *AJR Am J Roentgenol.* 2007;189(6):1502–1509.

22. Sommer OJ, Kladosek A, Weiler V, et al. Rheumatoid arthritis: a practical guide to state-of-the-art imaging, image interpretation, and clinical implications. *Radiographics.* 2005;25(2):381–398.

23. Koch AE. Review: angiogenesis: implications for rheumatoid arthritis. *Arthritis Rheum.* 1998;41(6):951–962.

24. Bianchi S, Della Santa D, Glauser T, et al. Sonography of masses of the wrist and hand. *AJR Am J Roentgenol.* 2008;191(6):1767–1775.

25. Filippucci E, Gabba A, Di Geso L, et al. Hand tendon involvement in rheumatoid arthritis: an ultrasound study. *Semin Arthritis Rheum.* 2012;41(6):752–760.

26. Kotob H, Kamel M. Identification and prevalence of rheumatoid nodules in the finger tendons using high frequency ultrasonography. *J Rheumatol.* 1999;26(6):1264–1268.

27. Wick MC, Weiss RJ, Arora R, et al. Enthesiopathy of the flexor carpi ulnaris at the pisiform: findings of high-frequency sonography. *Eur J Radiol.* 2011;77(2):240–244.

28. Nagaoka M, Matsuzaki H, Suzuki T. Ultrasonographic examination of de Quervain's disease. *J Orthop Sci.* 2000;5(2):96–99.

29. Jeyapalan K, Choudhary S. Ultrasound-guided injection of triamcinolone and bupivacaine in the management of De Quervain's disease. *Skeletal Radiol.* 2009;38(11):1099–1103.

30. Chhabra A, Soldatos T, Thawait GK, et al. Current perspectives on the advantages of 3-T MR imaging of the wrist. *Radiographics.* 2012;32(3):879–896.

31. Owers KL, Lee J, Khan N, et al. Ultrasound changes in the extensor pollicis longus tendon following fractures of the distal radius—a preliminary report. *J Hand Surg Eur Vol.* 2007;32(4):467–471.

32. Santiago FR, Plazas PG, Fernández JM. Sonography findings in tears of the extensor pollicis longus tendon and correlation with CT, MRI, and surgical findings. *Eur J Radiol.* 2008;66(1):112–116.

33. Kleinbaum Y, Heyman Z, Ganel A, et al. Sonographic imaging of mallet finger. *Ultraschall Med.* 2005;26(3):223–226.

34. Lopez-Ben R, Lee DH, Nicolodi DJ. Boxer knuckle (injury of the extensor hood with extensor tendon subluxation): diagnosis with dynamic US—report of three cases. *Radiology.* 2003;228(3):642–646.

35. Jeyapalan K, Bisson MA, Dias JJ, et al. The role of ultrasound in the management of flexor tendon injuries. *J Hand Surg Eur Vol.* 2008;33(4):430–434.

36. de Gautard G, de Gautard R, Celi J, et al. Sonography of Jersey finger. *J Ultrasound Med.* 2009;28(3):389–392.

37. Al-Qattan MM. Type 5 avulsion of the insertion of the flexor digitorum profundus tendon. *J Hand Surg Br.* 2001;26(5):427–431.

38. Klauser A, Frauscher F, Bodner G, et al. Finger pulley injuries in extreme rock climbers: depiction with dynamic US. *Radiology.* 2002;222(3):755–761.

39. Martinoli C, Bianchi S, Nebiolo M, et al. Sonographic evaluation of digital annular pulley tears. *Skeletal Radiol.* 2000;29(7):387–391.

40. Hauger O, Chung CB, Lektrakul N, et al. Pulley system in the fingers: normal anatomy and simulated lesions in cadavers at MR imaging, CT, and US with and without contrast material distention of the tendon sheath. *Radiology.* 2000;217(1):201–212.

41. Le Viet D, Rousselin B, Roulot E, et al. Diagnosis of digital pulley rupture by computed tomography. *J Hand Surg Am.* 1996;21(2):245–248.

42. Parellada JA, Balkissoon AR, Hayes CW, et al. Bowstring injury of the flexor tendon pulley system: MR imaging. *AJR Am J Roentgenol.* 1996;167(2):347–349.

43. Gabl M, Rangger C, Lutz M, et al. Disruption of the finger flexor pulley system in elite rock climbers. *Am J Sports Med.* 1998;26(5):651–655.

44. Bianchi S, Martinoli C, Abdelwahab IF. High-frequency ultrasound examination of the wrist and hand. *Skeletal Radiol.* 1999;28(3):121–129.

45. Tagliafico A, Resmini E, van Holsbeeck MT, et al. Sonographic depiction of trigger fingers in acromegaly. *J Ultrasound Med.* 2009;28(11):1441–1446.

46. Guerini H, Pessis E, Theumann N, et al. Sonographic appearance of trigger fingers. *J Ultrasound Med.* 2008;27(10):1407–1413.

47. Peters-Veluthamaningal C, van der Windt DA, Winters JC, et al. Corticosteroid injection for trigger finger in adults. *Cochrane Database Syst Rev.* 2009;21(1):CD005617.

48. Benson LS, Ptaszek AJ. Injection versus surgery in the treatment of trigger finger. *J Hand Surg Am.* 1997;22(1):138–144.

49. Rajeswaran G, Lee JC, Eckersley R, et al. Ultrasound-guided percutaneous release of the annular pulley in trigger digit. *Eur Radiol.* 2009;19(9):2232–2237.

50. Wright TW, Del Charco M, Wheeler D. Incidence of ligament lesions and associated degenerative changes in the elderly wrist. *J Hand Surg Am.* 1994;19(2):313–318.

51. Schweitzer ME, Brahme SK, Hodler J, et al. Chronic wrist pain: spin-echo and short tau inversion recovery MR imaging and conventional and MR arthrography. *Radiology.* 1992;182(1):205–211.

52. Timins ME, Jahnke JP, Krah SF, et al. MR imaging of the major carpal stabilizing ligaments: normal anatomy and clinical examples. *Radiographics.* 1995;15(3):575–587.

53. Schmid MR, Schertler T, Pfirrmann CW, et al. Interosseous ligament tears of the wrist: comparison of multidetector row CT arthrography and MR imaging. *Radiology.* 2005;237(3):1008–1013.

54. Zanetti M, Saupe N, Nagy L. Role of MR imaging in chronic wrist pain. *Eur Radiol.* 2007;17(4):927–938.

55. Griffith JF, Chan DP, Ho PC, et al. Sonography of the normal scapholunate ligament and scapholunate joint space. *J Clin Ultrasound.* 2001;29(4):223–229.

56. Jacobson JA, Oh E, Propeck T, et al. Sonography of the scapholunate ligament in four cadaveric wrists: correlation with MR arthrography and anatomy. *AJR Am J Roentgenol.* 2002;179(2):523–527.

57. Dao KD, Solomon DJ, Shin AY, et al. The efficacy of ultrasound in the evaluation of dynamic scapholunate ligamentous instability. *J Bone Joint Surg Am.* 2004;86-A(7):1473–1478.

58. Finlay K, Lee R, Friedman L. Ultrasound of intrinsic wrist ligament and triangular fibrocartilage injuries. *Skeletal Radiol.* 2004;33(2):85–90.

59. Boutry N, Lapegue F, Masi L, et al. Ultrasonographic evaluation of normal extrinsic and intrinsic carpal ligaments: preliminary experience. *Skeletal Radiol.* 2005;34(9):513–521.

60. Lacelli F, Muda A, Sconfienza LM, et al. High-resolution ultrasound anatomy of extrinsic carpal ligaments [in English, Italian]. *Radiol Med.* 2008;113(4):504–516.

61. Chiou HJ, Chang CY, Chou YH, et al. Triangular fibrocartilage of wrist: presentation on high resolution ultrasonography. *J Ultrasound Med.* 1998;17(1):41–48.

62. Keogh CF, Wong AD, Wells NJ, et al. High-resolution sonography of the triangular fibrocartilage: initial experience and correlation with MRI and arthroscopic findings. *AJR Am J Roentgenol.* 2004;182(2):333–336.

63. Heuck A, Bonél H, Stäbler A, et al. Imaging in sports medicine: hand and wrist. *Eur J Radiol.* 1997;26(1):2–15.

64. Klauser AS, Tagliafico A, Allen GM, et al. Clinical indications for musculoskeletal ultrasound: a Delphi-based consensus paper of the European Society of Musculoskeletal Radiology. *Eur Radiol.* 2012;22(5):1140–1148.

65. Moser T, Khoury V, Harris PG, et al. MDCT arthrography or MR arthrography for imaging the wrist joint? *Semin Musculoskelet Radiol.* 2009;13(1):39–54.

66. Watanabe A, Souza F, Vezeridis PS, et al. Ulnar-sided wrist pain. II. Clinical imaging and treatment. *Skeletal Radiol.* 2010;39(9):837–857.

67. Ebrahim FS, De Maeseneer M, Jager T, et al. US diagnosis of UCL tears of the thumb and Stener lesions: technique, pattern-based approach, and differential diagnosis. *Radiographics.* 2006;26(4):1007–1020.

68. Shinohara T, Horii E, Majima M, et al. Sonographic diagnosis of acute injuries of the ulnar collateral ligament of the metacarpophalangeal joint of the thumb. *J Clin Ultrasound.* 2007;35(2):73–77.

69. Noszian IM, Dinkhauser LM, Orthner E, et al. Ulnar collateral ligament: differentiation of displaced and nondisplaced tears with US. *Radiology.* 1995;194(1):61–63.

70. Descatha A, Huard L, Aubert F, et al. Meta-analysis on the performance of sonography for the diagnosis of carpal tunnel syndrome. *Semin Arthritis Rheum.* 2012;41(6):914–922.

71. Klauser AS, Halpern EJ, Faschingbauer R, et al. Bifid median nerve in carpal tunnel syndrome: assessment with US cross-sectional area measurement. *Radiology.* 2011;259(3):808–815.

72. Ghasemi-Esfe AR, Khalilzadeh O, Vaziri-Bozorg SM, et al. Color and power Doppler US for diagnosing carpal tunnel syndrome and determining its severity: a quantitative image processing method. *Radiology.* 2011;261(2):499–506.

73. Wilder-Smith EP, Therimadasamy A, Ghasemi-Esfe AR, et al. Color and power Doppler US for diagnosing Carpal tunnel syndrome and determining its severity. *Radiology.* 2012;262(3):1043–1044; author reply 104.

74. Pfirrmann CW, Zanetti M. Variants, pitfalls, and asymptomatic findings in wrist and hand imaging. *Eur.J.Radiol.* 2005;56(3):286–295.

75. Klauser AS, Halpern EJ, De Zordo T, et al. Carpal tunnel syndrome assessment with US: value of additional cross-sectional area measurements of the median nerve in patients versus healthy volunteers. *Radiology.* 2009;250(1):171–177.

76. Marshall S, Tardif G, Ashworth N. Local corticosteroid injection for carpal tunnel syndrome. *Cochrane Database Syst Rev.* 2007;18(2):CD001554.

77. El-Karabaty H, Heyzel A, Galla TJ, Horch RE, Lücking CH, Glocker FX. The effect of carpal tunnel release on median nerve flattening and nerve conduction. *Electromyogr Clin Neurophysiol* 2005;45(4):223–227.

78. Vögelin E, Nüesch E, Jüni P, et al. Sonographic follow-up of patients with carpal tunnel syndrome undergoing surgical or nonsurgical treatment: prospective cohort study. *J Hand Surg Am.* 2010;35(9):1401–1409.

79. Elias DA, Lax MJ, Anastakis DJ. Musculoskeletal images. Ganglion cyst of Guyon's canal causing ulnar nerve compression. *Can J Surg.* 2001;44(5):331–332.

80. Cooke R, Lawson I. Use of Doppler in the diagnosis of hypothenar hammer syndrome. *Occup Med (Lond).* 2009;59(3):185–190.

81. Felman AH, Fisher MS. The radiographic detection of glass in soft tissue. *Radiology.* 1969;92(7):1529–1531.

82. Horton LK, Jacobson JA, Powell A, et al. Sonography and radiography of soft-tissue foreign bodies. *AJR Am J Roentgenol.* 2001;176(5):1155–1159.

83. Bradley M. Image-guided soft-tissue foreign body extraction—success and pitfalls. *Clin Radiol.* 2012;67(6):531–534.

84. Jacobson JA, Powell A, Craig JG, et al. Wooden foreign bodies in soft tissue: detection at US. *Radiology.* 1998;206(1):45–48.

85. Rubin JM, Adler RS, Bude RO, et al. Clean and dirty shadowing at US: a reappraisal. *Radiology.* 1991;181(1):231–236.

86. Bianchi S, van Aaken J, Glauser T, et al. Screw impingement on the extensor tendons in distal radius fractures treated by volar plating: sonographic appearance. *AJR Am J Roentgenol.* 2008;191(5):W199–W203.

87. Teefey SA, Dahiya N, Middleton WD, et al. Ganglia of the hand and wrist: a sonographic analysis. *AJR Am J Roentgenol.* 2008;191(3):716–720.

88. Wang G, Jacobson JA, Feng FY, et al. Sonography of wrist ganglion cysts: variable and noncystic appearances. *J Ultrasound Med.* 2007;26(10):1323–1328.

89. Breidahl WH, Adler RS. Ultrasound-guided injection of ganglia with coricosteroids. *Skeletal Radiol.* 1996;25(7):635–638.

90. Kransdorf MJ, Murphey MD, Smith SE. Imaging of soft tissue neoplasms in the adult: benign tumors. *Semin Musculoskelet Radiol.* 1999;3(1):21–38.

91. Middleton WD, Patel V, Teefey SA, et al. Giant cell tumors of the tendon sheath: analysis of sonographic findings. *AJR Am J Roentgenol.* 2004;183(2):337–339.

92. De Schepper AM, Hogendoorn PC, Bloem JL. Giant cell tumors of the tendon sheath may present radiologically as intrinsic osseous lesions. *Eur Radiol.* 2007;17(2):499–502.

93. Murphey MD, Rhee JH, Lewis RB, et al. Pigmented villonodular synovitis: radiologic-pathologic correlation. *Radiographics.* 2008;28(5):1493–1518.

94. Bianchi S. Ultrasound of the peripheral nerves. *Joint Bone Spine.* 2008;75(6):643–649.

95. Reynolds DL Jr, Jacobson JA, Inampudi P, et al. Sonographic characteristics of peripheral nerve sheath tumors. *AJR Am J Roentgenol.* 2004;182(3):741–744.

96. Parizel PM, Simoens WA, Matos C, et al. Tumors of peripheral nerves. In: *Imaging of Soft Tissue Tumors.* 2nd ed. Berlin, Heidelberg, NY: Springer; 2006:301–330.

97. Baek HJ, Lee SJ, Cho KH, et al. Subungual tumors: clinicopathologic correlation with US and MR imaging findings. *Radiographics.* 2010;30(6):1621–1636.

98. Drapé JL, Idy-Peretti I, Goettmann S, et al. Subungual glomus tumors: evaluation with MR imaging. *Radiology.* 1995;195(2):507–515.

99. Hwang S, Adler RS. Sonographic evaluation of the musculoskeletal soft tissue masses. *Ultrasound Q.* 2005;21(4):259–270.

100. Fornage BD, Tassin GB. Sonographic appearances of superficial soft tissue lipomas. *J Clin Ultrasound.* 1991;19(4):215–220.

101. Inampudi P, Jacobson JA, Fessell DP, et al. Soft-tissue lipomas: accuracy of sonography in diagnosis with pathologic correlation. *Radiology.* 2004;233(3):763–767.

Adult Hip

Paul Mallinson
Philip Robinson

INTRODUCTION

Advances in sonographic technology and increasing awareness of its capabilities have led to a rapidly expanding role for ultrasound in assessing the adult hip. Ultrasound provides a valuable addition or alternative to other imaging modalities due to its dynamic capabilities, rapid scan times, exquisite soft tissue detail (even in the presence of metal implants), and ability to guide interventional procedures. This chapter describes the anatomy, scanning technique, and pathologies of the adult hip and pelvis. Advantages and limitations of ultrasound when compared with magnetic resonance imaging (MRI) are also discussed.

ANATOMY AND TECHNIQUE

The optimal probe for scanning the hip depends on the depth of the structure being imaged and the size of the patient. High-frequency linear transducers of the order of 17 MHz provide excellent superficial soft tissue detail in smaller patients, but 12 MHz, 9 MHz linear, or even 2 to 5 MHz curvilinear probe may be required for deeper structures in larger patients. Start with the highest frequency and then reduce as required.

Anatomy and scanning techniques are best considered as four quadrants: anterior, posterior, medial, and lateral.

Anterior

The anterior quadrant contains the anterior joint recess, iliopsoas tendon, rectus femoris, sartorius, and tensor fascia lata (TFL). (Examination of groin hernias is covered in the hernia section.) The examination is performed with the patient supine and transverse (TS) and longitudinal (LS) images are obtained **(Fig. 6.1)**. The *anterior joint recess* is evaluated with the probe aligned obliquely along the femoral neck to look for the presence of an effusion or large anterior labral injury in the normally hyperechoic labrum. The hyperechoic iliofemoral ligament can sometimes be seen overlying the anterior capsule **(Fig. 6.2A)**.

The iliopsoas muscle is scanned in true longitudinal and transverse views **(Figs. 6.2 and 6.3)**. It lies superficial to the capsule and lateral to the femoral neurovascular bundle. The hyperechoic iliopsoas tendon lies on the deep and medial aspect of the muscle and inserts distally on the lesser trochanter. The iliopsoas bursa lies between the anterior joint capsule and tendon, but is not seen unless bursitis or fluid are present. Superficial to iliopsoas is sartorius, which can be traced distally from the anterior superior iliac spine (ASIS). Tensor fascia lata is superficial and lateral and also originates from the ASIS and iliac crest **(Fig. 6.3)**. The TFL courses laterally to blend into the anterior aspect of the fascia lata. Superficial and medial to iliopsoas is rectus femoris, which originates from the anterior inferior iliac spine (AIIS). Longitudinal views of these muscles and tendons should be performed when evaluating for tendinopathy and muscle tears.

Posterior and Lateral

For anatomical purposes these two quadrants are considered together. They incorporate the gluteal muscles and tendons. The hamstring origins and sciatic nerve will also be considered here.

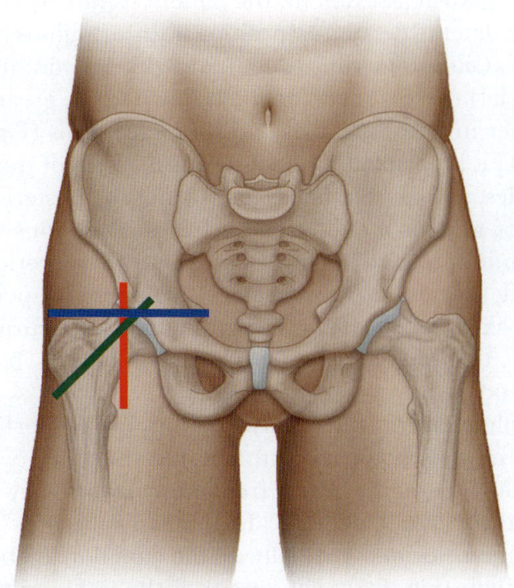

Figure 6.1. Anterior hip probe positions. The three probe positions for imaging the anterior hip are demonstrated by the three colored lines: True LS (*red*), longitudinal femoral neck (*green*), and TS (*blue*).

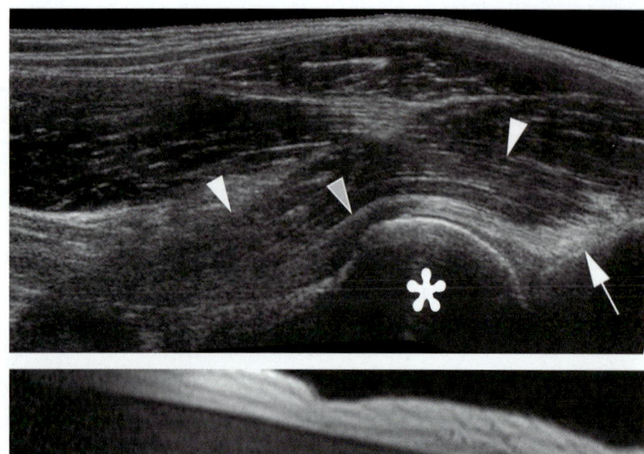

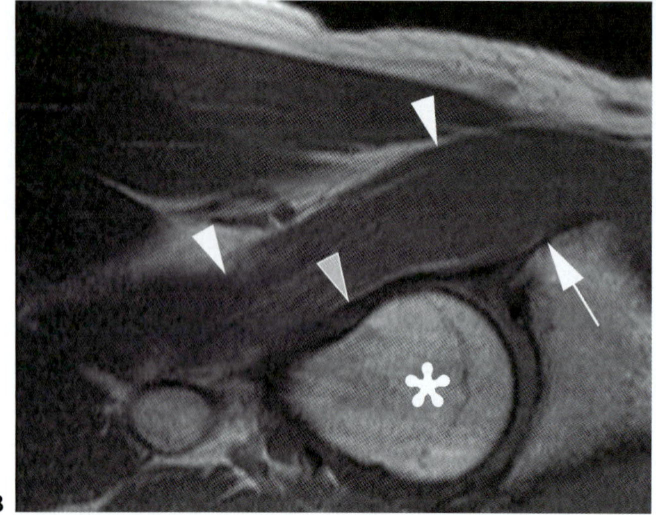

Figure 6.2. Normal LS views of the hip. **A:** Longitudinal sonogram and **B:** Sagittal T1-weighted (T1W) MRI show femoral head (*asterisk*), iliopsoas (*white arrowheads*), normal capsule (*gray arrowhead*) and acetabular rim (*white arrow*).

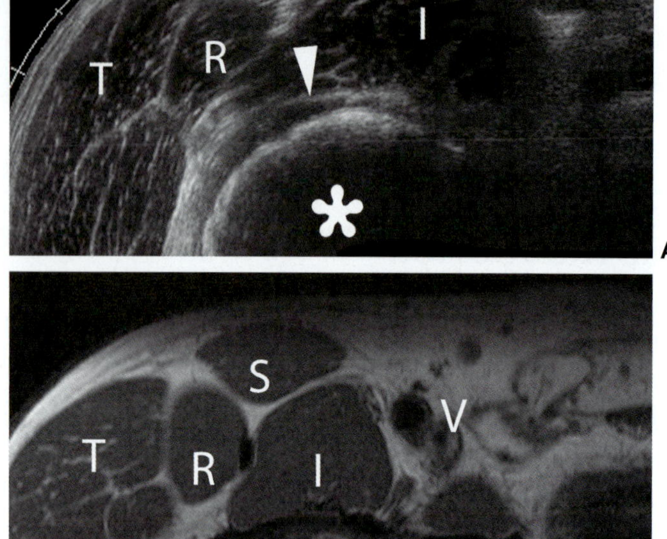

Figure 6.3. Normal TS views of the hip. **A:** Transverse sonogram and **B:** Axial T1W MRI show femoral head (*asterisk*), iliopsoas (*I*), TFL (*T*), rectus femoris (*R*), sartorius (*S*), femoral vessels (*V*), and capsule (*arrowhead*).

For gluteal assessment, the patient is initially scanned in the lateral decubitus position with a high-frequency probe. Gluteus medius (deep) and gluteus minimus (superficial) can be traced cranially down to the greater trochanter in both long-axis and short-axis scans **(Fig. 6.4)**. The TFL is adjacent to the anterior margins of these two muscles, and gluteus maximus overlies the posterior portion of gluteus medius. The echogenic tendons of gluteus minimus and medius insert into the anterior and lateral aspects of the greater trochanter, respectively. Long-axis and short-axis scans should be performed to detect tendinopathy and evidence of bursitis between the tendons and trochanter.

Evaluation of the hamstring origins is performed with the patient prone with the feet hanging over the end of the couch. Lower frequency probes may be required for larger patients. The ischial tuberosity is first identified, located medially at the junction of buttock and thigh **(Fig. 6.5)**. The origin of the ischiocrural tendons (semimembranosus, long head of biceps femoris, and semitendinosus) attaches laterally **(Fig. 6.6)**. They cannot always be appreciated separately at this level on

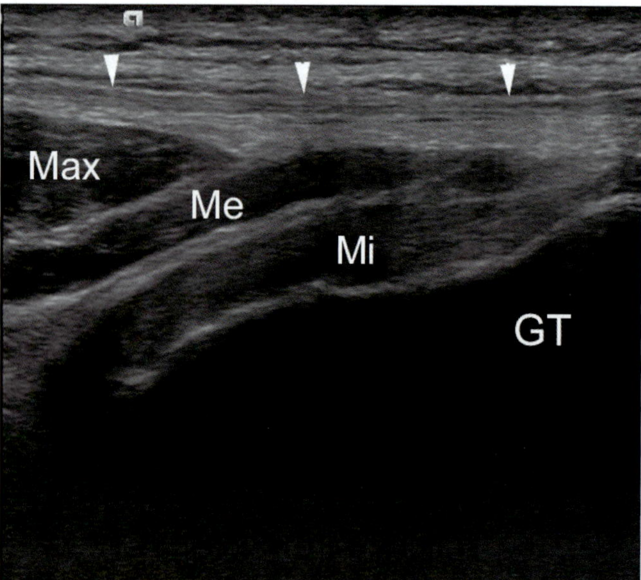

Figure 6.4. Longitudinal view of the greater trochanter. Longitudinal sonogram shows normal greater trochanter (*GT*), gluteus medius (*Me*), and minimus (*Mi*) muscles and tendons. The gluteus maximus (*Max*) is more superficial with overlying fibrillar fascia lata (*arrowheads*).

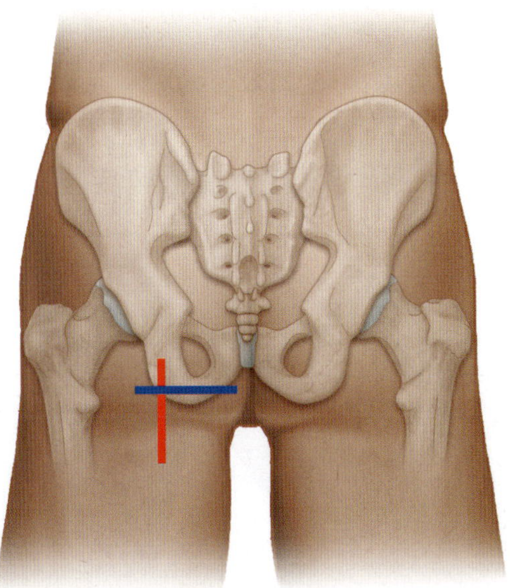

Figure 6.5. Posterior hip probe positions. The two probe positions for imaging the posterior hip are demonstrated by the two colored lines: LS (*red*) and TS (*blue*).

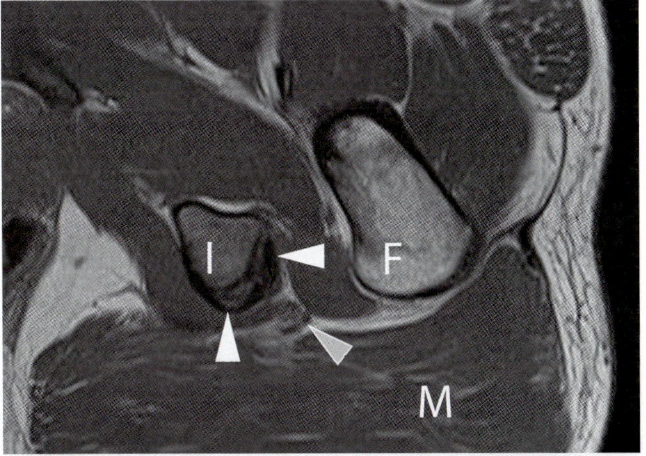

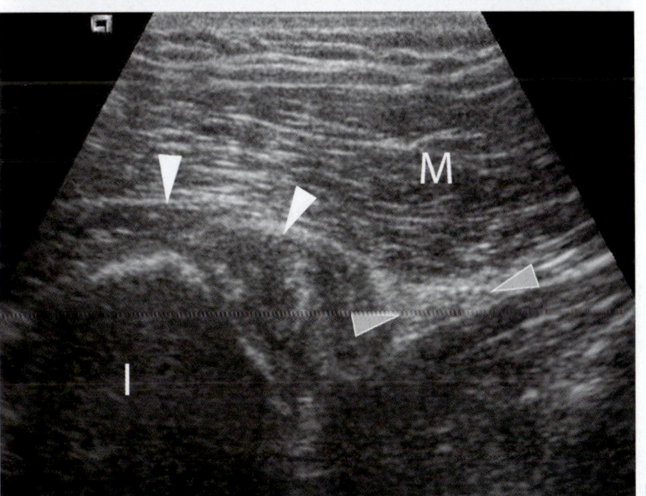

Figure 6.6.   Normal axial/TS views of the ischial tuberosity. **A:** Axial TW1 MRI and **B:** Transverse sonogram shows ischial tuberosity (*I*), femur (*F*), gluteus maximus (*M*), hamstring origins (*white arrowheads*) and sciatic nerve (*gray arrowheads*).

ultrasound, but individual tendons can be identified by tracing them caudally. They initially separate into the semimembranosus tendon (medial) and the conjoined tendon of semitendinosus and the long head of biceps femoris (superficial and lateral). The conjoined tendon then further divides into the muscle bellies of semitendinosus (medial) and biceps femoris (lateral). Evaluate them in longitudinal and transverse planes to assess for tendinopathy **(Fig. 6.7)**. Lateral to the ischiocrural tendon origin, the sciatic nerve has the characteristic neural fascicular pattern **(Fig. 6.6)**.

Medial

This quadrant contains the origins of the adductor muscles: longus, brevis, and magnus along with gracilis and the insertion of iliopsoas. The patient is scanned in the supine position with the thigh abducted and externally rotated and the knee flexed **(Fig. 6.8)**. The insertion of iliopsoas can be best assessed in this position using LS views, as anisotropy is a common problem, with the leg in the adducted position.

Place the probe over the anterior aspect of the medial muscle compartment, medial to the neurovascular bundle to reveal the three adductor muscles separated by hyperechoic fascial planes **(Fig. 6.9)**. Adductor longus is anterior, adductor brevis is intermediate, and adductor magnus lies posterior. Gracilis is found medial to adductor longus and superficial to adductor brevis. The muscles can be traced to their origin at the pubis to evaluate for tendinopathy and muscle tears using LS and TS views. Next, assess the

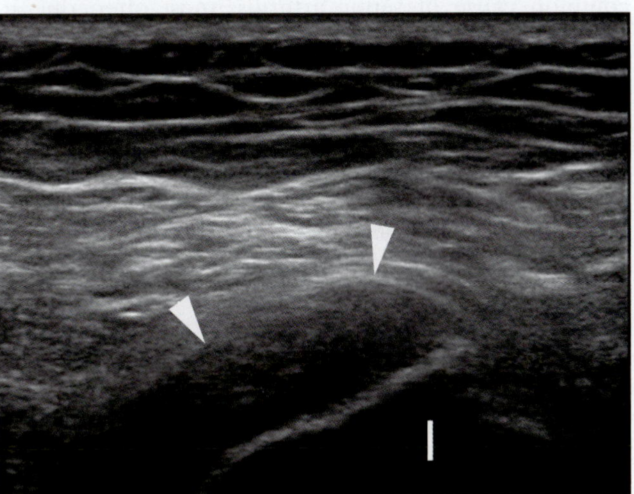

Figure 6.7. Overuse hamstring tendinopathy. Longitudinal sonogram shows hypoechoic thickened hamstring origin tendons (*arrowheads*) and adjacent ischial tuberosity (*I*).

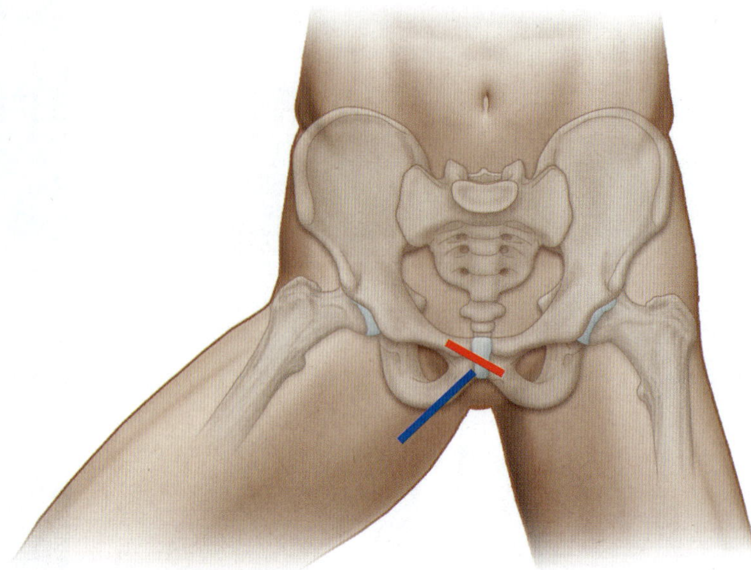

Figure 6.8.   Medial hip probe positions. The two probe positions for imaging the adductor area are demonstrated by the two colored lines: LS (*blue*) and TS (*red*).

symphysis pubis joint space, found medial to the adductor insertion, for arthropathic changes **(Fig. 6.10)**.

HIP JOINT EFFUSION

Effusions of the hip joint are almost always pathological, but are rarely detectable clinically owing to the depth of the hip joint. Ultrasound is rapid, portable, and effective[1–3], avoids unnecessary "dry" aspirations and joint contamination, and shows extra-articular collections. Power Doppler identifies coexisting inflammation. Ultrasound can be employed to guide diagnostic aspiration, biopsy, and therapeutic injections.[4]

Causes

Hematological seeding during bacteremia is the most common cause of septic arthritis, most often due to *Staphylococcus aureus*.[3] Risk factors include IV drug abuse, endocarditis, indwelling catheters, advanced age, immunosuppression, and preexisting joint injuries.[5] Other causes include adjacent surgery or direct extension of infection from the abdomen via iliopsoas. Rapid diagnosis is vital as delay worsens the prognosis.[3] Bacterial arthritis results in irreversible loss of joint function in 25% to 50% of patients and 5% to 15% fatality rates.[6] The appearances of the effusion in terms of complexity and echogenicity do not predict infectious or inflammatory nature.[7] Ultrasound cannot prove sepsis and if suspected, analysis of aspirated fluid is usually required. However, large joint effusions with extra-articular extension in painful prosthetic hips are strongly associated with infection.[8]

Inflammatory arthritides, both seropositive and seronegative, cause hip effusions. Immunosuppressive treatment increases the risk of avascular necrosis and infection, which themselves cause effusions. Increased synovial power Doppler flow suggests an inflammatory rather than noninflammatory cause, but does not differentiate between types of inflammation, for example, infective or noninfective.[9] Marginal erosions may rarely be seen at the bone–cartilage interface at the femoral head and neck in inflammatory arthropathy.

Benign tumors of bone and soft tissue, including synovial osteochondromatosis, pigmented villonodular synovitis, osteoid osteoma, and giant cell tumors of bone can be associated with hip effusions.[10] Effusions in association with malignant tumors of bone may indicate joint involvement or be a consequence of underlying pathological fracture, but MRI and plain radiographs provide the optimum method of assessment.

Effusions can occur in osteoarthritis. Synovitis and debris in the joint and underlying osteonecrosis may occur.[10] Osteophytes at the femoral head/neck junction can also be demonstrated, but are better shown on plain radiographs, computed tomography (CT), and MRI.[1]

For clinically suspected fracture not confirmed by radiographs, MRI is the investigation of choice. Ultrasound is not very sensitive or specific in these cases, but may occasionally show a femoral neck fracture. In addition to the resulting hip effusion/hemarthrosis, the fracture may be seen as a step or breach of the hyperechoic cortex.[1] An osteochondral injury could also result in effusion, but would not itself be visible on ultrasound.

Postsurgical complications such as infection, aseptic loosening, or wear debris can all result in effusion. Ultrasound appearances of hip replacement will be discussed later in the chapter.

Identifying Pathology on Ultrasound

An effusion appears as a hypoechoic layer between the hyperechoic bone cortex of the femoral neck and the

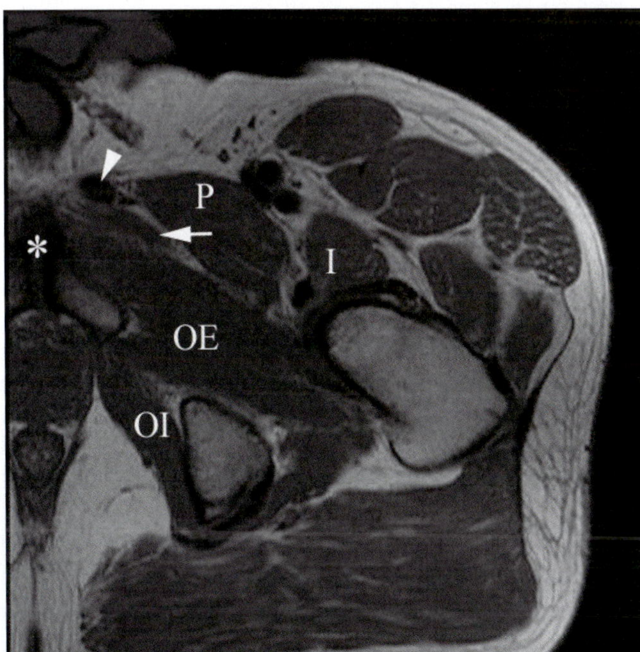

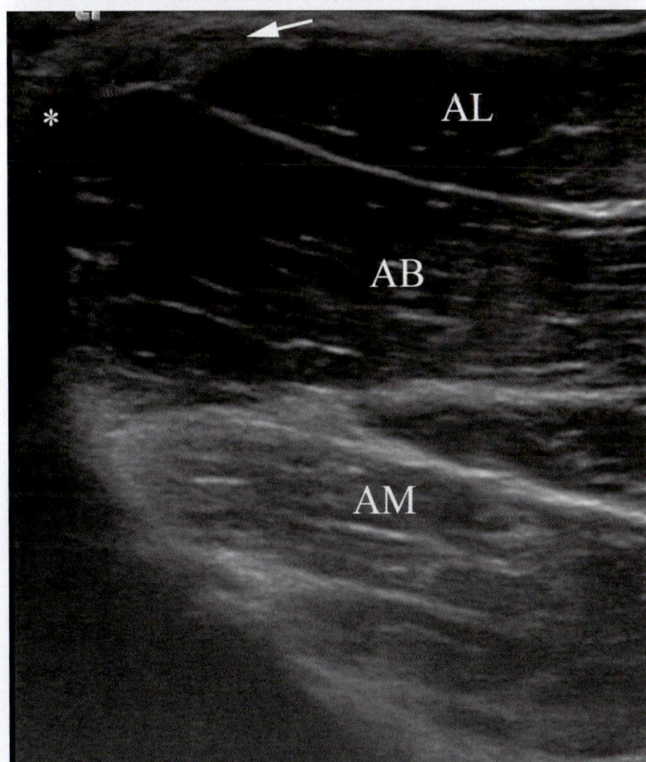

Figure 6.9. Normal views of the adductor origins. **A:** Axial T1W MRI shows the adductor origin, including adductor longus (*arrowhead*), brevis (*arrow*), and obturator externus (*OE*) with adjacent Iliopsoas (*I*), obturator internus (*OI*), pectineus (*P*), and pubic symphysis (*asterisk*). **B:** Short-axis sonogram of the thigh inferior to (**A**) shows the adductor longus tendon (*arrow*) and muscle (*AL*) with adductors brevis (*AB*) and magnus (*AM*) lying deep and pubic symphysis (asterisk) lying superficial.

overlying psoas muscle, extending along the anterior recess on the femoral neck (**Fig. 6.11**). The optimal probe position is an oblique longitudinal scan along the femoral

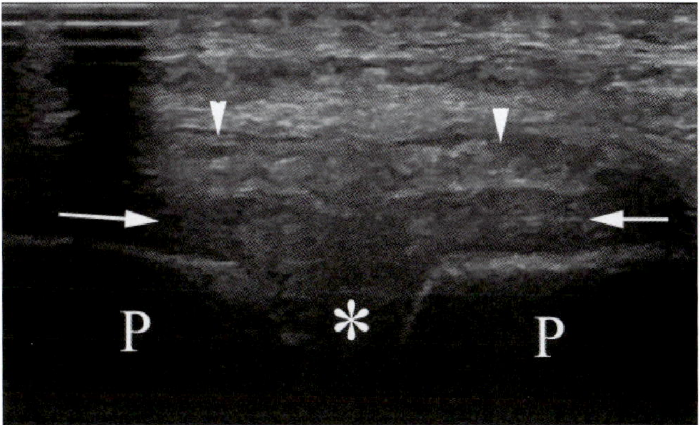

Figure 6.10. Normal pubic symphysis. Transverse sonogram shows pubic symphysis joint space and disc (*asterisk*), pubic bones (*P*), anterior capsule (*arrows*) and attachment of rectus abdominis muscles (*arrowheads*).

neck. Hip joint effusions as small as 1 to 2 mL may be identified,[11] although small effusions may "disappear" into the posterior recess and become undetectable on ultrasound.

Effusion can be difficult to distinguish from the synovial thickening. Under normal circumstances, synovium is not visible on ultrasound, and the fibrous layer is a thin hyperechoic band (**Fig. 6.11**). Aging, degenerative disease, synovitis, and surgery can result in thickening of the synovial layer or joint capsule, and this may be mistaken for an effusion (**Fig. 6.12**).

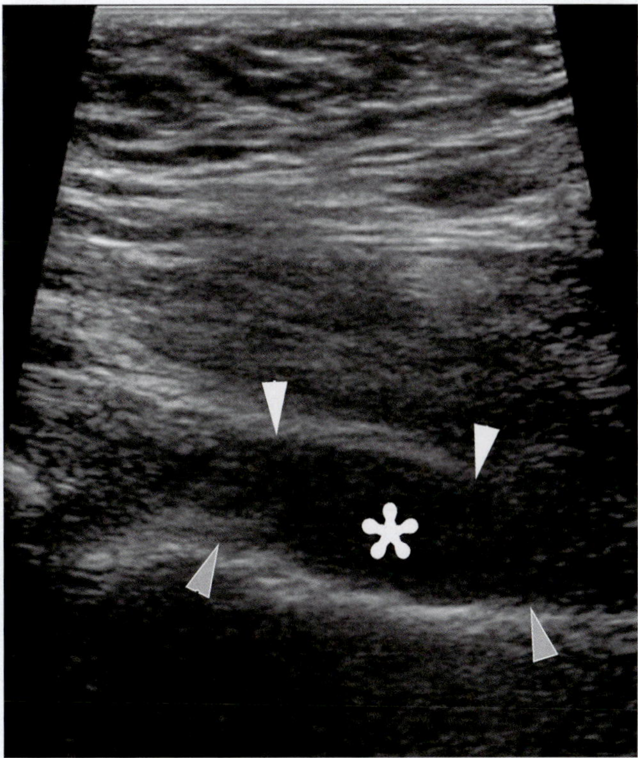

Figure 6.11. Hip effusion. Longitudinal sonogram shows anechoic hip effusion (*asterisk*) between the hyperechoic capsule (*white arrowheads*) and femoral neck (*gray arrowheads*).

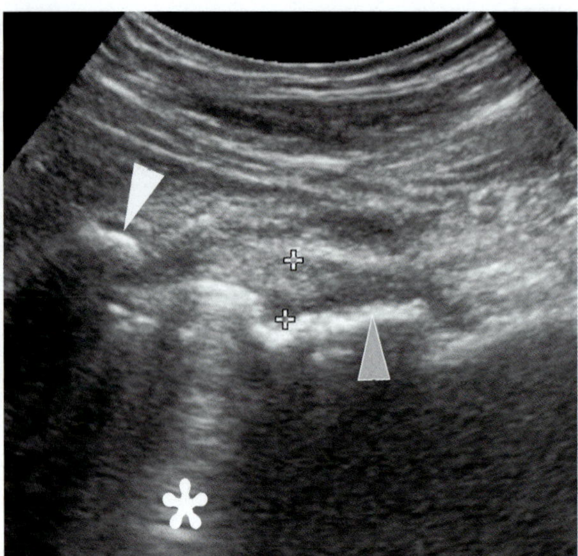

Figure 6.12. Normal sonographic appearances of a metallic hip. Longitudinal sonogram shows metal-on-metal resurfaced hip with the typical hyperechoic margin at the acetabulum (*white arrowhead*), femoral neck (*gray arrowhead*), and significant reverberation artifact. *Calipers* measure the capsule that shows typical thickening postsurgery.

Tips For Identifying an Effusion:
- Ensure the probe is perpendicular to avoid anisotropy artifact.
- Check the joint contour—a convex, bulging contour suggests effusion.
- Do not press too firmly with the probe or small effusions may be effaced.
- Measure the depth: capsular thickening or displacement of 5 to 10 mm are more significant.[10,12]
- Compare with the other hip. A discrepancy of 1 to 2mm or more has been described as significant,[12,13] but this needs to be interpreted with caution as surgery, aging, and previous synovitis may leave residual capsular thickening.[10]
- Use power Doppler: the presence of internal flow indicates thickened synovium rather than fluid.
- If still in doubt, a diagnostic tap can be performed to confirm the presence of fluid, with the advantage that a sample is then available for biochemical and microbiological analysis.

It is important to be aware that other pathologies may mimic effusions on USS.

- The iliopsoas bursa lies between the hip joint capsule and the iliopsoas muscle/tendon. The bursa is usually empty and not normally visible, but appears as an an-echoic/hypoechoic area anterior to the capsule if bursitis is present **(Fig 6.13A)**.
- Paralabral cysts can form near the anterior recess **(Fig 6.13B)**.
- Femoral artery aneurysms are identifiable by their pulsatile nature: check with Doppler for internal flow **(Fig 6.13C)**.

- Extra-articular abscesses/collections do not communicate with the joint and may demonstrate surrounding increased Doppler flow **(Fig 6.13D)**.

ASPIRATION AND INJECTION

Aspiration can show if bacteria or crystals are present and can relieve pain by decompressing large effusions. Ultrasound-guided aspirations reduce the risks of a "dry tap" or contamination of a sterile hip with the infected contents of an extra-articular collection compared with blind aspirations that rely on bony landmarks. The absence of ionizing radiation makes it preferable in pregnant women and children when compared to fluoroscopy or CT. A major concern when performing hip aspiration is to avoid iatrogenic septic arthritis. The risk is low (<1/1,000) provided that proper aseptic technique is observed,[14] but this should be discussed when obtaining consent from the patient. Ultrasound-guided joint injections can be diagnostic (contrast for arthrography, including MR arthrography) and diagnostic/therapeutic (local anesthetic and steroid for arthritis). Recent evidence has suggested that local anesthetic may be chondrotoxic and should be used with caution.[15] This is also discussed in Chapter 14 Interventional.

There are two methods for aspirating an effusion/suspected effusion from the hip. The first is to use ultrasound to mark the position of the target point on the skin, and then proceed "blind." The second method is to place the needle and aspirate under direct ultrasound vision. For both techniques, strict aseptic technique is essential. A sterile probe cover should be used for the direct vision method. A spinal needle of at least 18G caliber should be chosen, as pus may be thick and viscous, and a narrow needle may result in a "dry tap." The needle length should be at least 5 cm, but may need to be longer, depending on patient size. Pre-measurement of the skin-to-effusion distance with ultrasound is useful if in doubt. Infiltration with 1% lidocaine is advised for local anesthesia. Care should be taken to avoid the neurovascular structures medially.

Tip:
If the first aspiration attempt is unsuccessful, rotate the bevel clockwise or counterclockwise. If the needle becomes blocked with debris, reinsert the stylet, and this may resolve the problem. Gradual needle withdrawal while applying gentle suction may succeed where the bevel has become embedded in the periosteum. Viscous or small effusions can be difficult to aspirate, and in these cases injection of a small volume of sterile saline into the effusion may aid aspiration.[7] This is particularly useful in cases with a high clinical suspicion of infection but minimal effusion.

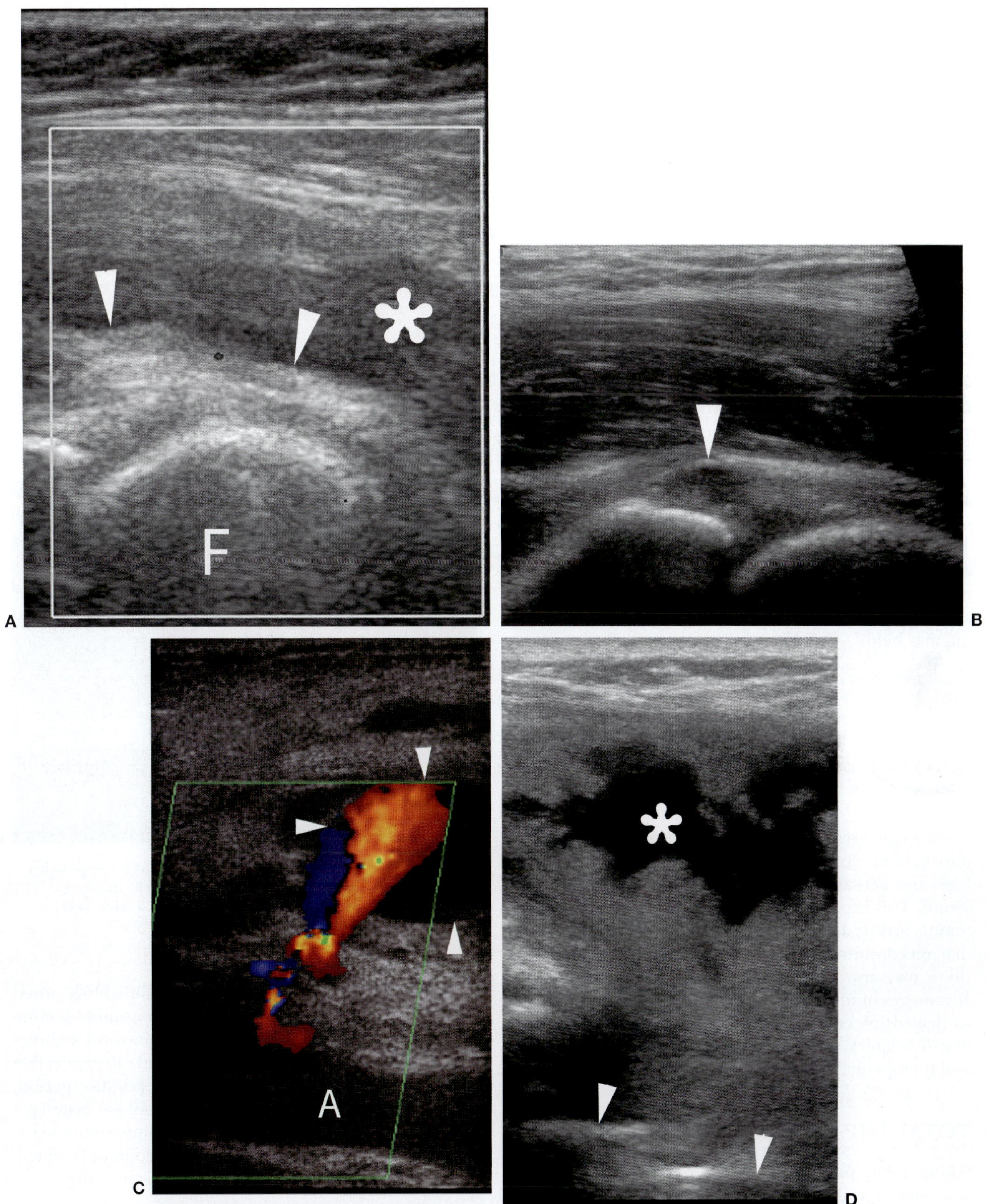

Figure 6.13.   Mimics of hips effusion. **A:** Longitudinal sonogram shows femoral head (*F*) and psoas bursa (*asterisk*). *Arrowheads* mark the hyperechoic capsule *deep to the* fluid. **B:** Longitudinal sonogram shows anechoic paralabral cyst (*arrowhead*) at the acetabular rim. **C:** Longitudinal sonogram shows femoral artery false aneurysm (*arrowheads*). Color Doppler shows communication with the underlying artery (*A*) and turbulent internal flow. **D:** Longitudinal sonogram shows extra-articular collection (*asterisk*) separate from the deeper femoral neck (*arrowheads*) and effusion.

Blind aspiration offers the advantage of a quick procedure for anxious/agitated patients and a simpler needle approach for deep joints in large patients. The probe is orientated along the femoral neck in longitudinal and/or transverse section, with the center of the footprint at the desired point of aspiration. The ends of the footprint are marked, followed by the center point, once the probe has been removed. Alternatively, the skin should be marked with the transducer oriented along both short and long axes of the femoral neck and the needle inserted at the point of intersection of the two lines. Following aseptic preparation and injection of local anesthetic, the needle is advanced through the skin vertically down to the femoral cortex, and aspiration is then performed. It is essential that the needle is vertically oriented.

The direct vision technique is useful for small effusions that can be difficult to target and for injections so that the position of the injectate can be confirmed. Transverse or longitudinal probe orientation is used with the transducer centered over the effusion. The end of the transducer is marked on the skin. After cleaning the skin and injecting local anesthetic, the needle is advanced obliquely under direct ultrasound guidance (**Fig. 6.14**). The needle should be inserted parallel or as close to parallel as possible to ensure maximum visualization of the needle tip. This may be difficult in larger patients, and altering transducer angulation or employing beam steering may help.

> **Tip:**
> If difficulty in needle visualization occurs, first check the alignment of the probe and needle, and reposition as necessary. Short, gentle needle motions can help reveal the location of the tip.

Magnetic resonance imaging provides additional information regarding the surrounding bone, cartilage, and peri-articular soft tissues compared with ultrasound. This is particularly useful in suspected infection, tumor, arthritides, and occult fracture. Small effusions that recede into the posterior recess in the supine position may also be more readily detected by MRI. The advantages of ultrasound as an initial test, particularly in suspected infections when speed is of the essence, are that it is quick, readily available, and offers diagnostic and therapeutic intervention.

TOTAL HIP REPLACEMENT

Sonographic imaging in the early postoperative period is a challenge due to difficulties recognizing "normal" postoperative changes from evolving pathologies such as major hematoma and associated infection. Clinical detection of these pathologies is often difficult, and ultrasound has been advocated[16, 17] as having superior sensitivity to

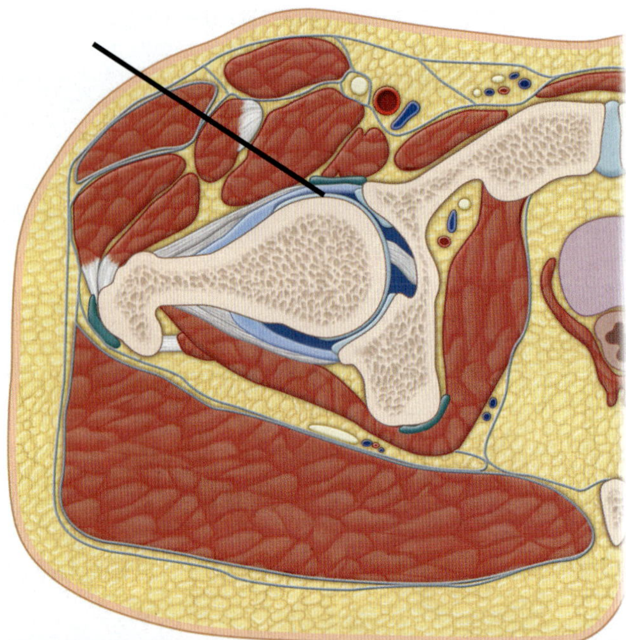

A

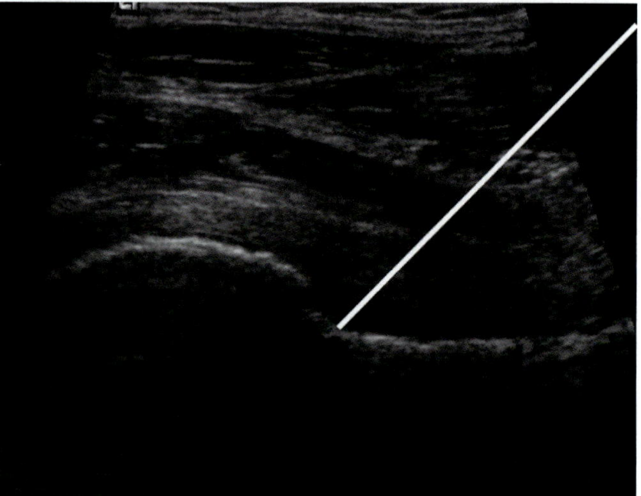

B

Figure 6.14.   Approaches to hip aspiration. The two approaches to aspirating a hip effusion are demonstrated. **A:** The transverse approach (*black line*). **B:** The longitudinal approach (*white line*).

clinical examination[18] and avoiding the difficulties posed by susceptibility artifact on MRI. Ultrasound demonstrates extra-articular collections not shown on arthrography. Where mobility is poor, ultrasound offers portable ward-based assessment. In the late postoperative period, ultrasound provides dynamic assessment of associated pathology such as gluteus minimus or medius tendon tears. Ultrasound can also guide aspiration of joint or fluid collections, capsular biopsy, and therapeutic injection.

Normal Postoperative Appearances

In the early postoperative period, a hypoechoic track extending from the skin incision to the hip represents the path of surgical access. Collections may routinely be identified along this path or around the prosthetic joint or the femur. The surface of the prosthesis is highly echogenic, more so than normal bone cortex, and may generate reverberation artifact (**Fig. 6.12**). A study of 47 postoperative hips at the second and fifth postoperative day concluded that a bone-to-capsule thickness of up to 6 mm, deep soft tissue fluid collections up to 21 mm, and superficial collections up to 28 mm were all considered to be normal.[16] Communication with the joint is an important distinction that is usually demonstrable by ultrasound, though it may be more readily demonstrated by arthrography.[19]

Subsequently, thickening of the joint capsule may be seen due to fibrosis and previous hemorrhage[10] (**Fig. 6.12**). Effusions and extra-articular collections are not normal after the first few weeks (**Fig. 6.13D**).

Complications

Mechanical loosening of the prosthesis is a common cause of pain after total hip arthroplasty. Infection is less frequent, but more serious. Preoperative diagnosis is important because prosthetic loosening is treated by revision arthroplasty, while infection often requires removal of the prosthesis followed by multistage revision procedures[8] and prolonged courses of antibiotics. Infection may occur years after arthroplasty, but typically occurs within 2 years of the initial operation, and may be due to hematological seeding from a remote site,[20,21] for example, urinary tract infection.

Distinguishing between loosening and infection using clinical assessment and radiographs alone is often not possible. Magnetic resonance imaging is limited by the artifact even when metal artifact reduction sequences are used, although large collections can be demonstrated. Ultrasound can identify and characterize fluid collections and effusions (**Fig. 6.15**). A study of 48 patients with total hip replacement (THR) found that infected hips have intra-articular fluid and fluid collections outside the pseudocapsule in most cases.[8] Guided aspiration can be performed in these cases to confirm or exclude infection. Prosthetic wear can also cause effusions in patients with replacement joints.[8]

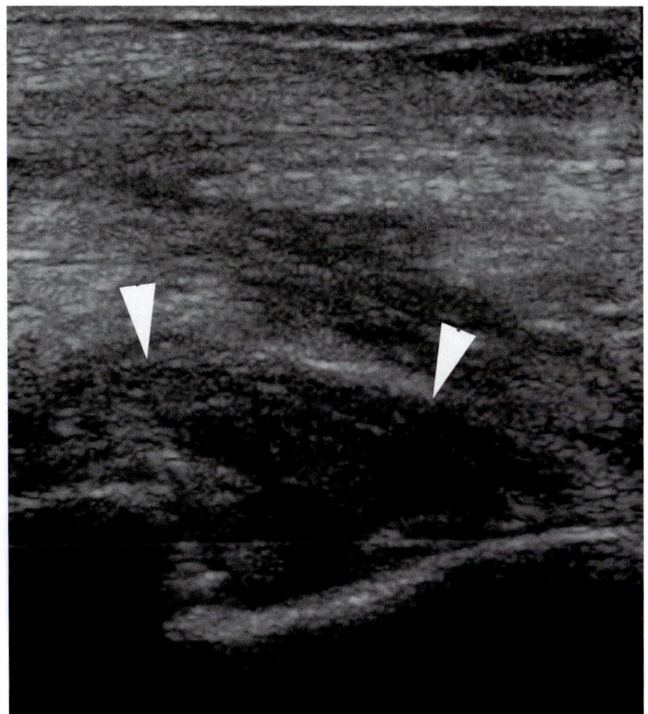

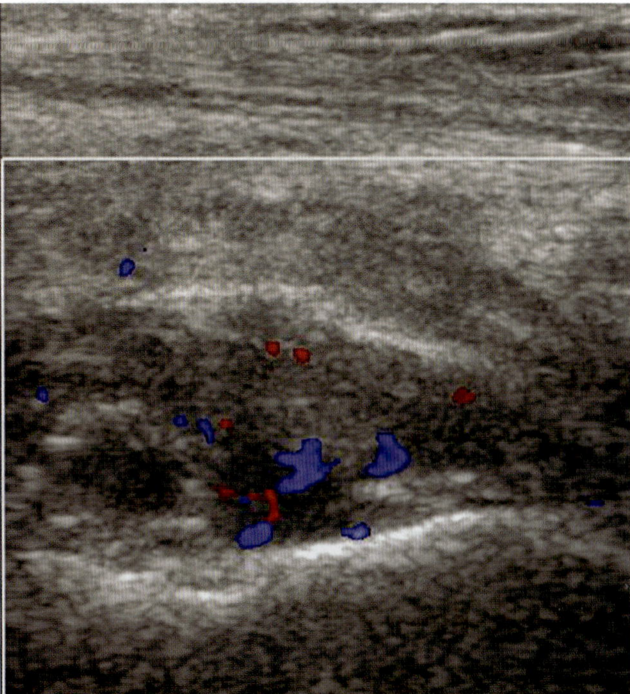

Figure 6.15. Infected Hip. Longitudinal sonogram shows **(A)** heterogeneous hypoechoic collection in a distended joint (*arrowheads*) and **(B)** Color Doppler demonstrates increased vascularity due to inflammation.

> **Tip:**
> If uncertainty exists regarding the communication between collection and joint, do not use the same needle to aspirate or penetrate both in the same pass, as infection may be disseminated between the two.

Communications between the bursae of the greater trochanter, iliopsoas bursa, and supra-acetabular region are common in patients with pain following hip arthroplasty[22] (**Fig. 6.16**). Bursitis can occur as a result of impingement of the prosthesis on the surrounding soft tissues, especially the acetabular cup; for example, bony spurs or cement may impinge on the rectus femoris tendon. Guided injection can offer diagnostic/therapeutic benefit in these cases. Care should be taken because of the increased susceptibility of prosthetic hips to iatrogenic infection.

Role of MRI in Pelvic Muscle Injury

The large field of view offered by MRI is of benefit when the location of the pathology is uncertain, for example, when the patient waves rather than points when asked to localize pain. MRI offers better evaluation of deep structures in large patients, for example, at the ischial tuberosity. Magnetic resonance imaging is also more sensitive than ultrasound in assessing minimally disruptive (Grade 1) injuries in the acute phase, and may be preferred in the professional athlete to detect subtle muscle edema.

The role of ultrasound in muscle and tendon assessment around the hip is for focused, dynamic examination with and without intervention.

HERNIAS

The role of ultrasound in hernia detection is to assist in cases where the clinical diagnosis is uncertain due to vague or conflicting examination findings. It also has a role in characterizing hernias and evaluating the contents of the sac. Accurate diagnosis is important, since hernias are associated with significant morbidity. Clinically obvious hernias do not require imaging. Where imaging is needed, several modalities exist.

Computed tomography is useful in acutely incarcerated hernias to confirm the diagnosis and assess for associated complication such as bowel obstruction. Valsalva CT has been used in the outpatient setting to identify hernias, which may reduce when the patient is supine and at rest. The disadvantages are the exposure to ionizing radiation and the inability to scan while the patient is standing. Dynamic MRI studies have also been reported, but are still not widely used in clinical practice.

In herniography, water soluble contrast is injected into the peritoneum, followed by patient maneuvers to fill the hernia sac, which is then demonstrated on fluoroscopy. The technique is invasive, and small hernias or those comprising only fat may not be demonstrated.[41]

Surgical exploration allows exclusion of nonreducing hernia and treatment, but has associated morbidity and can potentially miss hernias that have reduced while the patient lies relaxed in the supine position.

Ultrasound offers the advantages of easy dynamic assessment during Valsalva and posture changes. Sensitivities of 86% to 100% have been reported with 82% to 97% specificity, although accuracy for hernia classification is more varied (45% to 85%).[41] Hernias consisting only of fat are also more readily detected, but care must be taken not to misinterpret prominent fat or, more rarely, a lipoma as a hernia. The exquisite soft tissue detail also allows accurate diagnosis of differential diagnoses such as undescended testis, lymphadenopathy, neoplasm, and aneurysm. The various types of hernias found around the hip are now discussed.

Inguinal (Direct/Indirect)

The inguinal region, from deep to superficial, comprises the peritoneum, transversus abdominis, internal oblique, external oblique, subcutaneous fat, and skin **(Fig. 6.25)**. The inguinal canal has a roof, floor, and anterior and posterior walls. The floor is formed by the inguinal ligament, which runs from the ASIS to the pubic tubercle. The posterior wall is formed from the muscle and fascia of transversus abdominis and part of the internal oblique. The anterior wall is formed from the fascia of external oblique. The roof of the canal is formed from the arching fibers of transversus abdominis and internal oblique. The canal commences at the deep inguinal ring located halfway along the inguinal ligament, just lateral to the origin of the inferior epigastric vessels. It runs obliquely in a medial and inferior direction for about 4 cm, to terminate at the superficial inguinal ring just superior and lateral to the pubic tubercle. Normally it transmits vessels, nerves, and lymphatics between the abdomen and external genitalia, the spermatic cord in men, and the round ligament in women.

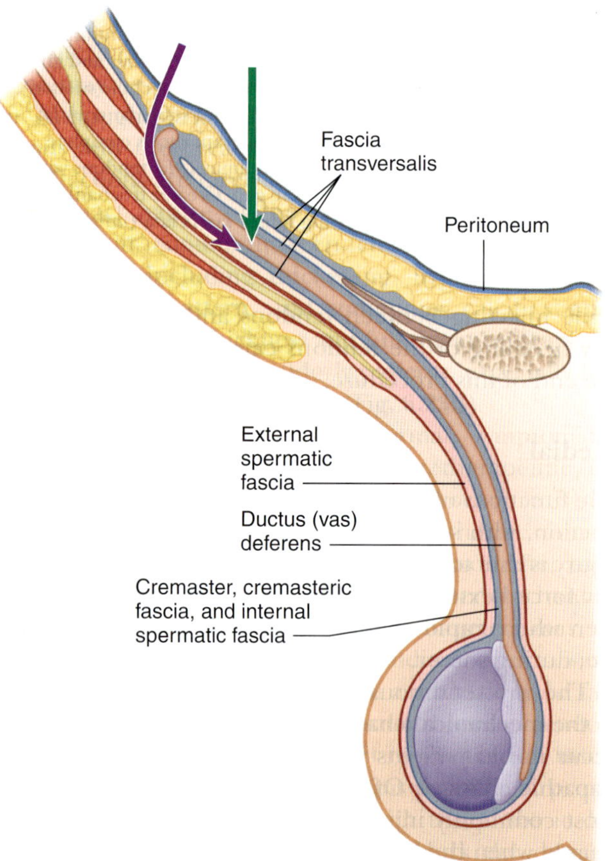

Figure 6.25.   Cross-sectional anatomy of the inguinal canal and inguinal hernias. The inguinal canal is shown in cross section with the paths of the two types of hernia demonstrated by the arrows, indirect (*purple arrow*) and direct (*green arrow*).

Posterior (deep) to the canal lie the femoral vessels, which give rise to the inferior epigastric vessels that course superior to the canal and deep to the rectus abdominis muscle. The origin of the inferior epigastric vessels **(Fig. 6.26)**, just medial to the deep inguinal ring, is an important landmark in inguinal hernia identification and classification. Inguinal hernias that arise lateral to the inferior epigastric vessels therefore pass through the deep inguinal ring and are indirect. Hernias arising medial are direct. The inferior epigastric vessels, along with the lateral margin of rectus abdominis and the inguinal ligament, form Hesselbach's triangle, where direct inguinal hernias will be seen to arise **(Fig. 6.26)**.

Scanning Technique

A linear probe of around 9 to 15 MHz is usually optimal, although higher frequencies provide better detail in slim patients.

Begin by identifying the inferior epigastric vessels **(Fig. 6.26)** deep to the rectus abdominis muscles and following them inferiorly to their origin. Alternatively, scan along the femoral vessels below the inguinal ligament in a cephalad direction until the origins appear. The second method may be easier in large patients where the abdominal apron can disrupt scanning. Once the origin is located, angle the probe parallel to the inguinal ligament, which will be visible superficial to the vessel origins.

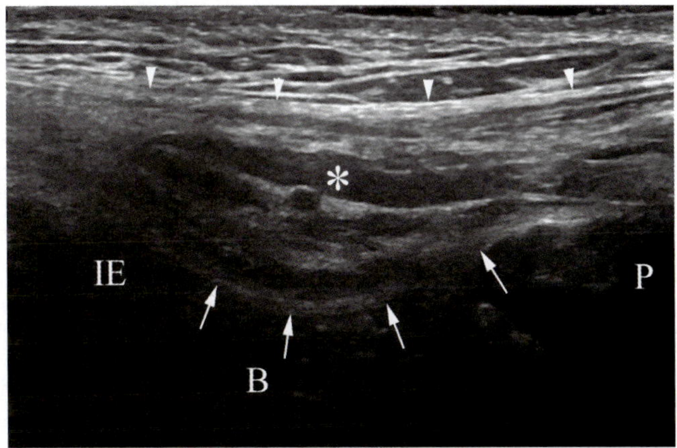

Figure 6.27. Normal inguinal canal (long axis). Longitudinal sonogram aligned parallel to the inguinal ligament demonstrates hyperechoic inguinal ligament (*white arrowheads*), inguinal canal contents (*asterisk*), inferior epigastric vessels (*IE*), and pubic tubercle (*P*). The hypoechoic area at the bottom of the picture represents bowel (*B*) deep to the posterior (deep) canal wall (*arrows*).

The inguinal ligament is a linear echogenic band with an echogenic internal fibrillar structure. The contents of the inguinal canal can be appreciated deep and superior to the ligament as a mixture of hypo and hyperechoic serpentine structures **(Figs. 6.27 and 6.28)**. They should be evaluated in long- and short-axis scans. Posterior and deep to the canal lie the psoas muscle, femoral vessels, and peritoneum. The peritoneum appears as an echogenic layer. The canal contents can be traced into the scrotum in males.

Both long- and short-axis evaluation is advised for inguinal hernias. Begin in the long axis. Unreduced hernias may be visible within the canal from the outset. The patient should be asked to perform a slow Valsalva

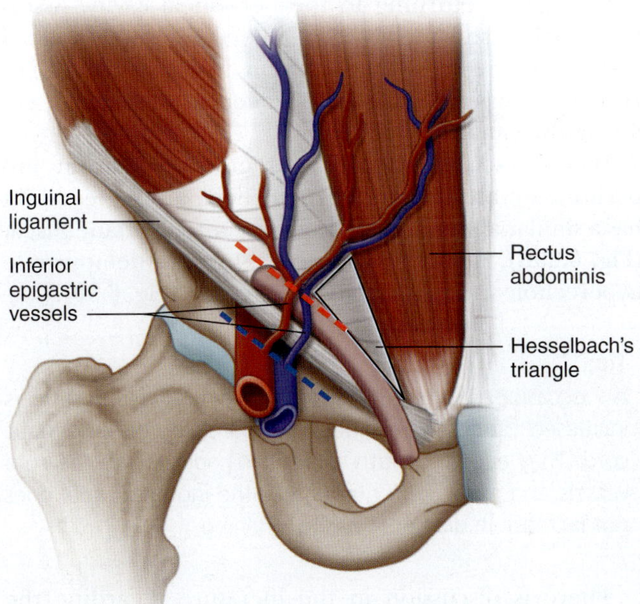

Figure 6.26. Anterior view of the inguinal canal and Hesselbach's triangle. The dotted lines show the optimal probe positions for imaging groin hernias. Inguinal hernias are best seen on the red dotted line and femoral hernias on the blue dotted line. The boundaries of Hesselbach's triangle, where direct hernias occur, are demonstrated; the lateral border of rectus abdominis, the inferior epigastric vessels, and the inguinal ligament.

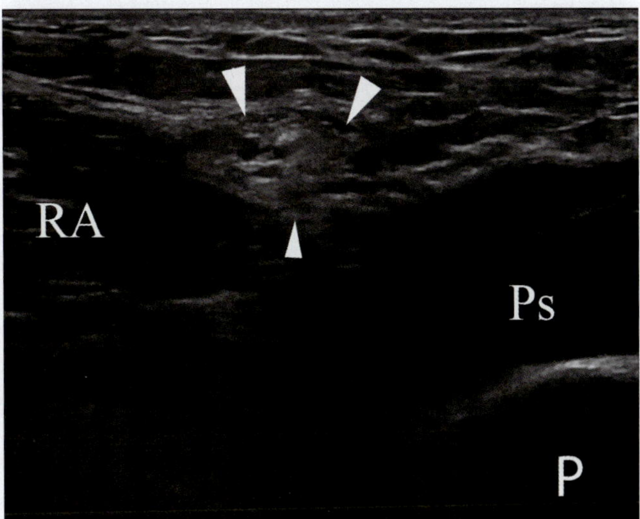

Figure 6.28. Normal inguinal canal (short axis). Transverse sonogram demonstrates the normal inguinal canal and contents (*arrowheads*). Iliopsoas muscle (*Ps*), rectus abdominis (*RA*), and pubic ramus (*P*).

maneuver. This can be achieved by gently raising their head from the bed or attempting to blow through their closed fist or an occluded straw. Avoid coughing, as this produces sudden motion that can be difficult to interpret.

Dilation of the femoral vein is indicative of an effective maneuver. Advise the clinician in the report if the patient is not able to perform this procedure effectively. Indirect inguinal hernias arise lateral to the inferior epigastric vessels and pass medially along the canal (**Fig. 6.29**). Direct inguinal hernias arise medially, bulge superficially toward the probe (**Fig. 6.30**), are seen within the boundaries of Hesselbach's triangle, and tend to be more localized.

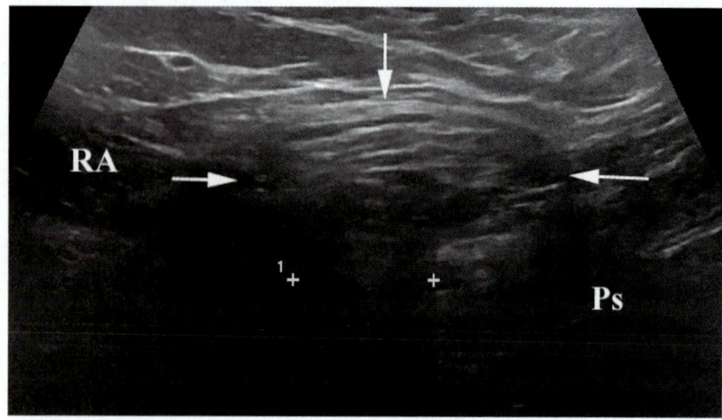

Figure 6.30.   Direct inguinal hernia. Transverse sonogram of the inguinal canal shows direct inguinal hernia (*arrows*) extending though a posterior wall defect (*calipers*) into the canal. Note the rectus abdominis (*RA*) and iliopsoas (*Ps*).

Some forward bulging of the peritoneal contents during Valsalva is normal but the inguinal canal should not be occluded. Bowel may approach the canal and cause a little prominence of the deep ring, but should not enter the canal. Mild vessel dilation and motion within the canal are also normal. The relaxation period after Valsalva can be an opportune moment to see the bowel slowly returning to the peritoneal cavity. Assess the canal in short axis next, looking for sudden canal distension with vessel effacement in indirect hernias. Direct hernias will bulge from deep to superficial, entering the canal.

When describing hernia contents, note that fat and peritoneum are relatively hyperechoic, and omental fat has a similar appearance to the adjacent subcutaneous fat (**Fig. 6.29B**). Bowel is hypoechoic, but can demonstrate hyperechoic mucosa/gas bubbles within (**Fig. 6.30**).

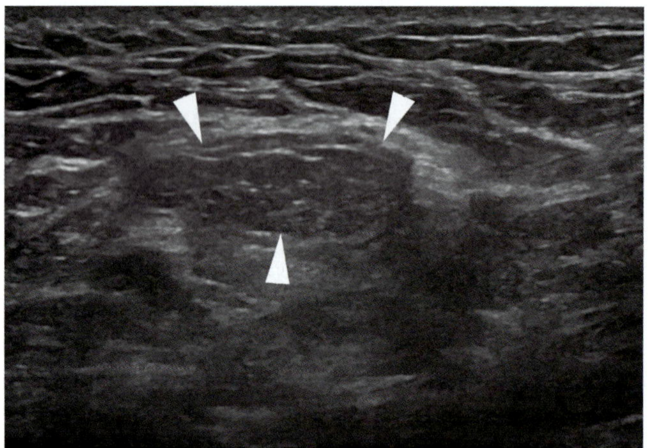

A

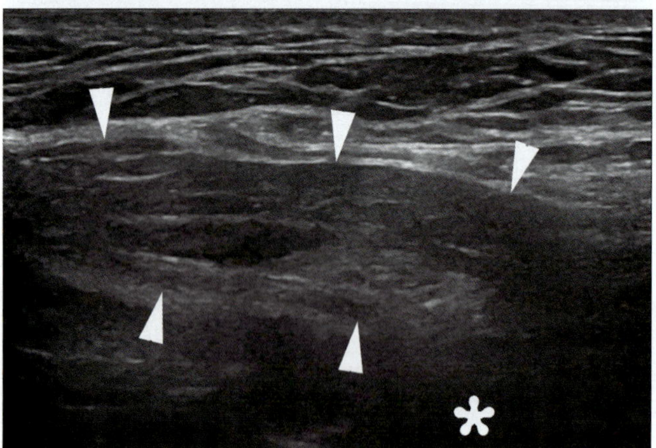

B

Figure 6.29.   Indirect inguinal hernia. Sonograms of the inguinal canal. **A:** Short axis during Valsalva shows hernia containing fat (*arrowheads*) expanding the canal and effacing contents. **B:** Long axis during Valsalva shows hernia containing fat (*arrowheads*). The location of the inferior epigastric vessels is marked (*asterisk*) with the hernia arising laterally.

There is discussion in the literature regarding the possible existence of a "pre-hernia" condition as a possible source of groin pain. This is characterized by bulging of the transversalis fascia such that the canal is almost occluded, but no actual herniation occurs. However, this has not been confirmed by ultrasound or herniography.[41] We advise caution when reporting such appearances.

Femoral

The femoral canal is a small compartment within the femoral sheath medial to the femoral vein. It is a potential space that ordinarily only contains fatty connective tissue and lymphatics. Hernias enter the canal via the femoral ring that lies superiorly and is bounded by the inguinal ligament anteriorly, pectineus and pectineus fascia posteriorly, lacunar ligament medially, and femoral vein laterally. Femoral hernias are most prevalent in middle-aged female patients, but even in this group they are less frequent than inguinal hernias. Femoral hernias may consist of preperitoneal fat only or include bowel. The narrow neck makes them prone to incarceration and strangulation.

Begin scanning at the level of inguinal ligament at the intersection with the femoral vessels and the probe parallel to the ligament (**Fig. 6.26**). Move just inferior to the ligament, and ask the patient to perform a Valsalva maneuver. Normally, the femoral vein will distend by expanding into the potential space of the canal. If a hernia is present within the canal, the femoral vein will fail to distend and may be compressed. The hernia itself may be visualized as hypoechoic bowel or just hyperechoic fat/peritoneum (**Fig. 6.31**).

Postoperative

The presentation of a lump at the site of surgery following hernia repair may be due to recurrent hernia, hematoma (**Fig. 6.32A**), seroma, or abscess. Ideally, ascertain prior to scanning whether the repair involved mesh, which

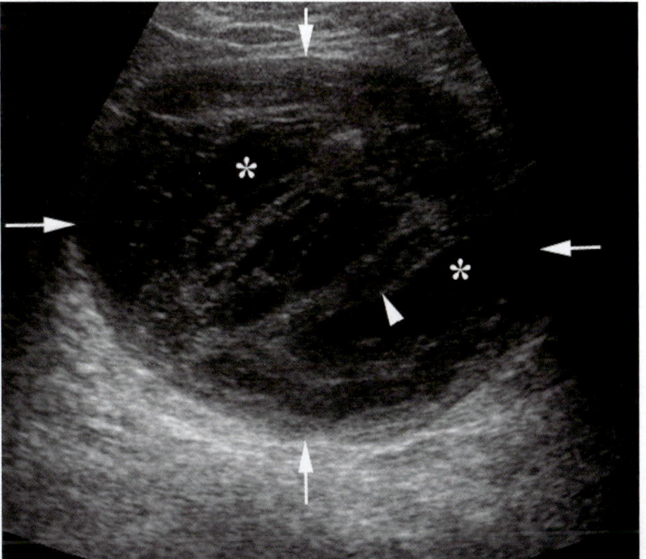

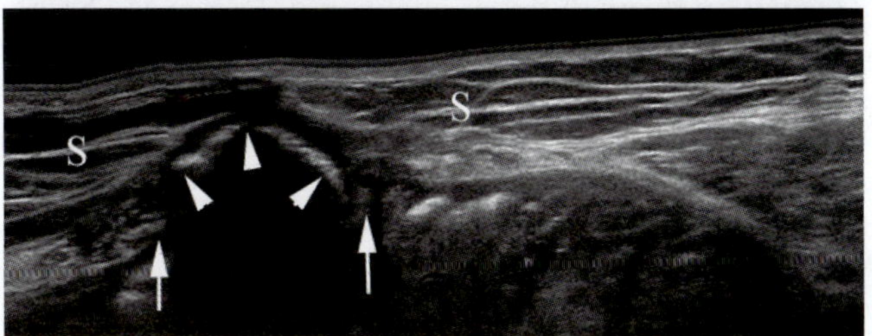

Figure 6.32. Postoperative changes. **A:** Transverse sonogram of the inguinal canal post direct hernia repair surgery shows hematoma (*arrows*) expanding the inguinal canal with echogenic stranding (*arrowhead*) and liquefied areas (*asterisk*). **B:** Longitudinal sonogram of a recurrent incisional hernia containing echogenic mesh (*arrowheads*) extending though a fascial defect (*arrows*) into the subcutaneous fat (*S*).

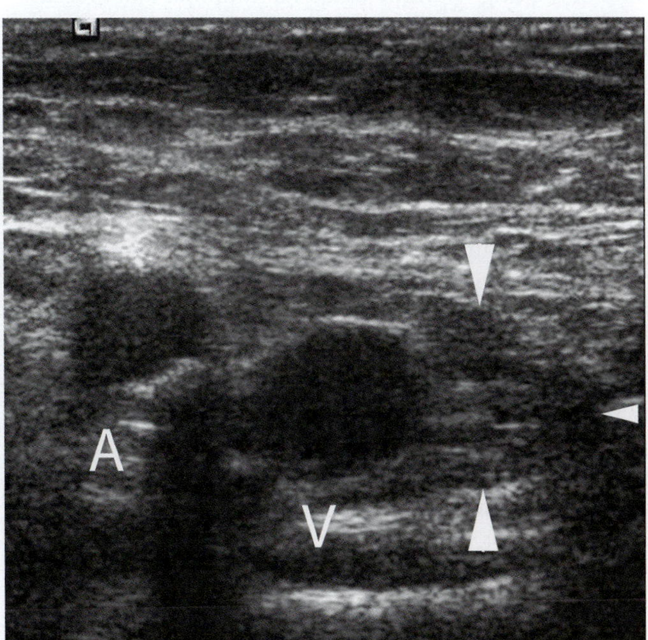

Figure 6.31. Femoral hernia. Transverse sonogram during Valsalva shows femoral hernia (*arrowheads*) medial to the femoral vein (*V*) and artery (*A*).

appears as a hyperechoic linear structure near the deep inguinal ring (**Fig. 6.32B**).

Fluid collections in the inguinal canal in the immediate postoperative period have an incidence of 0 to 17%, and are thought to be the result of surgical trauma or fluid in the hernia sac that remains after laparoscopic repair.[43] They can usually be left to reabsorb naturally unless they persist beyond 6 to 8 weeks, after which aspiration, or rarely resection, can be considered.[44] If a collection contains gas, it can be difficult to differentiate from hernia recurrence. In these cases, look for other ancillary features, such as herniated mesentery, the relationship of the mesh to the collection, and the presence of a hernia sac. CT with oral contrast may be useful.[45]

Sepsis rates after mesh repair have been reported as 0.2% to 0.8%.[43] The important distinction is whether or not any resulting collection involves the mesh, as this usually calls for mesh removal.

Spermatic cord thickening is a relatively frequent finding in the immediate postoperative period and usually resolves on follow-up.[43] Testicular complications such as pain, ischemia, epididymitis, and atrophy have been reported in 0.03% to 5.0% after laparoscopic repair.[44]

Other postoperative findings associated with groin pain and easily identified at ultrasound include neuromas and stitch granulomas.

Spigelian

Spigelian hernias are mostly acquired and are associated with raised intra-abdominal pressure, chronic obstructive pulmonary disease, obesity, collagen disorders, and laparoscopy, although congenital cases occur.[46–49] Presenting symptoms are varied, but pain with or without a palpable mass is the major presentation and may be provoked by a Valsalva maneuver. Detection and surgical correction are important due to the high incidence of strangulation (up to 21%).[47,50]

The Spigelian fascia is the aponeurotic layer between the lateral border of the rectus abdominis muscle and the medial border of the transversus abdominis muscle. Herniation through this aponeurosis is known as a Spigelian hernia **(Fig. 6.33)**. The majority occur within a 6-cm area inferior to the umbilicus.[47] They are particularly common where the inferior epigastric vessels penetrate the rectus sheath.[10] Scan with the probe transverse at the lateral margin of the rectus abdominis (linea semilunaris), from the level of the umbilicus, and move inferiorly. Careful attention should be given to the area just superior to where the inferior epigastric artery passes deep to the lateral border of rectus abdominis.[51] The report should comment on the size of any fascial defect and the nature of the contents where possible (i.e., fat or bowel).

Umbilical and Paraumbilical

These occur through and around the umbilicus in the midline, via defects in the linea alba and umbilical fascia. There is an association with abdominal distension (postpartum, ascites, and obesity). They may become more apparent if the patient is scanned while standing. Paraumbilical hernias are more common over the age of 35 years and in women than men. They are more prone to complications than true umbilical hernias and may be multiple.

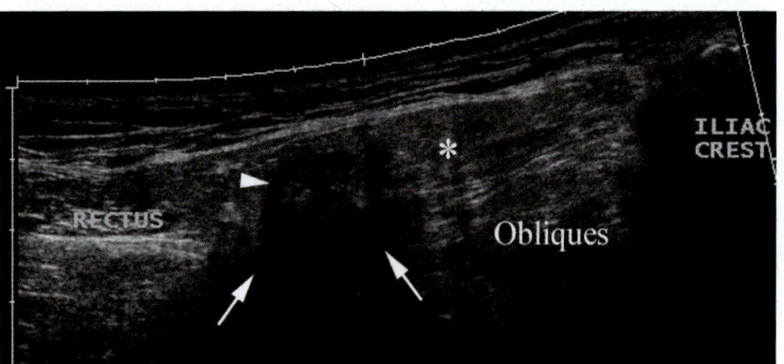

Figure 6.33. Spigelian hernia. Transverse sonogram shows Spigelian hernia of fat (*asterisk*) and edematous fat (*arrowhead*) emerging through the Spigelian fascia (*arrows*) between rectus and the oblique muscle group.

Incisional

Following surgery, the muscle and fascia commonly have residual weakness/ defects through which hernias may pass. Care should be taken not to confuse hypoechoic scar tissue and collections with hernia. Evaluate the relationship between the "hernia" and the deep fascia and any mesh present **(Fig. 6.32)**. If in doubt, CT can help, but is rarely needed unless there has been extensive surgery with an associated large fascial defect.

Sportsman's Hernia

"Sportsman's hernia" can also be known as athletic pubalgia, hockey groin, or "Gilmore's groin." These terms have arisen in association with chronic groin pain in athletes. The exact etiology and pathology are poorly understood, and there is no consensus as to what constitutes the diagnosis.[52]

Clinical presentation is typically groin pain that occurs during activity and is associated with stiffness following a rest period such as overnight sleep. Warm-up routines may provide relief, but more intense activities, such as kicking, exacerbate symptoms. Coughing, sneezing, and other sudden movements can also exacerbate the pain. Symptoms last for months and cause significant disruption to training schedules. Hip extension, twisting, turning, and sudden directional changes have all been implicated as biomechanical causes. Several potential underlying pathological processes have been proposed, with true hernia often being absent. Theories suggest that the injury occurs due to imbalance between the strong adductor muscles of the thigh and the weaker abdominal wall muscles.[53]

Gilmore described groin disruption comprising a combination of a torn external oblique aponeurosis with dilated superficial inguinal ring, torn conjoined tendon, and dehiscence between the inguinal ligament and conjoined tendon **(Fig. 6.34)**.[54] Several variations have been described.[52,54–57] A recent systematic review of the literature found that the most common surgical finding was posterior inguinal wall insufficiency resulting in an occult hernia that was not apparent on clinical examination.[52] Other proposed causes of groin pain include rectus abdominis insertion tears, osteitis pubis, pubic stress fractures, adductor enthesis injury, and entrapment of the ilioinguinal nerve. Referred pain from the spine, hip, or even knee may also manifest as groin pain.

Conservative treatments involve rest, strengthening, and stretching exercises and NSAIDs. Surgical treatments involve strengthening the abdominal wall musculature and fascia around the inguinal ligament and are variations of the traditional inguinal hernia repair. The literature favors surgical outcomes, but there is a lack of clinical trials.[10,52,58,53]

The role of ultrasound is to exclude true inguinal hernia and assess for signs of significant acute muscle or

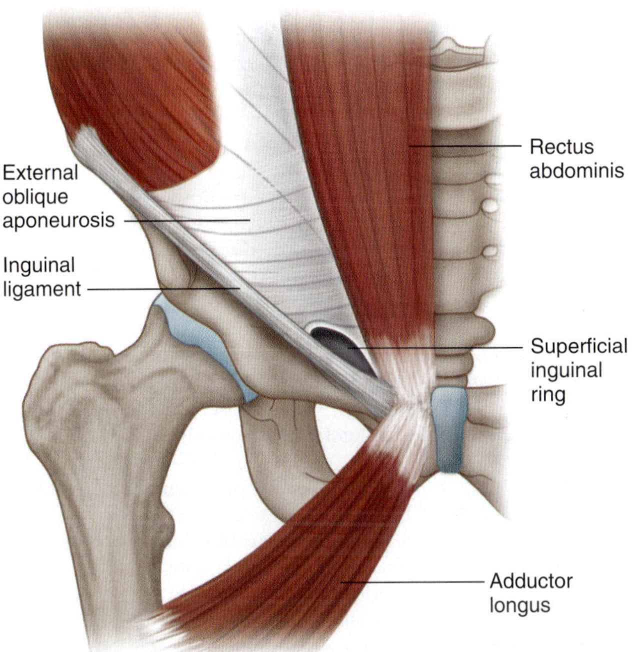

Figure 6.34. Anatomy of sportsman's hernias. The potentially affected areas of the inguinal region are shown: external oblique aponeurosis, superficial inguinal ring, inguinal ligament, rectus abdominis, and adductor longus junction at the symphysis pubis.

tendon injury such as edema, hematoma, or retraction **(Fig. 6.24A)**. However, these abnormalities are frequently absent at ultrasound in athletes with chronic pubalgia. Similarly, the adductor origin is usually "normal" at ultrasound. Tendon thickening and pubic cortical irregularity are commonly seen in athletes over the age of 20, making these findings nonspecific **(Fig. 6.24B)**. Patients with suspected sports hernias often go on to surgery/laparoscopy, which can identify small aponeurotic, muscular, or tendinous tears not seen at ultrasound. During the examination, note any focal areas of tenderness under transducer pressure, as this may give clues to the affected structure.

Diagnostic/therapeutic injections to the pubic symphysis and adductor origin have been used in the setting of groin pain.[59–61] Care should be taken to avoid the medial aspect of the inguinal canal.

The Role of MRI in Chronic Pubalgia

Magnetic resonance imaging is useful for detection of edema of the adductor enthesis and pubic symphysis, which are usually not apparent on ultrasound. The wide field of view is helpful in reviewing the multiple structures that may potentially be responsible, but inguinal canal abnormality is rarely demonstrated. Plain film may occasionally be useful in revealing suspected stress fractures, but degenerative symphyseal and remodeling changes are often seen in asymptomatic active

subjects.[10,40] Herniography has also been described in this clinical context.[62]

NERVE PATHOLOGY

Femoral

The femoral nerve courses down the lateral border of psoas major and runs in the groove between psoas and iliacus. It runs lateral to the femoral artery as it enters the thigh deep to the inguinal ligament, where it then divides into multiple branches in the femoral triangle. Injuries can occur during lower abdominal surgery, such as appendectomy and hernia repair, pelvic fractures, hematoma, penetrating wounds, abscesses, tumors, or diabetic neuropathy. Clinical presentation includes groin pain, weakness of hip flexion and knee extension, and anterior thigh sensory deficit. The saphenous nerve arises from the femoral nerve, and sensation medially below the knee may also be affected. Scanning the nerve transversely along its superficial course allows detection of scars and masses, which may be causing symptoms. In the event of deeper/pelvic pathology, CT or MRI offer superior views of the pelvic contents or nerve origins respectively.

Sciatic

Sciatic nerve pathology at the level of the hip may present as posterior hip pain radiating down the back of the thigh or in the case of serious injury, paralysis of the hamstrings and muscles below the knee and sensory loss of the posterior/lateral calf and sole of the foot. The most common cause of pathology at this level is trauma, either fracture dislocation of the hip or iatrogenic injury as a result of hip replacement. Acute nerve injuries occur due to instrumentation, hip dislocation, and traction during surgery, or as a consequence of the resulting hematoma, or leg lengthening. Scar and callus formation adjacent to the nerve following injuries, prolonged bed rest, and the piriformis muscle (piriformis syndrome) have also been implicated in sciatic nerve impingement.

The role of ultrasound is to identify abnormality in the nerve such as disruption of the normal fibrillar architecture, swelling, or edema, and to assess for adjacent sources of compression such as a mass or scarring. The symptoms can be mimicked by ischiogluteal bursitis, and this area should be evaluated during scanning. Magnetic resonance imaging offers a superior alternative for the identification of deeper and more proximal lesions such as piriformis anomalies and can identify pathology arising from the nerve roots.

Lateral Cutaneous Nerve of the Thigh

Entrapment of this nerve results in pain and paresthesia in the lateral and anterolateral aspects of the thigh.

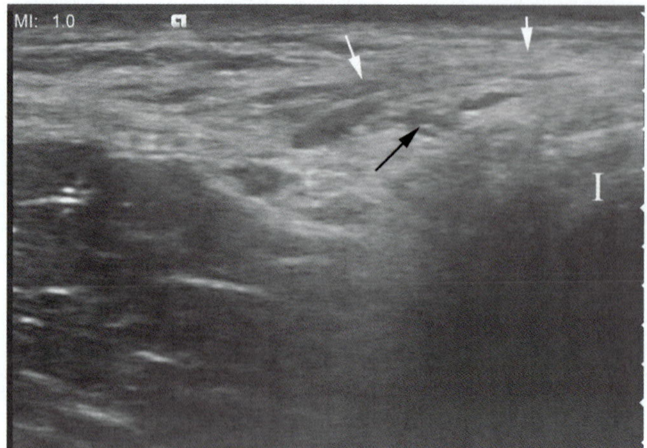

Figure 6.35. Lateral cutaneous nerve. Transverse sonogram shows normal lateral cutaneous nerve (*black arrow*) deep to the inguinal ligament (*white arrows*) inferior to the anterior superior iliac spine (*I*).

It arises from L2 to L4, forms within the psoas, and courses over the iliacus and travels posterior to the inguinal ligament **(Fig. 6.35)**. It is at this point that entrapment usually occurs. The nerve then continues over sartorius into the thigh. Nerve pathology may arise from intrapelvic causes such as masses or inflammatory processes like diverticulitis/appendicitis. Extrapelvic causes include trauma, for example, from seat belts in motor vehicle collisions and clothing (e.g., belts or pressure from obesity). Prolonged sitting and standing have also been implicated. Ultrasound may reveal the intrapelvic causes, though if these are suspected, CT/MRI may also be required. More superficially, the course of the nerve should be traced in transverse section as it is passed under the inguinal ligament, close to the ASIS, with a high-frequency probe. Look for hematomas, masses, and scarring in the adjacent tissue. However, appearances are often normal, but diagnostic injection can be performed with local anesthetic at the level of the ASIS just deep to the inguinal ligament. If positive, a more lasting effect may be achieved with steroid.

REFERENCES

1. Bianchi S, Martinoli C. *Ultrasound of the Musculoskeletal System.* 1st ed. New York, NY: Springer; 2007.
2. Bierma-Zeinstra SM, Bohnen AM, Verhaar JA, et al. Sonography for hip joint effusion in adults with hip pain. *Ann Rheum Dis.* 2000;59(3):178–182.
3. Bureau NJ, Chhem RK, Cardinal E. Musculoskeletal infections: US manifestations. *Radiographics.* 1999;19(6):1585–1592.
4. Van Holsbeeck MT, Introcaso JH. *Musculoskeletal Ultrasound.* 2nd ed. St. Louis, MO: Mosby; 2001.
5. Lin HM, Learch TJ, White EA, et al. Emergency joint aspiration: a guide for radiologists on call. *Radiographics.* 2009;29(4): 1139–1158.
6. Goldenberg DL. Septic arthritis. *Lancet.* 1998;351(9097): 197–202.
7. Fessell DP, Jacobson JA, Craig J, et al. Using sonography to reveal and aspirate joint effusions. *AJR Am J Roentgenol.* 2000;174(5):1353–1362.
8. Van Holsbeeck MT, Eyler WR, Sherman LS, et al. Detection of infection in loosened hip prostheses: efficacy of sonography. *AJR Am J Roentgenol.* 1994;163(2):381–384.
9. Breidahl WH, Newman JS, Taljanovic MS, et al. Power Doppler sonography in the assessment of musculoskeletal fluid collections. *AJR Am J Roentgenol.* 1996;166(6):1443–1446.
10. Allan PL, Baxter GM, Weston MJ. *Clinical Ultrasound.* 3rd ed. Philadelphia, PA: Churchill Livingstone; 2011.
11. Zieger MM, Dörr U, Schulz RD. Ultrasonography of hip joint effusions. *Skeletal Radiol.* 1987;16(8):607–611.
12. Koski JM, Anttila PJ, Isomäki HA. Ultrasonography of the adult hip joint. *Scand J Rheumatol.* 1989;18(2):113–117.
13. Nimityongskul P, McBryde AM Jr, Anderson LD, et al. Ultrasonography in the management of painful hips in children. *Am J Orthop (Belle Mead NJ).* 1996;25(6):411–414.
14. McNally EG. *Practical Musculoskeletal Ultrasound.* 1st ed. Philadelphia, PA: Churchill Livingstone; 2004.
15. Webb ST, Ghosh S. Intra-articular bupivacaine: potentially chondrotoxic? *Br J Anaesth.* 2009;102(4):439–441.
16. Hoefnagels EM, Obradov M, Reijnierse M, et al. Sonography after total hip replacement: reproducibility and normal values in 47 clinically uncomplicated cases. *Acta Orthop.* 2007;78(1):81–85.
17. Parrini L, Baratelli M, Parrini M. Ultrasound examination of haematomas after total hip replacement. *Int Orthop.* 1988;12(1):79–82.
18. Kong K, Jeyagopal N, Davies SJ. Should we still stitch the subcutaneous fat layer? A clinical and ultrasound assessment in 50 hip operations. *Ann R Coll Surg Engl.* 1993;75(1): 23–25.
19. Fang CS, Harvie P, Gibbons CL, et al. The imaging spectrum of peri-articular inflammatory masses following metal-on-metal hip resurfacing. *Skeletal Radiol.* 2008;37(8):715–722.
20. Marmery H, Ostlere S. Imaging of prosthetic joints. *Imaging.* 2007;19:299–309.
21. Tsukayama DT, Estrada R, Gustilo RB. Infection after total hip arthroplasty. A study of the treatment of one hundred and six infections. *J Bone Joint Surg Am.* 1996;78(4):512–523.
22. Berquist TH, Bender CE, Maus TP, et al. Pseudobursae: a useful finding in patients with painful hip arthroplasty. *AJR Am J Roentgenol.* 1987;148(1):103–106.
23. Lequesne M, Dang N, Montagne P, et al. Conflict between psoas and total hip prosthesis [in French]. *Rev Rhum Mal Osteoartic.* 1991;58(9):559–564.
24. Rezig R, Copercini M, Montet X, et al. Ultrasound diagnosis of anterior iliopsoas impingement in total hip replacement. *Skeletal Radiol.* 2004;33(2):112–116.
25. Jasani V, Richards P, Wynn-Jones C. Pain related to the psoas muscle after total hip replacement. *J Bone Joint Surg Br.* 2002;84(7):991–993.
26. Iorio R, Healy WL. Heterotopic ossification after hip and knee arthroplasty: risk factors, prevention, and treatment. *J Am Acad Orthop Surg.* 2002;10(6):409–416.
27. Malchau H, Herberts P, Eisler T, et al. The Swedish total hip replacement register. *J Bone Joint Surg Am.* 2002;84-A(suppl 2):2–20.
28. Willert H-G, Buchhorn GH, Fayyazi A, et al. Metal-on-metal bearings and hypersensitivity in patients with artificial hip joints. A clinical and histomorphological study. *J Bone Joint Surg Am.* 2005;87(1):28–36.
29. Mistry A, Cahir J, Donell ST, et al. MRI of asymptomatic patients with metal-on-metal and polyethylene-on-metal total hip arthroplasties. *Clin Radiol.* 2011;66(6):540–545.

30. Toms AP, Marshall TJ, Cahir J, et al. MRI of early symptomatic metal-on-metal total hip arthroplasty: a retrospective review of radiological findings in 20 hips. *Clin Radiol.* 2008;63(1):49–58.

31. Visuri T, Borg H, Pulkkinen P, et al. A retrospective comparative study of mortality and causes of death among patients with metal-on-metal and metal-on-polyethylene total hip prostheses in primary osteoarthritis after a long-term follow-up. *BMC Musculoskelet Disord.* 2010;11:78.

32. Adler RS, Buly R, Ambrose R, et al. Diagnostic and therapeutic use of sonography-guided iliopsoas peritendinous injections. *AJR Am J Roentgenol.* 2005;185(4):940–943.

33. Blankenbaker DG, De Smet AA, Keene JS. Sonography of the iliopsoas tendon and injection of the iliopsoas bursa for diagnosis and management of the painful snapping hip. *Skeletal Radiol.* 2006;35(8):565–571.

34. Jacobson T, Allen WC. Surgical correction of the snapping iliopsoas tendon. *Am J Sports Med.* 1990;18(5):470–474.

35. Pelsser V, Cardinal E, Hobden R, et al. Extraarticular snapping hip: sonographic findings. *AJR Am J Roentgenol.* 2001;176(1):67–73.

36. Bass CJ, Connell DA. Sonographic findings of tensor fascia lata tendinopathy: another cause of anterior groin pain. *Skeletal Radiol.* 2002;31(3):143–148.

37. Robinson P, Farrant JM, Bourke G, et al. Ultrasound and MRI findings in appendicular and truncal fat necrosis. *Skeletal Radiol.* 2008;37(3):217–224.

38. Parra JA, Fernandez MA, Encinas B, et al. Morel-Lavallée effusions in the thigh. *Skeletal Radiol.* 1997;26(4):239–241.

39. Connell DA, Bass C, Sykes CA, et al. Sonographic evaluation of gluteus medius and minimus tendinopathy. *Eur Radiol.* 2003;13(6):1339–1347.

40. Robinson P, Barron DA, Parsons W, et al. Adductor-related groin pain in athletes: correlation of MR imaging with clinical findings. *Skeletal Radiol.* 2004;33(8):451–457.

41. Robinson P, Hensor E, Lansdown MJ, et al. Inguinofemoral hernia: accuracy of sonography in patients with indeterminate clinical features. *AJR Am J Roentgenol.* 2006;187(5):1168–1178.

42. van den Berg JC, de Valois JC, Go PM, et al. Detection of groin hernia with physical examination, ultrasound, and MRI compared with laparoscopic findings. *Invest Radiol.* 1999;34(12):739–743.

43. Parra JA, Revuelta S, Gallego T, et al. Prosthetic mesh used for inguinal and ventral hernia repair: normal appearance and complications in ultrasound and CT. *Br J Radiol.* 2004;77(915):261–265.

44. Bendavid R. Complications of groin hernia surgery. *Surg Clin North Am.* 1998;78(6):1089–1103.

45. Lin BH, Vargish T, Dachman AH. CT findings after laparoscopic repair of ventral hernia. *AJR Am J Roentgenol.* 1999;172(2):389–392.

46. Read RC. Observations on the etiology of spigelian hernia. *Ann Surg.* 1960;152:1004–1009.

47. Vos DI, Scheltinga MR. Incidence and outcome of surgical repair of spigelian hernia. *Br J Surg.* 2004;91(5):640–644.

48. Al-Salem AH. Congenital spigelian hernia and cryptorchidism: cause or coincidence? *Pediatr Surg Int.* 2000;16(5–6):433–436.

49. Fitzgibbons RJ Jr, Greenburg AG, Nyhus LM. *Nyhus and Condon's Hernia.* Philadelphia, PA: Lippincott William & Wilkins; 2002.

50. Larson DW, Farley DR. Spigelian hernias: repair and outcome for 81 patients. *World J Surg.* 2002;26(10):1277–1281.

51. Jamadar DA, Jacobson JA, Morag Y, et al. Sonography of inguinal region hernias. *AJR Am J Roentgenol.* 2006;187(1):185–190.

52. Caudill P, Nyland J, Smith C, et al. Sports hernias: a systematic literature review. *Br J Sports Med.* 2008;42(12):954–964.

53. LeBlanc KE, LeBlanc KA. Groin pain in athletes. *Hernia.* 2003;7(2):68–71.

54. Williams P, Foster ME. 'Gilmore's groin'—or is it? *Br J Sports Med.* 1995;29(3):206–208.

55. Irshad K, Feldman LS, Lavoie C, et al. Operative management of "hockey groin syndrome": 12 years of experience in National Hockey League players. *Surgery.* 2001;130(4):759–766.

56. Joesting DR. Diagnosis and treatment of sportsman's hernia. *Curr Sports Med Rep.* 2002;1(2):121–124.

57. Paluska SA. An overview of hip injuries in running. *Sports Med.* 2005;35(11):991–1014.

58. Morelli V, Smith V. Groin injuries in athletes. *Am Fam Physician.* 2001;64(8):1405–1414.

59. Schilders E, Talbot JC, Robinson P, et al. Adductor-related groin pain in recreational athletes: role of the adductor enthesis, magnetic resonance imaging, and entheseal pubic cleft injections. *J Bone Joint Surg Am.* 2009;91(10):2455–2460.

60. Holt MA, Keene JS, Graf BK, et al. Treatment of osteitis pubis in athletes. Results of corticosteroid injections. *Am J Sports Med.* 1995;23(5):601–606.

61. O'Connell MJ, Powell T, McCaffrey NM, et al. Symphyseal cleft injection in the diagnosis and treatment of osteitis pubis in athletes. *AJR Am J Roentgenol.* 2002;179(4):955–959.

62. Smedberg SG, Broome AE, Gullmo A, et al. Herniography in athletes with groin pain. *Am J Surg.* 1985;149(3):378–382.

CHAPTER

7

Knee

David Connell
Guilio Comin

INTRODUCTION

Ultrasound (US) is frequently used to guide percutaneous intervention in and around the knee joint and for the diagnosis of juxta-articular tendinopathies. Beyond this, some may consider ultrasound of the knee to be rather limited, with little else to contribute. Magnetic resonance imaging (MRI) is often favored as a multipurpose tool for the evaluation of the knee, allowing an overall inspection of structures in and around the joint. However, ultrasound is often superior to MRI for the assessment of superficial structures such as tendons and is surprisingly capable for the assessment of deeper structures. As technology and operator experience have improved, the scope and application of diagnostic ultrasound have enlarged. Its utility has been demonstrated for the assessment of cartilage degeneration,[1-3] chondrocalcinosis,[4] anterior cruciate ligament rupture,[5] meniscal injuries,[6,7] impingement by intra-articular plicae,[8] "snapping" syndromes,[9] and other intra-articular pathology that are often considered the exclusive domain of MRI. Ultrasound has a major advantage over MRI when there has been a knee joint replacement, which usually results in substantial artifact, and has proven utility in diagnosis of postoperative complaints such as fibrous impingement[10] and prosthetic loosening.[11]

Aside from its capability in tendon imaging due to excellent near-field spatial resolution and useful technical applications such as color Doppler and elastography, the main advantages of ultrasound are the ability to perform focussed examinations at sites of interest, during dynamic movement, and in varying positions.

CLINICAL ASSESSMENT

Ultrasound of the knee is predicated on targeted and dynamic scanning. When performed without consideration for the clinical features, this advantage is lost and ultrasound becomes less fruitful. Clinical assessment is an integral component of ultrasound examination of the knee and commences before meeting the patient, with an evaluation of the patient's age. Children, young adults, and old adults are more likely to present with some specific pathologies than others. For example,

anterior knee pain in a young child raises suspicion of Osgood–Schlatter disease, in an older child or a young adult of patellar tendinopathy, in a middle-aged adult of fat pad impingement or plica syndromes, and in an older adult of patellofemoral osteoarthritis. The patient's stance and gait on entering the examination room give useful cues to the site and severity of pathology before any words have been spoken.

History Taking

The patient should be asked to recount current symptoms and concerns, recent and previous injuries, and previous surgery, and should be given time to do so without prompting or interruption, as valuable information can be brought to light that would otherwise be missed. The most important information to be gleaned includes:

- Acute injury versus gradual development.
- The nature of the injury or the activity(ies) that led to symptom development.
- The type of symptom: pain, swelling, locking or snapping, stiffness, etc.
- Region of symptoms. This can be grossly characterized as anterior, posterior, lateral, or medial, but patients are often able to localize pain with a fingertip, particularly in tendinopathies.
- Exacerbating and relieving factors.
- When pain is the predominant symptom, the type of pain: dull, sharp, burning, vague, etc.
- The patient's physical abilities and requirements: the type and "seriousness" of any sports played, the nature of their work, etc.
- History of surgery and/or prior treatments.

Physical Examination

This should be performed in the ultrasound room with the lights fully up to permit proper observation of sometimes subtle clinical findings such as swelling, redness, bruising, surgical scars, or muscle wasting. Palpation should be performed for confirmation of tenderness or lump. It is often useful to mark regions of interest with a pen. The dynamic part of the clinical examination is usually best done with the ultrasound probe. A number of tests have been described and validated. An in-depth discussion of their technique is beyond the scope of this chapter, but it may help sonologists to learn some of the more frequently used ones such as Apley, patella apprehension, Lachman, and anterior and posterior drawer tests.

Clinical Correlation

Perhaps the most important reason for ensuring that a good history and examination have been performed is to allow a final consideration of the ultrasound findings in light of the clinical presentation. Do the ultrasound abnormalities explain all of the patient's symptoms? If so, is the severity of the symptoms concordant with the severity of the ultrasound abnormality? If not, further investigation is required, perhaps with a different imaging modality, such as radiography or MRI, especially if there is suspicion of meniscal, bony, or chondral pathology.

ANATOMY

As ultrasound technology has improved, the anatomical knowledge required to perform and interpret ultrasound of the knee has increased. In the 1980s ultrasound involved a comparatively crude visualization of the juxtaarticular tendons and assessment for joint effusion or Baker cyst. Current scanners allow visualization and characterization of intra-articular structures such as meniscus and cartilage, discrimination of tendons and capsule into component parts, and identification of fine nerve and vessel branches.

As knowledge of knee mechanics and pathology has improved, there has been renewed interest in once obscure anatomical details, such as the vastus medialis insertion or the posterolateral capsular structures. The sonologist requires a wider and more intricate awareness of the normal location, function, and appearance of these structures.

Although a full description of this anatomy would require much more space than is available here, we will attempt to provide an overview and highlight the clinically and sonographically important points by breaking the anatomy down into its constituent parts:

Bone: Bone edges, periosteum, and tendon and ligament insertions.
Joint: Articular cartilage, meniscus and joint fluid.
Ligaments and Capsule
Tendons and Muscle
Bursae
Fat and fibrous layers
Nerves
Vessels

Bones

There are four or five bones at the knee joint: Femur, tibia, fibula, patella, and the inconsistently present fabella. The tibia and femur articulate at two surfaces or compartments: the medial femoral condyle with the medial tibial plateau, and the lateral femoral condyle with the lateral tibial plateau (**Figs. 7.1 and 7.2**). The medial articulation provides flexion and extension, while the

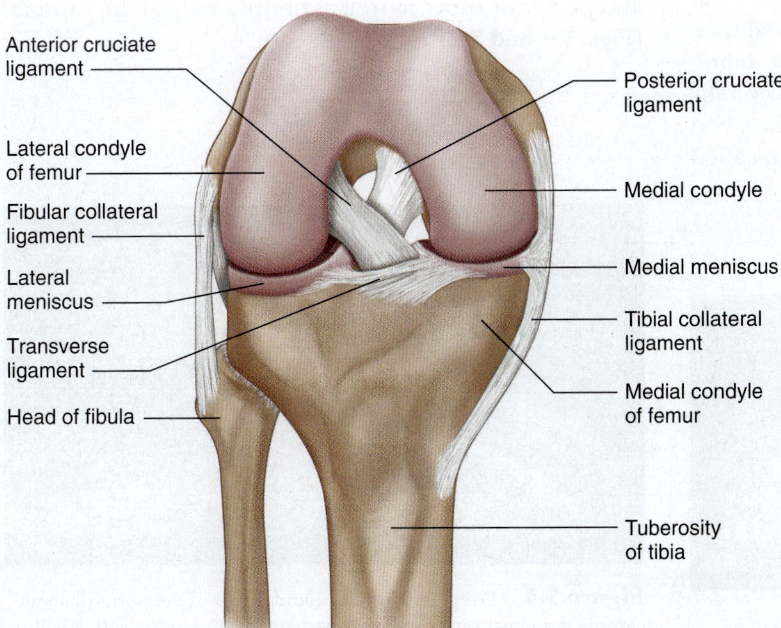

Figure 7.1. Deep dissection diagram of the anterior knee demonstrating the articular surfaces and the menisci.

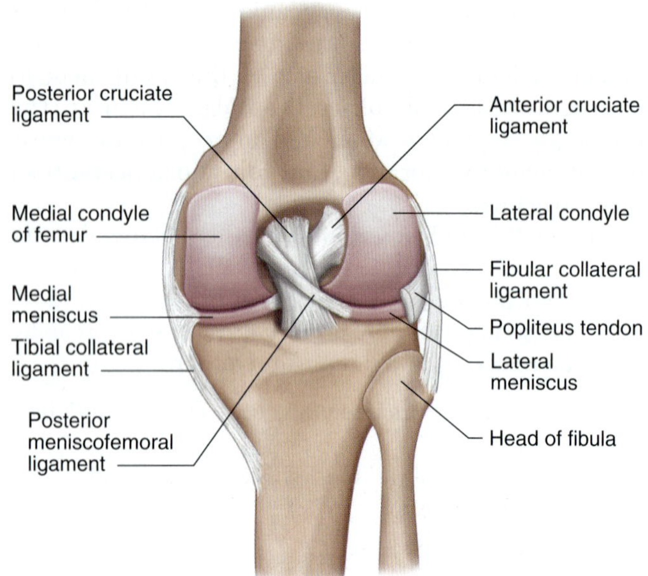

Figure 7.2.   Deep dissection diagram of the posterior knee demonstrating the articular surfaces and the menisci.

lateral articulation additionally provides some rotation and anterior/posterior translation.

The patella articulates with the trochlea of the femur, a V-shaped groove, with medial and lateral facets of variable inclination that articulate with the medial and lateral patellar facets, respectively. A third and small "odd" patellar facet lies most medially and only articulates with the trochlea beyond 90 degrees of flexion.[12]

A bipartite (or tripartite) patella is a variant that results from failure of fusion of an accessory ossification center(s) with the remainder of the patella **(Fig. 7.3)**. It occurs in 2% of the population, is more common in males than in females,[13] and is typically, but not always, superolaterally located. As well as potentially being mistaken for a fracture, a bipartite patella occasionally becomes symptomatic when the fibrous union between the ossified parts is placed under stress. The so-called

"dorsal defect of the patella" is a similar but incomplete bony defect in a superolateral position; it is unclear whether this is a related forme fruste of bipartite patella or an acquired lesion.

The base of the lateral tibial plateau articulates with the medial fibular head to form the proximal tibiofibular joint.

The fabella is a sesamoid bone that lies posteriorly, usually laterally, occasionally medially, and has a synovial articulation with the posterior femoral condyle. It is found, in varying states of ossification, in up to two-thirds of subjects,[14] and has a potentially important role in stabilization of the posterior (and particularly posterolateral) capsule. When lateral, it has a complex relationship with the lateral gastrocnemius **(Fig. 7.4)** and plantaris tendons, and the oblique popliteal, arcuate, and fabellofibular ligaments (see below).

Bony prominences around the knee joint that are important and reliable landmarks for tendon insertion include the tibial tuberosity (for the patellar tendon) and Gerdy tubercle (for the iliotibial band [ITB]).

Joints

There are three consistent and distinct articulations at the knee. The largest are the tibiofemoral joint, which is further divided into medial and lateral compartments, and the patellofemoral joint. They share a common synovial cavity. Their articular surfaces are covered by hyaline cartilage of varying thickness. The medial and lateral menisci are interposed between the respective tibiofemoral articular surfaces. Menisci are fibrocartilaginous structures and act as shock absorbers and distributors of force, helping to maintain stability of the joint. They are attached centrally to the tibia by their anterior and posterior roots, as well as peripherally to the capsule. **(Figs. 7.1 and 7.2)**

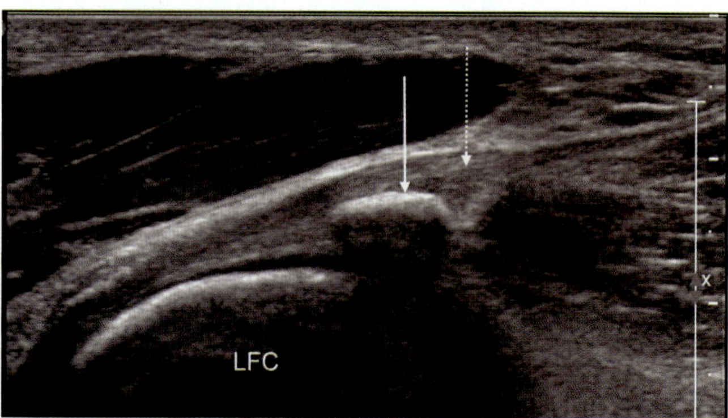

Figure 7.3.   Transverse ultrasound image of the patella demonstrating a bipartite patella (*arrows*).

Figure 7.4.   Longitudinal ultrasound image of the posterolateral capsule demonstrating the lateral gastrocnemius tendon with fabella (*arrow*). Lateral gastrocnemius tendon (*dashed arrow*).

Plicae are folds of synovium within the knee joint. They are remnants of embryological structures and have three common locations in the knee:

- Infrapatellar (ligamentum mucosum): Running obliquely in the intercondylar notch, in front of the anterior cruciate ligament (ACL).
- Suprapatellar: Running vertically in the suprapatellar recess.
- Mediopatellar: Running vertically at the medial aspect of the knee joint. When large, its free border can extend into the medial aspect of the patellofemoral joint, potentially resulting in symptomatic irritation.

The proximal tibiofibular joint is a separate, small joint and has its own synovial lining and hyaline cartilage surfaces.

Ligaments

The ligaments of the knee are classified as intra-articular or capsular.

The intra-articular ligaments are the cruciate ligaments and the variably present and thick meniscal and meniscofemoral ligaments.

The ACL originates from the posterolateral wall of the intercondylar notch and passes caudally, anteriorly, and medially to insert on the anterior tibial plateau, in front of the tibial spine **(Figs. 7.1 and 7.2)**. It has two principal components, named for their position at the tibial insertion: The larger posterolateral bundle and the smaller anteromedial bundle. The former resists anterior translation in extension, and the latter resists anterior translation in flexion.

The posterior cruciate ligament (PCL) arises from the anteromedial wall of the intercondylar notch and passes caudally, posteriorly, and laterally to insert on the posterior aspect of the tibia, inferior to the tibial plateau **(Figs. 7.1 and 7.2)**. It has two principal components: The larger anterolateral bundle and the smaller posteromedial bundle. The former resists posterior translation in flexion, and the latter resists posterior translation in extension.

The most anatomically consistent meniscal ligament is the transverse or meniscomeniscal ligament or intermeniscal ligament. The other meniscomeniscal ligaments are the posterior transverse ligament, connecting the posterior horns of the menisci, and the medial and lateral oblique ligaments, connecting the anterior and posterior horns. The meniscofemoral ligaments run from the posterior horn of the lateral meniscus to the posterolateral aspect of the medial femoral condyle, the ligament of Wrisberg posterior to the PCL and the ligament of Humphrey anterior to the PCL. There is no literature regarding ultrasound assessment of these structures, and they are not currently considered particularly clinically significant.

The capsular ligaments are focal condensations of the joint capsule and adjacent tissues. The largest are the medial and lateral collateral ligaments. They are thin elongated structures, are well defined, and have a lamellar appearance. The medial or tibial collateral ligament (MCL) arises from the medial femoral condyle and runs to insert on the medial edge of the tibia, well below the joint line **(Fig. 7.5)**. It acts as a restraint to valgus angulation and external rotation. It is a discrete structure on ultrasound but blends imperceptibly at its anterior and

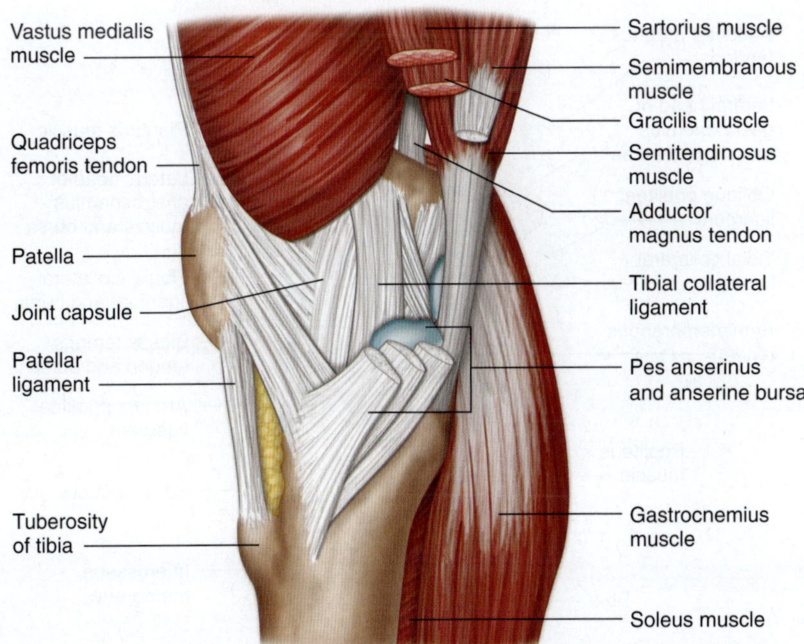

Figure 7.5. Superficial dissection diagram of the medial knee showing ligaments and bursa.

posterior borders with the adjacent superficial capsule. The superficial capsule at the anterior edge is composed of fibers from the MCL, fibers from the pes anserinus tendons (described below) and the so-called "crural" fascia. The superficial capsule at the posterior edge is composed of fibers from the MCL (the so-called posterior oblique ligament) and fibers from the semimembranosus tendon (described below) **(Fig. 7.6)**. At the deep surface of the MCL are ligamentous attachments to the meniscus and the adjacent bones at the level of the joint, the meniscofemoral and meniscotibial (or coronary) ligaments, which are all well seen at ultrasound.[15]

The lateral collateral ligament (LCL) arises from the lateral femoral epicondyle and runs posterolaterally to insert on the head of the fibula, often blending with the insertion of the biceps femoris **(Fig. 7.7)**. Anteriorly, it may blend with the ITB insertion. The LCL primarily resists varus angulation and internal rotation and is well seen at ultrasound.

The capsuloligamentous anatomy at the posterior edge of the LCL (dubbed the posterolateral corner [PLC]) is both complex and clinically important. The PLC is primarily a restraint against varus angulation and external rotation. Identifying injuries to this area has important implications for surgical repair. Ultrasound is useful,[16] and possibly superior to MRI, which is slightly handicapped by magic angle artifacts and the non-orthogonal orientation of the structures. The main components of the posterolateral corner are **(Fig. 7.6)**:

- Arcuate ligament: arises from the fibular tip and has a limb that passes posteriorly to form part of the posterior joint capsule, and a limb that passes superiorly to

the lateral femoral condyle, paralleling the course of the LCL.
- Popliteus tendon: runs from the popliteal groove of the lateral femoral condyle (an easy sonographic landmark), behind the joint and deep to the arcuate ligament, to the posteromedial tibia.
- Fabellofibular ligament: passes from fabella to fibular head.
- Popliteofibular ligament: passes from the popliteus to the fibular head.
- Meniscopopliteal ligament: passes from the popliteus to the lateral meniscus. This structure may be important in facilitating the important role of popliteus in stabilizing the lateral meniscus.

All except the meniscopopliteal ligament are visible by ultrasound.[17]

The ligaments vary in size between individuals. In particular, the size of the arcuate ligament is inversely proportional to the size of the fabellofibular ligament, which in turn is variably important depending on the presence or absence of the fabella.[18]

Tendons

The tendons around the knee are classified into three groups: Anterior, posteromedial, and lateral.

Anteriorly, the quadriceps tendon is formed by the confluence of fibers from rectus femoris, vastus lateralis, vastus medialis, and vastus intermedius. It has a trilaminar appearance, often appreciable on ultrasound with the superficial layer formed by fascicles from rectus femoris, the middle layer by fascicles from vastus medialis and

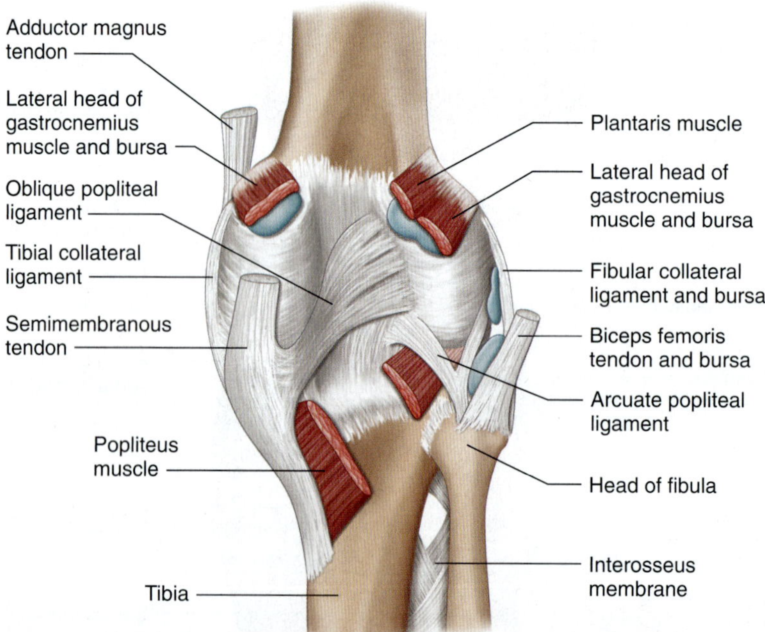

Figure 7.6. Superficial dissection diagram of the posterior knee showing posterior ligaments and bursa.

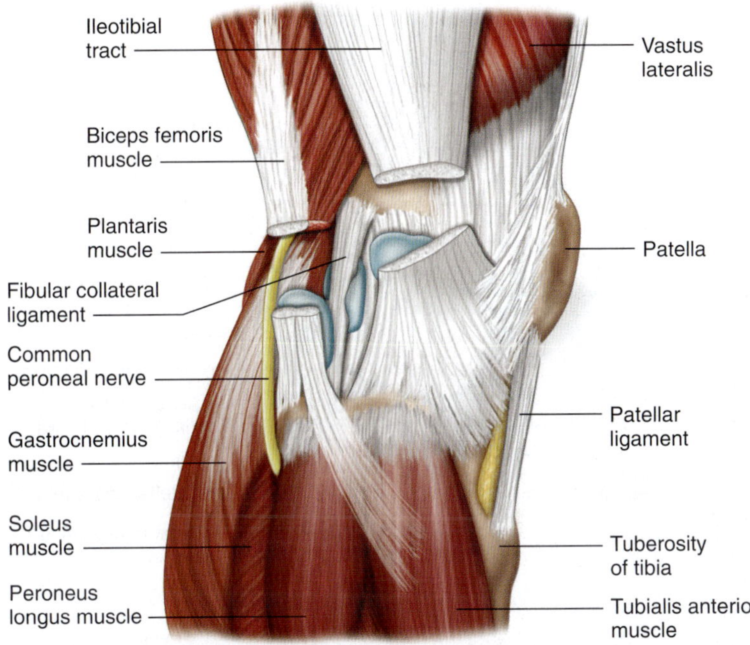

Figure 7.7. Superficial dissection diagram of the lateral knee showing ligaments and bursa.

vastus lateralis, and the deep layer by fascicles from vastus intermedius **(Fig. 7.8)**. The three layers are not completely fused and do have some degree of independent differential movement on knee extension. The quadriceps tendon inserts on the superior pole of the patella. The patellar tendon passes from the inferior pole of the patella to the tibial tubercle. Variable amounts of superficial quadriceps fibers run across the anterior surface of the patella and contribute to the patellar tendon. Strictly speaking, the non-quadriceps component of the patellar tendon is not a tendon as it connects bone with bone and should be more accurately described as a ligament.

The patellar tendon is contiguous on either side with the medial and lateral patellar retinacula, which are important in ensuring appropriate patellar tracking. The medial retinaculum is formed by condensation of the joint capsule, medial fibers of the vastus medialis tendon (the so-called vastus medialis obliquus [VMO], and the medial patellofemoral ligament (MPFL), which arises from the adductor tubercle. The VMO and MPFL are important structures, both visible at ultrasound.[19–21] The lateral retinaculum is formed by fibers from the vastus lateralis, ITB, and condensation of the joint capsule, and often has a bilaminar appearance

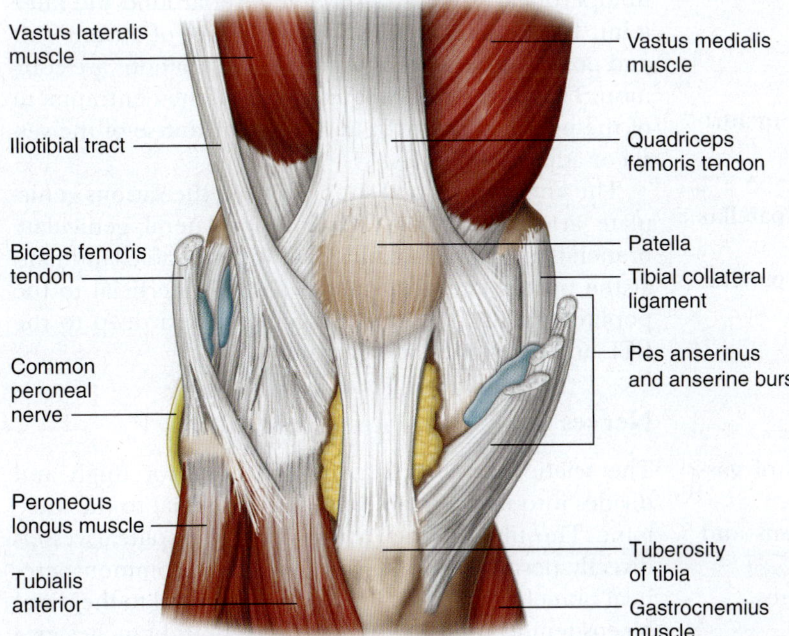

Figure 7.8. Superficial dissection diagram of the anterior knee showing the extensor mechanism.

on ultrasound.[22] The superficial layer is believed to be formed predominantly from the musculotendinous contributions, and the deep layer predominantly from the capsular contribution.

Posteromedially are the internal rotators and flexors (**Fig. 7.5**). The semimembranosus has a relatively wide insertion along the posterior and medial tibia near the joint line, and provides an important contribution to the posterior joint capsule (part of this contribution is named the oblique popliteal ligament (**Fig. 7.6**)), which is visible on ultrasound. The sartorius, gracilis, and semitendinosus tendons (or the "pes anserinus") insert more anteriorly and more distally, at the transverse level of the tibial tuberosity (**Fig. 7.5**). The medial head of gastrocnemius originates above the posterior aspect of the medial femoral epicondyle and passes superficial to the joint.

Laterally, the biceps femoris inserts on the fibular head, blending here with the LCL insertion (**Fig. 7.7**), while further fibers variably extend to the adjacent tibia. The ITB, a condensation and continuation of the deep fascia of the thigh, is an important lateral stabilizer of the knee. It passes over the lateral femoral condyle, where it can become irritated by repetitive contact/friction, and inserts on Gerdy tubercle, which lies anteriorly, on the lateral edge of the lateral tibial plateau (**Figs. 7.7 and 7.8**). The lateral head of gastrocnemius and the plantaris arise from above the posterior aspect of the lateral femoral condyle (**Fig. 7.7**).

Bursae

Bursae are synovial-lined, fluid-filled sacs that lubricate movement between adjacent structures. They can become inflamed independently or fill with fluid due to communications with the knee joint, either congenital or acquired (degenerative/traumatic).

The most common bursae are:

Anterior (Fig. 7.9)

1. Suprapatellar bursa (or recess): Deep to the quadriceps tendon and patella.
2. Prepatellar: Between patella and skin.
3. Deep infrapatellar: Between tibia and distal patellar tendon.
4. Subcutaneous infrapatellar bursa: Between patellar tendon and skin.
5. Pretibial: Between tibial tuberosity and skin.

Medial (Fig. 7.5)

1. Medial gastrocnemius: Between medial head of gastrocnemius and knee joint capsule.
2. Semimembranosus: Between semimembranosus and MCL.
3. Anserine bursa: Between MCL and pes anserinus.
4. Bursa between semimembranosus and tibia.

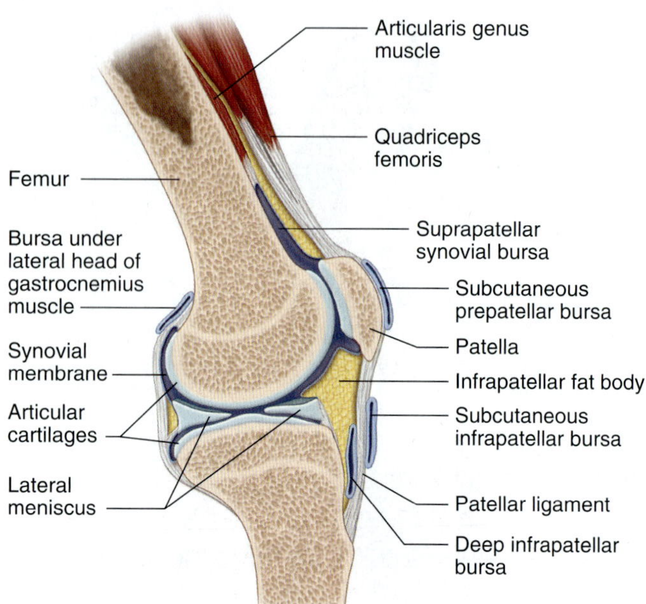

Figure 7.9. Mid-sagittal section diagram of the knee.

Lateral (Fig. 7.7)

1. Lateral gastrocnemius: Between the lateral head of gastrocnemius and knee joint capsule.
2. Fibular: Between LCL and biceps femoris.
3. Fibulopopliteal: Between LCL and popliteus tendon.
4. Subpopliteal: Between tendon of popliteus and lateral femoral condyle.

Vascular

The popliteal artery is the continuation of the femoral artery and passes posterior to the joint and the popliteus muscle. It branches into the anterior tibial artery and the tibioperoneal trunk at a variable level around the knee joint. The popliteal vein is the confluence of the anterior and posterior tibial veins. Anatomical variations are common. The most significant involves muscular entrapment of the popliteal artery by an abnormal course of the vessel or adjacent muscles.

The knee joint blood supply is from the various geniculate artery branches. The inferior lateral geniculate branch is an important and readily identifiable landmark at the posterolateral corner; it passes superficial to the popliteofibular and arcuate ligaments and deep to the LCL and fabellofibular ligament.

Nerves

The sciatic nerve runs along the posterior thigh and divides into its two main branches proximal to the knee joint. The tibial branch runs with the popliteal vessels directly posterior to the joint, while the common peroneal branch veers laterally to pass superficial to the distal biceps femoris and the fibular head. Both branches give off further superficial sural cutaneous branches that supply the skin around the knee, whereas the common peroneal nerve divides into deep and superficial branches distal to the head of the fibula.

The femoral nerve runs anteromedially in the thigh, giving off multiple branches along the way. The most distal of these is the saphenous nerve, which runs deep along the posteromedial aspect of the knee, behind the sartorius tendon, and then becomes subcutaneous, piercing the fascia between the sartorius and gracilis tendons. The saphenous nerve gives off the infrapatellar branch, which supplies the skin of the anterior knee and is sometimes injured at surgery.

All of these nerves can be visualized by ultrasound, particularly when pathological.

TECHNIQUE

Several transducers are required to perform a scan of the whole knee. Superficial structures should be examined with a high-frequency linear transducer. Deeper structures need lower frequency transducers; for example, a 3.5 MHz transducer may be required to examine the deepest aspects of the popliteal fossa, such as the PCL origin.

The core controls of gain, time gain compensation (TGC), depth, and focus should be continually adjusted to optimize the ultrasound image. Harmonic imaging provides improved contrast resolution at the cost of poorer spatial resolution, and is useful when scanning fluid-filled structures such as ganglia, joint effusions, collections, or fluid-filled muscle or meniscal tears. The fluid appears more obviously anechoic, and any true echoes within the fluid will be highlighted.

Compound imaging improves images by obtaining echoes from areas that previously were anechoic; for example, when there is anisotropy or acoustic shadowing from calcifications or wall edges, compound imaging can fill in these areas. The downside is that sometimes identification of these artifacts is required to make a diagnosis, for example, dense acoustic shadowing distal to foreign bodies and calcification or acoustic enhancement to confirm that a structure is fluid-filled.

Color Doppler imaging should be used since hyperemia is a sensitive marker for inflammation and tendinopathy. Accurate assessment requires skilled use of the Doppler controls. When examining superficial structures with Doppler, it may be worth switching transducers as lower frequency transducers show low-velocity blood flow better than high-frequency transducers. The pulse repetition frequency (PRF) and wall filter should be set low and the Doppler gain setting below the level of saturation. The knee should be extended to relax the quadriceps and patellar tendons, and only very light transducer pressure should be employed or vascularity may be obliterated. Comparison with the opposite side may help.

A complete knee scan that examines all four anatomical quadrants is rarely needed. Most ultrasound examinations of the knee are targeted to answer specific clinical questions, but a systematic approach to each quadrant is desirable so that all relevant anatomy is scanned. This text describes a uniform approach to positioning and examination that should be adapted to meet the needs of the individual patient.

Anterior Knee Assessment

Ultrasound assessment of the extensor mechanism can be considered as a three-part examination, starting superiorly and finishing inferiorly. First, the suprapatellar structures of the quadriceps tendon, suprapatellar recess and the trochlea of the femur are examined; second, the patella and associated structures including the retinacula; and third, the patella tendon and bursae (e.g., prepatellar and infrapatellar bursa).

The anterior knee also includes the slightly off-midline structures of the ITB and the pes anserine insertion.

The examination starts with a higher frequency transducer. Two patient positions are used:

1. The examination commences with the knee in 30 degrees of flexion (**Fig. 7.10**) to ensure that the quadriceps and patellar tendons are stretched and the risk of anisotropy artifact reduced. Careful scanning in longitudinal and transverse planes should be performed. For the quadriceps, this is from the distal third of the thigh to the insertion on the patella. Due to the large area to be covered, this is achieved by multiple sweeps, scanning each of the four muscles

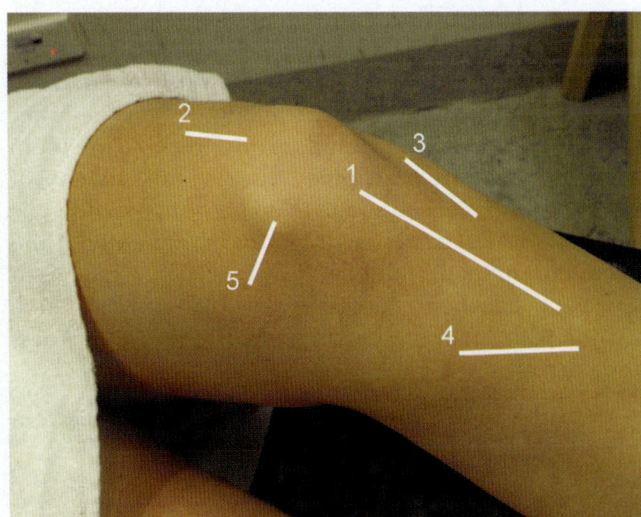

Figure 7.10. Image planes for the anteromedial knee. (*1*). Longitudinal plane of the patella tendon. (*2*). Longitudinal plane of the quadriceps tendon. (*3*). Longitudinal plane of the ITB insertion. (*4*). Longitudinal plane of the pes anserine insertion. (*5*). Transverse plane of the medial patellar retinaculum.

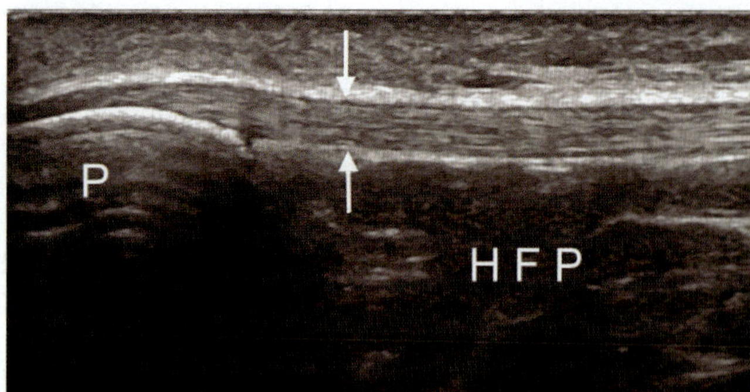

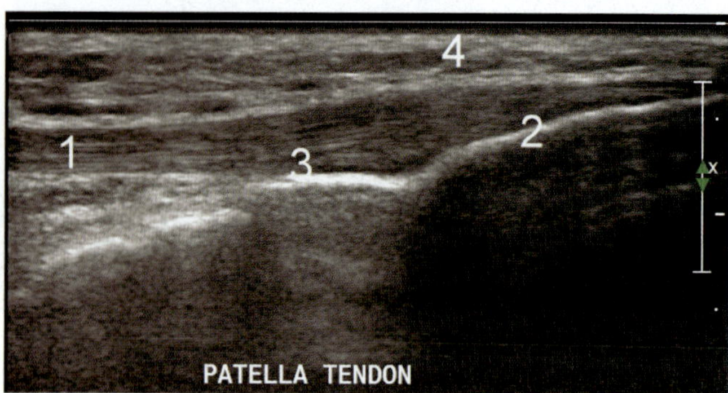

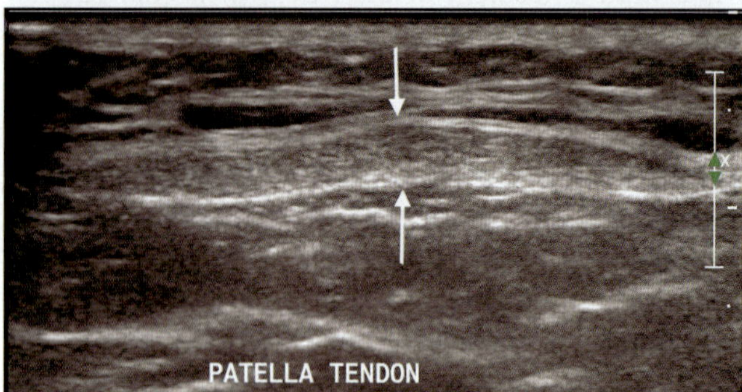

Figure 7.11. **A:** Normal longitudinal ultrasound image of the proximal patella tendon (*arrows*). P, patella; HFP, Hoffa fat pad. The tendon is well-defined and is uniform in caliber and texture. **B:** Normal longitudinal ultrasound image of the distal patella tendon (*1*). Tibial insertion of patella tendon (*2*). Deep infrapatellar bursa (*3*). Subcutaneous infrapatellar bursa (*4*). The tendon expands slightly as it runs to its insertion and often appears hypoechoic due to anisotropy. **C:** Transverse image demonstrating a normal patellar tendon (*arrows*). Note fine fascicle pattern.

separately into their tendon and down to the patellar insertion. The contours of the patella and the retinaculum should be included in the examination to look for retinacular thickening or tears.

The patellar tendon is scanned from its origin on the patella to its insertion on the tibial tuberosity in longitudinal and transverse planes **(Fig. 7.11 A–C)**. As pathology here can be subtle, the contralateral tendon should be scanned for comparison. The structures seen superficial and deep to the tendon should also be assessed. Some may only present when pathological, such as the prepatellar or pretibial bursae. The infrapatellar fat pad of Hoffa **(Fig. 7.11A)** lies deep to the patellar tendon. There is normally clear demarcation between the lower level echoes of fat lobules and the hyperechoic interconnecting fascia. The remaining infrapatellar structures of the ITB and pes anserinus should also be assessed.

Parts of the femoral cartilage can be examined if the knee is positioned in full flexion **(Fig. 7.12)**. Changes in its usual hypoechoic echogenicity should be noted. Comparison with the opposite knee helps to assess thickness and contour.

2. With the knee fully extended and relaxed, the tendons and fat pads are assessed with color Doppler.

The suprapatellar space can be examined for excess fluid in varying degrees of knee flexion to increase sensitivity for knee joint fluid.[23]

While these are the minimum two positions required for the anterior knee, scanning in other degrees of flexion may produce more fluid in or around structures or open up defects/tears in retinacula, ligaments, or tendons.)

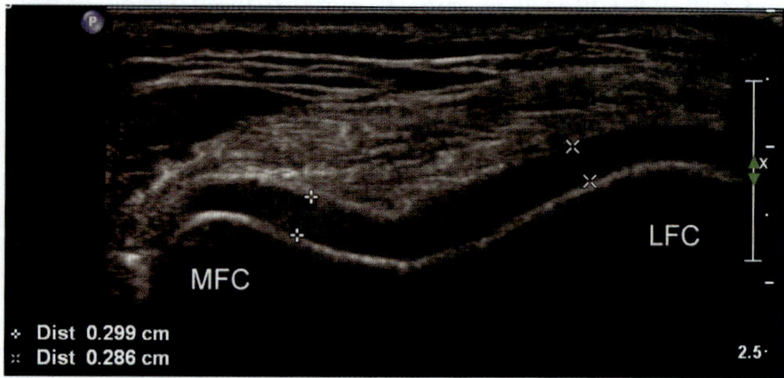

Figure 7.12. Transverse ultrasound image of the distal femur demonstrating the anechoic articular cartilage of the distal femur with measurements (*calipers*). MFC, medial femoral condyle; LFC, lateral femoral condyle.

Medial Knee Assessment

The patient is positioned as in **Figure 7.13**, lying on the side to be examined with the knee partly flexed. The MCL, medial meniscus, pes anserinus tendons and their muscles, and the semimembranosus tendon are examined. Each structure should be scanned in longitudinal and transverse planes, optimized by adjusting the degree of knee flexion to elongate the fibers maximally. Assessment of the menisci by ultrasound is limited as a large proportion of the meniscus is intra-articular and not readily seen[24] (**Fig. 7.14**). Nevertheless, there can be clinical value in scanning the peripheral margins of the menisci to look for cysts, degenerative changes (**Fig. 7.15**), and, on occasion, meniscal tears.

Lateral Knee Assessment

The patient is positioned as in **Figure 7.16**, lying on the opposite side and the knee partly flexed. The lateral knee has more complicated anatomy than the medial side and takes longer to assess. The key structures to examine in both longitudinal and transverse planes are the insertions of the biceps femoris tendon, LCL and ITB, and the lateral meniscus and popliteus tendon (**Fig. 7.17**) in varying degrees of knee flexion and extension. Care should be taken in examining the biceps femoris insertion as the junction with the LCL can create areas of anisotropy or a heterogeneous echo pattern that can be mistaken for pathology such as a tear or tendinosis (**Fig. 7.18**). Examining the arcuate ligament complex[25] is best done with direct comparison with the opposite knee to detect subtle changes in the echo pattern or size of the ligament (**Figs. 7.19 and 7.20**). Other structures to examine are the common peroneal nerve as it passes around the fibula, and the superior tibiofibular joint looking for joint effusion or capsular thickening. The lateral meniscus appears similar to the medial meniscus.

Posterior Knee Assessment

The patient should be prone with the knee extended, as in **Figure 7.21**.

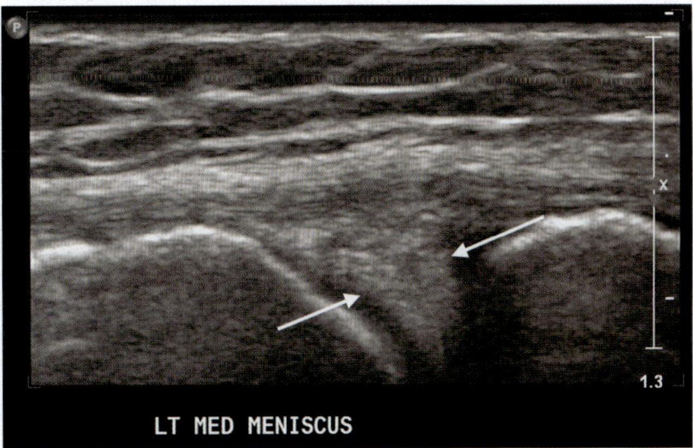

Figure 7.14.   Longitudinal image of a normal medial meniscus (*arrows*).

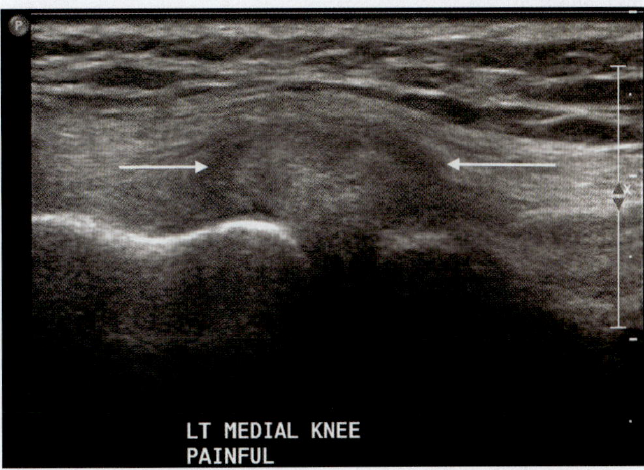

Figure 7.15.   Longitudinal image of the medial knee demonstrating a bulging medial meniscus (*arrows*). The normal meniscus is usually flush with the line between the femur and the tibia.

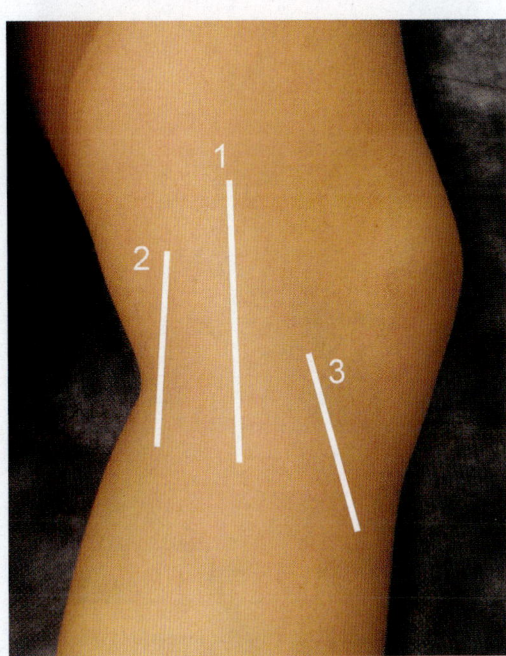

Figure 7.13.   Image planes for the medial knee. (*1*). Longitudinal plane of the MCL. (*2*). Longitudinal plane of the distal semimembranosus tendon and insertion. (*3*). Longitudinal plane of the pes anserinus.

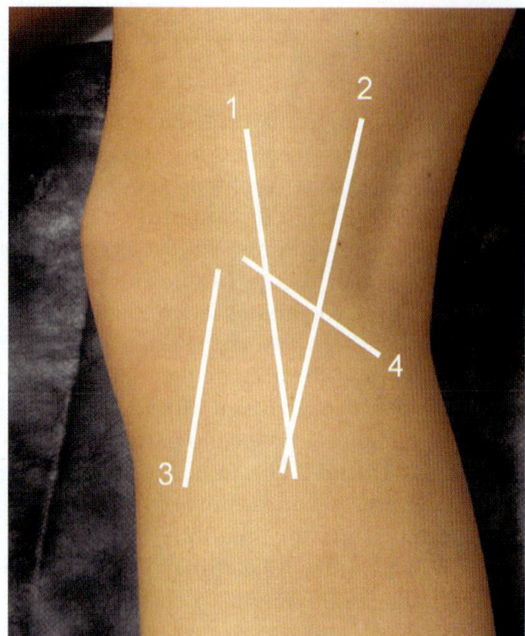

Figure 7.16. Image planes for the lateral knee. (*1*). Longitudinal plane of the LCL. (*2*). Longitudinal plane of the biceps femoris insertion on the fibula. (*3*). Longitudinal plane of the ITB insertion. (*4*). Longitudinal plane along the popliteus tendon origin.

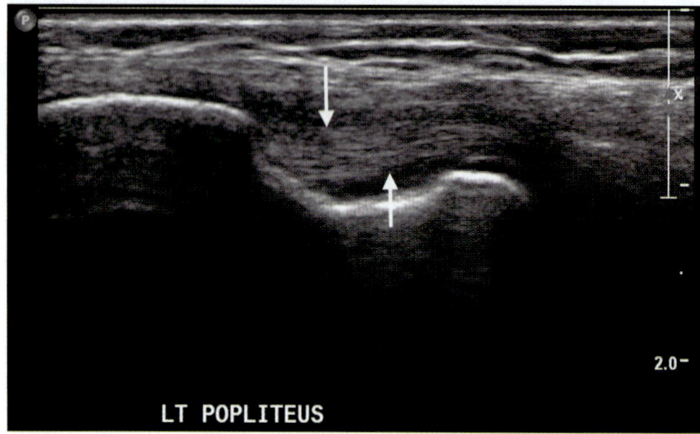

Figure 7.17. Longitudinal image of the origin of a normal popliteus tendon (*arrows*).

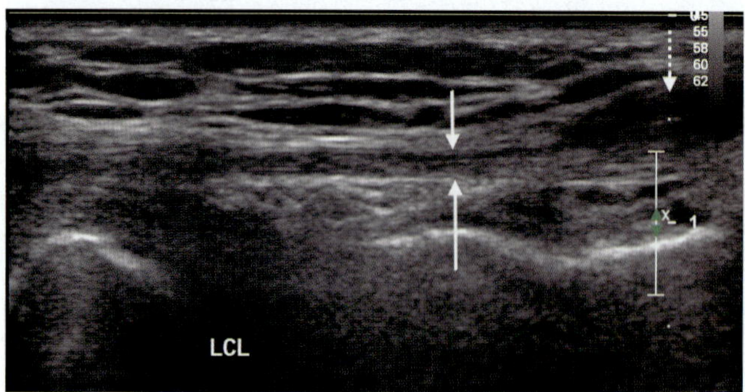

Figure 7.18. Longitudinal image of the normal LCL (*solid arrows*). Dashed arrow indicates biceps femoris insertion, which is hypoechoic due to anisotropy.

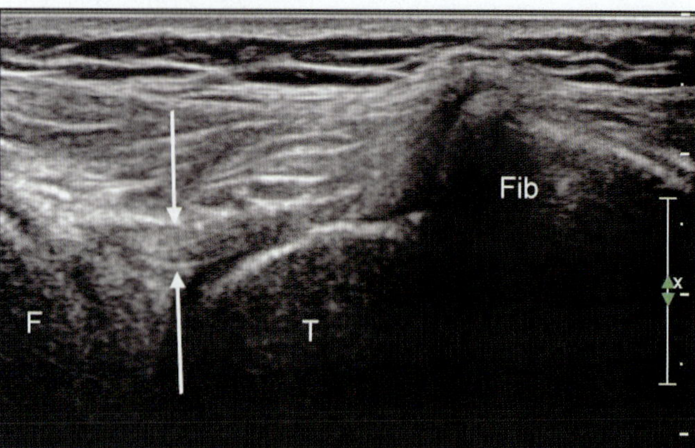

Figure 7.19. Longitudinal image of the arcuate ligament (*arrows*). F, femur; T, tibia; Fib, fibula.

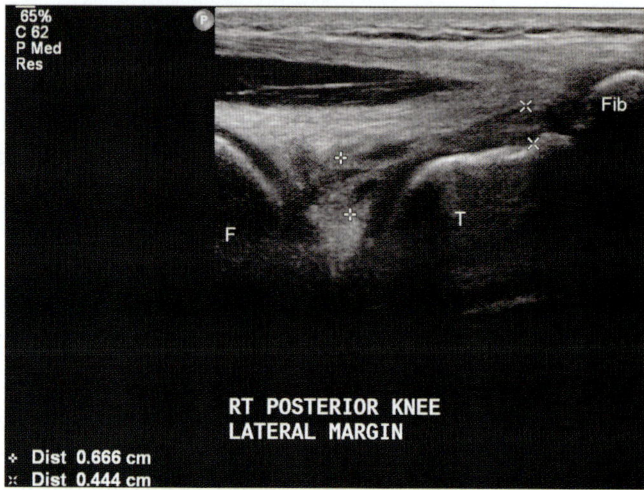

Figure 7.20. Longitudinal oblique ultrasound image of a scarred arcuate ligament (*caliper marks*). F, femur; T, tibia; Fib, fibula.

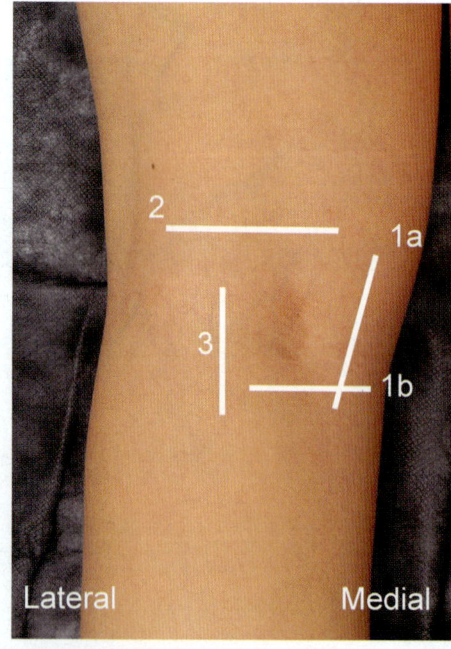

Figure 7.21. Imaging planes for the posterior knee. (*1a*). Longitudinal plane of the distal semimembranosus tendon and insertion. (*1b*). Transverse plane of the semimembranosus tendon insertion. (*2*). Transverse plane of the intercondylar notch for assessing the ACL origin. (*3*). Longitudinal image of the PCL insertion.

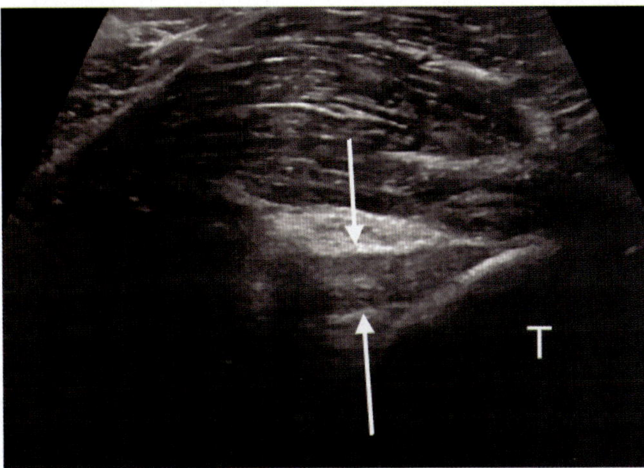

Figure 7.22.   Longitudinal image of the PCL insertion into the tibia (*arrows*). T, tibia.

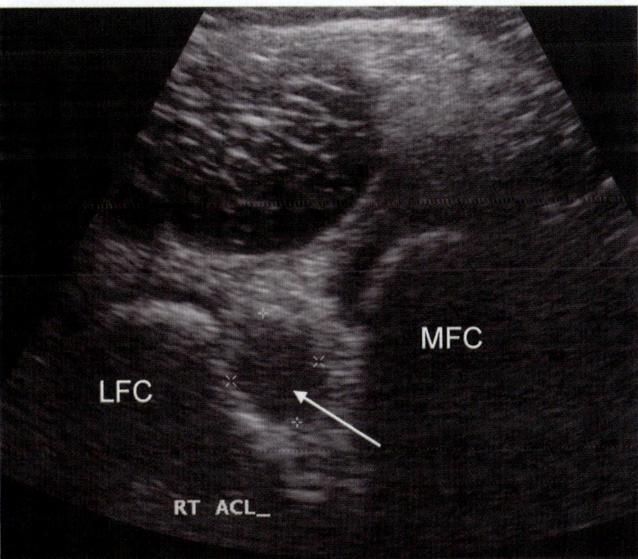

Figure 7.23.   Transverse image demonstrating a hematoma at the site of the torn ACL (*arrow and calipers*). LFC, lateral femoral condyle; MFC, medial femoral condyle.

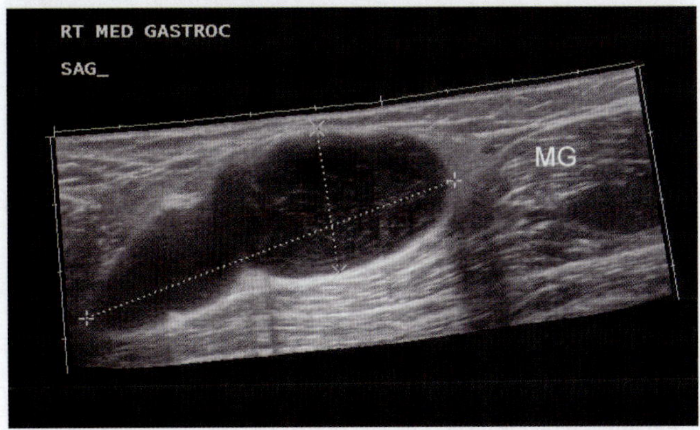

Figure 7.24.   Extended field of view, longitudinal image demonstrating a Baker cyst (*calipers*) with low-level internal echoes and distal acoustic enhancement. MG, medial gastrocnemius muscle.

The posterior knee examination requires multiple transducers of varying frequency to visualize structures at variable depth. Using a high-frequency transducer, the popliteal artery and vein and sciatic and tibial nerves are inspected. Next, a lower frequency linear, or even curvilinear, transducer is used to assess the deeper structures, for example, the PCL insertion on the tibia (**Fig. 7.22**), the lateral margin of the intercondylar notch looking for a hematoma as a marker for an ACL tear (**Fig. 7.23**), or a Baker cyst (**Fig. 7.24**).

While this four-quadrant approach covers most clinical problems, the sonologist should also listen to the patient. If the patient points to the mid thigh or mid calf, this region should also be scanned.

PATHOLOGY

Anterior/Extensor Mechanism

Anterior/extensor mechanism–related knee pain is perhaps the most common indication for ultrasound of the knee. Pathology includes patellar tendinosis, quadriceps tendinosis, patellar maltracking, medial plica syndrome, and bursitis.

Patellar and Quadriceps Tendinosis (or Tendinopathy)

Tendinosis is common at the patellar tendon and can affect the quadriceps tendon, with similar clinical, pathological, and sonographic manifestations. Tendinosis generally results from overuse. Histology shows disruption of normal collagen architecture with deposition of mucoid ground substance and sometimes dystrophic ossification.[26] Clinically, tendinosis manifests with pain, particularly on activity, tenderness, and swelling. In the patellar tendon, it occurs most commonly at the proximal end of the tendon, in the midline, known as "jumper's knee." In its most subtle form, there is minimal sonographic abnormality with reduction in echogenicity and some blurring of the normal fiber pattern. As tendinosis becomes more severe, the tendon becomes swollen with reduction of echogenicity and loss of the normal fibrillar pattern[27] **(Fig. 7.25)**. Neovascularity on Doppler examination is a sensitive sign of tendinosis[28] **(Fig. 7.26)**. Discrete defects or tears in the tendon are important and have prognostic and treatment implications (such as whether autologous blood or platelet-rich plasma [PRP] injections are to be used). Examination of the patellar tendon should extend to the fat pad of Hoffa. In moderate-to-significant tendinosis, the fat pad has increased echogenicity and there are blurring of fascial planes **(Fig 7.27)** and increased Doppler vascularity. At the chronic end of the disease spectrum, tendinosis is associated with enthesopathy, and minor bony contour changes, hyperostosis, or large bony excrescences are seen[29] **(Fig 7.25)**. Intratendinous calcifications (dystrophic ossification) can also be seen in chronic tendinosis.[30]

Most of these sonographic abnormalities are frequently found in the patellar tendons of asymptomatic individuals, particularly those who engage in regular or strenuous athletic activity.[31] Although many of the changes may be adaptive rather than pathological, the presence of focal hypoechoic changes has some predictive value for the future development of symptoms.[32]

PRP and autologous whole blood are often used to treat patellar tendinosis. Both utilize the theoretical ability of platelet-related growth factors to encourage healing of tendon tissue. The best technique for their administration and the overall efficacy of therapy remain controversial.[33] We have anecdotally found the following protocol effective in treatment of patellar tendinopathy:

Five milliliters of blood is drawn from the patient's antecubital vein and centrifuged in a test tube for 3 to 5 minutes. This yields a three-layered appearance: The supernatant and middle platelet layer are aspirated from the test tube using a 3 mL syringe, while the precipitant of red cells is discarded. A 25G needle is placed in the abnormal part of the tendon, under ultrasound guidance. We most often use a transverse approach, entering the patellar tendon from lateral or medial, with the probe held longitudinally along the planned course of the needle. The contents of the 3 mL syringe are gently injected under ultrasound visualization. There should be little resistance to injection, and injected material should be observed entering small clefts (often running longitudinally along the tendon and therefore out of the original transverse plane of the probe). If this is not the case, the needle can be minimally repositioned until this occurs. Distension of the tendon and small clefts often results in discomfort for several days after the procedure, and the patient should be warned about this. Following completion of the procedure, the patient is counseled to rest for several days before recommencing any rehabilitative exercise. The patient is also counseled not to expect an immediate improvement, and that a further treatment may be required in 4 to 6 weeks.

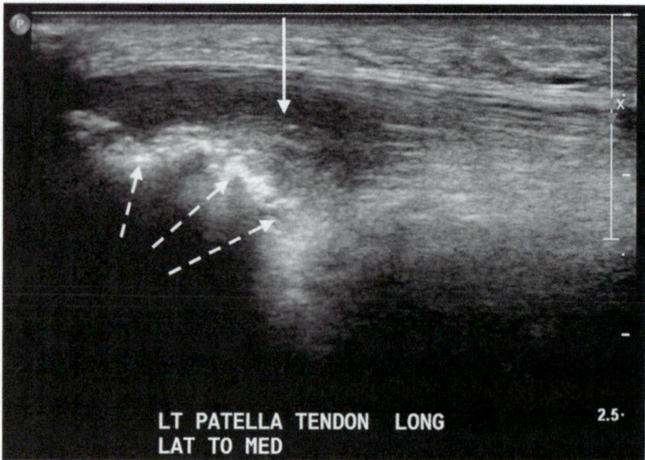

Figure 7.25.   Longitudinal image of the proximal patella tendon demonstrating severe chronic patellar tendinosis and enthesopathy of the patella. Note the loss of normal tendon architecture and reduced echogenicity (*solid arrow*). *Dashed arrows* depict enthesopathy/hyperostosis of the patella.

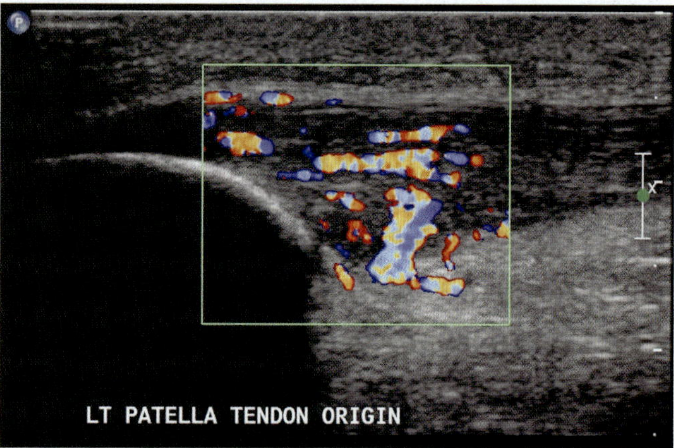

Figure 7.26.   Longitudinal color Doppler image of the proximal patella tendon demonstrating severe tendinosis with marked hyperemia.

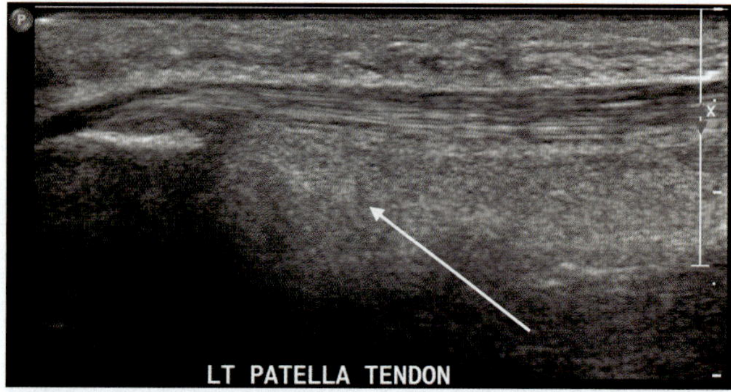

Figure 7.27.   Longitudinal image of the proximal patella tendon and Hoffa fat pad (*arrow*). The fat pad has increased echogenicity and has lost the normal fascial lines that demarcate the individual fat lobules, indicative of inflammation.

A similar technique can be applied to the treatment of tendinopathy elsewhere in the body. Variations on the substance used (PRP vs. whole blood), the amount injected, and the location of injection (intratendinous vs. peritendinous) are common among different practitioners.

Quadriceps and Patellar Tendon Tears

Tears of these tendons are unusual and are far less common than tendinosis of the same tendons or tears of other tendons, such as the Achilles or supraspinatus. Tears often result from relatively minor trauma in tendons that are already severely degenerated from connective tissue disease or old age/disuse. They are readily recognized sonographically as a focal discontinuity of tendon fibers; the interval is often filled with hematoma or granulation tissue that is amorphous and hypointense, lacking the normal organized appearance of parallel tendon fibers. The most common type of tears are intratendinous delaminations that occur in the proximal and deep surfaces of the patellar tendon. Anechoic foci may evolve, which may breech the deep surface of the tendon. Neovascularity and hyperemia are common.

Patellar Maltracking

Abnormalities of the patellofemoral articulation are extremely common and result from abnormalities of trochlear and patellar morphology, malposition of the tibial tubercle, muscular imbalances of the quadriceps muscles, or abnormal tension of the patellar retinacula. Maltracking manifests as the patellofemoral pain syndrome and includes pain from chondral wear and impingement of juxtapatellar fat. Chondral damage is difficult to visualize sonographically because the patellar articular surface lies deep to and is obscured by the patella itself.[34] Impingement of the fat is readily appreciated sonographically as increased echogenicity and color Doppler vascularity, which, if identified, suggest maltracking. This can be further assessed with radiographs, computed tomography, or MRI.[35]

Medial Plica Syndrome

The medial patellar plica is a remnant embryological structure of variable size and extent. Its role in the development of knee symptoms and patellofemoral chondral wear is controversial,[36] as the plica is commonly present in asymptomatic individuals. Symptomatic patients usually present with chronic anterosuperior knee pain, and sometimes snapping or local tenderness medially. Ultrasound complements MRI by showing friction of the plica against the patella or femoral condyle during dynamic movement[37] and thickening.[38]

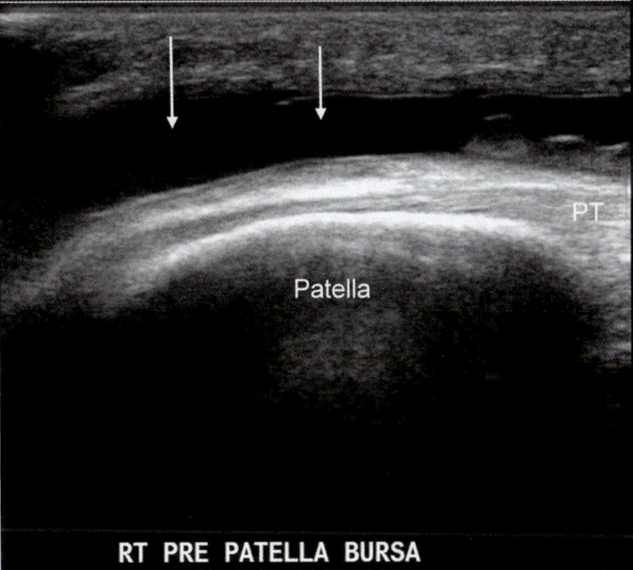

Figure 7.28. Longitudinal image of a distended fluid-filled prepatella bursa (*arrows*).

Bursitis

Inflammation of the prepatellar bursa is most often seen after acute (e.g., a fall on to the knee) or repetitive (e.g., prolonged kneeling) trauma. The soft tissues superficial to the patella are thickened and edematous, or there may be an effusion in the bursa **(Fig. 7.28)** with prominent neovascularity. The transducer must be applied very lightly to the skin as the sonographic changes are easily obliterated by even light pressure and may be embarrassingly missed. The suprapatellar bursa is often distended when there is a joint effusion, and is a sensitive location to look for joint fluid and synovial thickening either just proximal to the patella or in the medial or lateral gutters **(Fig. 7.29)**. The infrapatellar bursae may be inflamed and distended if there is adjacent patellar tendinopathy **(Fig. 7.30)**.

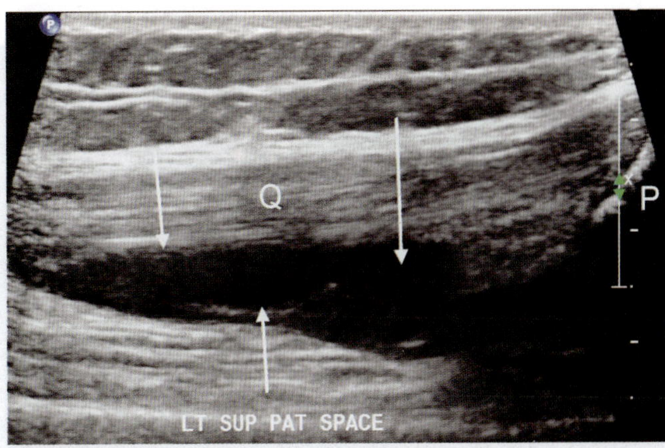

Figure 7.29. Longitudinal ultrasound image demonstrating fluid in the suprapatellar recess (*arrows*). Q, quadriceps tendon; P, patella.

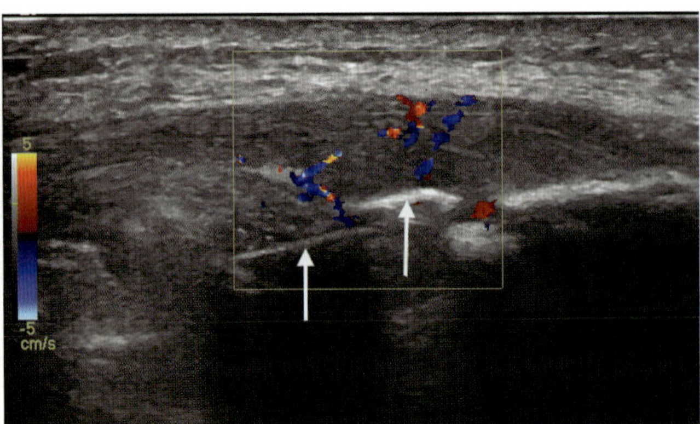

Figure 7.37. Longitudinal image of the ITB insertion demonstrating tendinosis (reduced echogenicity and hyperemia). Also note this patient has had an arthroplasty (*arrows*).

Pes Anserinus Bursitis

Inflammation of the bursa that is interposed between the tibia and the distal pes anserinus tendons is seen in athletes and older sedentary individuals, who often have diabetes or connective tissue disease.[47] Ultrasound shows the fluid-distended bursa between the MCL and the pes anserinus tendons. It sometimes has a thickened and hypervascular wall[48] **(Fig. 7.38)**. As for ITBFS, the diagnosis is often apparent clinically, and ultrasound has an additional important role in guiding injections into the bursa[49] using the same technique and materials as for ITBFS.

Semimembranosus Tendinopathy

This is seen occasionally in young athletic patients, more commonly in less active older patients. It often coexists with degenerative changes in the knee,[50] and is more

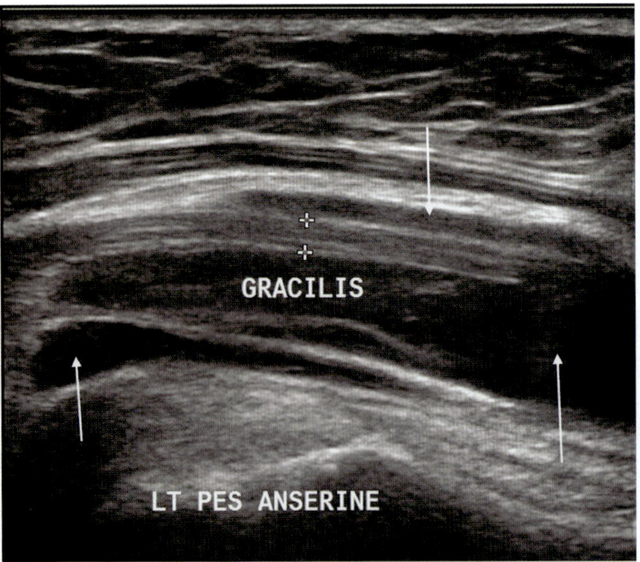

Figure 7.38. Longitudinal image of the pes anserinus in the presence of a large pes anserinus bursitis (*arrows*). Note separation of tendons such that gracilis is clearly seen (*calipers*).

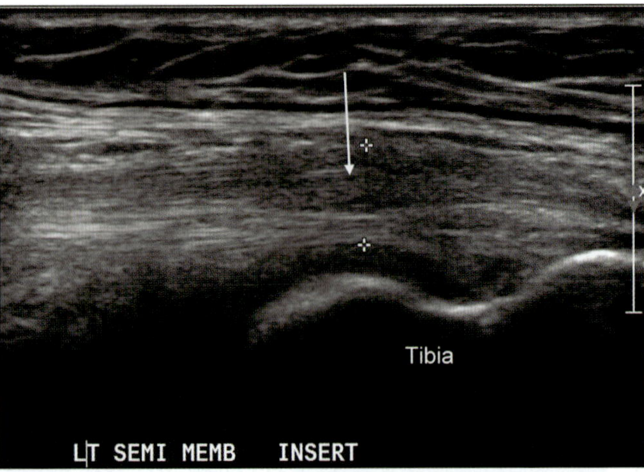

Figure 7.39. Longitudinal image of the distal semimembranosus tendon. The tendon is focally swollen and hypoechoic with loss of the normal fibrillary architecture due to tendinosis (*arrow*).

common in women.[51] It may be related to abnormal valgus orientation and friction at the adjacent medial joint line (with osteophytes possibly creating additional friction). Pain and discomfort occur more posteriorly and proximally than in pes anserinus bursitis. Ultrasound shows typical tendinopathy **(Fig. 7.39)**.

CRUCIATE LIGAMENTS

Cruciate ligament injuries occur when there is substantial overextension or overrotation of the knee, generally in sports or motor vehicle accidents. Diagnosis is important as surgical repair is often performed acutely, particularly in young and active patients.

The ACL is normally not identifiable with ultrasound, but degenerative injury may be inferred by the presence of ganglia,[52] and acute injury by a joint effusion and hematoma in the intercondylar notch[53] **(Fig. 7.23)** or by small variations in ultrasound measurements of tibial translation.[54] The PCL is identifiable,[55] **(Fig. 7.22)** particularly in those with a slim body habitus, and ultrasound has reasonable accuracy in detecting injury.[56,57] Frank disruption or thickening and loss of the normal architectural pattern can be seen in the accessible distal portion of the tendon.[58] Comparison should be made with the opposite side.

Ultrasound has very limited utility in the assessment of cruciate injuries, especially when compared with MRI, which has the substantial advantage of being able to identify associated injuries. MRI is the preferred examination for acute knee injuries.

CARTILAGE ASSESSMENT

Osteoarthritis is one of the most significant causes of morbidity in the western world.[59] Its pathology and etiology are complex. Genetic factors likely play a role,[60] but the condition is generally due to acute or chronic mechanical cartilage injury that triggers an inflammatory response. Manifestations include loss of cartilage thickness, surface uniformity and quality, meniscal degeneration, osteophyte formation, and adjacent capsular and synovial inflammation that progress gradually over years, causing generalized pain and disability.

MRI cartilage mapping techniques are rapidly developing for the quantification and qualification of cartilage damage in osteoarthritis.[61] In comparison, ultrasound currently has a limited role, although patellar and femoral cartilage can be assessed directly for thickness and qualitative surface changes such as loss of sharpness. Previous studies have shown reasonable correlation with arthroscopic[62] and MRI evaluation.[63] Secondary changes such as marginal osteophytes and neovascularity from associated synovitis can be detected and may correlate with severity of symptoms and be equivalent to MRI or radiography for this purpose.[64,65] Ultrasound may be useful in patients who present with symptomatic flares.

Calcium pyrophosphate deposition disease (CPPD) is a metabolic arthropathy of unknown etiology that is particularly common in the knee.[66] It may be asymptomatic or present with acute symptoms similar to gout or chronic symptoms similar to osteoarthritis. The diagnosis in acute cases is usually made by aspiration of joint fluid and detection of characteristic crystals by polarized light microscopy. However, CPPD crystals can also be detected by ultrasound as punctate or band-like hyperechoic foci in hyaline cartilage, that is, deep to the surface of the cartilage. Ultrasound is highly accurate, superior to radiography.[67]

NERVES

Neural lesions appreciable on ultrasound include post-traumatic neuromas and neoplasms. They produce focal thickening or enlargement of the nerve, often with a fusiform appearance that is usually elliptically elongated along the axis of the nerve (**Fig. 7.40**). They are particularly common after knee arthroscopy or arthroplasty.

Compressive lesions of the nerves around the knee are also common. These include: Compression of the tibial nerve by popliteal artery aneurysm,[68] and compression or invasion of the common peroneal nerve by superior tibiofibular joint ganglion[69] (see also Chapter 9, p 206 and Chapter 12, p 288).

MUSCLES

Muscle tears around the knee most commonly involve the quadriceps (especially the rectus femoris) and gastrocnemius muscles. Tears of the medial gastrocnemius at the aponeurosis with soleus are termed "tennis leg."[70] The clinical presentation of a muscle tear is usually sufficient to make the diagnosis, but ultrasound is important to localize the injury to a particular muscle and quantify its severity. Clinically, muscle injuries are graded from I to III depending on the presence or absence of pain, weakness, or loss of function. Ultrasound shows hematoma, peri- and interfascial fluid, and discontinuity of muscle fibers[71] (**Fig. 7.41**). Tears most commonly occur at the myotendinous junction. It is important to look for associated tendinous injury, which can occur at the proximal and distal "free" ends of the tendon as well as at the intramuscular portion.[72]

BAKER CYST

A "Baker cyst" is a distended medial gastrocnemius–semimembranosus bursa. The bursa usually communicates with the knee joint. The communication may be congenital, or due to degeneration of the relatively thin joint capsule[73] that occurs with aging, possibly accelerated by degenerative conditions such as osteoarthritis. Baker cysts are extremely common. They are frequently found incidentally during deep vein thrombosis (DVT)

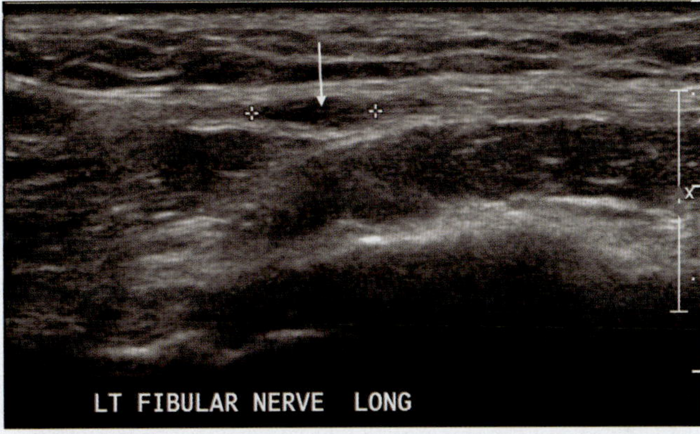

Figure 7.40. Longitudinal image of a small neuroma in the fibular nerve (*arrow and calipers*).

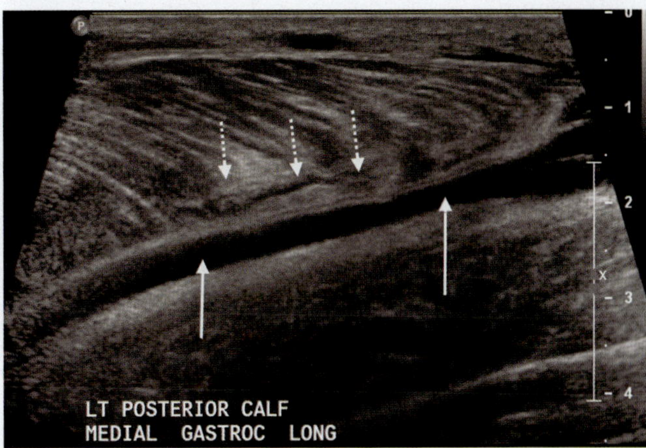

Figure 7.41. Longitudinal image of a medial gastrocnemius tear (tennis leg). *Solid arrows,* fluid (blood). *Dashed arrow,* myotendinous junction tear.

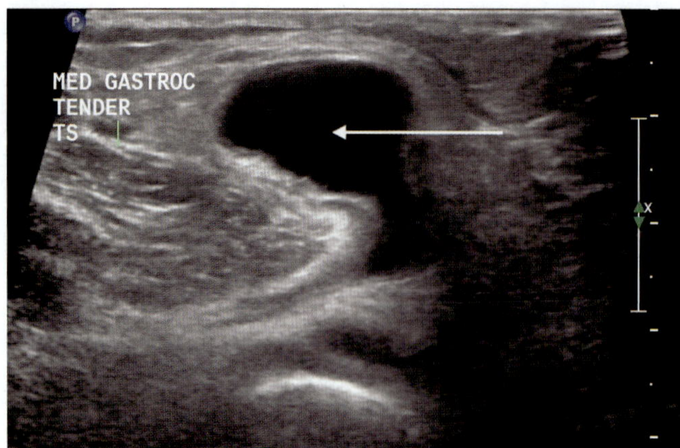

Figure 7.42.   Transverse image of a simple Baker cyst. *Arrow,* anechoic fluid in the cyst. The echogenic and comma-shaped medial head of gastrocnemius marks the lateral margin of the neck of the cyst.

scans[74] or present as asymptomatic popliteal masses, but they may present with acute, severe calf pain and swelling due to rupture or with local pressure effects causing pain, nerve compression (tibial or rarely common peroneal),[75] or vascular occlusion (popliteal vein or rarely artery).[76] They are markers for knee joint effusion, which is in turn a marker for knee joint pathology.[77]

Usually, the bursa is an anechoic thin-walled round structure, filled with simple fluid **(Fig. 7.42)** and has a narrow neck or stalk between the medial head of gastrocnemius and the semimembranosus and more posterior semitendinosus tendons. However, when hemorrhage occurs in the joint or bursa, the fluid becomes echogenic and particulate. Inflammation causes thickening and indistinctness of the normally thin and sharply defined bursal wall, internal echoes due to synovial proliferation and hypervascularity **(Fig. 7.43)**. Bursal rupture causes acute calf pain and swelling and can mimic gastrocnemius muscle tear, DVT, or even Achilles tendon tear. The ruptured bursa may deflate, but typically has an elongated inferior margin and extensive fluid tracks along fascial planes.

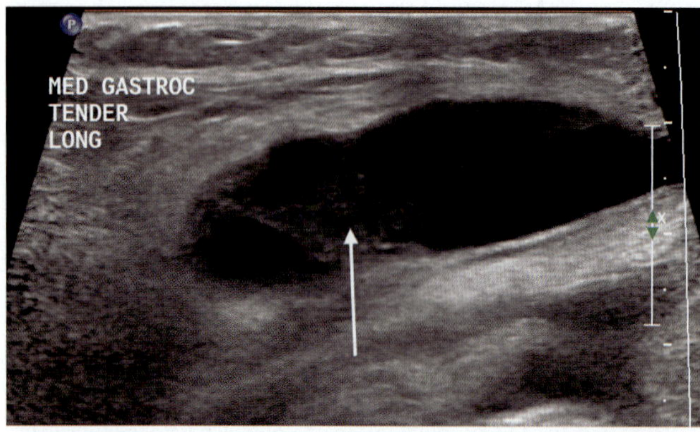

Figure 7.43.   Transverse image of a Baker cyst. The internal echoes (*arrow*) are due to hemorrhage.

The stalk of a Baker cyst lies between the comma-shaped medial head of gastrocnemius and the more medial semimembranosus and semitendinosus tendons.

PEDIATRIC KNEE

Ultrasound of the pediatric musculoskeletal system is described in more detail in Chapter 13.

The pediatric knee differs from the adult knee in several respects. The epiphyses, epiphyseal plates, apophyses, and apophyseal plates are not yet fully formed or fused, and are of variable appearance depending on their maturity. Tendon origins and insertions are not fully matured and have transitional zones of fibrocartilage **(Fig. 7.44)**. The fibrocartilage and physeal echogenicity is quite variable in appearance depending on maturity, and ranges from totally anechoic to almost the echogenicity of tendon.

The epiphysis and tendon insertions can be very echo poor and should not be mistaken for fluid or tears. Careful scanning should be performed when diagnosing fluid or a tear, including scanning of the opposite side.

The most common sonographic abnormality of the pediatric knee is traction apophysitis, an overuse injury at the osteotendinous junction. There are two eponymously named syndromes:

Osgood–Schlatter disease: this is a traction osteochondritis of the tibial tubercle, at the distal patellar tendon insertion. It is diagnosed clinically by swelling and tenderness at the tuberosity. Ultrasound in conjunction with plain radiographs determines severity and acuity by demonstrating color Doppler hyperemia at and around the fragmented apophysis **(Figs. 7.45–7.47)**.

Sinding-Larsen–Johansson disease: this is a traction apophysitis of the inferior patella involving the tendinous attachment of the patellar tendon. It typically occurs in early adolescence in athletic children and manifests as tenderness and swelling. Ultrasound shows abnormal

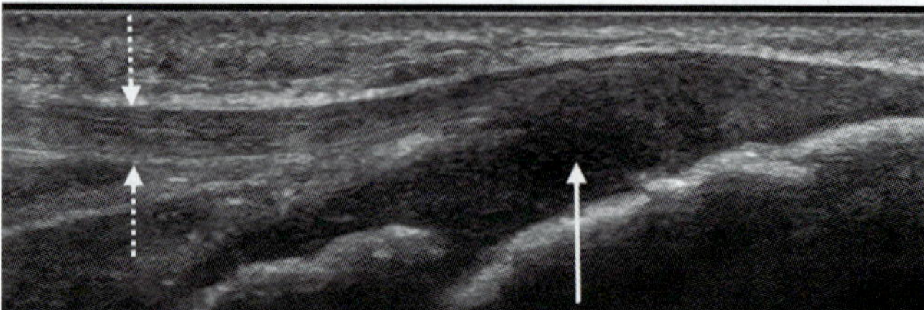

Figure 7.44.   Longitudinal scan of the patellar tendon insertion of an adolescent. The epiphysis and the apophysis where the tendon inserts have not fully ossified. *Solid arrow,* fibrocartilage that will subsequently ossify. *Dashed arrow,* distal patella tendon.

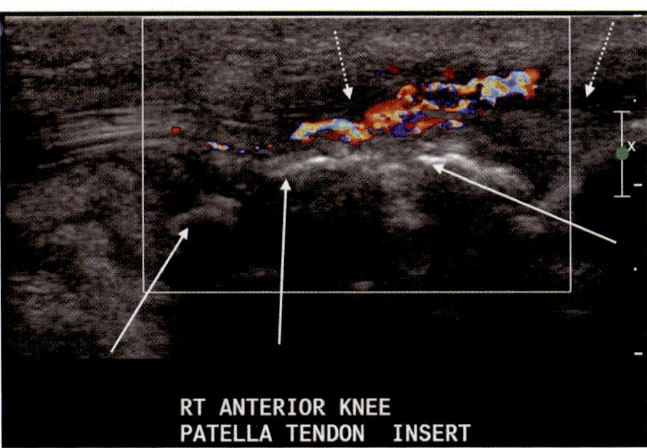

Figure 7.45. Longitudinal color Doppler image of the patellar tendon insertion in Osgood–Schlatter disease. *Solid arrow,* fragmented tibial apophysis. *Dashed arrow,* swollen tendon and hyperemia.

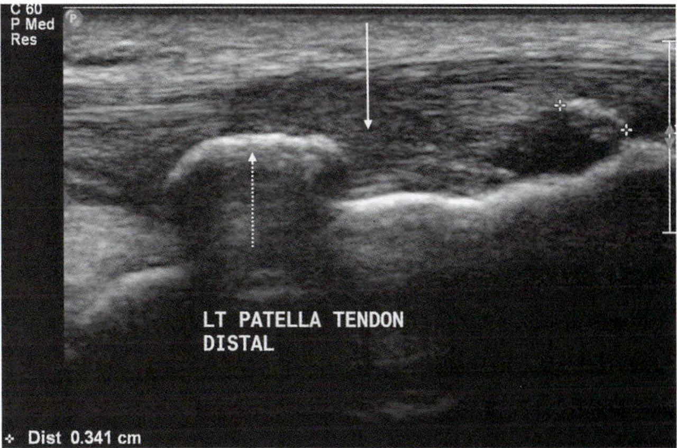

Figure 7.47. Longitudinal image of the patellar tendon insertion in Osgood–Schlatter disease. *Solid arrow,* tendon change with loss of echogenicity and architecture. *Dashed arrow,* fragmented apophysis. *caliper,* bony avulsion from tibia.

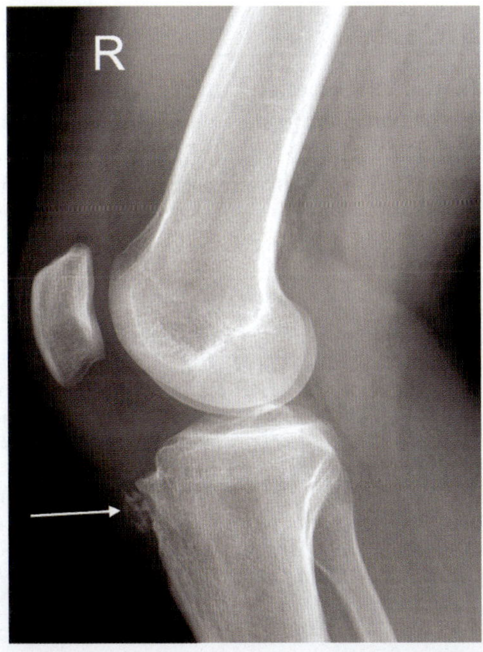

Figure 7.46. Same patient as in Figure 7.45; lateral radiograph demonstrating fragmentation at tibial apophysis (*arrow*).

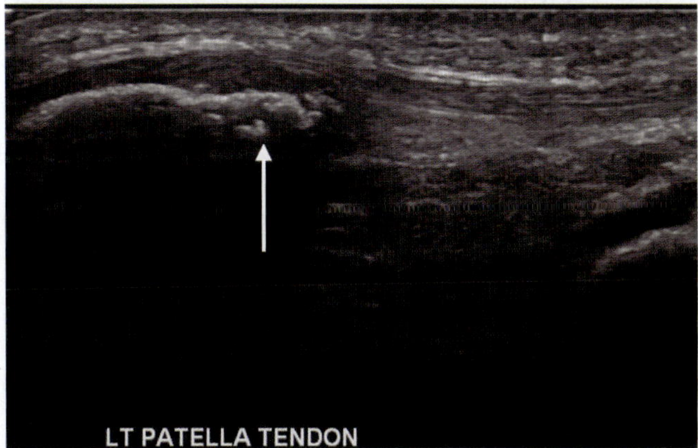

Figure 7.48. Longitudinal image of the patella apex and patella tendon origin in Sinding-Larsen–Johansson disease. *Arrow,* fragmentation of the patella apex. The adjacent patellar tendon is thickened and hypoechoic in keeping with tendinosis.

thickening of the superior part of the tendon, and irregularity and fragmentation of the adjacent inferior patella **(Fig. 7.48)**.

Other pediatric knee conditions seen on ultrasound include joint effusions that are important in suspected sepsis; Baker cysts, which may be an early sign of juvenile rheumatoid arthritis but are also seen in otherwise normal pediatric knees; bursitis; and tendinopathy in athletic children.

VASCULAR ABNORMALITIES

Vascular abnormalities around the knee are few and are generally isolated to the popliteal fossa.

Popliteal Aneurysm

The ultrasound diagnosis of popliteal artery aneurysm is sometimes a surprise finding in what may have been clinically considered as a Baker cyst. The artery is dilated, shows turbulent flow on color Doppler, and may contain hypoechoic thrombus.

If an aneurysm is found, the opposite side and the aorta should be examined as there is a high incidence of coexistent aneurysms. Measurements should be taken and a note made of complications such as mural thrombus, dissection, or leakage. Large popliteal aneurysms can cause calf swelling from venous obstruction and may lead to DVT **(Fig. 7.49)**.

Deep Vein Thrombosis

Some patients with calf pain may have a DVT, and the popliteal vein should be assessed for compressibility and for augmentation when the calf is squeezed.

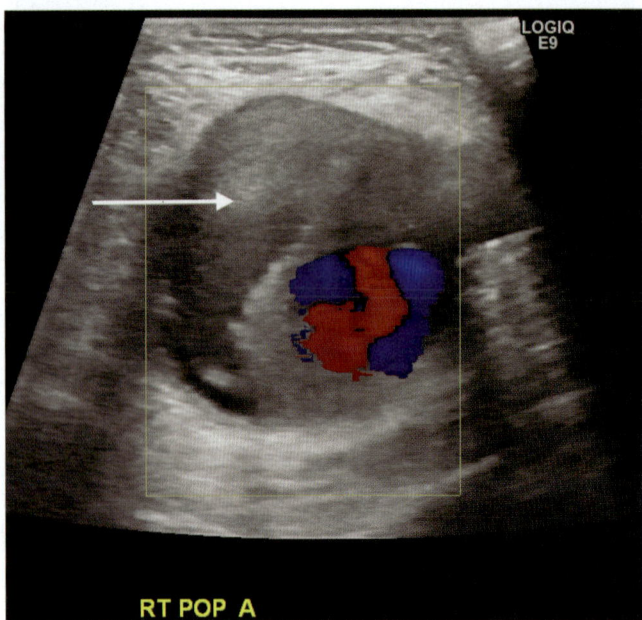

Figure 7.49. Transverse image demonstrating a large popliteal aneurysm with dissection. *Arrow,* region of dissection. Color Doppler demonstrates patent lumen.

Popliteal Artery Entrapment Syndrome

Popliteal artery entrapment syndrome (PAES) presents clinically with claudication symptoms during exercise in young, otherwise healthy patients (usually males). It is due to anatomical variation(s) in the popliteal fossa, either an abnormal course of the artery or abnormal slips of the medial head of gastrocnemius.[78]

PAES has been well described as a clinical entity, but anatomical abnormality can also occur in the absence of symptoms, and clinical correlation is required to make the diagnosis.

Although MRI/MRA or catheter angiography are usually employed, ultrasound may be superior.[79] It can be used dynamically and demonstrates the vascular stenosis and, with sufficient operator skill, the causal anatomical abnormality. The ultrasound examination commences with a full arterial study of the leg to ensure that the arterial supply is normal. With the patient prone and the knee slightly flexed by a bolster under the ankle, the popliteal fossa is scanned, noting the relative positions of the popliteal artery and the gastrocnemius and popliteus muscles. Comparison should be performed with the other side.

The patient is then asked to plantar flex the foot against resistance provided by an assistant. The resistance should be sufficient to prevent flexion beyond 90 degrees. As this is occurring, the sonologist should note the diameter of the popliteal artery and measure flow velocity. There is normally a small degree of narrowing of the artery with slight elevation of velocities. In PAES, the artery narrows or occludes (**Fig. 7.50**). The opposite leg should be examined for comparison.

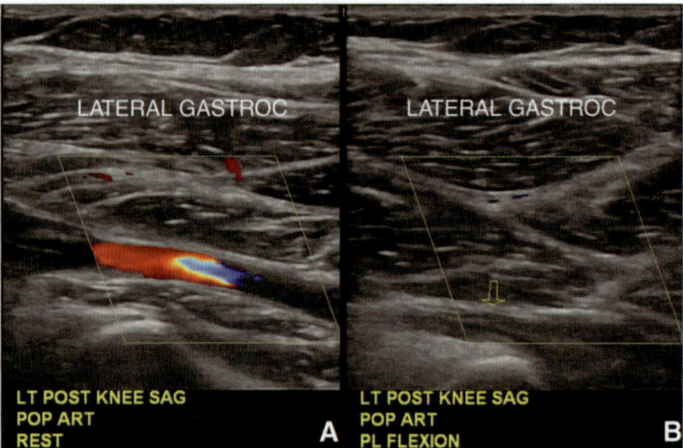

Figure 7.50. Color Doppler images demonstrating PAES. **A:** Color Doppler flow is seen in the popliteal artery at the level of the tibial plateau at rest. **B:** No flow is seen in the popliteal artery during resisted plantar flexion.

CONCLUSION

Proficiency and experience with ultrasound of the knee, a deceptively complex joint, is hard-earned but rewarding. Tendon, muscle, nerve, and intra-articular pathologies are common and well assessed with ultrasound.

REFERENCES

1. Iagnocco A, Perricone C, Scirocco C, et al. The interobserver reliability of ultrasound in knee osteoarthritis. *Rheumatology (Oxford).* 2012;51(11):2013–2019.
2. Yoon CH, Kim HS, Ju JH, et al. Validity of the sonographic longitudinal sagittal image for assessment of the cartilage thickness in the knee osteoarthritis. *Clin Rheumatol.* 2008;27(12):1507–1516.
3. Ohashi S, Ohnishi I, Matsumoto T, et al. Measurement of articular cartilage thickness using a three-dimensional image reconstructed from B-mode ultrasonography mechanical scans feasibility study by comparison with MRI-derived data. *Ultrasound Med Biol.* 2012;38(3):402–411.
4. Ellabban AS, Kamel SR, Omar HA, et al. Ultrasonographic diagnosis of articular chondrocalcinosis. *Rheumatol Int.* 2012;32(12):3863–3868.
5. Ptasznik R, Feller J, Bartlett J, et al. The value of sonography in the diagnosis of traumatic rupture of the anterior cruciate ligament of the knee. *AJR Am J Roentgenol.* 1995;164(6):1461–1463.
6. Casser HR, Sohn C, Kiekenbeck A. Current evaluation of sonography of the meniscus. Results of a comparative study of sonographic and arthroscopic findings. *Arch Orthop Trauma Surg.* 1990;109(3):150–154.
7. Khan Z, Farugui Z, Ogyunbiyi O, et al. Ultrasound assessment of internal derangement of the knee. *Acta Orthop Belg.* 2006;72(1):72–76.
8. Paczesny L, Kruczynski J. Medial plica syndrome of the knee: diagnosis with dynamic sonography. *Radiology.* 2009;251(2):439–446.
9. Marchand AJ, Proisy M, Ropars M, et al. Snapping knee: imaging findings with an emphasis on dynamic sonography. *AJR Am J Roentgenol.* 2012;199(1):142–150.
10. Okamoto T, Futani H, Atsui K, et al. Sonographic appearance of fibrous nodules in patellar clunk syndrome: a case report. *J Orthop Sci.* 2002;7(5):590–593.

11. Sofka CM, Adler RS, Laskin R. Sonography of polyethylene liners used in total knee arthroplasty. *AJR Am J Roentgenol.* 2003;180(5):1437–1441.

12. Goodfellow J, Hungerford DS, Zindel M. Patello-femoral joint mechanics and pathology. 1. Functional anatomy of the patello-femoral joint. *J Bone Joint Surg Br.* 1976;58(3):287–290.

13. Oohashi Y, Koshino T, Oohashi Y. Clinical features and classification of bipartite or tripartite patella. *Knee Surg Sports Traumatol Arthrosc.* 2010;18(11):1465–1469.

14. Kawashima T, Takeishi H, Yoshitomi S, et al. Anatomical study of the fabella, fabellar complex, and its clinical implications. *Surg Radiol Anat.* 2007;29(8):611–616.

15. De Maeseneer M, Lenchik L, Starok M, et al. Normal and abnormal medial meniscocapsular structures: MR imaging and sonography in cadavers. *AJR Am J Roentgenol.* 1998;171:969–976.

16. Seiya JK, Swaringen JC, Wojtys EM, et al. Diagnostic ultrasound evaluation of posterolateral corner knee injuries. *Arthroscopy.* 2010;26(4):494–499.

17. Barker RP, Lee JC, Healy JC. Normal sonographic anatomy of the posterolateral corner of the knee. *AJR Am J Roentgenol.* 2009;192(1):73–79.

18. Minowa T, Murakami G, Kura H, et al. Does the fabella contribute to the reinforcement of the posterolateral corner of the knee by inducing the development of associated ligaments? *J Orthop Sci.* 2004;9(1):59–65.

19. Phornphutkul C, Sekiya JK, Wojtys EM, et al. Sonographic imaging of the patellofemoral medial joint stabilizing structures: findings in human cadavers. *Orthopedics.* 2007;30(6):472–478.

20. Trikha SP, Acton D, O'Reilly M, et al. Acute lateral dislocation of the patella: correlation of ultrasound scanning with operative findings. *Injury.* 2003;34(8):568–571.

21. Engelina S, Robertson CJ, Moggridge J, et al. Using ultrasound to measure the fibre angle of vastus medialis oblique: a cadaveric validation study. *Knee.* 2012 July 20 [Epub ahead of print].

22. Starok M, Lenchik L, Trudell D, et al. Normal patellar retinaculum: MR and sonographic imaging with cadaveric correlation. *AJR Am J Roentgenol.* 1997;168(6):1493–1499.

23. Mandl P, Brossard M, Aegerter P, et al. Ultrasound evaluation of fluid in knee recesses at varying degrees of flexion. *Arthritis Care Res (Hoboken).* 2012;64(5):773–779.

24. Azzoni R, Cabitza P. Is there a role for sonography in the diagnosis of tears of the knee menisci? *J Clin Ultrasound.* 2002;30(8):472–476.

25. Sekiya JK, Jacobson JA, Wojtys EM. Sonographic imaging of the posterolateral structures of the knee: findings in human cadavers. *Arthroscopy.* 2002;18(8): 872–881.

26. Cook JL, Purdam CR. Is tendon pathology a continuum? A pathology model to explain the clinical presentation of load-induced tendinopathy. *Br J Sports Med.* 2009;43(6):409–416.

27. Malliaras P, Purdam C, Maffulli N, et al. Temporal sequence of greyscale ultrasound changes and their relationship with neovascularity and pain in the patellar tendon. *Br J Sports Med.* 2010;44(3):944–947.

28. Cook JL, Malliaras P, De Luca J, et al. Neovascularization and pain in abnormal patellar tendons of active jumping athletes. *Clin J Sport Med.* 2004;14(5):296–299.

29. Kamel M, Eid H, Mansour R. Ultrasound detection of knee patellar enthesitis: a comparison with magnetic resonance imaging. *Ann Rheum Dis.* 2004;63(2):213–214.

30. Gohr CM, Fahey M, Rosenthal AK. Calcific tendonitis: a model. *Connect Tissue Res.* 2007;48(6):286–291.

31. Cook JL, Khan KM, Harcourt PR, et al. Patellar tendon ultrasonography in asymptomatic active athletes reveals hypoechoic regions: a study of 320 tendons. Victorian Institute of Sport Tendon Study Group. *Clin J Sport Med.* 1998;8(2):73–77.

32. Comin J, Cook JL, Malliaras P, et al. The prevalence and clinical significance of sonographic tendon abnormalities in asymptomatic ballet dancers: a 24-month longitudinal study. *Br J Sports Med.* 2013;47(2):89–92.

33. Engebretsen L, Steffen K, Alsousou J, et al. IOC consensus paper on the use of platelet-rich plasma in sports medicine. *Br J Sports Med.* 2010;44(15):1072–1081.

34. Katchburian MV, Bull AM, Shih YF, et al. Measurement of patellar tracking: assessment and analysis of the literature. *Clin Orthop Relat Res.* 2003;(412):241–259.

35. McNally EG. Imaging assessment of anterior knee pain and patellar maltracking. *Skeletal Radiol.* 2001;30(9):484–495.

36. Ewing JW. Plica: pathologic or not? *J Am Acad Orthop Surg.* 1993;1(2):117–121.

37. Paczesny L, Krucyznski J. Medial plica syndrome of the knee: diagnosis with dynamic sonography. *Radiology.* 2009;251(2):439–446.

38. García-Valtuille R, Abascal F, Cerezal L, et al. Anatomy and MR imaging appearances of synovial plicae of the knee. *Radiographics.* 2002;22(4):775–784.

39. Schein A, Matcuk G, Patel D, et al. Structure and function, injury, pathology, and treatment of the medial collateral ligament of the knee. *Emerg Radiol.* 2012;19(6):489–498.

40. Marchant MH Jr, Tibor LM, Taylor D, et al. Management of medial-sided knee injuries, part 1: medial collateral ligament. *Am J Sports med.* 2011;39(5):1102–1113.

41. Hughston JC, Andrews JR, Cross MJ, et al. Classification of knee ligament instabilities. Part I. The medial compartment and cruciate ligament. *J Bone Joint Surg Am.* 1976;58(2):159–172.

42. Sekiya JK, Swaringen JC, Wojtys EM, et al. Diagnostic ultrasound evaluation of posterolateral corner knee injuries. *Arthroscopy.* 2010;26(4):494–499.

43. Rutten MJ, Collins JM, van Kampen A, et al. Meniscal cysts: detection with high-resolution sonography. *AJR Am J Roentgenol.* 1998;171(2):491–496.

44. Shetty AA, Tindall AJ, James KD, et al. Accuracy of hand-held ultrasound scanning in detecting meniscal tears. *J Bone Joint Surg Br.* 2008;90(8):1045–1048.

45. Kawaguchi K, Enokida M, Otsuki R, et al. Ultrasonographic evaluation of medial radial displacement of the medial meniscus in knee osteoarthritis. *Arthritis Rheum.* 2012;64(1):173–180.

46. Kirk KL, Kuklo T, Klemme W. Iliotibial band friction syndrome. *Orthopedics.* 2000;23(11):1209–1214.

47. Alvarez-Nemegyei J. Risk factors for pes anserinus tendinitis/bursitis syndrome: a case control study. *J Clin Rheumatol.* 2007;13(2):63–65.

48. Unlu Z, Ozmen B, Tarhan S, et al. Ultrasonographic evaluation of pes anserinus tendino-bursitis in patients with type 2 diabetes mellitus. *J Rheumatol.* 2003;30(2):352–354.

49. Finnoff JT, Nutz DJ, Henning PT, et al. Accuracy of ultrasound-guided versus unguided pes anserinus bursa injections. *P M R.* 2010;2(8):732–739.

50. Ray JM, Clancy WG Jr, Lemon RA. Semimembranosus tendinitis: an overlooked cause of medial knee pain. *Am J Sports Med.* 1988;16(4):347–351.

51. Weiser HI. Semimembranosus insertion syndrome: a treatable and frequent cause of persistent knee pain. *Arch Phys Med Rehabil.* 1979;60(7):317–319.

52. Lunhao B, Yu S, Jiashi W. Diagnosis and treatment of ganglion cysts of the cruciate ligaments. *Arch Orthop Trauma Surg.* 2011;131(8):1053–1057.

53. Skowgaard Larsen LP, Rasmussen OS. Diagnosis of acute rupture of the anterior cruciate ligament of the knee by sonography. *Eur J Ultrasound.* 2000;12(2):163–167.

54. Palm HG, Bergenthal G, Ehry P, et al. Functional ultrasonography in the diagnosis of acute anterior cruciate ligament injuries: a field study. *Knee.* 2009;16(6):441–446.

55. Stickel WH. Sonographic appearance of the normal posterior cruciate ligament (PCL). *J Ultrasound Med.* 2000;19(1):6.

56. Sorrentino F, Iovane A, Nicosia A, et al. Role of high-resolution ultrasonography without and with real-time spatial compound imaging in evaluating the injured posterior cruciate ligament: preliminary study [in English, Italian]. *Radiol Med.* 2009;114(2):312–320.

57. Miller TT. Sonography of injury of the posterior cruciate ligament of the knee. *Skeletal Radiol.* 2002;31(3):149–154.

58. Cho KH, Lee DC, Chhem RK, et al. Normal and acutely torn posterior cruciate ligament of the knee at ultrasound evaluation: preliminary experience. *Radiology.* 2001;219(2):375–380.

59. Lawrence RG, Felson DT, Helmick RC, et al. Estimates of the prevalence of arthritis and rheumatic conditions in the United States. Part I. *Arthritis Rheum.* 2008;58(1):15–25.

60. Valdes AM, Loughlin J, Oene MV, et al. Sex and ethnic differences in the association of ASPN, CALM1, COL2A1, COMP, and FRZB with genetic susceptibility to osteoarthritis of the knee. *Arthritis Rheum.* 2007;56(1):137–146.

61. Roemer FW, Crema MD, Trattnig S, et al. Advances in imaging of osteoarthritis and cartilage. *Radiology.* 2011;260(2):332–354.

62. McCune WJ, Dedrick DK, Aisen AM, et al. Sonographic evaluation of osteoarthritic femoral condylar cartilage. Correlation with operative findings. *Clin Orthop Relat Res.* 1990;(254):230–235.

63. Yoon CH, Kim HS, Ju JH, et al. Validity of the sonographic longitudinal sagittal image for assessment of the cartilage thickness in the knee osteoarthritis. *Clin Rheumatol.* 2008;27(12):1507–1516.

64. Monteforte P, Rovetta G. Sonographic assessment of soft tissue alterations in osteoarthritis of the knee. *Int J Tissue React.* 1999;21(1):19–23.

65. Iagnocco A, Perricone C, Scirocco C, et al. The interobserver reliability of ultrasound in knee osteoarthritis. *Rheumatology (Oxford).* 2012;51(11):2013–2019.

66. Ea H, Lioté F. Calcium pyrophosphate dehydrate and basic calcium phosphate crystal-induced arthropathies: update on pathogenesis, clinical features, and therapy. *Curr Rheumatol Rep.* 2004;6(3):221–227.

67. Ellabban AS, Kamel SR, Omar HA, et al. Ultrasonographic diagnosis of articular chondrocalcinosis. *Rheumatol Int.* 2012;32(12):3863–3868.

68. Beaudry Y, Stewart JD, Errett L. Distal sciatic nerve compression by a popliteal artery aneurysm. *Can J Neurol Sci.* 1989;16(3):352–353.

69. De Schriver F, Simon JP, De Smet L, et al. Ganglia of the superior tibiofibular joint: report of three cases and review of the literature. *Acta Orthop Belg.* 1998;64(2):233–241.

70. Kwak HS, Han YM, Lee SY, et al. Diagnosis and follow-up ultrasound evaluation of ruptures of the medial head of the gastrocnemius ("tennis Leg"). *Korean J Radiol.* 2006;7(3):193–198.

71. Lee JC, Healy J. Sonography of lower limb muscle injury. *AJR Am J Roentgenol.* 2004;182(2):341–351.

72. Comin J, Malliaras P, Baquie P, et al. Return to competitive play after hamstring injuries involving disruption of the central tendon. *Am J Sports Med.* 2013;41(1):111–115.

73. Labropoulos N, Shifrin DA, Paxinos O. New insights into the development of popliteal cysts. *Br J Surg.* 2004;91(10):1313–1318.

74. Volteas SK, Labropoulos N, Leon M, et al. Incidence of ruptured Baker's cyst among patients with symptoms of deep vein thrombosis. *Br J Surg.* 1997;84(3):342.

75. Nakano KK. Entrapment neuropathy from Baker's cyst. *JAMA.* 1978;239(2):135.

76. Gordon GV, Edell S, Brogadir SP, et al. Baker's cysts and true thrombophlebitis. Report of two cases and review of the literature. *Arch Intern Med.* 1979;139(1):40–42.

77. Miller TT, Staron RB, Koenigsberg T, et al. MR imaging of Baker cysts: association with internal derangement, effusion, and degenerative arthropathy. *Radiology.* 1996;201(1):247–250.

78. Insua JA, Young JR, Humphries AW. Popliteal artery entrapment syndrome. *Arch Surg.* 1970;101(6):771–775.

79. Keen HI, Wakefield RJ, Conaghan PG. A systematic review of ultrasonography in osteoarthritis. *Ann Rheum Dis.* 2009;68(5):611–619.

Foot and Ankle

Ryan Lee
James Griffith

INTRODUCTION

The superficial location of most soft tissue and surface bone lesions of the ankle and foot makes this area readily accessible to high frequency (>10 MHz) ultrasound. The high resolution and clinical efficacy of ultrasound ensure that it is a comparable, and in many respects better, imaging modality than magnetic resonance imaging (MRI) when assessing most soft tissues of the foot and ankle. Imaging anatomy and pathology are best approached by arbitrarily dividing the ankle into anterior, posterior, medial, and lateral regions, whereas the foot is best approached by separately considering the hindfoot, midfoot, and forefoot.

PATIENT POSITION

For the anterior, medial, and lateral ankle and dorsal foot, the patient should be supine with the knee semiflexed. The knee is rotated medially and the ankle slightly inverted for the lateral ankle, and the knee rotated laterally with the ankle slightly everted for the medial ankle. For the posterior ankle and sole of the foot, the patient is best examined prone with the foot hanging freely or in a dorsiflexed position over the edge of the examination couch.

ULTRASOUND APPEARANCES OF LIGAMENTS, TENDONS, AND NERVES

The ultrasound appearances of ankle and foot ligaments, tendons, and nerves are similar to those in other parts of the body. In general, ligaments are seen as thin, regular, hyperechoic fibers aligned in parallel with a well-defined border and attached to bone at both ends. Ankle ligaments are best examined with the transducer aligned with the long axis of the ligament and the ligament stretched. Tendons have a thicker, tightly packed linear fibrillar echotexture when scanned longitudinally and have a speckled echogenic dot appearance on transverse scanning. Most tendons and nerves around the ankle joint are best examined in a transverse plane. Extended longitudinal views of the curved ankle tendons

are difficult to obtain. Ankle tendons are prevented from "bowstringing" by overlying thin fibrous retinacula, which also serve as fulcra for the pulley action of the tendons. All ankle and foot ligaments and tendons are anisotropic and appear hypoechoic if the transducer is not perpendicular to their fibers. Anisotropy can be used to identify a tendon or ligament by distinguishing it from adjacent tissues. For example, tilting the transducer to make the anterior talofibular ligament (ATFL) appear hypoechoic accentuates the conspicuity of the ligament against the adjacent echogenic fat. Conversely, tendon or ligament echogenicity should always be interpreted in the light of anisotropy. Nerves are also tubular echogenic fascicular structures. They have a slightly coarser fibrillar echotexture than tendons and are found in predictable locations, typically in neurovascular bundles. If doubt exists, nerves can be differentiated from tendons by tracing their course proximally or distally, while scanning in short axis.

> **Tip:**
> In general, most ankle and foot tendons or ligaments are best assessed with ultrasound except for those on the plantar aspect of the foot, which are best assessed with MR imaging

RELEVANT ULTRASOUND ANATOMY

Anterior Ankle

Anterior Ligaments

The anterior inferior tibiofibular ligament is a strong multifascicular fan-shaped ligament that lies between the anterior aspect of the distal tibia (Tillaux-Chaput tubercle) and the adjacent fibula (**Fig. 8.1**). It runs slightly obliquely upward and medially from the anteromedial aspect of the distal fibula at the upper margin of the ankle joint and is widest at the tibial insertion (**Fig. 8.1**). Moving the transducer proximally in a transverse plane from the ankle joint shows the anterior tibiofibular ligament (**Fig. 8.2**). Ligament conspicuity can be improved by slight angulation of the transducer or by rotating the tibial end of the transducer slightly more cranially.

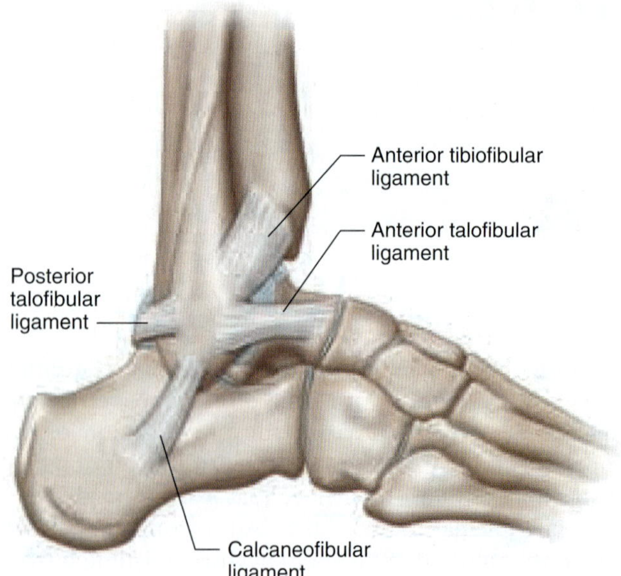

Figure 8.1.   Schematic diagram of the ankle showing lateral and anterior ankle ligaments.

The ligament is <2-mm wide at its mid-portion and provides major support to the distal tibiofibular syndesmosis.[1] The distal interosseous membrane is seen as a thin, hyperechoic (almost isoechoic to bone) line between the tibia and the fibula[2] proximal to the anterior tibiofibular ligament.

Anterior Tendons

The anterior ankle tendons comprise the tibialis anterior, extensor hallucis longus (EHL), and extensor digitorum longus (EDL) from medial to lateral **(Fig. 8.3)**. They can

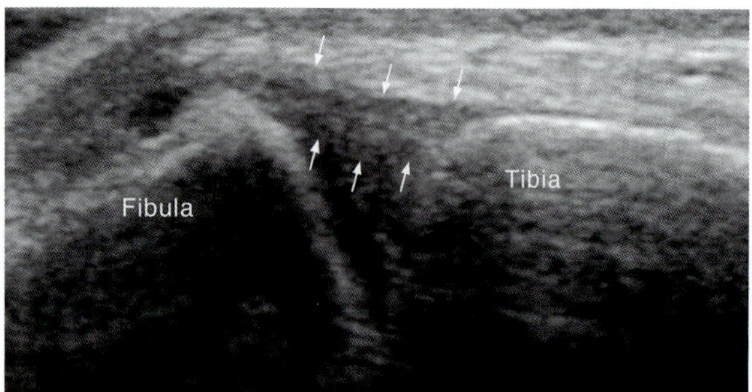

Figure 8.2.   Transverse ultrasound showing normal anterior inferior tibiofibular ligament (*arrows*) with a wider attachment to the tibia than the fibula.

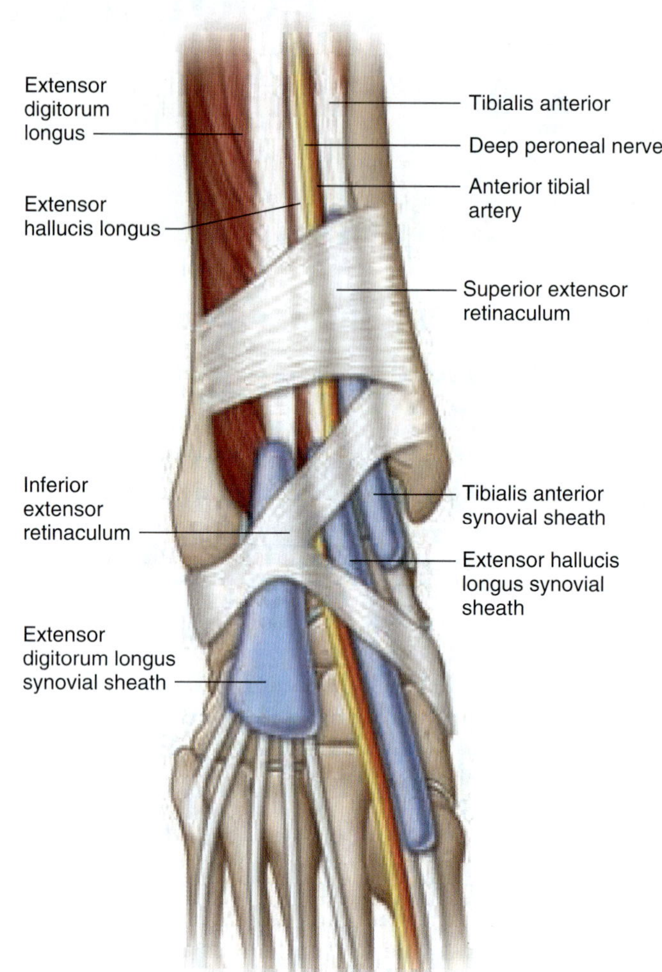

Figure 8.3.   Schematic diagram of the anterior aspect of the ankle showing tendons running deep to the superior and inferior extensor retinacula. Note how the dorsalis pedis neurovascular bundle runs between the FDL and the flexor pollicis longus tendons. The deep branch of the peroneal nerve lies alongside the FHL tendon. FDL, flexor digitorum longus; FHL, flexor hallucis longus.

be memorized by "Tom Has a Date Perhaps" from medial to lateral (Tom = Tibialis anterior, Has = extensor Hallucis longus, A = Anterior tibial artery/vein and deep peroneal nerve, Date = extensor Digitorum longus, and Perhaps = Peroneus tertius). They are covered by retinaculum. The superior extensor retinaculum extends from the lateral malleolus to the medial malleolus and is continuous with the flexor retinaculum medially and superior peroneal retinaculum laterally. The inferior extensor retinaculum is Y-shaped. The stem of the Y lies on the lateral aspect of the retinaculum and divides into superomedial and inferomedial limbs, which attach to the medial malleolus and navicular-cuneiform area, respectively.

The tibialis anterior tendon is the strongest, largest, and most superficial of the anterior tendons. It begins at the junction of the lower and middle-thirds of the tibia. At the level of the ankle joint, it lies medial to the midline and then runs toward the medial border of the foot, where it attaches to the superomedial aspect of the medial cuneiform and the first metatarsal[3,4] (**Fig. 8.3**). The tendon is ovoid proximally and becomes flatter distally, measuring <5 mm in width at 3 cm from its insertion.[5]

The EHL tendon lies just lateral to the tibialis anterior tendon and inserts dorsally on the base of the distal phalanx of the hallux. The anterior tibial artery, anterior tibial vein, and deep peroneal nerve lie just lateral to EHL. In the distal leg, the deep peroneal nerve lies on the medial side of the anterior tibial artery. At the ankle, the nerve crosses over the artery to lie on its lateral side (**Fig. 8.3**). This arrangement is important to note during aspiration of an ankle joint effusion using an anterior approach.

The EDL tendon is the most lateral of the anterior tendons, and branches at the anterior ankle joint line into separate tendons to the second to fifth toes (**Fig. 8.3**). The peroneus tertius tendon crosses the ankle joint lateral to the EDL tendon to insert into the dorsal surface of the fifth metatarsal base. It is absent in about 10% of individuals.

> **Tip:**
> All extensor tendons of the ankle have their own individual tendon sheath at the level of the inferior retinaculum.

The deep and superficial peroneal nerves arise from the common peroneal nerve at the level of the fibular neck and run distally deep to the peroneus longus muscle. At the ankle, the deep peroneal nerve runs deep to the extensor retinaculum initially medial to and then lateral to the anterior tibial artery. Just distal to the retinaculum it divides into a medial sensory branch, which supplies the first digital interspace, and a lateral motor branch, which supplies the extensor digitorum brevis muscle. It can become trapped between the extensor digitorum brevis muscle and the head of the talus.[6] The superficial peroneal nerve separates from the deep peroneal nerve 10 to 15 cm above the ankle. It pierces the investing fascia about 9 cm proximal to the lateral malleolus, where it is prone to injury,[7] then runs anterolateral to the lateral malleolus, superficial to the superior and inferior extensor retinacula, before dividing into medial and intermediate dorsal cutaneous nerves. It provides sensory innervation to the skin on the dorsum of the foot and most of the toes.

> **Tip:**
> The deep peroneal nerve lies initially medial to and then lateral to the anterior tibial artery at the ankle joint.

Anterior Ankle Joint

The anterior ankle joint is best assessed in the longitudinal plane with the ankle in slight plantar flexion. The

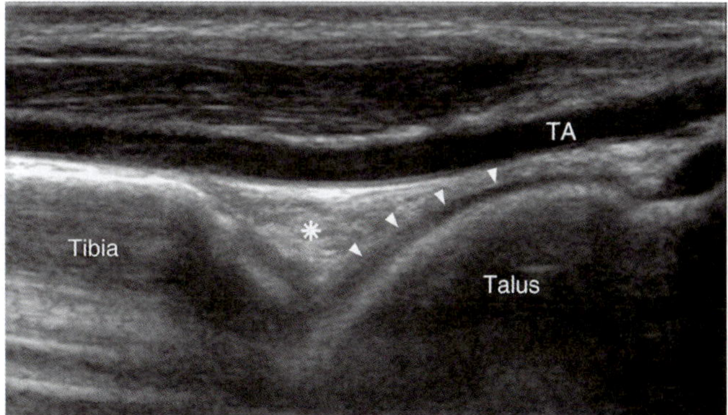

Figure 8.4. Longitudinal ultrasound of normal anterior aspect of ankle joint at the level of tibialis anterior artery (TA). Note the distal tibia and hypoechoic articular cartilage (*arrowheads*) on anterior aspect of the talar dome. Note the subcapsular triangular-shaped anterior fat pad (*asterisk*) segregating the anterior recess into smaller superior and larger inferior recesses.

anterior joint capsule is attached along the distal margin of the tibia and fibula approximately 10 mm from the ankle joint and extends to the neck of the talus.[8] High-resolution imaging is needed to distinguish the capsule from the triangular-shaped fat pad that lies slightly deeper and divides the anterior recess of the ankle into smaller superior and larger inferior recesses (**Fig. 8.4**). A small amount of joint fluid is normal and best appreciated in the medial and lateral recesses. Larger quantities of fluid distend the anterior and posterior recesses. Increased fluid in the anterior recess displaces the fat pad anteriorly. A thin (approximately 2 mm), hypoechoic layer of articular cartilage covers the anterior aspect of the talar dome when the ankle is plantar flexed and should not be confused with joint fluid. Articular cartilage in the central and posterior ankle joint cannot be seen with ultrasound.

The anterolateral recess or gutter is bounded laterally by the fibula, medially by the talus and tibia, anteriorly by the tibiotalar joint capsule, the anterior talofibular and tibiofibular ligaments, anteroinferiorly by the calcaneofibular (CFL) ligament, and superiorly by the tibial plafond and distal tibiofibular syndesmosis.[9] The anterolateral and anteromedial recesses should be routinely assessed on ultrasound of the ankle joint as fluid, crystal aggregates, synovial proliferation, and other pathologies may be visible, although not apparent in the anterior recess.

Lateral Ankle

Lateral Ligaments

The lateral ankle ligaments, or lateral collateral ligaments, comprise the anterior talofibular, CFL, and posterior talofibular ligaments (**Fig. 8.1**).

Anterior Talofibular Ligament (ATFL)

The ATFL is a condensation of the ankle capsule similar to the glenohumeral ligaments in the shoulder.[10] It extends from the anterosuperior aspect of the distal fibula at the level of the malleolar fossa to the lateral aspect of the neck of talus. It is best visualized with the ankle in a relaxed position (about 20 degrees plantar flexed, i.e., with the sole of the foot flat on the examination couch) and the ligament almost parallel to the ankle joint. The transducer is placed just anterior to the lateral malleolus and oriented horizontally. The distal end of the transducer is then turned slightly caudally.[11] The normal thickness of the ATFL is 2 mm, and it is about 20 mm in length.[12] The ligament is best seen when straight and taut **(Fig. 8.5)** by plantar flexing the ankle joint.

Tip:
The ATFL is best seen by scanning almost transversely when the foot is slightly plantar flexed just distal to the ankle joint.

Calcaneofibular Ligament

The CFL ligament extends posteroinferiorly from the inferior tip of the fibula to insert on the lateral aspect of the calcaneal body. It lies deep, almost at right angles to the peroneal tendons **(Fig. 8.1)**, and has a curved alignment akin to a hammock when relaxed. The normal ligament is about 2 mm wide and 2 mm thick and can be seen deep to the peroneal tendons when the tendons are scanned transversely[12] **(Fig. 8.6)**. The ligament is best seen with the ankle in dorsiflexion as this stretches the ligament and reduces its curvature. The transducer is positioned with its proximal end at the inferior tip of the lateral malleolus and its distal end aligned posteriorly and slightly toward the heel.[12] The ligament is hyperechoic in the distal two-thirds only. The curved proximal portion of the ligament usually appears hypoechoic due to anisotropy.

Tip:
The CFL ligament is best seen deep to the inframalleolar peroneal tendons when these tendons are scanned in a transverse plane.

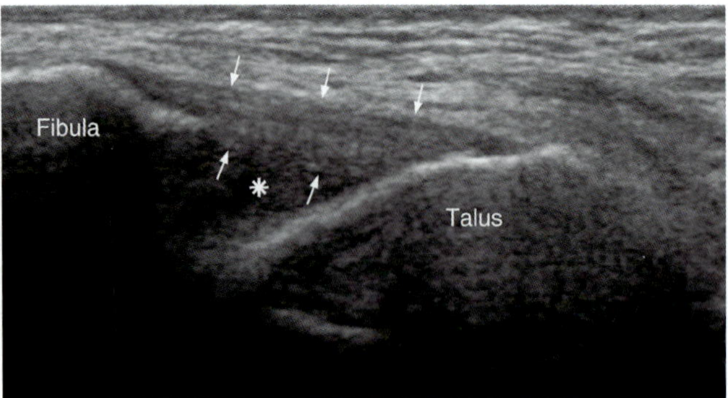

Figure 8.5.   Transverse ultrasound showing normal ATFL (*arrows*). There is a small amount of fluid in the anterolateral ankle recess (*asterisk*). ATFL, anterior talofibular ligament.

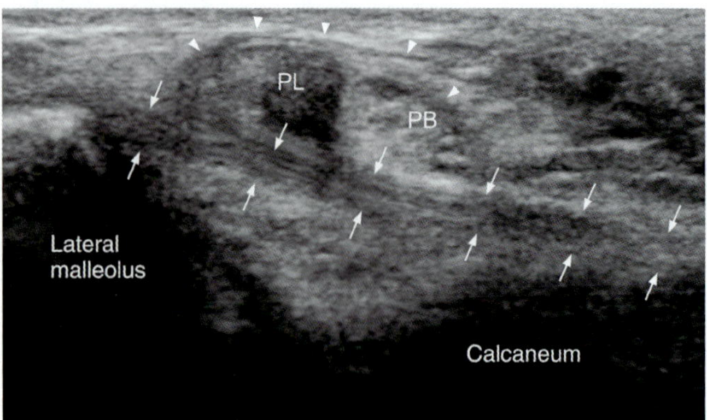

Figure 8.6.   Transverse oblique ultrasound showing the CFL (*arrows*) extending between the fibular tip and the calcaneum. The ligament lies deep to the peroneus longus (*PL*) and brevis (*PB*) tendons. Note also the inferior extensor retinaculum (*arrowheads*) overlying the peroneal tendons at this location. CFL, calcaneofibular ligament.

Posterior Talofibular Ligament

This ligament is partially obscured by the fibula and is difficult to see in its entirety on ultrasound. It is orientated in a similar plane to the ATFL and extends from the distal aspect of the malleolar fossa and to the lateral tubercle of the posterior process of the talus. It is best seen with the patient prone.

Lateral Tendons

The tendons posterior to the lateral malleolus are the peroneus brevis and peroneus longus tendons **(Fig. 8.7)**. The peroneus longus tendon starts about 4 cm above the level of the ankle joint and peroneus brevis more distally. Both tendons run posterior and then inferior to the lateral malleolus where they share a common supramalleolar and retromalleolar synovial sheath. They lie within the fibro-osseous retromalleolar groove of the fibula covered by the superior peroneal retinaculum. The groove is lined by fibrocartilage and varies in width and depth. The superior peroneal retinaculum is about 1mm thick, 1- to 2 cm wide; extends from the posterolateral edge of the distal fibula to the lateral wall of the calcaneum, although variations of this insertion exist[13]; and is the primary restraint to peroneal tendon subluxation. The peroneus longus tendon lies posterolateral to the brevis tendon in the retromalleolar groove and takes the longer route around the inferior aspect of the malleolus (remembered by the peroneus *longus* takes the *longer* route round the malleolus or peroneus *brevis* lies closer to the *bone*). The peroneus longus is marginally (10% to 15%) larger in cross-sectional area than the peroneus brevis tendon.[10]

Tip:
The peroneus longus tendon is slightly larger than the peroneus brevis tendon in cross-sectional area.

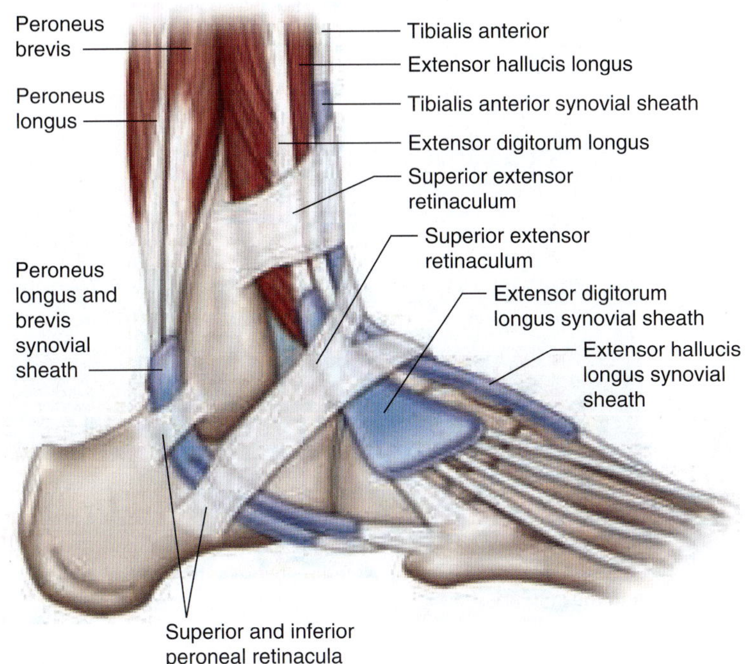

Figure 8.7.   Schematic diagram of the tendons and retinacula on the anterior and lateral aspects of the ankle joint.

The common peroneal tendon sheath divides just proximal to the peroneal tubercle of the calcaneus, and the tendons run anteriorly in their respective tendon sheaths. Peroneus brevis runs dorsal and peroneus longus plantar to the peroneal tubercle, deep to the inferior peroneal retinaculum. The tubercle varies in size from a clearly palpable and distinct tubercle to a barely discernible one. As peroneus longus moves around the peroneal tubercle, it may become irritated when the tubercle is hypertrophied. Small amounts of fluid in the peroneal tendon sheaths are normal, particularly in the dependent inframalleolar region. The peroneus brevis tendon extends horizontally from the peroneal tubercle to insert on the base of the fifth metatarsal.

Peroneus longus passes into the sole of the foot running in a groove on the cuboid (the cuboid tunnel) before turning sharply and running obliquely across the midfoot to insert onto the undersurface of the medial cuneiform and the base of the first metatarsal. The os peroneum is a sesamoid bone located in the peroneus longus tendon just proximal to the cuboid tunnel in up to 30% of adults, bilateral in 60% of cases, bipartite in about 10%,[14] and seen as a small (5 to 15 mm) hyperechoic body with posterior acoustic shadowing. The primary function of the peroneus longus tendon is plantar flexion of the medial forefoot. Along with the peroneus brevis, it also everts and stabilizes the ankle joint.

Tip:
The os peroneum is located within the peroneus longus tendon and is sometimes associated with focal tendinosis of the peroneus longus and fracture.

An accessory peroneus quartus muscle, present in about 10% of subjects, lies medial and posterior to the peroneus brevis and longus. Its tendon runs in the common peroneal tendon sheath and usually inserts into the retrotrochlear eminence of the calcaneus, which is often hypertrophied, just posterior to the peroneal tubercle.[15] Other insertions include the peroneus longus and brevis tendons, the base of the fifth metatarsal, and the cuboid.[16] Occasionally, the muscle belly inserts directly into the retrotrochlear eminence.

The sural nerve runs initially between the Achilles tendon and the peroneal tendons accompanied by the small saphenous vein, then inferior to the peroneal tendons. It bifurcates into terminal lateral and medial branches at the base of the fifth metatarsal and provides sensory supply to the lateral ankle, foot, and the small toe. It anastomoses with branches of the superficial peroneal nerve.

Medial Ankle

Medial Ligament

Deltoid Ligament

The deltoid ligament is a strong, fan-shaped ligament extending from the medial malleolus to insert on the posterior talus, sustentaculum tali of the calcaneum, anterior talus, and navicular (**Fig. 8.8A**). It has superficial and deep components that are separable on ultrasound. The superficial fibers extend to the navicular bone, spring ligament, and calcaneum, and are known as the tibionavicular, tibiospring, and tibiocalcaneal fibers, respectively. The stronger and shorter deep fibers extend

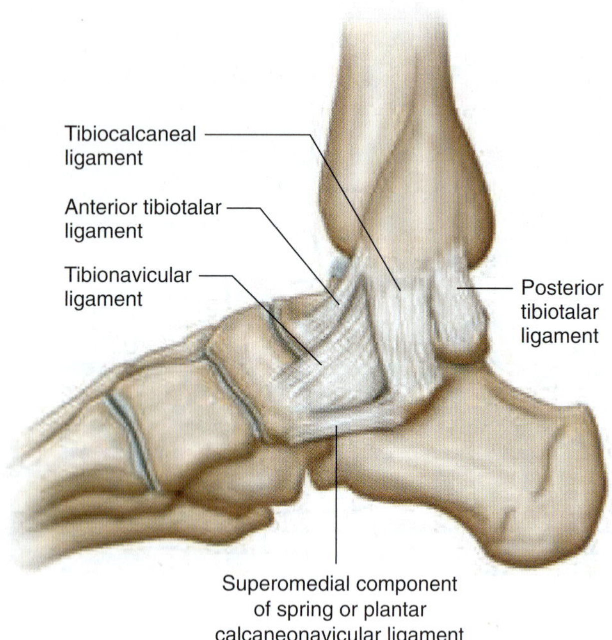

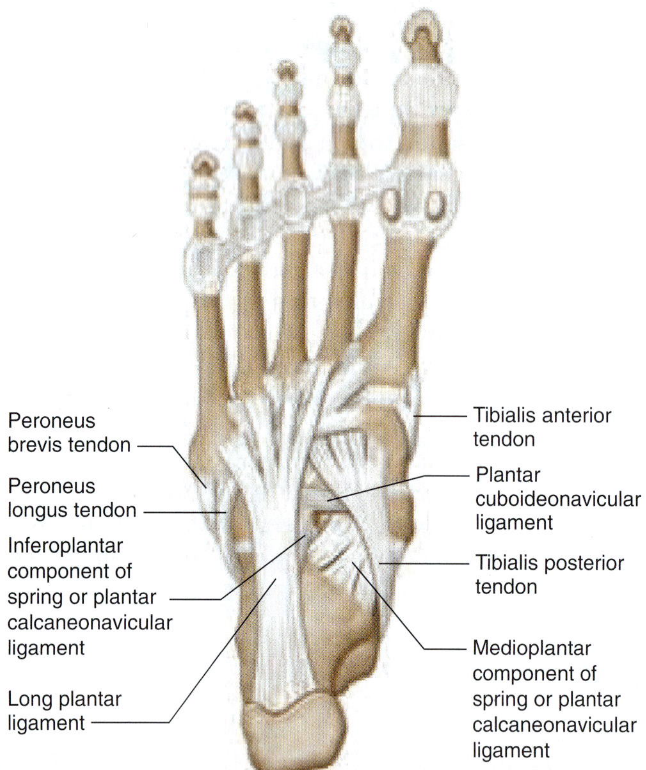

Figure 8.8.   **A:** Schematic diagram of the medial aspect of ankle showing components of deltoid ligament. The superomedial component of the calcaneonavicular component is also shown. **B:** Schematic diagram of the plantar aspect of foot showing tendon insertions, and plantar components of spring ligament (inferoplantar and medioplantar components).

to the talus and are known as the anterior and posterior tibiotalar fibers. While the superficial and deep fibers are identifiable as separate structures, the individual

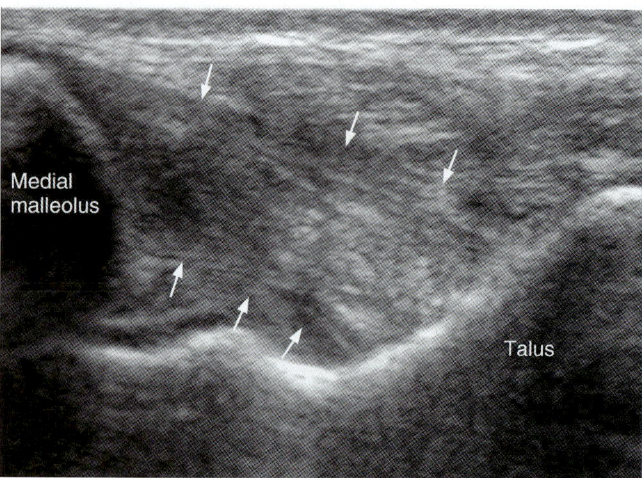

Figure 8.9.   Longitudinal ultrasound showing normal fan-shaped deltoid ligament. The five different components of the deltoid ligament (*arrows*) are not readily distinguishable on ultrasound. The posterior fibers of the ligament extending between the medial malleolus and the talus are shown.

components of the superficial and deep layers are seen as a continuum. In general, the superficial fibers tend to be located more anteriorly, though considerable overlap does occur. The deltoid ligament is best visualized in a longitudinal plane with the ankle slightly dorsiflexed and the hindfoot everted. The proximal end of the probe is placed on the medial malleolus, while the distal end of the probe is moved in a fan-shaped manner to show all components **(Fig. 8.9)**. The anterior and mid-fibers are not as consistently well visualized as the posterior fibers which run posteriorly and inferiorly to the talus.[17] The deltoid ligament is normally 4- to 5 mm thick in its mid-portion.[18] On transverse scanning, the tibialis posterior tendon crosses the superficial component of the deltoid ligament.

Tip:
The deltoid ligament is composed of superficial and deep fibers. The separate components of the fibers are inseparable on ultrasound.

Spring Ligament Complex

The spring (plantar calcaneonavicular) ligament complex is located between the calcaneus and navicular on the medial and inferoplantar aspects of the foot. It helps to support the head of the talus and, with the tibialis posterior tendon, forms a crucial support for the medial longitudinal arch[19] **(Figs. 8.8A, B)**. It has superomedial, oblique medioplantar, and inferoplantar components (also known respectively as the medial, intermediate, and lateral components). The superomedial fibers are functionally the most important, and extend from the sustentaculum tali, over the surface of talar head, to insert onto the superomedial aspect of the navicular. There is a "gliding layer" of fibrocartilage between these fibers and the overlying posterior tibial tendon, though this gliding layer is not seen as a discrete separate structure on ultrasound imaging. There are also some connecting collagenous fibers between the posterior tibial tendon and the superomedial fibers of the spring ligament. The superomedial fibers are seen as an echogenic band just deep to the posterior tibial tendon,[20] best demonstrated by placing the probe with one end over the sustentaculum tali and the other over the talar head and medial aspect of the navicular bone.[20] The superomedial component of the spring ligament can also be seen deep to the posterior tibial tendon just proximal to the tendon insertion when the tendon is scanned transversely. Proximally, the normal thickness of the superomedial component of the spring ligament is 4 mm overlying the talar head.[21] The medioplantar and inferoplantar components of the spring ligament are functionally less important and not consistently seen on ultrasound **(Fig. 8.8B)**.

Medial Tendons

The tendons that run posterior to the medial malleolus are from anterior to posterior (or medial to lateral), the posterior tibial (tibialis posterior), flexor digitorum longus (FDL), and flexor hallucis longus (FHL) tendons. The neurovascular bundle, comprising the posterior tibial vessels and tibial nerve, lies between the FDL and FHL tendons **(Fig. 8.10)**. The arrangement can be memorized by "Tom, Dick, And Harry" from anterior to posterior (Tom = *Tibialis posterior*, Dick = FDL, And = posterior tibial *Artery*, concomitant veins and tibial nerve, and Harry = FHL). In the retromalleolar region, they are covered by the flexor retinaculum to form a fibro-osseous tarsal tunnel.[22] The retinaculum is a thin (<1 mm) echogenic band extending from the medial malleolus to the posterosuperior aspect of the calcaneus. The proximal tunnel is covered by a deep aponeurosis of the leg and has an osseous floor formed by the tibia and the talus. The more distal tunnel is covered by the flexor retinaculum and the fascial covering of the abductor hallucis muscle and has an osseous floor formed by the calcaneus, sustentaculum tali, and inferomedial navicular.

The tibial nerve trifurcates about 1.5 cm proximal to the tip of the medial malleolus.[23] Its first branch is the sensory medial calcaneal nerve, which arises proximal to the flexor retinaculum in 40% of subjects. When it does so, sensory deficit due to compression of the tibial nerve in the tarsal tunnel tends to spare the heel.[24] The tibial nerve then divides into the medial and lateral plantar nerves, deep to the flexor retinaculum and separated by the interfascicular septum. The medial plantar nerve runs with the posterior tibial tendon along the medial

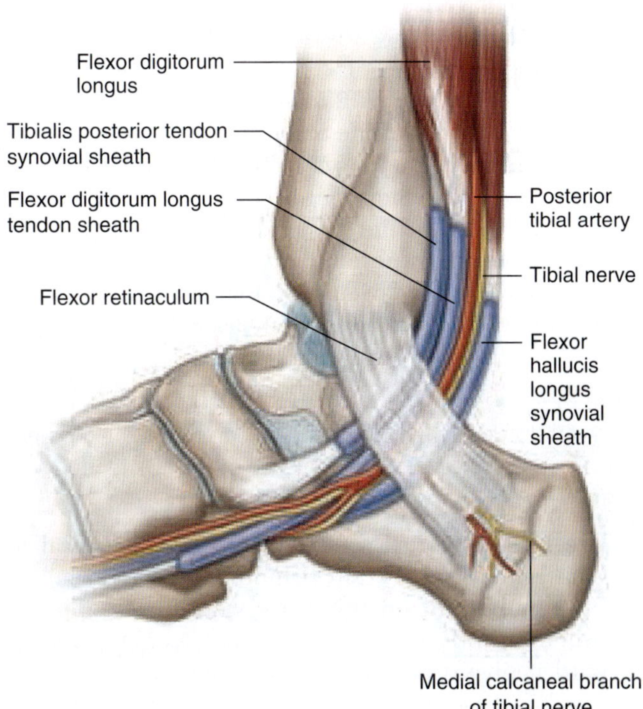

Figure 8.10. Schematic diagram showing "Tom, Dick, and Harry" arrangement of tendons on medial aspect of the ankle. The tibial nerve divides into the medial and lateral plantar nerves just distal to the medial retinaculum. The sensory medial calcaneal nerve often originates just proximal to or within the retinaculum.

aspect of the foot to innervate the small muscles (abductor hallucis, flexor hallucis brevis, flexor digitorum brevis, and the first lumbrical muscles). The lateral plantar nerve descends under the midfoot to innervate the small muscles on the lateral side of the foot (abductor digiti minimi, abductor hallucis, quadratus plantae, interosseous muscles, second to fifth lumbricals).

The posterior tibial tendon is held against the posteromedial aspect of the medial malleolus by the flexor retinaculum. It courses around the inferior tip of the medial malleolus. The inframalleolar segment of the tendon runs over the deltoid ligament and the body of the calcaneum before inserting on the plantar aspects of the medial pole of the navicular, the cuneiforms, and the second to fourth metatarsal bases. Its tendon sheath extends from just distal to the musculotendinous junction to 1 to 2 cm proximal to the navicular insertion. The tendon sheath is usually dry, but a trace of fluid (<2 mm in thickness and not circumferential) is normal. The posterior tibial tendon is best examined in short axis in the supra-, retro-, and inframalleolar regions. Distally, it is best examined in long axis as this allows easier evaluation of the insertion. The posterior tibial tendon normally fans out near its insertion, leading to thickening and hypoechogenicity that may mimic a tendon tear or tendinosis. It may insert into an elongated (cornuate) medial pole of the navicular or an accessory navicular. The normal cross-sectional area/mean width of the posterior tibial tendon are: retromalleolar <0.16 cm^2/<2 mm; inframalleolar <0.18 cm^2/<2.5 mm; and pre-insertional <0.27 cm^2/<3.5 mm. The retromalleolar and inframalleolar segments of the posterior tibial tendon are about twice the size of the adjacent FDL tendons. The largest variability in size of the posterior tibial tendon is the most distal portion where it flares out to insert onto the undersurface of the navicular medially, the three cuneiforms, and the medial metatarsal bases.[25]

> **Tip:**
> The retromalleolar and inframalleolar portions of the posterior tibial tendon are about twice the size of the EDL tendon.

The FDL tendon lies immediately posterolateral to the posterior tibial tendon behind the medial malleolus. It is important on transverse scanning to appreciate whether both tendons are present, as FDL can slip forward if tibialis posterior is ruptured and simulate a normal tibialis posterior tendon. In the inframalleolar region, FDL separates from the posterior tibial tendon and runs superficial to the sustentaculum tali. The normal caliber of the FDL is approximately half that of the tibialis posterior. Usually, there is no detectable fluid within the FDL tendon sheath on ultrasound.[26]

The FHL tendon is the most posterior and deepest ankle tendon in the medial ankle. The fleshy muscle belly extends to the level of the ankle joint. The tendon originates behind the ankle joint and lies in a fibro-osseous inframalleolar groove between the medial and lateral talar tubercle. The tendon is covered by the retinaculum and may become entrapped by reactive changes affecting the posterior talar process. Distally, the tendon courses inferior to the sustentaculum tali before inserting on the base of the distal phalanx of the hallux. Due to its deep location, it is less easily appreciated than the other medial ankle tendons on ultrasound. The retromalleolar portion is best seen on sagittal scanning medial to the Achilles tendon. Passive flexion and extension of the big toe during scanning help to confirm continuity of the FHL. In the hindfoot, FHL crosses the tendon of FDL to which it is connected by a thin fibrous slip. In 20% of normal individuals, the FHL tendon sheath communicates with the ankle joint, and an ankle effusion may result in considerable fluid distension of the FHL tendon sheath.

> **Tip:**
> Scanning in a sagittal plane medial to the Achilles tendon while flexing the big toe will help confirm continuity of FHL tendon.

Posterior Ankle

Posterior Ligaments

The posterior inferior tibiofibular and posterior intermalleolar ligaments are deep, not entirely accessible by ultrasound and better assessed by MRI. The posterior tibiofibular ligament is a short ligament between the posterior tibia and fibula. The posterior intermalleolar ligament is present in half of normal subjects and extends obliquely from the superior margin of the medial malleolus to the superior margin of the fibular malleolar fossa where it attaches just proximal to the posterior talofibular ligament.[27]

Posterior Tendon Groups

The Achilles tendon, the largest tendon in the human body, is a merger of the tendons of the triceps surae (i.e., gastrocnemius and soleus muscles) **(Fig. 8.11)**. The gastrocnemius muscle ends in the mid-calf, soleus more distally. The Achilles tendon inserts via a broad attachment on the posterosuperior aspect of the calcaneus[28] **(Fig. 8.12)**. There is a narrow band of fibrocartilage binding the tendon to the bone. The tendon is moderately echogenic with fine parallel echogenic lines on longitudinal scanning. It is generally oval-shaped with a flat or concave anterior border on transverse scanning and is covered by an incomplete tendon sheath or paratenon that envelops the dorsum and sides of the tendon. The paratenon is a thin echogenic band that outlines the moderately echogenic tendon. Anterior to the distal tendon is an echogenic fat pad known as

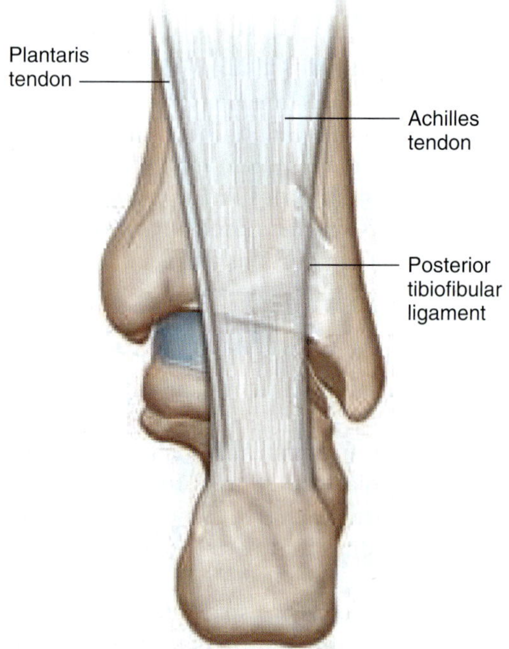

Figure 8.11. Schematic diagram of the posterior tendons showing the Achilles tendon and the plantaris tendon medially. The posterior tibiofibular ligament is also shown.

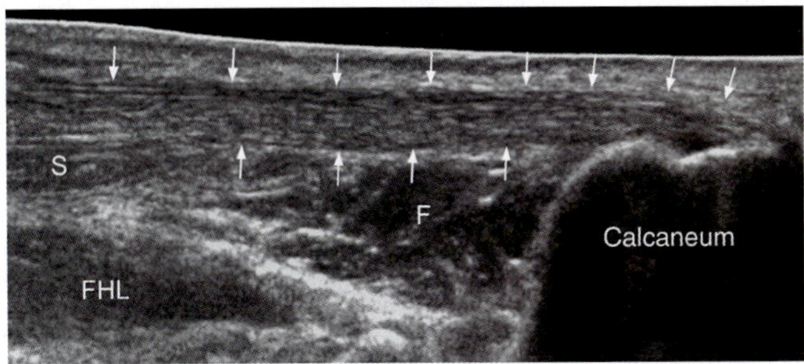

Figure 8.12. Longitudinal ultrasound showing normal Achilles tendon (*arrows*) attached to the posterosuperior aspect of the calcaneum. Note how the soleus muscle (*S*) joins the undersurface of the Achilles tendon. The gastrocnemius muscle joins the more superficial aspect of the tendon more proximally in the leg (not shown). Also shown are Kager fat pad (F) and the flexor hallucis longus (*FHL*) muscle.

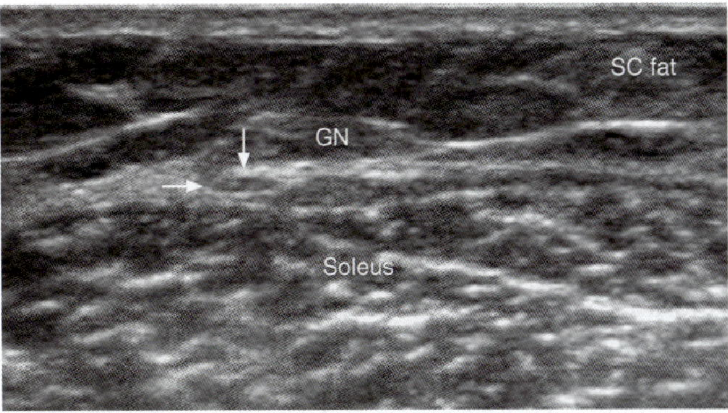

Figure 8.13. Transverse ultrasound of calf showing the ovoid-shaped plantaris tendon (*arrows*) between the medial belly of gastrocnemius muscle (GN) and the soleus muscle. SC fat, subcutaneous fat.

Kager's fat. There are two bursae at the insertion. The retrocalcaneal bursa is a comma-shaped hypoechoic structure (2 to 3 mm in depth) between the tendon and the calcaneus. A subcutaneous bursa lies between the tendon and the skin. It is usually not distended or visible. Focal tendon calcification, fluid in the retrocalcaneal bursa, and bony contour abnormalities at the calcaneal insertion are seen in 2%, 35%, and 63% of asymptomatic subjects.[28] The normal Achilles tendon is 4 to 6 mm (mean 5.3 mm) wide and 5 to 6 cm long, although size is greater in taller and heavier subjects, and in men.[24,25] Achilles tendon measurements are best made on transverse scanning as measurements made on longitudinal scanning tend to be overestimations due to tendon obliquity. Vascularity on Doppler ultrasound is normally minimal or absent.[28] The middle third of the tendon is almost avascular,[28] while the proximal and distal portions are better vascularized from the soleus muscle belly and calcaneal periosteum, respectively. The Achilles tendon receives its sensory nerve supply from the nerves innervating the adjacent muscles and from cutaneous nerves, such as the sural nerve.[29]

> **Tip:**
> Measurements of the Achilles tendon are best made on transverse sections.

The plantaris muscle, which is present in about 90% of the population, has a short (7 to 10 cm) muscle belly arising from the lateral supracondylar region of the femur superficial to the origin of the lateral head of gastrocnemius.[30] The long slender plantaris tendon runs inferomedially, deep to the medial belly of gastrocnemius, to the medial side of the Achilles tendon, and either fuses with the Achilles tendon or inserts into the flexor retinaculum or the calcaneus. The myotendinous junction of plantaris is in the upper calf region.[31] The tendon is a thin ribbon-like structure between the medial head of gastrocnemius and the soleus muscle proximally, medial

to the Achilles tendon distally **(Fig. 8.13)**. It is best identified just proximal to the Achilles myotendinous junction, deep to the medial belly of gastrocnemius, as a small oval hyperechoic structure with an internal fibrillar appearance **(Fig. 8.13)**. The whole course of the tendon may be traced, although it is more difficult to trace proximally than distally. Plantaris should be distinguished from an accessory soleus muscle and tendon. The accessory soleus muscle is a larger more fleshy structure, usually located at the anteromedial aspect of the Achilles tendon, and its tendon inserts into the medial side of the calcaneum.

Posterior Ankle Joint

Fluid distension of the posterior recess of the ankle joint is best appreciated with the patient prone and can lead to unusual configurations such as an inverted "figure of 3" shape due to fluid bulging between the posterior tibiofibular and tibiotalar ligaments.

The posterior talocalcaneal articulation is continuous with the ankle joint in about 20% of normal subjects. The posterior talar process originates from a secondary ossification center that mineralizes between 7 and 14 years and fuses with the talar body within a year to form the lateral talar tubercle. If elongated, it is called a trigonal (Stieda) process. Failure of fusion occurs in approximately 25% of subjects, and the resulting ossicle, or os-trigonum, articulates via a synchondrosis with the talus. Ultrasound cannot usually distinguish between an os-trigonum and a Stieda process as acoustic shadowing precludes assessment of any synchondrosis.

> **Tip:**
> All the tendons crossing the ankle joint are enclosed in a tendon sheath except for the Achilles tendon (which has a paratenon) and the plantaris tendon. Only the Achilles paratenon can be seen in normal subjects on ultrasound. The synovial sheaths of the other ankle tendons cannot be seen in normal subjects.

Foot

Plantar Foot

The plantar fascia is examined with the patient prone or supine. The plantar fascia is not strictly fascial but can be regarded as a common tendon aponeurosis for the superficial layer of the intrinsic plantar foot muscles. It is a thin structure that arises from the medial and lateral inferior calcaneal tubercles and attaches to the plantar plates of the metatarsophalangeal joints and the proximal phalangeal bases. It is a homogeneous echogenic band with internal linear interfaces on longitudinal scans, normally 2- to 3.6-mm thick near its calcaneal origin (**Fig. 8.14**), becoming thinner (1 to 2 mm) and more superficial distally. It comprises a thicker central cord and smaller medial and lateral cords that are not distinct entities but merge indistinguishably with each other. The plantar fascia is the main supporting structure for the longitudinal arches of the foot, connecting the posteroinferior calcaneus and the proximal phalanges.

The intertarsal joints, tarsometatarsal joints, metatarsophalangeal and interphalangeal joints, and their ligaments are assessed individually. The Lisfranc ligament extends obliquely between the lateral aspect of the medial cuneiform and the medial aspect of the second metatarsal base and is an important stabilizer of the tarsometatarsal joints, although it is not assessable by ultrasound. The normal joint space between the medial cuneiform and second metatarsal base is <1.0 mm.[32]

The sinus tarsi is an area bounded by the talus, calcaneum, talonavicular joint, and the posterior compartment of the subtalar joint. It contains the cervical and talocalcaneal interosseous ligaments, inferior extensor retinaculum, fat, and nerve endings of the deep peroneal nerve. The interosseous ligaments cannot be seen on ultrasound as they are deep, partially obscured by bone, and surrounded by adjacent echogenic sinus fat.

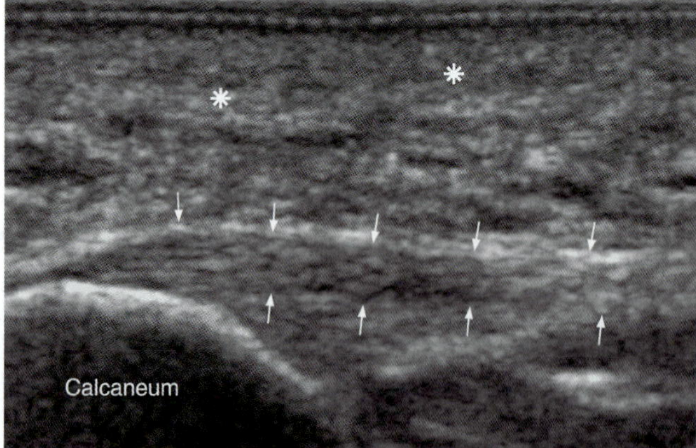

Figure 8.14. Longitudinal ultrasound showing normal plantar fascia (*arrows*) attached to the anteroinferior aspect of the calcaneum. As a general guide, the normal plantar fascia is <4-mm thick at the medial calcaneal tuberosity. Asterisks, heel fat pad.

The sinus tarsi region can be assessed by placing the probe anteroinferior to the tip of the lateral malleolus and angling toward the anterior subtalar joint.

Small plantar digital nerves and their accompanying vessels run between the metatarsal bones. The diameter of the normal plantar digital nerve is 1 to 2 mm at the level of the intermetatarsal heads, and the nerve can be seen on high-resolution (>10 MHz) ultrasound. The intermetatarsal bursa is normally present in each interspace, dorsal to the deep transverse intermetatarsal ligament and neurovascular bundle, and just proximal to the metatarsal head.[33] The bursa may reach ≤3 mm in asymptomatic subjects.[34]

The capsulo-ligamentous-sesamoid complex on the plantar aspect of the first metatarsophalangeal joint includes the joint capsule, collateral ligaments, fibrous plantar plate, and the flexor hallucis brevis, abductor hallucis, and adductor hallucis tendons. Flexor hallucis brevis originates on the cuboid and lateral cuneiform and splits beneath the first metatarsal into medial and lateral tendons that blend with the medial and lateral sesamoid bones just proximal to inserting into the proximal phalanx. The sesamoids are paired oval hyperechoic structures with posterior acoustic shadowing. The sesamoids are embedded in the medial and lateral tendon slips of the flexor hallucis brevis muscle and in the tendon of abductor hallucis muscle. Between the sesamoid bones runs the FHL tendon and deep to this, the thick interconnecting intersesamoid ligament. The sesamoids are bipartite in about 10% of subjects. In this situation, the summated width of the two bipartite ossicles is more than the width of the normal adjacent sesamoid allowing the distinction of bipartite sesamoid to be made.

The plantar plate is a triangular thick biconcave hyperechoic fibrocartilaginous structure on the plantar aspect of the metatarsophalangeal joints. It is firmly attached to the proximal phalanx and extends posteriorly to cover the articular cartilage on the plantar aspects of the metatarsal heads. The plantar plates are connected at the sides to the collateral ligaments of the metatarsophalangeal joints. The long and short toe flexors, invested in a synovial sheath, run just superficial to the plantar plates within a common fibrous sheath. In full-thickness tears of the plantar plate, the tendon sheath may communicate with the metatarsophalangeal joint.

Dorsal Foot

The tibialis anterior, EHL, and the four slips of the EDL tendons can be identified on the dorsal aspect of the midfoot (**Fig. 8.3**). The most medial tendon is the tibialis anterior tendon, which tapers distally to insert on the anteromedial aspect of the first cuneiform and the base of the first metatarsal bone. The distal portion of this tendon is more medial than dorsal and may normally show a mild longitudinal separation just prior to insertion. This should not be confused with a longitudinal split tear. The EHL tendon is thin and more easily appreciated by passive flexion and extension of the big toe. The four diverging slips of EDL insert onto the middle and distal phalanges of the toes. Peroneus tertius may be seen as an accessory fifth lateral slip of the EDL extending toward the base of the fifth metatarsal bone. The dorsal pedis artery and medial branch of the deep peroneal nerve both run between EHL and EDL distal to the ankle joint. The medial branch of the deep peroneal nerve lies just lateral to the dorsalis pedis artery.

The intertarsal, tarsometatarsal, metatarsophalangeal, and interphalangeal joints and corresponding ligaments are assessed individually. A small amount of fluid in the dorsal recess of the metatarsophalangeal or interphalangeal joints is normal. Extensor digitorum brevis and extensor hallucis brevis are the only muscles on the dorsal foot. They extend from the superolateral aspect of the calcaneus (just lateral to sinus tarsi) to the toes, the flat muscle belly lying deep to the EDL tendons.[34] The extensor hallucis brevis muscle is on the medial aspect of the extensor digitorum brevis muscle belly and may be indistinguishable from it. The extensor digitorum tendons insert into the lateral aspects of the EDL tendons.

> **Tip:**
> A small effusion in the dorsal recesses of the small joints of the toes is normal and should not be misinterpreted as synovitis.

ANKLE PATHOLOGY

Tendon Pathology

Anterior Tendons

The anterior tendons are the least prone of all the ankle tendons to tendinosis or tenosynovitis, and of these the tibialis anterior is the most commonly affected (**Fig. 8.15**).

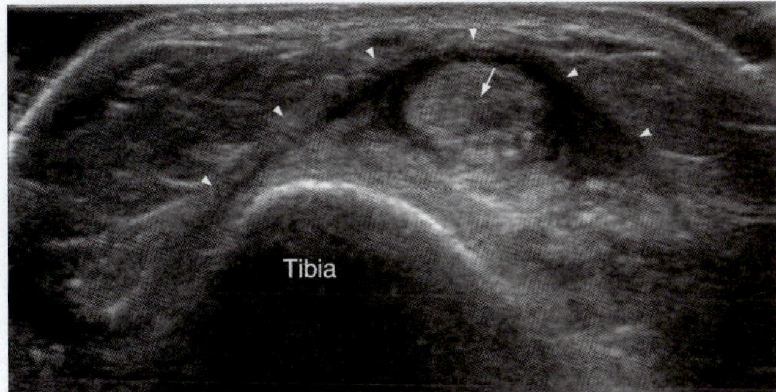

Figure 8.15. Transverse ultrasound of the ankle joint showing a severe tendinosis of the tibialis anterior tendon (*arrow*) with diffuse tendon thickening and a surrounding tendon sheath effusion and peritendinitis. Note the overlying thickened superior retinaculum (*arrowheads*).

It is the strongest dorsiflexor of the ankle and also assists foot inversion. As it runs a relatively straight course within a fibrous tunnel, the mechanical demands on the tendon are low. Complete tears are rare but can result from acute injury or spontaneous rupture of a chronically degenerate tendon.[3] Acute rupture usually presents in younger patients and acute-on-chronic spontaneous rupture in elderly patients, predominantly males.[35,36] Predisposing factors include diabetes mellitus, inflammatory arthropathy, gout, and local steroid injections. The distal tendon is relatively avascular, and this, together with friction against the retinaculum, may explain why most tears occur distally. Ruptures occur at the medial cuneiform, beneath the superomedial limb of the inferior extensor retinaculum, or just distal to the superior extensor retinaculum. Ultrasound shows complete fiber discontinuity. The proximal end of the tendon usually retracts, appears moderately enlarged and hypoechoic, and is typically located deep to the superomedial limb of the inferior retinaculum. It may manifest clinically as a soft tissue mass anterior to the ankle joint. The distal end of the tendon tends not to swell or retract to the same degree and is not as well seen.

The next most common disorder of the tibialis anterior tendon is tendinosis of the distal tendon, which results in a swollen, hypoechoic tendon.[5] Partial tears can occur on a background of tendinosis, usually located near the superomedial limb of the inferior retinaculum.[3,37] The tendon is focally swollen to a moderate degree and hypoechoic. Surface fraying or a discrete partial tear may be visible. Small partial tendon tears may be too small to detect, although swelling and hypoechogenicity are apparent.

Tenosynovitis, tears precipitated by large dorsal osteophytes, and cortical avulsion at the distal insertion are occasionally encountered in EHL and EDL.

> **Tip:**
> Tears of the tibialis anterior tendon may present as a mass anterior to the ankle joint.

Lateral Tendons

The peroneus longus and brevis tendons primarily evert the foot and stabilize the ankle. After the Achilles and posterior tibial tendons, disorders of the peroneal tendons are the next most common.

Tenosynovitis and Tendinosis

Tenosynovitis and tendinosis are the most frequent abnormalities. Tenosynovitis is primarily a disease of the tendon sheath with secondary involvement of the tendon, while tendinosis is primarily a disease of the tendon with secondary involvement of the tendon sheath. In most ankle tendons, one or other predominates, but in the peroneal tendons, a mixed picture with features of both

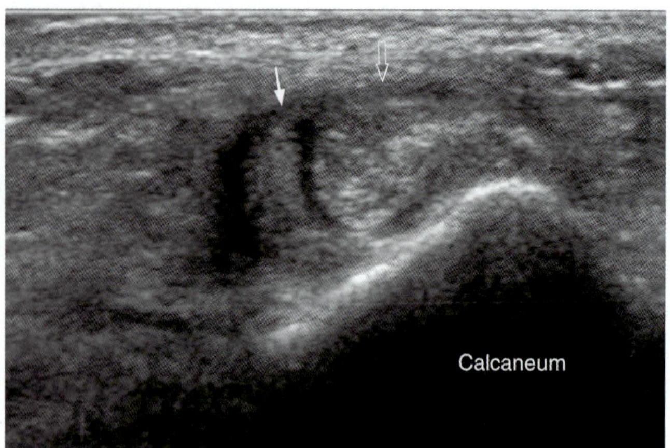

Figure 8.16. Transverse ultrasound lateral aspect of the hindfoot just distal to lateral malleolus. The peroneus longus (PL) tendon is moderately swollen, consistent with moderate-severity tendinosis (*open arrow*). Normally, the PL tendon is about one-third larger than the peroneus brevis tendon. The peroneus brevis tendon (*closed arrow*) is of normal size.

tends to occur. Tenosynovitis produces distension of the tendon sheath with synovial proliferation ± fluid, peritendinous hyperemia, and a relatively unaffected tendon. Tendinosis manifests as tendon thickening, hypoechogenicity, intratendinous tears, and a variable degree of peritendinitis **(Fig. 8.16)**. The more severe the tendinosis, the greater the likelihood of a tendon tear **(Fig. 8.17)**. Tendons are prone to tendinosis at areas of greatest physical stress, and for the peroneal tendons this occurs at the tip of the lateral malleolus, around the peroneal tubercle and in the cuboid groove (for peroneus longus). Several anatomical variants predispose to tendinosis. A low-lying

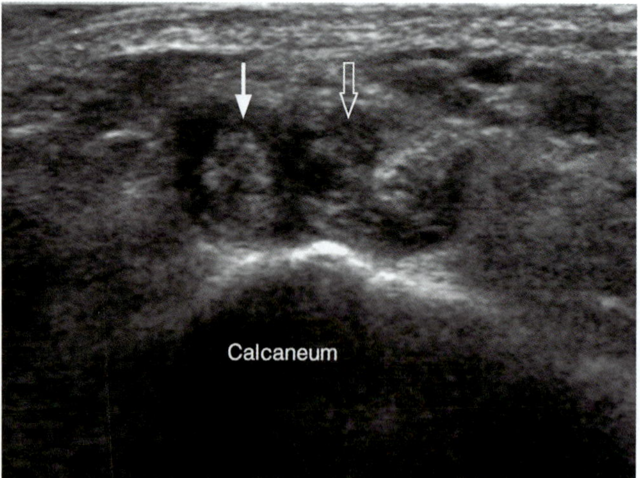

Figure 8.17. Transverse ultrasound lateral aspect of the hindfoot just distal to lateral malleolus. There is moderate to severe tendinosis of the peroneus longus (*open arrow*) and peroneus brevis tendons with tendon enlargement, heterogeneity, longitudinal tears (*closed arrow*), and irregular margin.

peroneus brevis muscle belly or an accessory peroneus quartus muscle can lead to stenosis within the fibro-osseous retromalleolar tunnel and stretching of the superior peroneal retinaculum. Hypertrophy of the peroneal tubercle, particularly if >5 mm in height, or a varus hindfoot alignment increase stress on the tendons.

Peroneal Tendon Tear

Most peroneal tendon tears are longitudinal, intrasubstance partial-thickness tears, or split tears[38] **(Fig. 8.17)**. Complete tears are uncommon and are transverse[39]. Tears of a healthy tendon may occur during acute ankle inversion. More commonly longitudinal tears, usually 2- to 5-cm long, occur in middle-aged patients on a background of tendinosis. Predisposing factors include tendon subluxation, a bony spur at the lateral malleolus, distal fibular or calcaneal fracture, or an os peroneum. Peroneus brevis tends to tear in the retromalleolar sulcus where it may be compressed by the overlying peroneus longus tendon. With more severe tears, peroneus brevis assumes a horseshoe shape on transverse scanning into which insinuates the peroneus longus tendon. Peroneus brevis may eventually split into two tendons, resulting in three apparent tendons being visible instead of the normal two in the retromalleolar region,[40,41] not to be confused with a concurrent peroneus quartus tendon, which usually inserts onto the retrotroclear eminence of the calcaneus. An effusion of the common peroneal tendon sheath is often present, and helps in visualization of the tendon tear. Dynamic examination with plantar or dorsiflexion may also accentuate any longitudinal tendon splits. Occasionally, multiple splits may occur, and the tendon looks like a horsetail at surgery.

> **Tip:**
> The peroneus brevis tendon is more prone to tear. Tears normally occur near the fibular tip and extend proximally and distally. Three rather than two tendons may be seen than peroneus longus.

Peroneus longus tends to tear near the peroneal tubercle and the cuboid groove. An os peroneum predisposes peroneus longus to tendinosis, partial splits, and complete tears, and the combination is known as os peroneum syndrome. An os peroneum is prone to fracture or stress reaction. A fracture is seen as a large gap in the ossicle with irregular margins usually associated with a full-thickness peroneus longus tendon tear.[13] The tendons and bone fragments retract ≥6 mm and have irregular margins, surrounding soft tissue swelling and tenderness on transducer pressure.[10,13] In an undisplaced os peroneum fracture or bipartite os peroneum, the gap is usually <2 mm. Stress reaction of the os peroneum and cuboid marrow edema in peroneal tendinosis are best seen on MRI.[1,10]

Peroneal tendon tears tend to be underdiagnosed on ultrasound as the split fibers do not clearly separate (and even at surgery, tears may only be identified by probing the tendon). A high index of suspicion is needed. Partial tears are best visualized in short axis as thin hypoechoic splits in the tendon. A complete tear produces a distinct transverse gap with retraction of both ends of the tendon. Occasionally, the torn margins remain quite closely apposed, and in this situation separation can be increased by ankle dorsiflexion and inversion.

> **Tip:**
> In general, ultrasound tends to underestimate the presence and extent of peroneal tendon tears.

Peroneal Tendon Subluxation

Subluxation of one or both peroneal tendons from the retromalleolar groove is uncommon[42,43] and results from a tear or attenuation of the superior peroneal retinaculum or, more typically, cortical avulsion or periosteal stripping of the retinaculum from its fibular attachment due to an acute inversion injury. Predisposing factors include a shallow fibular groove, congenital absence or laxity of the superior peroneal retinaculum, and crowding of the peroneal groove by a low-lying peroneus brevis muscle or an accessory peroneus quartus muscle. Ultrasound, particularly dynamic ultrasound with the foot in resisted eversion and dorsiflexion,[44] shows one or both peroneal tendons moving anteriorly and laterally over the lateral malleolus. The superior peroneal retinaculum may be thickened or torn. Sometimes, a small avulsed bony fragment (the "fleck sign") attached to the superior peroneal retinaculum can be identified. Recurrent subluxation usually leads to tendon degeneration and longitudinal splitting.[44]

In some subjects with a sensation of subluxation or a click, the retinaculum is intact and the tendons do not sublux from the retromalleolar groove, but their relationship in the groove changes. Either peroneus longus moves deep to the peroneus brevis or peroneus brevis splits longitudinally and subluxes around the peroneus longus tendon.[10] Intra-sheath subluxation shares some clinical features with true peroneal tendon subluxation such as retrofibular pain and a clicking sensation on ankle movement.[45]

Medial Tendons

Posterior Tibial Tendon Abnormality

The posterior tibial tendon plantar flexes and inverts the foot and, with the spring ligament and sinus tarsi ligaments, helps maintain the medial longitudinal plantar arch. Posterior tibial tendon dysfunction is a progressive spectrum characterized by degeneration of the tendon

and acquired flat foot (pes planus). The tendon is prone to tendinosis rather than tenosynovitis. Tendinosis manifests by progressive tendon thickening, intrasubstance tears and hyperemia, and a variable degree of peritendinitis, usually involving the inframalleolar and distal tendon **(Figs. 8.18A, B)**. Noting the degree of peritenditis is important since peritendinitis will respond to anti-inflammatory medication. The tendon should be examined in cross section from the supramalleolar region to the insertion. A cross-sectional area >20 mm^2 in the retro- and inframalleolar tendon indicates tendinosis. The tendon normally widens at its insertion, and cross-sectional measurements of the distal tendon are larger and more variable. Intratendinous vascularity on Doppler imaging

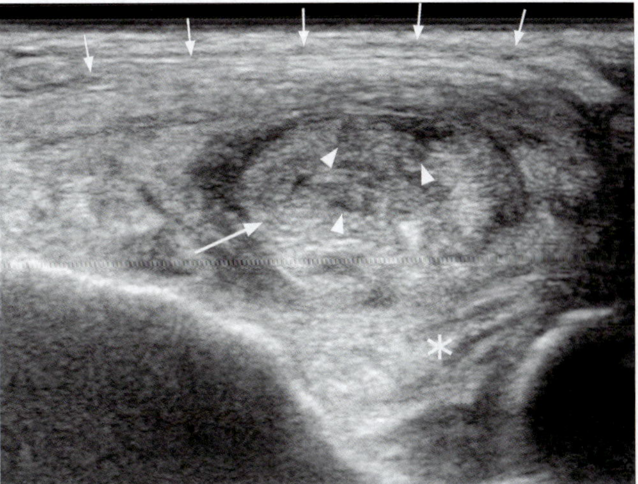

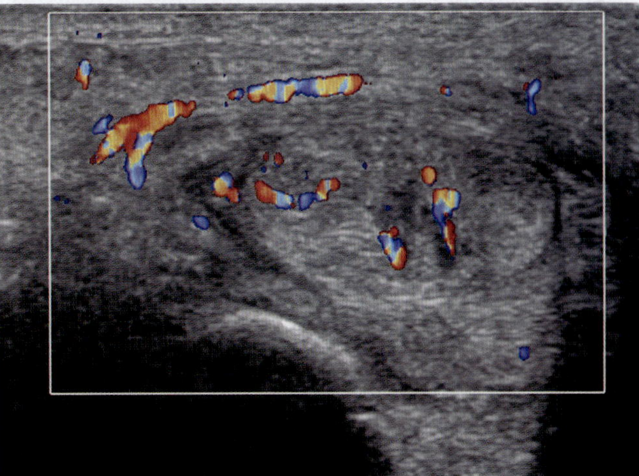

Figure 8.18. **A:** Transverse ultrasound of inframalleolar region showing moderate to severe tendinosis of posterior tibialis tendon (*long arrow*). The tendon is thickened, slightly hypoechoic with many small linear hypoechoic foci (*arrowheads*) representing small intrasubstance micro tears. The surface of the tendon is also irregular and frayed. There is moderate associated peritendinitis with surrounding soft tissue swelling, including the flexor retinaculum (*arrows*). Note the deltoid ligament (*asterisk*) deep to the tendon. **B:** Color Doppler imaging at a similar position to (**A**) showing mild peritendinous and intratendinous hyperemia.

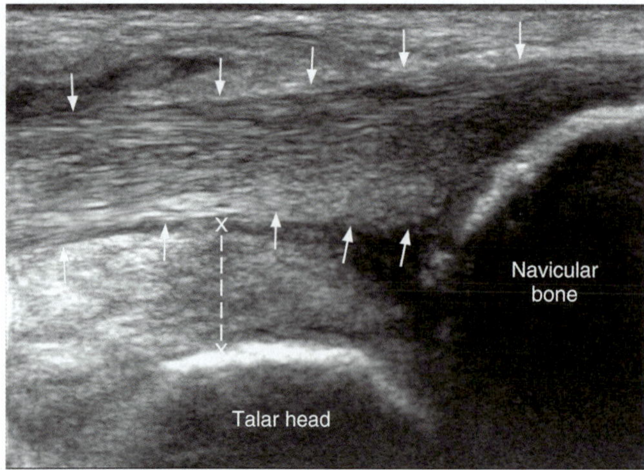

Figure 8.19. Longitudinal ultrasound medial aspect of midfoot showing mild insertional tendinosis of posterior tibialis tendon with thickening (*arrows*). There is also moderate thickening (*dotted line*) of the superomedial component calcaneonavicular (or spring) ligament deep to the posterior tibialis tendon. The ligament is 6.4-mm thick, while the normal ligament thickness should be <4.0 mm.

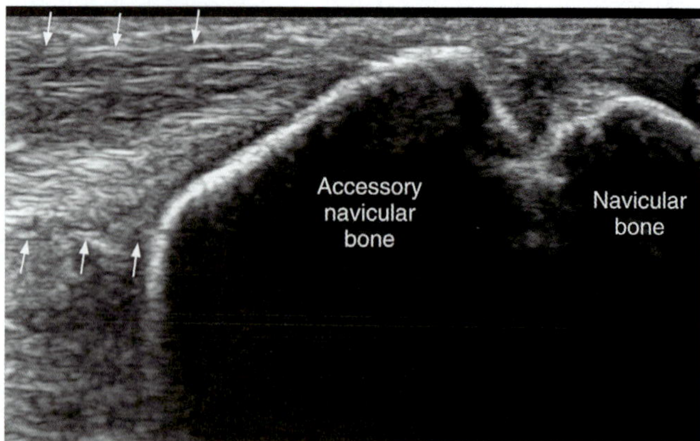

Figure 8.20. Longitudinal ultrasound medial aspect of the midfoot showing a quite large accessory navicular bone with attached posterior tibialis tendon (*arrows*) fibers. The junction with the main navicular bone is also shown.

is always abnormal.[46–48] Always examine an apparent longitudinal split with Doppler imaging as occasionally, a large vessel traversing the tendon may simulate a tear. Tendinosis (**Fig. 8.19**) is strongly associated with an accessory navicular bone (**Fig. 8.20**). Subclinical tendinosis is common, so seeing the same appearance on the opposite side is not always a reliable sign of normality.

Complete rupture is uncommon, while short segment intrasubstance longitudinal tears are frequent.[4] Early diagnosis and treatment of posterior tibial dysfunction may prevent later disability and surgery.[46,47] An intact FDL tendon may move forward into the retromalleolar groove following posterior tibial rupture and mimic a normal posterior tibial tendon.

The vertical or superomedial component of the spring ligament complex becomes thickened with posterior tibial tendinosis/tears (in pes planus) (**Fig. 8.19**). The normal thickness of the superomedial portion of the spring ligament measured deep to the posterior tibialis tendon at the level of the talar neck is <4 mm. Superomedial component thickness of 4 to 5 mm is borderline, while thickness of >5 mm is generally abnormal.

Rarely, an accessory navicular may separate at the synchondrosis with the navicular, leading to retraction of the posterior tibial tendon.

Posterior Tibial Tendon Subluxation

Subluxation or dislocation of the posterior tibial tendon is due to forced dorsiflexion of the ankle with hindfoot supination and external rotation of the leg.[49] Patients may present late.[50] The flexor retinaculum tears or its medial malleolar attachment is avulsed, resulting in anteromedial dislocation of the tendon. Dislocation is

readily appreciated on ultrasound, accentuated, if necessary, by ankle dorsiflexion and supination.[40,41]

> **Tip:**
> Subclinical tendinosis of the posterior tibial tendon, is common so you cannot necessarily rely on the contralateral side as a normal standard.

Posterior Tendons

Plantaris Tendon Pathology

The plantaris muscle is a weak flexor of the knee and ankle. Its tendon is thin and prone to acute tear, which is typically complete.[51] Isolated tears of the plantaris tendon are relatively uncommon. Tears usually occur in the mid-calf, and with tears of the medial head of gastrocnemius, constitute "tennis leg," which usually affects middle-aged "weekend warriors" who present with acute calf pain and swelling. More distal plantaris tendon tears are usually associated with Achilles tendon tears.

Plantaris tears present with calf pain and may mimic deep vein thrombosis, ruptured Baker cyst, Achilles tendon tear, or medial belly of gastrocnemius tear.[30,31,51,52] Hemorrhagic and serous fluid around the tear can be mistaken for a myofascial tear of gastrocnemius or a leaking Baker cyst as the fluid tracks between gastrocnemius and soleus, but these can be excluded by recognition of the normal half-arrowhead configuration of the distal medial belly of gastrocnemius and the absence of a Baker cyst, or a crisply defined inferior margin to the cyst if a Baker cyst is present.[51,52] The injured tendon is typically swollen and hypoechoic. The proximal end retracts, thickens, and has irregular margins. There is usually a thin hematoma in the gap and around the ends of the tendon.[52] In chronic rupture, the gap is filled by hypoechoic granulation tissue or more mature fibrous tissue.

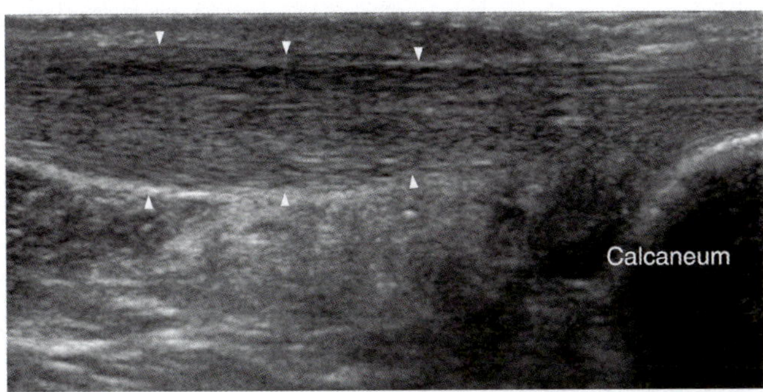

Figure 8.21. Longitudinal ultrasound showing moderate mid-portion Achilles tendinosis with moderate fusiform swelling and slight hypoechogenicity of the mid-third of the Achilles tendon (*arrowheads*). Color Doppler imaging (not shown) revealed mild intratendinous hyperemia. The distal one-third of the Achilles tendon is more normal in caliber and echo-texture.

Achilles Tendon Pathology

The Achilles tendon is the ankle tendon most prone to degeneration or tear. Pathology ranges from mild peritenonitis to a full-thickness tear.[53] Tendinosis, the most common Achilles tendon disorder, is characterized by pain and swelling, usually in mid-tendon **(Fig. 8.21)** or near the calcaneal insertion (insertional tendinosis) **(Fig. 8.22)**. The incidence of Achilles tendinosis is rising as a result of greater participation in sports such as running, racquet sports, track and field, basketball, volleyball, and soccer.[54] Runners are about 10 times more likely than age-matched controls to develop Achilles tendinosis, and elite runners have a lifetime prevalence of up to 10%.[55] About one-third of subjects are nonathletes.[54] Histologically, tendinosis has features of a failed healing response with haphazard tenocyte proliferation, tenocyte degeneration, disruption of collagen fibers, and increase in proteoglycan matrix.[54] Tendon vascularity is typically increased. Vessels are arranged haphazardly and are generally perpendicular to the collagen fibers. Inflammatory lesions and granulation tissue are infrequent and,

when present, are usually associated with partial tears. Vascular proliferation with an inflammatory infiltrate is common in the paratenon.[56] Tendinosis is characterized by progressive tendon thickening, hypoechogenicity with loss of the normal fibrillar pattern, and increase in tendon vascularity **(Figs. 8.21 and 8.22)**. There may be a variable degree of paratenonitis manifested by swelling, edema, increased echogenicity, and hyperemia of the Achilles paratenon. Depending on the conspicuity of these features, the severity of Achilles tendinosis and paratenonitis can be graded as mild, moderate, or severe.

The size of the Achilles tendon varies considerably,[28] and diagnosis should be based on an impression of overall tendon size and echotexture rather than relying on size measurements alone. Cross-sectional area can be compared with the opposite side or used to provide a baseline for longitudinal studies and is best measured at: (1) the soleus musculotendinous junction, (2) the mid-portion of the tendon, and (3) the calcaneal insertion. The normal cross-sectional areas are at level 1: 0.54 ± 0.11 cm^2; at level 2: 0.54 ± 0.12 cm^2,[28] and at level 3: 0.72 ± 0.15 cm^2.

The severity of tendinosis and paratenonitis do not necessarily parallel each other; for example, there may be a severe degree of tendinosis but only a mild degree of paratenonitis, or there may be paratenonitis with no evidence of tendinosis **(Figs. 23A, B)**. The distinction is clinically relevant as active paratenonitis responds to anti-inflammatory medication, whereas tendinosis does not.[57] Tendon calcification, fluid in the retrocalcaneal bursa, and bony contour abnormalities at the calcaneal insertional are seen in 2%, 35%, and 63%, respectively, of normal asymptomatic subjects, although they occur with greater frequency in subjects with insertional Achilles tendinosis[28] **(Fig. 8.24)**. Tendinosis usually leads to diffuse or fusiform swelling of the tendon, although occasionally focal nodular expansion occurs due to localized accumulation of proteoglycans, partial tendon tears, or focal reparative fibrosis.[53] Partial tears are seen as focal discontinuity of the fibrillar echogenic fibers on a background of tendinosis. Small partial tears are an inherent part of any moderate to severe tendinosis, and ultrasound is not able to distinguish them from background tendinopathic changes. Tendon vascularity seems to be associated more with duration and chronicity of physical activity and severity of tendinosis than pain.[57]

> **Tip:**
> The degree of paratenonitis as well as the degree of Achilles tendinosis should be assessed independently.

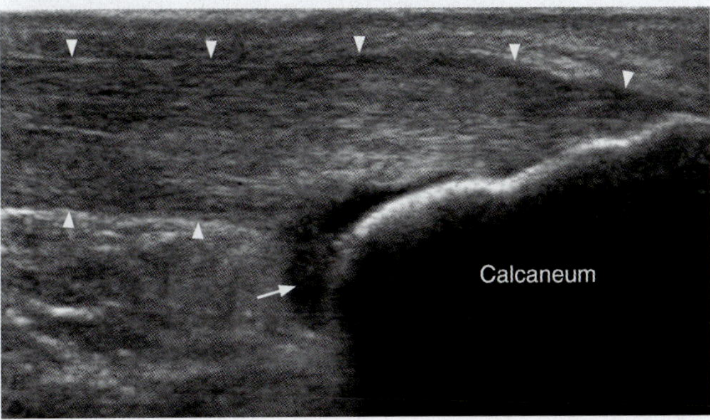

Figure 8.22. Longitudinal ultrasound of posterior aspect of ankle showing diffusely thickened distal Achilles tendon (*arrowheads*) consistent with moderate-severity tendinosis. There is a mildly distended retrocalcaneal bursa (*arrow*). In this patient, no cortical irregularity of the calcaneal insertional area is present.

Asymptomatic pre-existing tendinosis is often present in Achilles tendons that rupture.[58] Tears typically affect middle-aged men, often overweight and engaged in physical activity above their level of fitness.[59] The tear

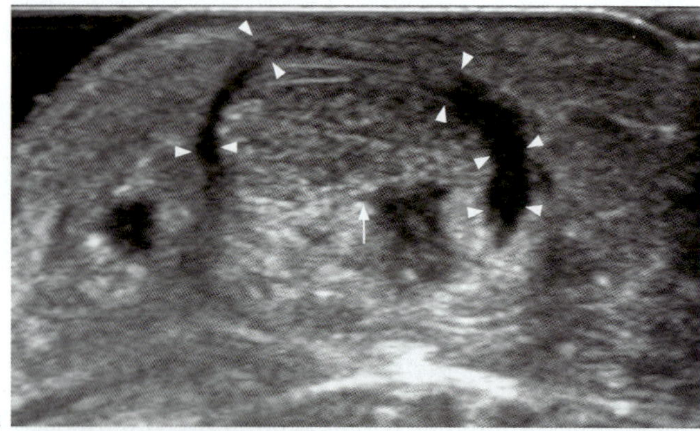

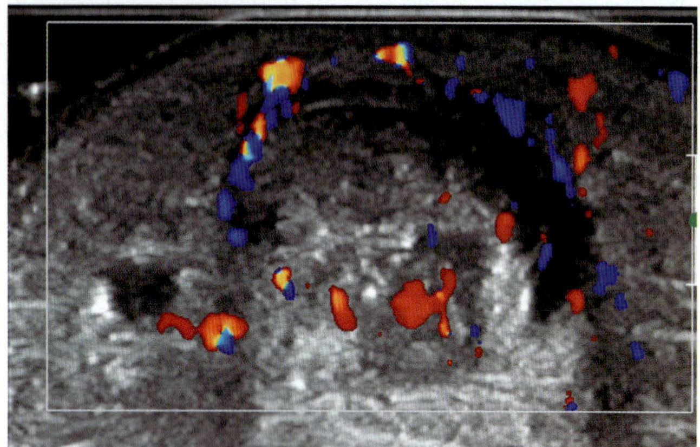

Figure 8.23. Transverse ultrasound of Achilles tendon (*arrow*) showing (**A**) a hypoechoic rim (*arrowheads*) around the sides and dorsal surface of the Achilles tendon due to a thickened paratenon. The Achilles tendon is normal. **B:** Color Doppler imaging shows a marked hyperemia around and, to a lesser degree, within this distended paratenon overall consistent with chronic paratenonitis.

is usually 2 to 6 cm from the calcaneal insertion where the tendon is relatively avascular.[28] It is important to differentiate full-thickness from partial-thickness tears as full-thickness tears may benefit from surgical repair. Distinguishing mild-to-moderate partial tears from

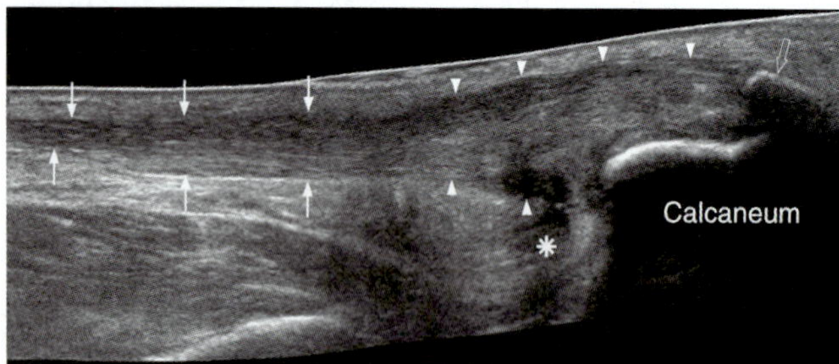

Figure 8.24. Longitudinal extended-field-of-view ultrasound showing severe insertional Achilles tendinosis. The distal one-third of the Achilles tendon (*arrowheads*) is thickened and hypoechoic with disruption of the normal fibrillar pattern. Color Doppler imaging (not shown) revealed mild peri- and intratendinous hyperemia. The tendon gradually tapers to a more normal caliber in the mid- to proximal one-third (*arrows*). Note mild distension of the retrocalcaneal bursa (*asterisk*) and a large posterior plantar calcaneal spur (*open arrow*).

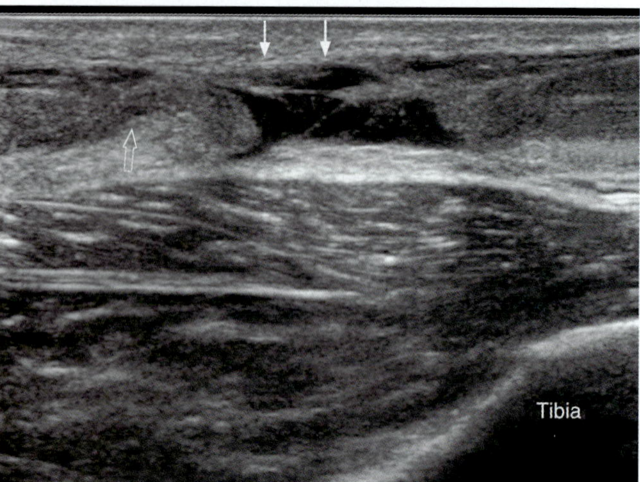

Figure 8.25. Longitudinal ultrasound showing complete Achilles tendon tear (*arrows*) just distal to the musculotendinous junction (*open arrow*). The tendon gap is filled with fluid.

tendinosis is less important as both are treated conservatively. A complete tear is seen as discontinuity in the tendon, with distraction and posterior acoustic shadowing of the tear edges[60] (**Fig. 8.25**). The tear should be evaluated comprehensively by moving the transducer from medial to lateral and superior to inferior to avoid misdiagnosis of partial tear as complete tear. In acute tears, a mixture of blood products, debris, and herniated fat leads to variable echogenicity in the gap. An intact plantaris tendon may run across the medial aspect of the tear (**Fig. 8.26**). Dynamic ultrasound examination is valuable. Dorsiflexion of the foot may accentuate a tear by separating the tear edges and creating or widening the gap between them. Normally the tendon moves as one unit on plantar/dorsiflexion, but with a complete tear paradoxical movement may be seen: The distal segment of the

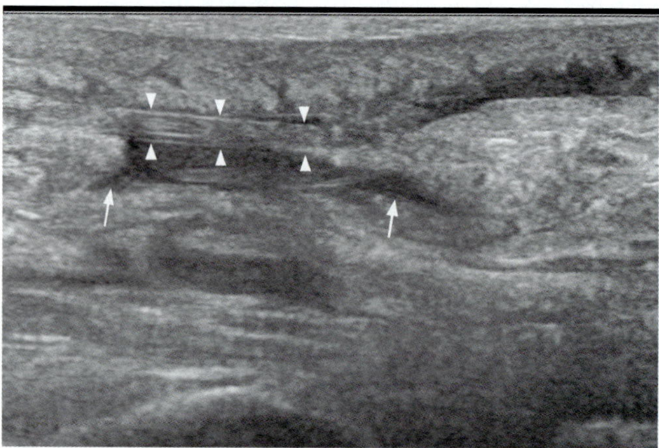

Figure 8.26. Longitudinal ultrasound of complete Achilles tendon tear, medial edge. The retracted ends of the tendon are shown (*arrows*) with the tendon gap filled with fluid. There is also an intact slightly swollen plantaris tendon (*arrowheads*) traversing the tendon gap. Do not confuse this with intact Achilles tendon fibers.

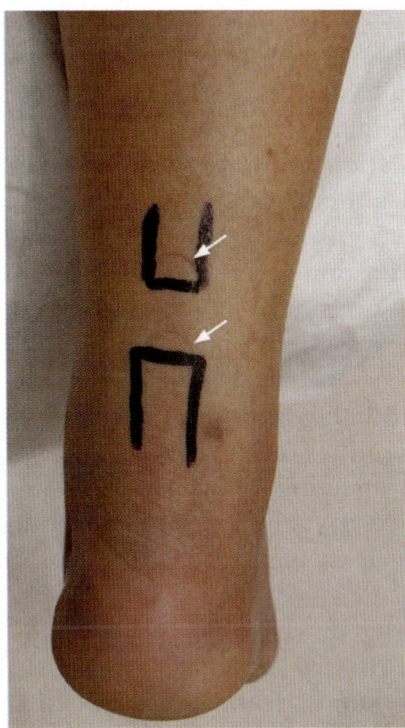

Figure 8.27.   Clinical image showing how the edges of the Achilles tendon tear are marked on the skin. The rounded depressions (*arrows*) on the skin were made with the top of the marker pen prior to the ultrasound gel being removed for ink marking of the tendon rupture site.

tendon moves normally and inferiorly and the proximal tendon is retracted superiorly on dorsiflexion, whereas on plantar flexion, the two segments move toward each other. Plantar flexion can also be used to assess whether conservative management in an equinus cast is appropriate: The edges of the tendon should become apposed. Most surgeons will operate if the gap is ≥1 cm. Marking the site of the tear on the skin is helpful for surgical planning **(Fig. 8.27)**. In chronic or missed Achilles tendon tears, isoechoic or hypoechoic granulation or fibrous tissue may fill or partially fill the gap **(Fig. 8.28)**. Injuries at the insertion are normally avulsive, and the tendon remains attached to an avulsed bone fragment **(Fig. 8.29)**.

An intact plantaris tendon can mimic residual intact fibers of the Achilles tendon in complete Achilles tendon tear.

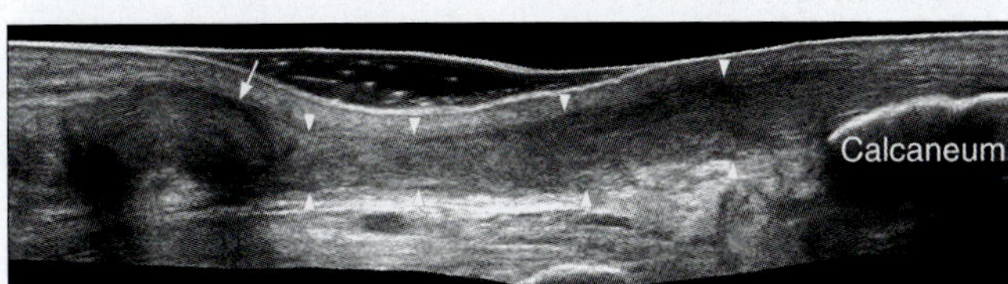

Figure 8.28.   Longitudinal extended-field-of-view ultrasound of partial chronic Achilles tendon tear. The Achilles tendon (*arrowheads*) is elongated, although still continuous with a retracted tendon mass (*arrow*) close to the musculotendinous junction.

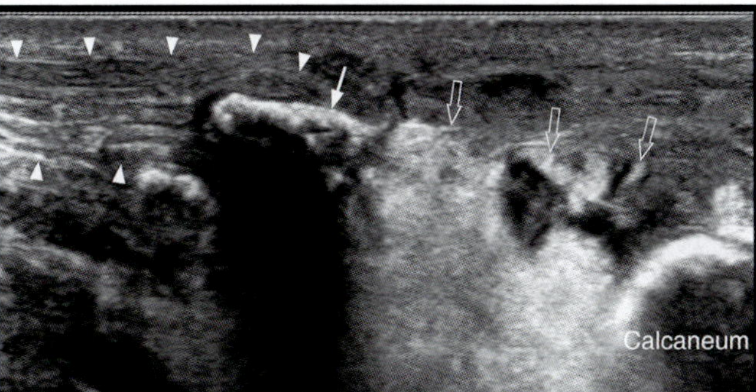

Figure 8.29.   Longitudinal ultrasound showing Achilles fracture avulsion from calcaneal insertion. The Achilles tendon (*arrowheads*) is attached to a large fragment of bone (*closed arrow*) avulsed from the calcaneum. The intervening gap is filled with echogenic fat and hematoma (*open arrows*).

Ultrasound can assess Achilles tendon repairs. The postoperative tendon is normally moderately to severely diffusely swollen with an irregular contour **(Fig. 8.30)**. The swelling increases postoperatively for the first year and decreases thereafter.[59] The site of repair varies from a hypoechoic to a mixed hypoechoic/hyperechoic appearance.[53] Large sutures such as a Krachow whip stitch can also be seen. The tendon ends should be closely apposed and reparative granulation tissue fills any gap. Occasionally, calcification occurs at the site of repair. In re-rupture, the repaired ends separate and sutures traverse the gap.[59]

In patients with familial hypercholesterolemia, the Achilles tendon can be diffusely swollen to a severe degree due to cholesterol deposition, and this can appear very similar to Achilles tendinosis[61,62] **(Fig. 8.31)**. Less frequently, focal deposition of cholesterol results in discrete intratendinous xanthomas **(Fig. 8.31)**. Recognizing a family history of hypercholesterolemia, the cutaneous stigmata of hypercholesterolemia, or the involvement of other tendons, particularly the extensor tendons of the digits and, less frequently, the patellar tendons, is helpful.

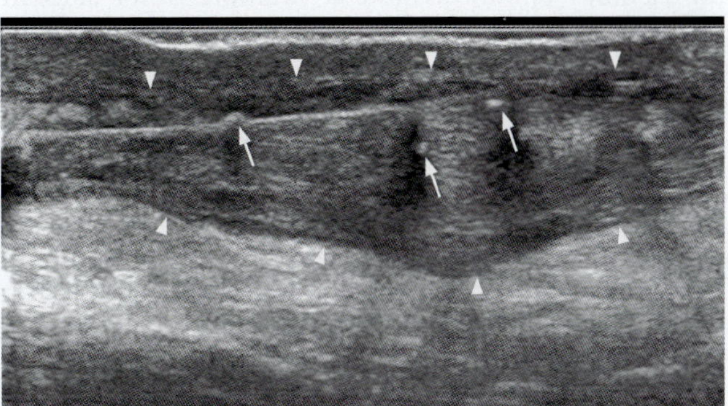

Figure 8.30.   Postoperative appearances of Achilles tendon. The appearances vary according to the site and type of repair performed, although typically the tendon (*arrowheads*) remains thickened with clearly recognizable suture material (*arrows*). No re-tear is present.

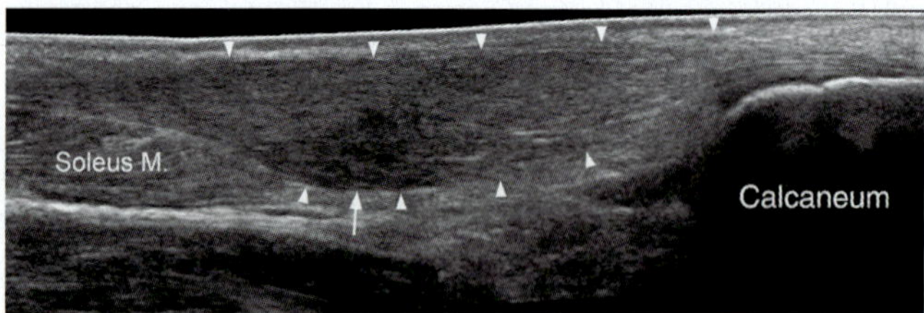

Figure 8.31. Longitudinal extended-field-of-view ultrasound showing diffusely thickened Achilles tendon (*arrowheads*) in patient with familial hypercholesterolemia. The tendon thickening is due to deposition of cholesterol-rich material between the collagen fibers. There is a more discrete hypoechoic area of cholesterol deposition on the deeper aspect of the mid-tendon, which could be termed a "xanthoma" (*arrow*).

Haglund syndrome

The Haglund syndrome is a constellation of bony and soft tissue abnormalities[63–65] characterized by a bony protuberance at the posterosuperior border of the calcaneus (Haglund deformity), Achilles tendinosis, and retrocalcaneal bursitis. The Achilles tendinosis and retrocalcaneal bursitis can be secondary to the bony deformity or occur together primarily. Ultrasound shows the bony prominence, abnormal thickening/heterogeneity of the tendon and distension, wall thickening, internal debris, or hyperemia of the bursa. Ultrasound-guided injection of local anesthetic and steroid into the bursa is both diagnostic and therapeutic. A short-axis approach and injection of 20 to 40 mg of methylprednisolone and 0.5 to 1 mL of 0.5% bupivacaine are appropriate. Pain relief is of variable duration. Recently, it has been proposed that the use of Haglund deformity or Haglund syndrome is inappropriate as the bony prominence is just as common in asymptomatic subjects,[66] and terminology such as Achilles tendinosis or tendinopathy, paratenonitis or retrocalcaneal bursitis is preferred.

Achilles tendon injection

Ultrasound-guided percutaneous interventions are used for Achilles tendinosis and at multiple other sites in the foot and ankle.[45,67–79] Ultrasound-guided treatment ensures accurate needle placement, avoids nerves and vessels,[45,67–79] and is employed when conservative methods have failed.[72] Treatments can be broadly divided into those designed to (1) obliterate tendon and paratenon neovascularity such as sclerotherapy, electrocoagulation, or high-volume saline injection,(2) stimulate a healing response such as dry needling, autologous blood injection, and hyperosmolar dextrose injection, or (3) control local inflammation, that is, anesthetic/steroid injection.

Neovascularity (and accompanying nociceptive fiber formation) is thought to be related to pain; hence methods such as sclerotherapy, electrocoagulation, and high-volume saline injection have been developed to reduce tendon and paratenon vascularity.[72] Sclerotherapy

by ultrasound-guided injection of phenol or polidocanol into peritendinous (not tendon) vessels results in reduced vascularity. There is some evidence of clinical benefit,[73] although multiple treatments may be needed. Electrocoagulation requires specialized equipment and is performed under local anesthesia. The electrocoagulation needle is placed against vessels entering the tendon under ultrasound guidance. Potential complications include infection, sural nerve damage, and tendon rupture. Brisement is high-volume injection (20 to 40 mL) of normal saline and local anesthetic between the Achilles tendon and the paratenon to strip the paratenon and break any adhesions.[72] A short-axis approach is best. High-volume injection of saline, local anesthetic, and steroid between the Achilles tendon and Kager fat pad[80] has been reported to improve pain scores, function, and symptoms.[74]

Dry needling by repeated fenestrations of the area of tendinosis precipitates intratendinous bleeding and is thought to stimulate healing and inflammation via deposition of blood-borne stem cells and inflammatory mediators. Autologous blood or platelet-rich plasma (PRP) injections contain various growth factors that are thought to promote healing. About 3 mL of PRP or autologous blood are injected into the area of tendinosis.

Prolotherapy (or regenerative injection therapy) involves ultrasound-guided injection of a small volume of irritant such as hyperosmolar dextrose in or around the tendon insertion to initiate a local inflammatory response.

Steroid injections remain the most frequently used percutaneous treatment of Achilles tendinosis, usually administered blindly, although ultrasound guidance can ensure accurate needle placement. Generally, peritendinous injections of 30 to 40 mg of methylprednisolone or triamcinolone mixed with lidocaine and/or bupivacaine are performed. Favored positions include deep to the paratenon adjacent to tendinosis or into the deep retrocalcaneal bursa. A short-axis approach is appropriate for both. Peritendinous injections often provide good short-term relief, but relapse, especially with vigorous rehabilitation, and soft tissue atrophy are common. Intratendinous injections are usually avoided because of the potential for tendon rupture, although good results have been reported for intratendinous injection of 40 mg of methylprednisolone.[72]

Ligament Pathology

The ultrasound appearances of ligament injury are dependent on the age and severity of injury. In acute partial tears, the ligament is swollen with an anechoic or hypoechoic zone due to edema or hematoma and disorganization of the normal internal echogenic fibrillar pattern. In complete tears, there is swelling and discontinuity of the ligament, sometimes with heterogenous

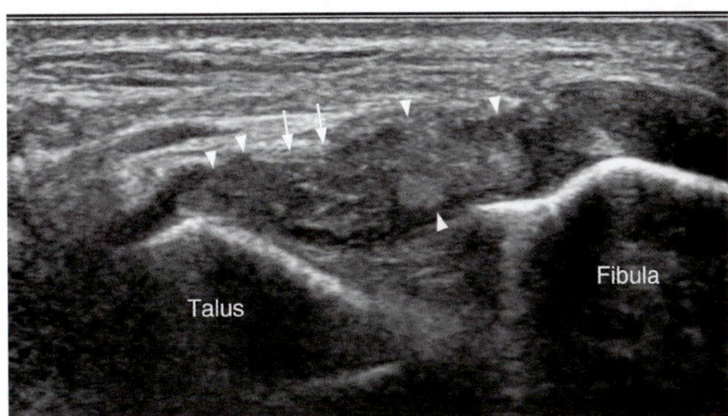

Figure 8.32.   Longitudinal ultrasound lateral aspect of ankle showing complete tear of ATFL. The ligament (*arrowheads*) is very swollen with a complete tear (*arrows*) close to the talar attachment.

hematoma filling the gap **(Fig. 8.32)**. Avulsion of the bony insertion may be seen. There may be a hyeprechoic rim of quite intense edema surrounding any ligament tear with swelling of the adjacent soft tissues. As a tear heals, the gap fills in and becomes hyperechoic and heterogeneous, and the ligament appears thicker. Thickening continues for a long time after injury **(Fig. 8.33)**. There is sometimes elongation of the ligament. Ligament continuity is usually eventually restored even after complete tears. Less frequently, the retracted torn ends undergo attrition and become reabsorbed, or the ligament heals in an attenuated fashion. Calcification or ossification rarely occur.[12] Stressing the ligament may be helpful when assessing acute or chronic ligament tears.

Lateral Collateral Ligament Injury

The lateral collateral ligaments are the most commonly injured ankle ligaments, the ATFL most frequently followed by the CFL, and rarely the posterior talofibular ligaments. They are injured during ankle inversion. Isolated ATFL injuries comprise up to 70% of ankle injuries.[1] Ultrasound is not usually indicated as the accuracy of clinical examination is high. Ligament tear can be divided into three types based on the severity of injury. A "sprain" is when the ligament is swollen indicative of ligament micro tear without visible ligament disruption. A partial-thickness tear is when a discrete tear presents in conjunction with some residual intact fibers. In full-thickness tears, the ligament substance is either completely torn or the ligament is completely avulsed from either its fibular or talar attachment, often with a thin slither of bone. In full-thickness tears, there is usually capsular rupture with leakage of synovial fluid into the soft tissues.[40,41] Anteriorly drawing the inverted and slightly plantar-flexed foot forward over the edge of the examination bed (the anterior drawer test) while scanning longitudinally over the ATFL can help distinguish between partial and complete tear of the ATFL.

Tip:
Performing the anterior drawer test during ultrasound scanning can help differentiate partial and complete ATFL tears.

With healing of complete ATFL tears, ligament continuity can be spontaneously restored with the ligament being thickened, continuous, and functionally competent. This ligament thickening can remain for years. If ligament continuity is not restored, the free ligament will usually undergo progressive attrition and resorption.

The CFL nearly always tears in conjunction with an ATFL tear. In acute severe tears of the CFL, there is usually fluid distension of the common peroneal tendon sheath, and there may be free communication between the ankle joint and the peroneal tendon sheath.[40,41] During dorsiflexion, the normal CFL elevates the peroneal tendons toward the probe, while in complete CFL tears, the peroneal tendons remain close to the calcaneus **(Fig. 8.34)**.

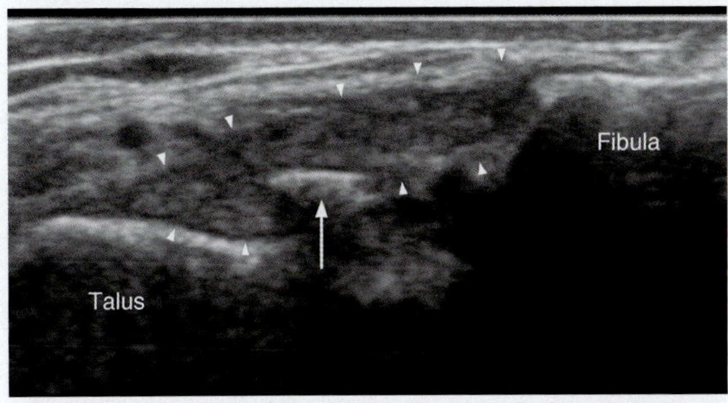

Figure 8.33.   Longitudinal ultrasound anterolateral aspect of ankle. There is a healing tear of the ATFL with moderate ligament thickening (*arrowheads*) and a small avulsion fracture (*arrow*) most likely from the fibular tip. Overall, ligament continuity is maintained.

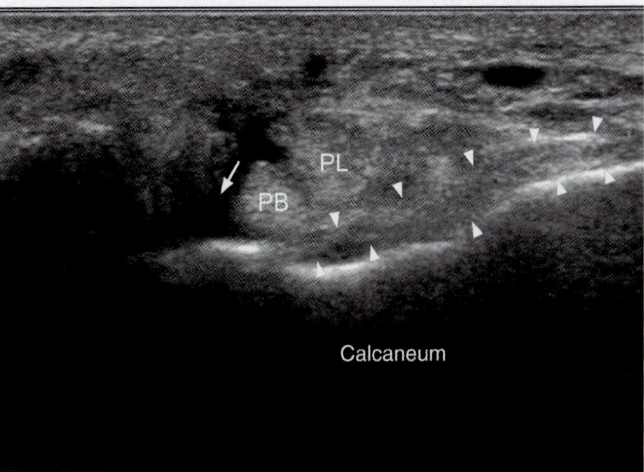

Figure 8.34.   Longitudinal ultrasound of the lateral inframalleolar region. There is a complete tear (*arrow*) of the CFL from its fibular attachment. The torn ligament (*arrowheads*) has lost its normal "hammock effect" and is lying against the calcaneum deep to the peroneus longus (*PL*) and peroneus brevis (*PB*) tendons.

Injury to the ATFL can also lead to synovial thickening on the deep aspect of the ligament, giving rise to anterolateral impingement syndrome.[9] This is discussed in the section on anterolateral impingement syndrome below.

> **Tip:**
> Isolated tears of the CFL ligament are very rare.

Syndesmotic Ligament Injury

The distal tibiofibular syndesmosis is strengthened by the anterior inferior tibiofibular ligament, the posterior inferior tibiofibular ligament, the interosseous ligament, and the transverse tibiofibular ligament. The anterior tibiofibular ligament is the most commonly injured syndesmotic ligament, known as "high ankle strain," and is often diagnosed late clinically. The injury leads to pain and tenderness at the anterolateral ankle, particularly on weight bearing.[1] Tears usually occur in the absence of any visible syndesmotic diastasis. Tears of the anterior inferior tibiofibular ligament usually occur as a result of an eversion injury, often in conjunction with deltoid ligament injury. Severe syndesmotic injury may involve the distal portion of the interosseous membrane between the tibia and the fibula. A torn distal interosseous membrane appears abnormally hypoechoic and poorly defined.[81] Usually the substance of the interosseous membrane is intact, although its periosteal attachment is stripped, mostly on the tibial side.

Medial Collateral Ligament (Deltoid Ligament)

The deltoid ligament is stronger than the lateral collateral ligament and less frequently torn.[1] Complete tears are rare and typically occur during severe eversion injury, often in association with lateral malleolar fracture and lateral displacement of the talus.[40,41] If there is rupture of the deltoid ligament, the posterior tibial tendon moves deeper, toward the articular and bony surface. In acute complete tears, the hematoma, joint effusion, and extension of joint fluid into the para-articular soft tissues give a similar appearance to severe acute lateral collateral ligament injuries.

Sinus Tarsi Ligament Injury

Tear of the sinus tarsi ligaments can manifest as a hypoechoic reparative mass on the lateral aspect of the ankle at the tarsal sinus level, although the ligaments themselves are not easily seen on ultrasound.[1] The sinus tarsi is best assessed on MRI, which shows replacement of the normal sinus tarsi fat on T1-weighted images and periligamentous edema on T2-weighted fat-suppressed images.

Spring Ligament Complex Injury

Isolated tears of the spring ligament are rare. Spring ligament insufficiency is commonly associated with posterior tibial tendon dysfunction and pes planus, which lead to repeated loading of the spring ligament. As a result of accelerated attrition, the ligament becomes lax or ruptures, resulting in acquired flat foot. Healing of partial ligament tears is characterized by thickening and hypoechogenicity.[19,21] Thickness >4 mm of the superomedial component of the spring ligament measured at its mid-portion deep to the posterior tibial tendon is considered abnormal.[20] The degree of posterior tibial tendinosis and thickening of the superomedial spring ligament do not necessarily parallel each other; for example, there may be only a mild degree of tendinosis but marked thickening of the ligament; hence each component should be individually assessed **(Fig 8.19)**.

> **Tip:**
> As the degree of posterior tibial tendinosis, peritendinitis, and superomedial component of spring ligament thickening do not necessarily parallel each other, each component should be individually assessed and graded.

Ankle Impingement

Posterior Impingement

Posterior ankle impingement syndrome is caused by compression of the posterior process of the talus and adjacent soft tissue between the tibia and the calcaneum on repeated or forced ankle plantar flexion. It is also termed "os-trigonum syndrome," "talar compression syndrome," "posterior block," or "posterior tibial talar impingement syndrome."[82,83] It is characterized by posterior ankle pain in plantar flexion and commonly occurs in athletes, particularly ballet dancers, soccer players, downhill runners, and activities that involve regular forceful plantar flexion of the ankle.

The most common bony association is a large os-trigonum, less commonly a downward sloping posterior tibial margin ("posterior malleolus") or prominent superior surface of the calcaneum. Soft tissue impingement involves the posterior recesses, posterior talofibular, posterior intermalleolar, and posterior tibiofibular ligaments that become inflamed, thickened, and fibrosed. Synovial thickening and swelling may be appreciated at the posterior recesses of the tibiotalar and posterior talocalcaneal articulations, superior and inferior to the posterior talar process, respectively. Ultrasound may reveal a prominent posterior talar process, nodular hypoechoic thickening of the posterior recesses, and an intact but thickened posterior talofibular ligament. The posterior intermalleolar and talofibular ligaments are deep and not easily accessed by ultrasound. The FHL tendon is particularly likely to be affected. Tenosynovitis or stenosing tenosynovitis may occur with increased fluid in the tendon sheath as well as more generalized adjacent soft tissue inflammation. In stenosing tenosynovitis, dynamic ultrasound may demonstrate tethering of the FHL tendon within the fibro-osseous tunnel behind the talus during flexion and extension of the great toe.[83] Ultrasound-guided injection of steroid and long-acting anesthetic provides a safe and effective treatment for posterior impingement symptoms.[76,84,85] A short-axis approach with the needle lateral and the transducer medial to the Achilles tendon avoids the tibial neurovascular bundle. A test injection of local anesthetic ensures that the needle is in the tendon sheath, and 20 to 40 mg of methylprednisolone is then injected.

Posteromedial Impingement

Posteromedial ankle impingement typically occurs 4 to 6 weeks after inversion injury and should be distinguished from tibialis posterior pathology, which has similar symptoms. The posteromedial tibiotalar capsule and posterior tibiotalar ligament become thickened and compressed between the talus and the medial malleolus.[27,83] Ultrasound shows thickening of the posteromedial capsule deep to the medial tendons that are displaced superficially.[86,87]

Anterior Impingement

Anterior impingement is a relatively common cause of anterior ankle pain due to impingement of hypertrophied soft tissue and anterior osteophytes of the distal tibia and talar neck. It is often associated with hypertrophic osteoarthritis and also commonly seen in soccer players. The osseous component forms a more significant part of the impinging mass, although the soft tissue component is also critical in producing the clinical syndrome. Capsular thickening, synovitis, and bony spurs are seen at the anterior margin of the ankle joint.

Anterolateral Impingement

Anterolateral impingement is caused by entrapment and inflammation of hypertrophied soft tissues within the anterolateral recess of the ankle and occurs most commonly in young athletes. Repeated inversion injuries and partial tears of the anterior talofibular and tibiotalar ligaments result in reparative hypertrophy of the anterolateral capsule and the ligaments without substantial instability. Chronic synovial-capsular thickening and inflammation leads to a hyalinized connective tissue mass termed a "meniscoid lesion"[9,27] that replaces fluid in the gutter. Marginal osteophytes can have a similar effect. Obliteration of the anterolateral gutter does not invariably imply that clinical impingement is present.[9]

Ultrasound shows thickened synovial tissue (>1 cm) of mixed echogenicity and nodular contour.[9,88] The mass bulges anteriorly, particularly with manual compression of the distal fibula against the tibia. Rarely soft tissue calcification and mild vascularity on Doppler imaging are seen.[9] The ATFL usually shows features of previous injury and is better seen if there is fluid in the anterolateral gutter. If ultrasound is negative or there is no improvement following injection therapy, MRI is recommended, particularly to assess for possible talar dome osteochondral injury.

Anteromedial Impingement

Anteromedial impingement is thought to be related to inversion injury, perhaps with a rotational component, leading to tearing of the anteromedial capsule, and is relatively uncommon.[27] Repeated microtrauma leads to synovitis and capsular thickening,[83] and there is usually a bony component. Findings include irregular anteromedial capsular thickening, synovitis, thickening of the anterior fibers of the deltoid ligament, and occasionally an anteromedial osteophyte.[83,89] If the ultrasound findings are not consistent with the presenting symptoms, MR is helpful in excluding a medial talar dome osteochondral lesion.

Tarsal Tunnel Syndrome

Tarsal tunnel syndrome is characterized by entrapment of the tibial nerve and/or its branches in the tarsal tunnel. Proximal entrapment occurs in the retromalleolar region, and distal entrapment in the inframalleolar region. Symptoms depend on the nerves affected and typically include pain or paresthesia along the medial aspect of the ankle radiating to the medial and/or lateral plantar aspects of the foot and toes. External compression from ill-fitting footwear or a tight plaster cast is the most common cause. Other causes include space-occupying lesions such as ganglia; talocalcaneal coalition; foot deformities such as heel varus or valgus; anomalous tendon and muscle such as an accessory FDL; schwannoma; or lipoma.[23,90,91] Ultrasound can trace the course of the tibial nerve and its branches and detect space-occupying lesions. A beak-shaped bony prominence protruding from the talus or calcaneus is due to talocalcaneal coalition. Local fusiform thickening of the tibial nerve, loss of the normal fascicular pattern, and size discrepancy between the medial and lateral branches suggest nerve compression within the tarsal tunnel.[78] Even small changes in nerve caliber can be detected by ultrasound.[22]

BONE AND JOINT DISORDERS

MRI or computed tomography (CT) is more sensitive in detecting radiographically occult fractures around the ankle and foot than ultrasound. However, ultrasound may show focal cortical disruption, callus, hematoma, or

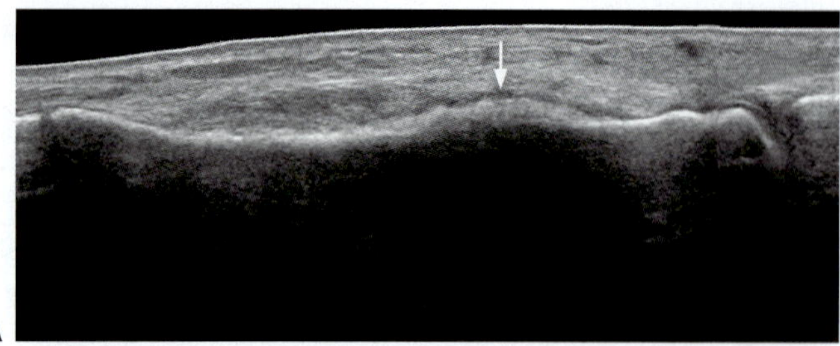

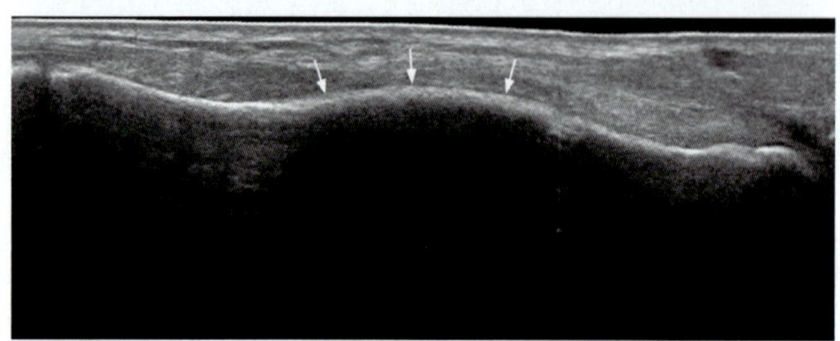

Figure 8.35.   Longitudinal ultrasound of forefoot showing **(A)** an active fracture of the second metatarsal shaft with callus (*arrow*) and mild surrounding soft tissue swelling. **B:** On the contralateral foot, there is a healed fracture of the second metatarsal shaft with bone enlargement (*arrows*), no active callus, and no soft tissue swelling.

soft tissue swelling **(Figs. 8.35A, B)**. Ultrasound is particularly useful in children where fractures may occur in unossified bone or in patients with osteoporosis who may have radiographically occult fractures.[92,93]

Because of their location, most osteochondral lesions of the talar dome are not visible on ultrasound. However, in patients with chronic ankle pain, a moderate or large ankle joint effusion without extra-articular ligament injury should raise the suspicion of an osteochondral lesion.[94]

Joint Disease

Ultrasound can detect as little as 2 mL of fluid in the ankle joint.[94] Plantar flexion of the ankle helps to show fluid in the anterior recess. A simple effusion is almost always anechoic **(Fig. 8.36)**. Increased

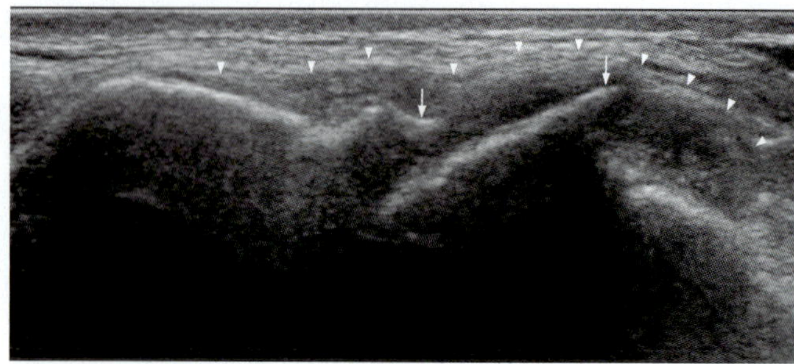

Figure 8.37.   Longitudinal ultrasound anterolateral aspect of ankle showing quite severe osteoarthrosis with joint space narrowing, marginal osteophytosis (*arrows*), together with moderate capsular thickening (*arrowheads*).

echogenicity suggests inflammation or hemarthrosis. Small echogenic foci with comet tail artifacts in joint fluid or attached to the synovium or cartilage suggest crystal arthropathy. It is not always possible to differentiate reactive synovitis, other inflammatory arthritis, infective arthritis, or hemarthrosis on ultrasound, although clinical correlation narrows the differential diagnosis **(Figs. 8.37 and 8.38)** and ultrasound usually distinguishes between joint fluid and synovitis. Chronic synovial proliferation is echogenic. Acute synovial proliferation is usually hypoechoic and can look similar to slightly echogenic joint fluid, but thickened folds of synovium and hyperemia on color or power Doppler distinguish acute synovitis from fluid.

Ultrasound-guided joint aspiration or synovial biopsy may be helpful. Ultrasound ensures accurate needle placement, avoids nerves and vessels, and helps to minimize the risk of cross contamination, for example, between joints and tendon sheaths.[45,67–79] A longitudinal anterior approach with the foot plantar flexed provides the best visualization of anterior tibiotalar joint. Remember that the deep peroneal nerve lies just lateral to the dorsalis pedis artery.

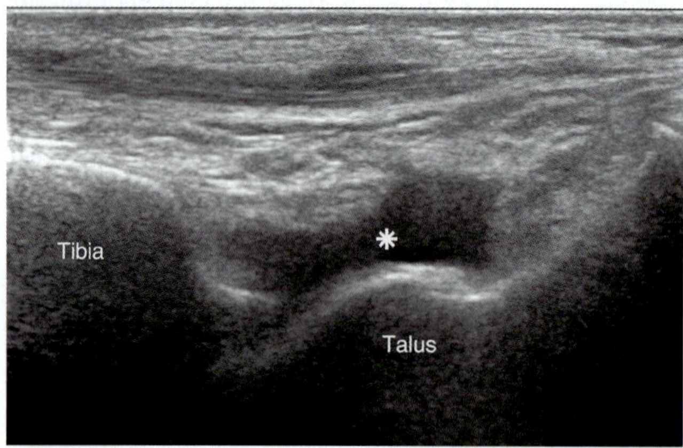

Figure 8.36.   Longitudinal ultrasound anterior aspect of ankle. There is a moderate ankle joint effusion (*asterisk*) displacing the anterior fat pad.

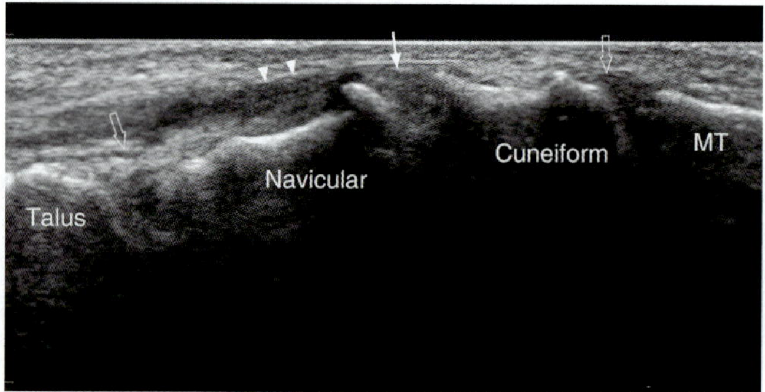

Figure 8.38.   Longitudinal ultrasound dorsum of foot showing moderate osteoarthrosis of navicular:cuneiform articulation (*arrow*) with marginal osteophytosis and adjacent soft tissue thickening (*arrowheads*). MT, metatarsal. Open arrows point to talo-navicular and tarso-metatarsal joints.

ANKLE/FOOT MASSES OR FOREIGN BODY

Ganglia

Ganglia are the most common soft tissue masses at the ankle and foot **(Fig. 8.39)**. They contain gelatinous material of variable viscosity and have a fibrous capsule without a synovial lining.[95] Ganglia usually communicate with an adjacent joint or, less commonly, tendon sheath, although this communication is often not identified.[96] Ganglia around the ankle are generally more symptomatic and larger than at the wrist. They appear cystic with anechoic or hypoechoic contents and posterior acoustic enhancement. Septations and a lobulated border are more common than at the wrist.[97] Small comet tail artifacts may be seen, particularly in larger ganglia, due to aggregations of colloid.

> **Tip:**
> Most ganglia arise from adjacent joints. A track is usually present from the ganglion pointing toward or extending toward an adjacent joint rather than a clear continuity with the joint.

Other Ankle and Foot Masses

Other common ankle masses include lipomas, nerve sheath tumors, abscesses, and tophi.[96] Lipomas are usually subcutaneous, well defined, easily compressible, have variable internal echogenicity, and lack vascularity on power Doppler imaging.[98] Nerve sheath tumors are well defined, fusiform, and have low-to-mixed echogenicity, increased through-transmission, and moderate intrinsic vascularity on color Doppler[97] **(Fig. 8.40)**. Continuity

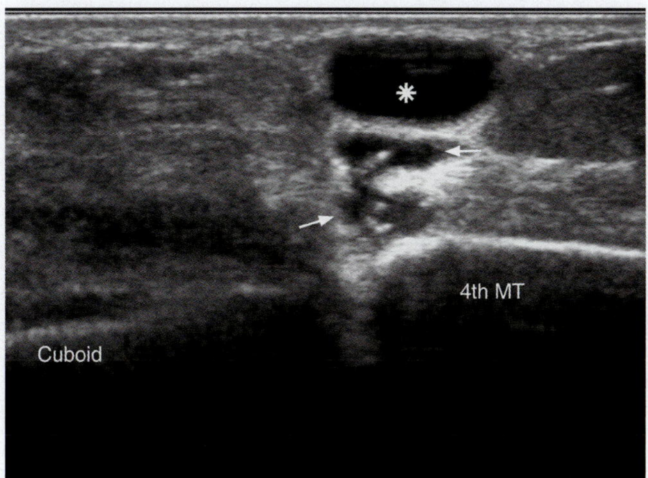

Figure 8.39.   Longitudinal ultrasound of dorsum of foot showing medium-sized ganglion cyst (*asterisk*) with serpiginous track (*arrows*) leading to cuboid: 4th metatarsal (*4th MT*) articulation.

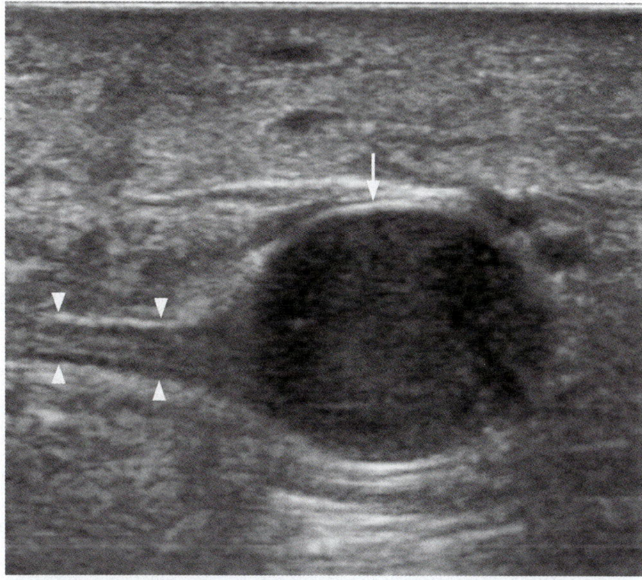

Figure 8.40.   Longitudinal ultrasound of medial ankle showing a nerve sheath tumor (*arrow*) of the tibial nerve. The thickened entering nerve is shown (*arrowheads*). The exiting nerve is not visible in this image plane.

with and/or thickening of the entering/exiting nerve are confirmatory, although tumors arising from small peripheral nerves are often not associated with nerve thickening. The ultrasound appearances of gouty tophi depend on chronicity.[99] The early "soft tophus" appears as a hypoechoic mass with some internal echogenic foci, through-transmission, and surrounding edematous soft tissues. In the intermediate stage, more discrete and larger echogenic foci are visible within a hypoechoic tophus, and there is more acoustic shadowing. In the late stage akin to a "hard tophus," a dense echogenic mass with strong posterior acoustic shadowing is due to calcification.[99] Gouty arthropathy is more common in the foot than isolated tophi **(Figs. 8.41A, B)**. Other common masses include epidermoid cyst, glomus tumor, and vascular leiomyoma **(Fig. 8.42)**.

Foreign Body

Ultrasound detects radiolucent foreign bodies such as wood. Wood splinters tend to be narrow and elongated. They are echogenic, and the transducer may have to be rotated to show the full length of the splinter, which may have a halo.[100] A hyperechoic halo occurs acutely due to surrounding inflammatory tissue. A hypoechoic halo occurs later due to reactive granulation tissue and increases conspicuity of the foreign body. In the acute setting, if a foreign body is not visible on first inspection, it is useful to repeat the ultrasound about a week later when a halo may increase conspicuity. Ultrasound is also useful in localizing and guiding retrieval of foreign bodies.

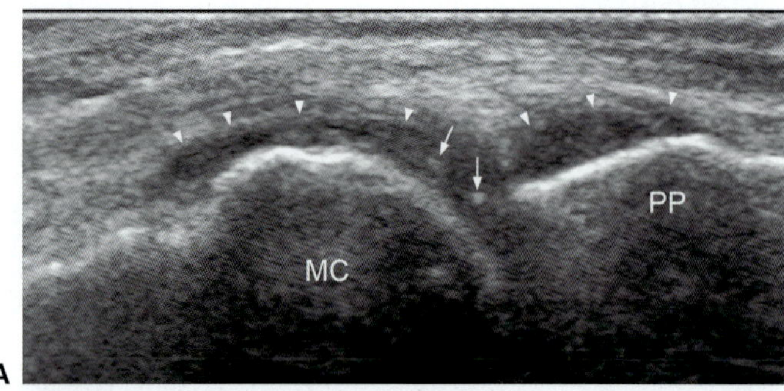

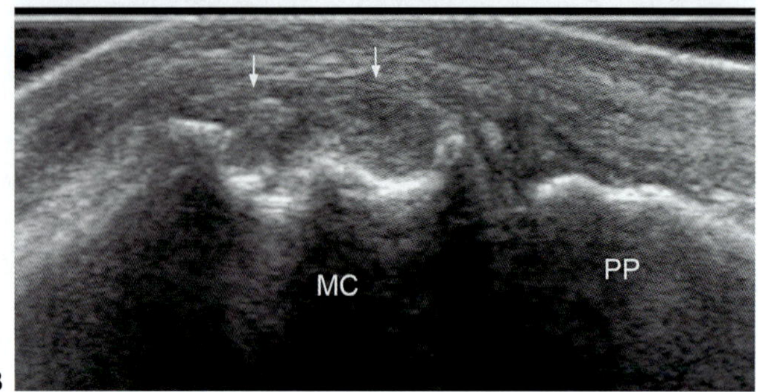

Figure 8.41. Longitudinal ultrasound of first metatarsophalangeal joint. **A:** Dorsal aspect of joint showing a small to moderate-sized effusion/synovial proliferation (*arrowheads*). There are several discrete echogenic foci within the joint consistent with crystal aggregates (*arrows*). **B:** Medial aspect of the joint. There is a wide deep erosion (*arrows*) with overhanging edges consistent with a gouty or crystal arthropathy. MC, metacarpal; PP, proximal phalanx.

FOOT PATHOLOGY

Tibialis Anterior and Extensor Tendon Abnormalities

Longitudinal splits of the distal tibialis anterior tendon have been noted in asymptomatic subjects.[101] Tendinosis of tibialis anterior tends to occur within 3 cm of the

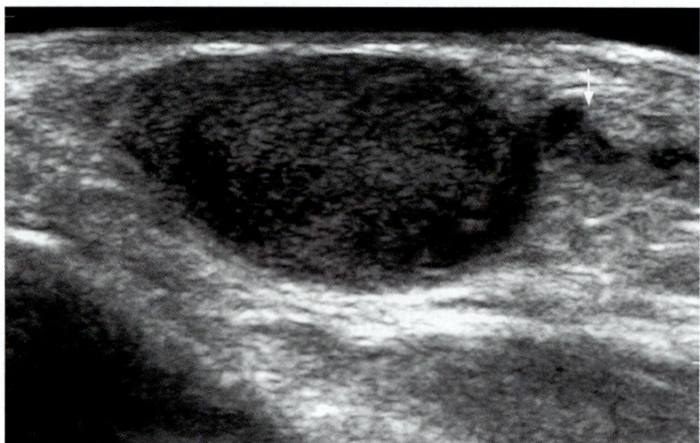

Figure 8.42. Longitudinal ultrasound dorsum of forefoot showing an ovoid hypoechoic mass in the subcutaneous tissues contiguous with a small artery distally (*arrow*). Histology revealed a vascular leiomyoma.

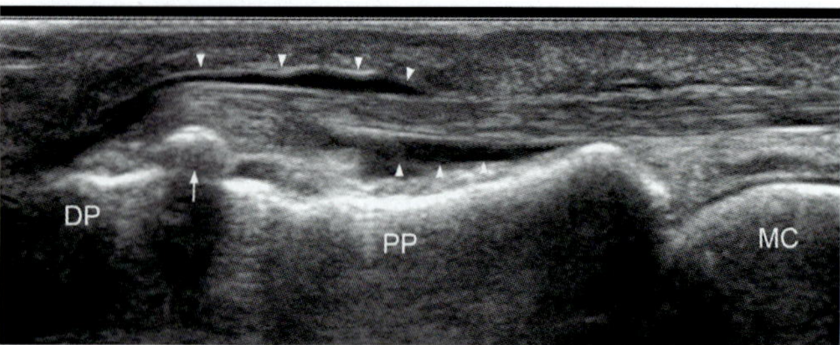

Figure 8.43. Longitudinal ultrasound of the big toe showing a moderate tenosynovitis (*arrowheads*) of the FHL tendon with a tendon sheath effusion surrounding a mildly swollen but otherwise normal tendon. Note the sesamoid bone (*arrow*) overlying the distal interphalangeal joint. MC, metatarsal; PP, proximal phalanx; DP, distal phalanx.

insertion on the medial cuneiform and first metatarsal. The extensor hallucis and extensor digitorum tendons are less prone to tendinosis or injury, and tears are usually secondary to direct trauma to the dorsum of the foot. All tendon pathology in the foot is readily seen with ultrasound **(Fig. 8.43)**, except for the flexor tendons and peroneus longus tendon deep in the midfoot region when MRI should be employed.

Plantar Hindfoot and Midfoot

Plantar Fasciitis

Plantar fasciitis is the most common cause of inferior heel pain and affects mainly middle-aged women and younger male runners.[102] It is related to overuse and repeated microtrauma, or occasionally associated with systemic enthesopathy, and involves the plantar fascia at its calcaneal insertion. Obesity is a risk factor.[103] Patients usually complain of heel pain, particularly on weight bearing, and there is deep tenderness at the medial calcaneal tuberosity. Thickening and hypoechogenicity of the fascia near its medial calcaneal insertion are the most consistent ultrasound findings[80,104] **(Fig. 8.44A)**. Plantar fascia thickness <4 mm can be considered unequivocally normal, between 4 and 5 mm is borderline, and >5 mm unequivocally abnormal. A very thick plantar fascia has a slightly convex plantar contour **(Fig. 8.44B)**. If symptoms are severe, there may be loss of definition of the fascia and perifascial edema close to the calcaneal insertion.[105] Calcaneal spurs may occur just deep to the calcaneal insertion. Intrafascial calcification is rare. Focal bony erosions and localized hyperemia at the attachment site may be seen with systemic enthesopathy.

Tip:
Plantar fascial thickness should be assessed at the medial leading edge of the calcaneum. Subclinical plantar fasciitis with plantar fascial thickening is not uncommonly present on the opposite, asymptomatic side.

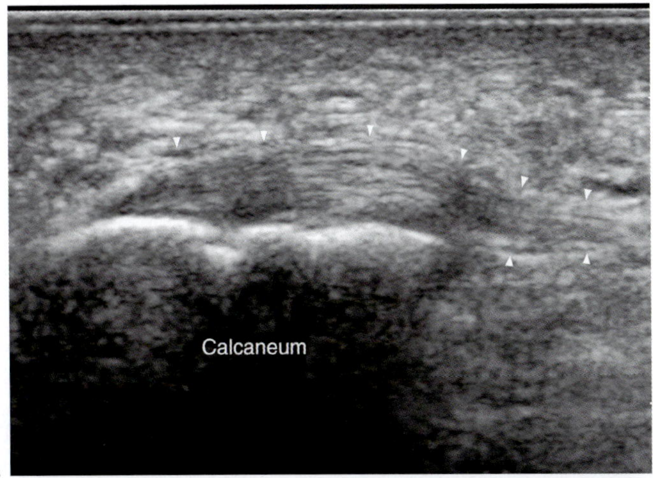

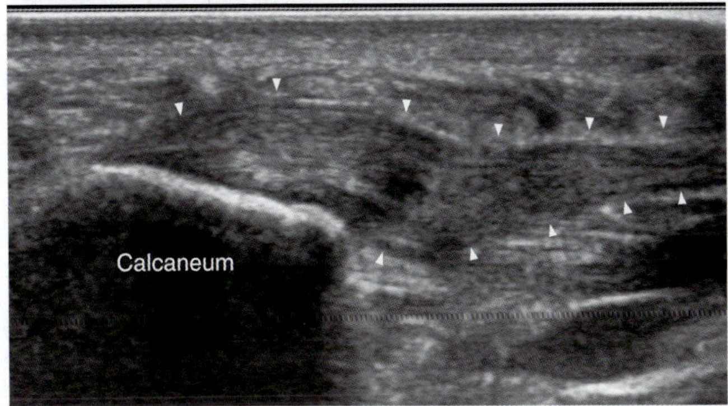

Figure 8.44. Longitudinal ultrasound of plantar heel. **A:** Mild (4.3 mm) thickening of the plantar fascia (*arrowheads*) at the leading edge of medial calcaneal tuberosity is present consistent with plantar fasciitis, although this degree of thickening can also be found in asymptomatic subjects. **B:** More marked (8.7 mm) thickening of the plantar fascia (*arrowheads*) is present, indicative of severe plantar fasciitis.

One treatment option is corticosteroid injection. Blind injections using bony landmarks have been associated with rupture of the fascia.[69] Ultrasound guidance minimizes direct intrafascial injection.[69,70,78] A longitudinal plantar approach is painful because of the thick skin on the sole of the foot. A medial, short-axis approach allows local anesthetic to be injected into the skin and is better tolerated. Dry needling may be performed initially and a steroid and local anesthetic mixture then injected deep and/or superficial but not into the fascia. Because of the risk of atrophy of the heel fat pad, short-acting steroids such as dexamethasone, or methylprednisolone of the long-acting steroids are preferred in a total dose of about 40 mg.

Plantar Fibromatosis

Plantar fibromatosis is a benign focal proliferation of fibrous tissue in the plantar fascia, and is most common between 30 and 50 years, affecting women almost twice as frequently as men.[106] Patients usually present with a slow-growing mass that is painful on weight bearing. Most lesions are solitary and unilateral, although about one-third are bilateral and one-quarter are multiple.[107] There is an increased prevalence in patients with Dupuytren contracture, penile fibromatosis (Peyronie disease), or those prone to keloid formation.[108] Ultrasound shows discrete fusiform or nodular thickening of the plantar fascia aligned along its long axis. Most swellings are avascular, well defined, hypoechoic without acoustic enhancement, <20 mm in length, and involve the central and medial portions of the fascia distal to the calcaneal insertion[106–109] **(Fig. 8.45)**. They tend to bulge more from the superficial aspect of the fascia than deeply. Larger lesions are more rounded.[109] Plantar fibromatosis is readily differentiated from plantar fasciitis by morphology and position. Differentiation from a chronic partial tear is more difficult, although tears are less common. A visible tear, perifascial edema, and a history of preceding trauma favor the diagnosis of a partial tear. Aggressive plantar fibromatosis is a different disease and is associated with an enlarging locally invasive irregular fibrotic mass that can grow to a large size deep into the soft tissues of the midfoot and forefoot.

> **Tip:**
> Plantar fibromatosis is often multiple and bilateral. Both feet should be examined.

Forefoot

Metatarsal Stress Fracture and Freiberg Disease

Metatarsal stress fractures are among the most common fractures in the forefoot[110] and usually involve the second and third metatarsal shafts. Ultrasound shows cortical irregularity, periosteal thickening, and callus formation. Usually, a clear fracture line is not visible,

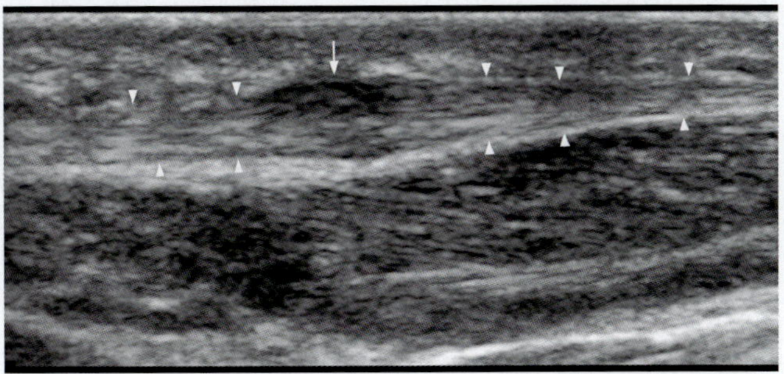

Figure 8.45. Longitudinal ultrasound of plantar aspect of foot showing medium-sized plantar fibroma (*arrow*) seen as fusiform, slightly hypoechoic swelling along the plantar fascia (*arrowheads*).

but soft tissue swelling and inflammation and occasionally small fluid collections in the adjacent soft tissues are seen.[40,41]

Freiberg disease is avascular necrosis of a metatarsal head. Ultrasound can identify the metatarsal head collapse and widening of the joint space, though this condition is usually diagnosed radiographically.

Plantar Plate Disruption ("Turf Toe")

Turf toe is a hyperextension injury to the capsulo-ligamentous-sesamoid complex on the plantar aspect of the first metatarsophalangeal joint, involving first the capsule and then the plantar plate. The injury manifests as a hypoechoic, discontinuous swelling on the plantar aspect of the metatarsophalangeal joint. Usually the capsule or the plantar plate is injured close to the metatarsal head since this attachment is weaker than at the proximal phalanx.[40,41] Plantar plate injury is associated with synovitis, joint effusion, and periarticular soft tissue swelling. Dynamic scanning during flexion or extension of the toe accentuates visibility by widening the separation gap. Sesamoid fracture or displacement can be an associated feature.

Lisfranc Ligament Injury

Lisfranc injury comprises a fracture dislocation of the tarsometatarsal articulation and may result in premature osteoarthrosis and chronic foot pain.[32] Assessment of the Lisfranc ligament proper is not possible on ultrasound. However, assessment of the dorsal ligament between the medial cuneiform and the second metatarsal base and bony alignment can indirectly indicate a Lisfranc ligament injury. The normal dorsal ligament is 0.9- to 1.2-mm thick with a hyperechoic echotexture.[32] Non-visualization of this ligament and a distance between the medial cuneiform and the second metatarsal base of 2.5 mm or greater are indirect signs of a Lisfranc ligament tear.[32]

Morton Neuroma

Morton neuroma is a common cause of forefoot pain. It is a non-neoplastic fusiform enlargement of the plantar digital nerve, almost always between the second and third or third and fourth metatarsal heads. It is due to perineural fibrosis probably caused by chronic repetitive low-grade trauma[62] and is not a true neuroma. Women are particularly susceptible to Morton neuroma possibly due to tight-fitting high-heeled shoes. Patients present with pain or paresthesiae radiating from the midfoot to the toes, often exacerbated by tight shoes or walking. Tinel sign or Mulder sign (a palpable or audible click when squeezing the metatarsals heads) can be elicited clinically. Most Morton neuromas are round or oval, hypoechoic nodules. They sometimes contain an anechoic

area due to an adjacent intermetatarsal bursa.[33] The neuroma is usually located more toward the plantar aspect of the intermetatarsal space at the level of the metatarsal heads or else midway between the metatarsal heads, typically on either side of the third metatarsal head. The intermetatarsal bursa may be difficult to distinguish from a neuroma on ultrasound, but its presence can be inferred if the mass shrinks when squeezed. Conspicuity of the neuroma can be improved by placing the transducer on the plantar aspect of the foot and applying finger pressure to the dorsal aspect of the intermetatarsal space. The neuroma is generally aligned parallel with the metatarsal shafts. Continuity with the plantar digital nerve is the most specific feature but is frequently not visible. Ultrasound-guided injections can be performed in cases refractory to the conservative treatment.[69,70,77] A dorsal approach is preferable as it is less painful than a plantar approach. Although the needle is placed in the mass, the injection sometimes shows swirling flow as the adjacent intermetatarsal bursa fills. Steroid injections, typically 40 mg of methylprednisolone along with bupivacaine, are the best first-line treatment options, often providing several months of pain relief.[111] After 3 months, if appreciable symptomatic relief from the first injection, a second steroid injection can be given. If the neuroma is large (>5 mm width) or does not respond to steroid injection, neuroablative therapy with alcohol injection may help to relieve symptoms.[112]

INFECTION

Ultrasound can assess soft tissue infection in the foot and distinguish between cellulitis, infective tenosynovitis, abscess, and joint infection (**Fig. 8.46**). MR should be used if osteomyelitis is suspected as ultrasound has low sensitivity for bone infection.

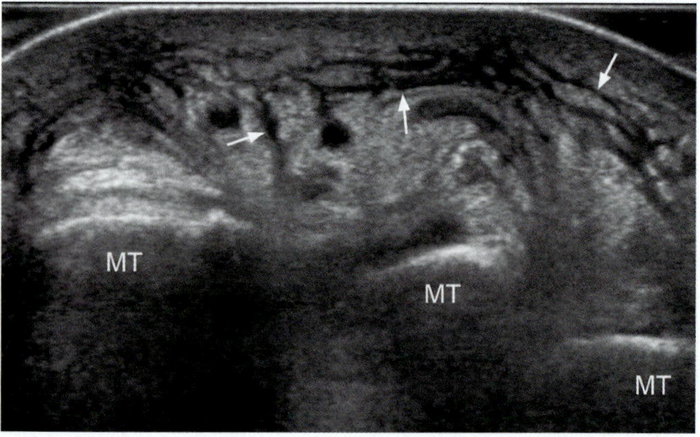

Figure 8.46. Transverse ultrasound of dorsum of forefoot. Severe edema of the subcutaneous fat is present with edematous thickening of the interlobular septa (*arrows*). Moderate hyperemia was present on color Doppler imaging. No discrete collection. Overall appearances are consistent with severe cellulitis. MT, metatarsal bones.

REFERENCES

1. Peetrons PA, Silvestre A, Cohen M, et al. Ultrasonography of ankle ligaments. *Can Assoc Radiol J.* 2002;53(1):6–13.
2. Friedrich JM, Schnarkowski P, Rübenacker S, et al. Ultrasonography of capsular morphology in normal and traumatic ankle joints. *J Clin Ultrasound.* 1993;21(3):179–187.
3. Lee MH, Chung CB, Cho JH, et al. Tibialis anterior tendon and extensor retinaculum: imaging in cadavers and patients with tendon tear. *AJR Am J Roentgenol.* 2006;187(2):W161–W168.
4. Morvan G, Busson J, Wybier M, et al. Ultrasound of the ankle. *Eur J Ultrasound.* 2001;14(1):73–82.
5. Mengiardi B, Pfirrmann CW, Vienne P, et al. Anterior tibial tendon abnormalities: MR imaging findings. *Radiology.* 2005;235(3):977–984.
6. Kennedy JG, Brunner JB, Bohne WH, et al. Clinical importance of the lateral branch of the deep peroneal nerve. *Clin Orthop Relat Res.* 2007;459:222–228.
7. Canella C, Demondion X, Guillin R, et al. Anatomic study of the superficial peroneal nerve using sonography. *AJR Am J Roentgenol.* 2009;193(1):174–179.
8. Lee PT, Clarke MT, Bearcroft PW, et al. The proximal extent of the ankle capsule and safety for the insertion of percutaneous fine wires. *J Bone Joint Surg Br.* 2005;87(5):668–671.
9. McCarthy CL, Wilson DJ, Coltman TP. Anterolateral ankle impingement: findings and diagnostic accuracy with ultrasound imaging. *Skeletal Radiol.* 2008;37(3):209–216.
10. Choudhary S, McNally E. Review of common and unusual causes of lateral ankle pain. *Skeletal Radiol.* 2011;40(11):1399–1413.
11. Milz P, Milz S, Putz R, et al. 13 MHz high-frequency sonography of the lateral ankle joint ligaments and the tibiofibular syndesmosis in anatomic specimens. *J Ultrasound Med.* 1996;15(4):277–284.
12. Peetrons P, Creteur V, Bacq C. Sonography of ankle ligaments. *J Clin Ultrasound.* 2004;32(9):491–499.
13. Numkarunarunrote N, Malik A, Aguiar RO, et al. Retinacula of the foot and ankle: MRI with anatomic correlation in cadavers. *AJR Am J Roentgenol.* 2007;188(4):W348–W354.
14. Brigido MK, Fessell DP, Jacobson JA, et al. Radiography and ultrasound of os peroneum fractures and associated peroneal tendon injuries: initial experience. *Radiology.* 2005;237(1):235–241.
15. Chepuri NB, Jacobson JA, Fessell DP, et al. Sonographic appearance of the peroneus quartus muscle: correlation with MR imaging appearance in seven patients. *Radiology.* 2001;218(2):415–419.
16. Wang XT, Rosenberg ZS, Mechlin MB, et al. Normal variants and diseases of the peroneal tendons and superior peroneal retinaculum: MR imaging features. *Radiographics.* 2005;25(3):587–602.
17. Brasseur JL, Luzzati A, Lazennec JY, et al. Ultrasono-anatomy of the ankle ligaments. *Surg Radiol Anat.* 1994;16(1):87–91.
18. Chen PY, Wang TG, Wang CL. Ultrasonographic examination of the deltoid ligament in bimalleolar equivalent fractures. *Foot Ankle Int.* 2008;29(9):883–886.
19. Harish S, Kumbhare D, O'Neill J, et al. Comparison of sonography and magnetic resonance imaging for spring ligament abnormalities: preliminary study. *J Ultrasound Med.* 2008;27(8):1145–1152.
20. Harish S, Jan E, Finlay K, et al. Sonography of the superomedial part of the spring ligament complex of the foot: a study of cadavers and asymptomatic volunteers. *Skeletal Radiol.* 2007;36(3):221–228.
21. Mansour R, Teh J, Sharp RJ, et al. Ultrasound assessment of the spring ligament complex. *Eur Radiol.* 2008;18(11):2670–2675.
22. Kotnis N, Harish S, Popowich T. Medial ankle and heel: ultrasound evaluation and sonographic appearances of conditions causing symptoms. *Semin Ultrasound CT MR.* 2011;32(2):125–141.
23. Delfaut EM, Demondion X, Bieganski A, et al. Imaging of foot and ankle nerve entrapment syndromes: from well-demonstrated to unfamiliar sites. *Radiographics.* 2003;23(3):613–623.
24. Oh SJ, Meyer RD. Entrapment neuropathies of the tibial (posterior tibial) nerve. *Neurol Clin.* 1999;17(3):593–615, vii.
25. Bing IP, Griffith JF. Paper presented at: HRCR Annual Congress of Radiology; 2011; Aberdeen, Hong Kong.
26. Fessell DP, Vanderschueren GM, Jacobson JA, et al. Ultrasound of the ankle: technique, anatomy, and diagnosis of pathologic conditions. *Radiographics.* 1998;18(2):325–340.
27. Hopper MA, Robinson P. Ankle impingement syndromes. *Radiol Clin North Am.* 2008;46(6):957–971, v.
28. Leung JL, Griffith JF. Sonography of chronic Achilles tendinopathy: a case-control study. *J Clin Ultrasound.* 2008;36(1):27–32.
29. Tumia N, Kader D, Arena B, et al. Achilles tendinopathy during pregnancy. *Clin J Sport Med.* 2002;12(1):43–45.
30. Bianchi S, Sailly M, Molini L. Isolated tear of the plantaris tendon: ultrasound and MRI appearance. *Skeletal Radiol.* 2011;40(7):891–895.
31. Helms CA, Fritz RC, Garvin GJ. Plantaris muscle injury: evaluation with MR imaging. *Radiology.* 1995;195(1):201–203.
32. Woodward S, Jacobson JA, Femino JE, et al. Sonographic evaluation of Lisfranc ligament injuries. *J Ultrasound Med.* 2009;28(3):351–357.
33. Quinn TJ, Jacobson JA, Craig JG, et al. Sonography of Morton's neuromas. *AJR Am J Roentgenol.* 2000;174(6):1723–1728.
34. Ansede G, Lee JC, Healy JC. Musculoskeletal sonography of the normal foot. *Skeletal Radiol.* 2010;39(3):225–242.
35. Trout BM, Hosey G, Wertheimer SJ. Rupture of the tibialis anterior tendon. *J Foot Ankle Surg.* 2000;39(1):54–58.
36. Kausch T, Rütt J. Subcutaneous rupture of the tibialis anterior tendon: review of the literature and a case report. *Arch Orthop Trauma Surg.* 1998;117(4–5):290–293.
37. Bianchi S, Zwass A, Abdelwahab IF, et al. Evaluation of tibialis anterior tendon rupture by ultrasonography. *J Clin Ultrasound.* 1994;22(9):564–566.
38. Grant TH, Kelikian AS, Jereb SE, et al. Ultrasound diagnosis of peroneal tendon tears. A surgical correlation. *J Bone Joint Surg Am.* 2005;87(8):1788–1794.
39. Smania L, Craig JG, von Holsbeeck M. Ultrasonographic findings in peroneus longus tendon rupture. *J Ultrasound Med.* 2007;26(2):243–246.
40. Martinoli C, Bianchi S. Ankle. In: *Ultrasound of the Musculoskeletal System.* Berlin, Germany: Springer; 2007:773–834.
41. Bianchi S, Martinoli C. Foot. In: *Ultrasound of the Musculoskeletal System.* Berlin, Germany: Springer; 2007:835–888.
42. Neustadter J, Raikin SM, Nazarian LN. Dynamic sonographic evaluation of peroneal tendon subluxation. *AJR Am J Roentgenol.* 2004;183(4):985–988.
43. Diaz GC, van Holsbeeck M, Jacobson JA. Longitudinal split of the peroneus longus and peroneus brevis tendons with disruption of the superior peroneal retinaculum. *J Ultrasound Med.* 1998;17(8):525–529.
44. Raikin SM. Intrasheath subluxation of the peroneal tendons. Surgical technique. *J Bone Joint Surg Am.* 2009;91(suppl 2, pt 1):146–155.
45. Sofka CM, Adler RS, Saboeiro GR, et al. Sonographic evaluation and sonographic-guided therapeutic options of lateral ankle pain: peroneal tendon pathology associated with the presence of an os peroneum. *HSS J.* 2010;6(2):177–181.
46. Kong A, Van Der Vliet A. Imaging of tibialis posterior dysfunction. *Br J Radiol.* 2008;81(970):826–836.
47. Nallamshetty L, Nazarian LN, Schweitzer ME, et al. Evaluation of posterior tibial pathology: comparison of sonography and MR imaging. *Skeletal Radiol.* 2005;34(7):375–380.

48. Premkumar A, Perry MB, Dwyer AJ, et al. Sonography and MR imaging of posterior tibial tendinopathy. *AJR Am J Roentgenol.* 2002;178(1):223–232.

49. Prato N, Abello E, Martinoli C, et al. Sonography of posterior tibialis tendon dislocation. *J Ultrasound Med.* 2004;23(5):701–705.

50. Goucher NR, Coughlin MJ, Kristensen RM. Dislocation of the posterior tibial tendon: a literature review and presentation of two cases. *Iowa Orthop J.* 2006;26:122–126.

51. Leekam RN, Agur AM, McKee NH. Using sonography to diagnose injury of plantaris muscles and tendons. *AJR Am J Roentgenol.* 1999;172(1):185–189.

52. Jamadar DA, Jacobson JA, Theisen SE, et al. Sonography of the painful calf: differential considerations. *AJR Am J Roentgenol.* 2002;179(3):709–716.

53. Fornage BD. Achilles tendon: ultrasound examination. *Radiology.* 1986;159(3):759–764.

54. Longo UG, Ronga M, Maffulli N. Acute ruptures of the Achilles tendon. *Sports Med Arthrosc.* 2009;17(2):127–138.

55. Ames PR, Longo UG, Denaro V, et al. Achilles tendon problems: not just an orthopaedic issue. *Disabil Rehabil.* 2008;30(20–22):1646–1650.

56. Magra M, Maffulli N. Nonsteroidal antiinflammatory drugs in tendinopathy: friend or foe. *Clin J Sport Med.* 2006;16(1):1–3.

57. Malliaras P, Richards PJ, Garau G, et al. Achilles tendon Doppler flow may be associated with mechanical loading among active athletes. *Am J Sports Med.* 2008;36(11):2210–2215.

58. Tallon C, Maffulli N, Ewen SW. Ruptured Achilles tendons are significantly more degenerated than tendinopathic tendons. *Med Sci Sports Exerc.* 2001;33(12):1983–1990.

59. Blei CL, Nirschl RP, Grant EG. Achilles tendon: ultrasound diagnosis of pathologic conditions. Work in progress. *Radiology.* 1986;159(3):765–767.

60. Hartgerink P, Fessell DP, Jacobson JA, et al. Full- versus partial-thickness Achilles tendon tears: sonographic accuracy and characterization in 26 cases with surgical correlation. *Radiology.* 2001;220(2):406–412.

61. Jarauta E, Junyent M, Gilabert R, et al. Sonographic evaluation of Achilles tendons and carotid atherosclerosis in familial hypercholesterolemia. *Atherosclerosis.* 2009;204(2):345–347.

62. Bureau NJ, Roederer G. Sonography of Achilles tendon xanthomas in patients with heterozygous familial hypercholesterolemia. *AJR Am J Roentgenol.* 1998;171(3):745–749.

63. Sofka CM, Adler RS, Positano R, et al. Haglund's syndrome: diagnosis and treatment using sonography. *HSS J.* 2006;2(1):27–29.

64. Sella EJ, Caminear DS, McLarney EA. Haglund's syndrome. *J Foot Ankle Surg.* 1998;37(2):110–114.

65. Blankstein A, Cohen I, Diamant L, et al. Achilles tendon pain and related pathologies: diagnosis by ultrasonography. *Isr Med Assoc J.* 2001;3(8):575–578.

66. Panchbhavi VK. Re: a biomechanical analysis of a tensioned suture device in the fixation of the ligamentous Lisfranc injury by Pelt et al: Foot Ankle Int. 32(4): 422–431, 2011. *Foot Ankle Int.* 2012;33(1):88.

67. Khosla S, Thiele R, Baumhauer JF. Ultrasound guidance for intra-articular injections of the foot and ankle. *Foot Ankle Int.* 2009;30(9):886–890.

68. Smith J, Finnoff JT, Henning PT, et al. Accuracy of sonographically guided posterior subtalar joint injections: comparison of 3 techniques. *J Ultrasound Med.* 2009;28(11):1549–1557.

69. Sofka CM, Adler RS. Ultrasound-guided interventions in the foot and ankle. *Semin Musculoskelet Radiol.* 2002;6(2):163–168.

70. Morvan G, Vuillemin V, Guerini H. Interventional musculoskeletal ultrasonography of the lower limb. *Diagn Interv Imaging.* 2012;93(9):652–664.

71. Reach JS, Easley ME, Chuckpaiwong B, et al. Accuracy of ultrasound guided injections in the foot and ankle. *Foot Ankle Int.* 2009;30(3):239–242.

72. Wijesekera NT, Chew NS, Lee JC, et al. Ultrasound-guided treatments for chronic Achilles tendinopathy: an update and current status. *Skeletal Radiol.* 2010;39(5):425–434.

73. Ryan M, Wong A, Taunton J. Favorable outcomes after sonographically guided intratendinous injection of hyperosmolar dextrose for chronic insertional and midportion Achilles tendinosis. *AJR Am J Roentgenol.* 2010;194(4):1047–1053.

74. Deans VM, Miller A, Ramos J. A prospective series of patients with chronic Achilles tendinopathy treated with autologous-conditioned plasma injections combined with exercise and therapeutic ultrasonography. *J Foot Ankle Surg.* 2012;51(6):706–710.

75. Muir JJ, Curtiss HM, Hollman J, et al. The accuracy of ultrasound-guided and palpation-guided peroneal tendon sheath injections. *Am J Phys Med Rehabil.* 2011;90(7):564–571.

76. Mehdizade A, Adler RS. Sonographically guided flexor hallucis longus tendon sheath injection. *J Ultrasound Med.* 2007;26(2):233–237.

77. Hassouna H, Singh D, Taylor H, et al. Ultrasound guided steroid injection in the treatment of interdigital neuralgia. *Acta Orthop Belg.* 2007;73(2):224–229.

78. McNally EG, Shetty S. Plantar fascia: imaging diagnosis and guided treatment. *Semin Musculoskelet Radiol.* 2010;14(3):334–343.

79. Redborg KE, Sites BD, Chinn CD, et al. Ultrasound improves the success rate of a sural nerve block at the ankle. *Reg Anesth Pain Med.* 2009;34(1):24–28.

80. Karabay N, Toros T, Hurel C. Ultrasonographic evaluation in plantar fasciitis. *J Foot Ankle Surg.* 2007;46(6):442–446.

81. Durkee NJ, Jacobson JA, Jamadar DA, et al. Sonographic evaluation of lower extremity interosseous membrane injuries: retrospective review in 3 patients. *J Ultrasound Med.* 2003;22(12):1369–1375.

82. Karasick D, Schweitzer ME. The os trigonum syndrome: imaging features. *AJR Am J Roentgenol.* 1996;166(1):125–129.

83. Datir A, Connell D. Imaging of impingement lesions in the ankle. *Top Magn Reson Imaging.* 2010;21(1):15–23.

84. Robinson P. Impingement syndromes of the ankle. *Eur Radiol.* 2007;17(12):3056–3065.

85. Robinson P, Bollen SR. Posterior ankle impingement in professional soccer players: effectiveness of sonographically guided therapy. *AJR Am J Roentgenol.* 2006;187(1):W53–W58.

86. Messiou C, Robinson P, O'Connor PJ, et al. Subacute posteromedial impingement of the ankle in athletes: MR imaging evaluation and ultrasound guided therapy. *Skeletal Radiol.* 2006;35(2):88–94.

87. Koulouris G, Connell D, Schneider T, et al. Posterior tibiotalar ligament injury resulting in posteromedial impingement. *Foot Ankle Int.* 2003;24(8):575–583.

88. Cochet H, Pelé E, Amoretti N, et al. Anterolateral ankle impingement: diagnostic performance of MDCT arthrography and sonography. *AJR Am J Roentgenol.* 2010;194(6):1575–1580.

89. Robinson P, White LM. Soft-tissue and osseous impingement syndromes of the ankle: role of imaging in diagnosis and management. *Radiographics.* 2002;22(6):1457–1469.

90. Martinoli C, Bianchi S, Gandolfo N, et al. Ultrasound of nerve entrapments in osteofibrous tunnels of the upper and lower limbs. *Radiographics.* 2000;20 Spec No:S199–S213.

91. Nagaoka M, Matsuzaki H. Ultrasonography in tarsal tunnel syndrome. *J Ultrasound Med.* 2005;24(8):1035–1040.

92. Hsu CC, Tsai WC, Chen CP, et al. Ultrasonographic examination for inversion ankle sprains associated with osseous injuries. *Am J Phys Med Rehabil.* 2006;85(10):785–792.

93. Wang CL, Shieh JY, Wang TG, et al. Sonographic detection of occult fractures in the foot and ankle. *J Clin Ultrasound.* 1999;27(8):421–425.

94. Chen HS, Chen SC, Wang HJ, et al. Ultrasonographic findings and clinical characteristics of two patients with talar osteochondritis dissecans. *J Ultrasound Med.* 2011;19(8):47–51.

95. Ortega R, Fessell DP, Jacobson JA, et al. Sonography of ankle Ganglia with pathologic correlation in 10 pediatric and adult patients. *AJR Am J Roentgenol.* 2002;178(6):1445–1449.

96. Jacobson JA, Andresen R, Jaovisidha S, et al. Detection of ankle effusions: comparison study in cadavers using radiography, sonography, and MR imaging. *AJR Am J Roentgenol.* 1998;170(5):1231–1238.

97. Pham H, Fessell DP, Femino JE, et al. Sonography and MR imaging of selected benign masses in the ankle and foot. *AJR Am J Roentgenol.* 2003;180(1):99–107.

98. Lin CS, Wang TG, Shieh JY, et al. Accuracy of sonography in the diagnosis of superficial ganglion cyst and lipoma. *J Ultrasound Med.* 2009;17(2):107–113.

99. Chu CH, Chen WS, Wang TG. Ultrasonographic presentations of tophi-like masses at atypical locations. *J Ultrasound Med.* 2006;14(2):35–39.

100. Rockett MS, Gentile SC, Gudas CJ, et al. The use of ultrasonography for the detection of retained wooden foreign bodies in the foot. *J Foot Ankle Surg.* 1995;34(5):478–484.

101. Fessell DP, Jacobson JA. Ultrasound of the hindfoot and midfoot. *Radiol Clin North Am.* 2008;46(6):1027–1043.

102. Sabir N, Demirlenk S, Yagci B, et al. Clinical utility of sonography in diagnosing plantar fasciitis. *J Ultrasound Med.* 2005;24(8):1041–1048.

103. Akfirat M, Sen C, Günes T. Ultrasonographic appearance of the plantar fasciitis. *Clin Imaging.* 2003;27(5):353–357.

104. Gibbon WW, Long G. Ultrasound of the plantar aponeurosis (fascia). *Skeletal Radiol.* 1999;28(1):21–26.

105. Cardinal E, Chhem RK, Beauregard CG, et al. Plantar fasciitis: sonographic evaluation. *Radiology.* 1996;201(1):257–259.

106. Haun DW, Cho JC, Kettner NW. Symptomatic plantar fibroma with a unique sonographic appearance. *J Clin Ultrasound.* 2012;40(2):112–114.

107. Griffith JF, Wong TY, Wong SM, et al. Sonography of plantar fibromatosis. *AJR Am J Roentgenol.* 2002;179(5):1167–1172.

108. Reed M, Gooding GA, Kerley SM, et al. Sonography of plantar fibromatosis. *J Clin Ultrasound.* 1991;19(9):578–582.

109. Bedi DG, Davidson DM. Plantar fibromatosis: most common sonographic appearance and variations. *J Clin Ultrasound.* 2001;29(9):499–505.

110. Rogers CJ, Cianca J. Musculoskeletal ultrasound of the ankle and foot. *Phys Med Rehabil Clin N Am.* 2010;21(3):549–557.

111. Thomson CE, Beggs I, Martin D, et al. Methylprednisolone injections for the treatment of Morton neuroma. A patient-blinded randomized trial. *J Bone Joint Surg Am.* 2013;95(9):790-798.

112. Fanucci E, Masala S, Fabiano S, et al. Treatment of intermetatarsal Morton's neuroma with alcohol injection under ultrasound guide: a 10-month follow-up. *Eur Radiol.* 2004;14(3):514–518.

Soft Tissue Masses

Jon A. Jacobson
David P. Fessell

INTRODUCTION

Ultrasound is routinely used to evaluate palpable soft tissue masses.[1] Ultrasound differentiates cystic from solid masses, which often require biopsy to exclude malignancy,[2] and can identify superficial soft tissue tumor margins and local tumor spread.[3] Limitations primarily relate to evaluation of deep soft tissue structures, bone, and masses that calcify or ossify, casting acoustic shadows that obscure deeper structures.

Advantages of ultrasound include direct correlation of symptoms and physical examination with imaging. Palpation during ultrasound imaging, "sonopalpation," is the ultrasound correlate of physical examination. Additional history gained during the ultrasound examination often adds insight to narrow the differential diagnosis. Ultrasound is less expensive and more accessible than magnetic resonance imaging (MRI). Color and power Doppler may help distinguish between cystic and solid masses and characterize malignant masses and lymph nodes. Ultrasound can guide percutaneous biopsy, particularly useful with masses near neurovascular structures or the pleura where real-time imaging during biopsy is necessary.

While ultrasound is primarily used to discriminate between cystic and solid masses, there are often features that can limit the differential diagnosis. The first critical distinction is to determine whether the mass originates from a synovial space (joint, bursa, or tendon sheath), as such masses are likely benign and related to a synovial process. A mass that originates in other soft tissues could be benign or malignant. Most malignant masses are predominantly hypoechoic, usually with low-level echoes or heterogeneity, and well defined as they have pseudocapsules. As a malignant mass enlarges, especially if high grade, it becomes more heterogeneous with hypoechoic areas of internal necrosis and increased flow on color and power Doppler imaging. Tumors with a significant myxoid component (myxoid liposarcoma, intramuscular myxoma) can be predominantly hypoechoic and have the appearance of a heterogeneous cyst. Many solid masses demonstrate increased through-transmission, simulating complex cysts.[4] The presence of an echogenic and shadowing focus requires radiography to evaluate for calcification or ossification. Ultrasound is accurate in the diagnosis of sarcoma and melanoma local recurrence.[5–7]

Color Doppler imaging has been used to characterize masses and tumor vascularity.[8] Aggressive tumors tend to have more flow on color and power Doppler imaging than benign tumors. However, hypervascular benign tumors such as peripheral nerve sheath tumors do occur.[9,10] Extreme vascularity of a hypoechoic soft tissue mass in the absence of necrosis is characteristic of lymphoma. Increased flow is also characteristic of vascular malformations and vascular tumors. Because of the overlap between lesions on Doppler, including spectral Doppler, ultrasound cannot reliably differentiate between benign and malignant masses.[11] Ultrasound contrast agents have been used to characterize the vascularity of soft tissue tumors,[12] but no role has been established for contrast agents.

In evaluating a soft tissue mass of the extremity, a differential diagnosis can be organized based on location of the mass and age of the patient,[13,14] and a short list of probable etiologies can be generated. This information is helpful when characterizing the mass with imaging, as imaging features are often in part explained by the histology of the tumor. The World Health Organization (WHO) classifies tumors by their histologic differentiation.[15,16] The ultrasound description of masses in the subsequent text will in part follow this classification scheme.

ULTRASOUND TECHNIQUE

Diagnostic

Examination technique is important when performing ultrasound of a soft tissue mass. Hold the transducer at its footprint, and anchor the probe to the patient with the side of the hand or fingers. This will stabilize the transducer, allow fine movements, and help to assess how much pressure is being placed with the transducer. Excessive pressure may obscure the margins of a soft tissue mass or compress a fluid component. Ideally, a variety of probe pressures should be used. Floating the transducer on a thick layer of gel helps to demonstrate soft tissue swelling or a very superficial mass. The application of pressure can show if a mass is pliable (such as a lipoma) and differentiates a fluid component (which is compressible) from an area of heterogeneous soft tissue. When assessing vascularity with color or power Doppler imaging, the application of pressure via the transducer may also obscure flow.

> **Tip:**
> - Use pressure to distinguish fluid (which is compressible and can be displaced) from solid tissue.
> - Avoid heavy pressure when performing Doppler examinations, or vascularity may be effaced or reduced.

Interventional

While a complete review of interventional techniques as they relate to soft tissue masses is beyond the scope of this chapter, several general points deserve emphasis. Ultrasound is ideal for guiding soft tissue biopsy or aspiration, especially when the mass is small and superficial[17,18] or adjacent to a vital structure, such as an artery, where real-time imaging during the biopsy is important.[19] While there are various techniques to guide needles with ultrasound, the in-plane approach with the needle parallel to the transducer is most accurate and shows the full length of the needle and its trajectory in real time. Needle visualization is improved when the sound beam is perpendicular to the needle to eliminate anisotropy. Typically three to five samples are obtained from various regions of the mass including the center and periphery, typically with a 16G or 18G needle. Fine needle aspiration generally does not provide diagnostic material, but may be helpful when performing a biopsy of a necrotic tumor, where soft tissue cores may not yield solid tissue, when the soft mass is small or in a critical location such as a pleural mass, or when recurrent or metastatic tumor is suspected. Discussion with the surgical oncologist prior to the biopsy is essential with regard to the approach and needle path as surgery often occurs along the biopsy needle path, which is also resected. Many centers perform local MRI staging prior to biopsy.

> **Tip:**
> - Do not biopsy a soft tissue mass without first discussing the needle approach with the surgical oncologist.

Confirmation of a malignant tumor typically initiates staging with thoracic computed tomography (CT) and possibly an isotope bone scan to identify potential metastases. Positron emission tomography (PET) scanning is generally restricted to a few rare tumors such as alveolar rhabdomyosarcoma that metastasize to unusual sites. Staging and histology help to determine whether and what type of surgery and adjuvant radiation or chemotherapy are employed.

SOFT TISSUE MASSES

Lipomatous Tumors

Lipoma

Lipomas are benign fatty tumors. They are common, have a prevalence of 2.1%, and account for nearly half of all soft tissue masses.[20] Frequent locations include the shoulder region and back.[20] Lipomas are often present for many years with little or no growth. Malignant transformation is nonexistent with no metastatic potential.[20] A lipoma may become clinically apparent when a patient loses weight and the surrounding fat decreases. Most lipomas occur in the subcutaneous fat and are <5 cm in diameter.[20] Intramuscular or intermuscular lipomas, referred to as deep lipomas, are less common.[20] Lipomas are multiple in 5% to 15% of cases, typically in males.[20]

In general, a lipoma is a discrete and homogeneous fatty mass that has similar imaging features to adjacent subcutaneous fat (**Fig. 9.1**). Superficial lipomas are usually encapsulated, while deep lipomas may have microscopic invasion of adjacent muscle tissue.[20] Other than fatty elements, a lipoma may contain thin fibrous septations.

Ultrasound evaluation largely depends on the location of the lipoma. Superficial lipomas are typically oval or oblong, well defined, compressible, and show no flow on color or power Doppler imaging (**Fig. 9.2**). Echotexture varies from hypoechoic to hyperechoic relative to the surrounding subcutaneous fat. Pure fat is essentially free of echoes.[21] Echogenicity is related to the fibrous component that increases the echogenic interfaces (**Figs. 9.3 and 9.4**).[22] A blood vessel coursing through a lipoma should not be interpreted as neovascularity. Any unusual features on imaging, history, or physical examination warrant MR imaging. Otherwise, ultrasound may be considered as a follow-up if symptoms change.

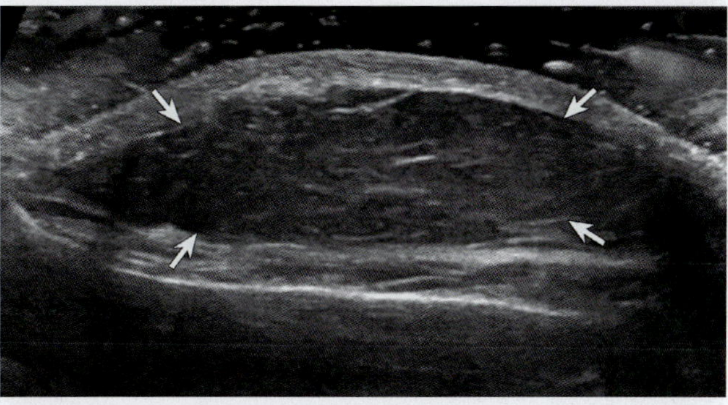

Figure 9.1. Lipoma. Ultrasound image shows oval hypoechoic subcutaneous lipoma (*arrows*) with internal linear hyperechoic fibrous tissue.

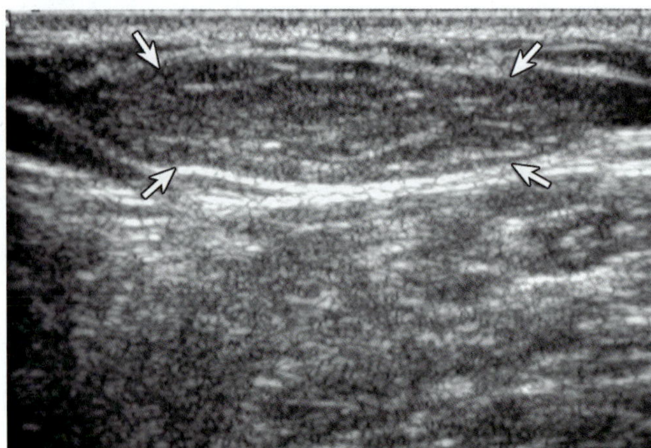

Figure 9.2.   Lipoma. Ultrasound image shows oval hyperechoic subcutaneous lipoma (*arrows*) with internal linear hyperechoic fibrous tissue.

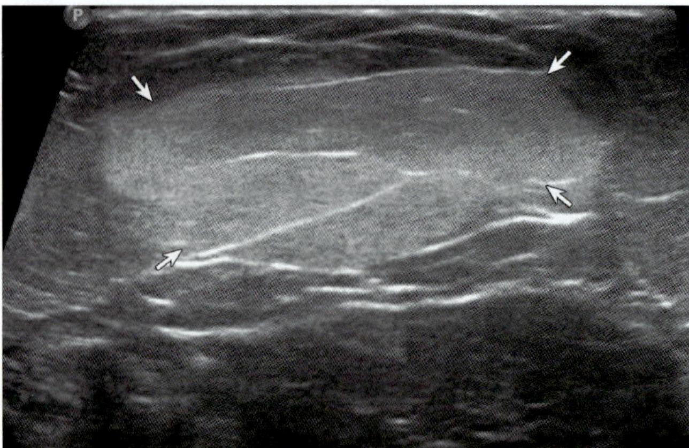

Figure 9.4.   Lipoma. Ultrasound image shows oval hyperechoic subcutaneous lipoma (*arrows*) with internal linear hyperechoic fibrous tissue (pathologically proven).

Tip:
- Superficial lipomas are typically elliptical, well defined, pliable, and avascular.
- Lipoma echotexture varies from hypoechoic to hyperechoic relative to subcutaneous fat, but is homogeneous.

The ultrasound features of deeper lipomas are more variable and diagnosis less accurate.[23] This is related to lower resolution of deeper structures, the inability of ultrasound to identify internal septations in well-differentiated liposarcomas, and the higher prevalence of liposarcomas in deeper soft tissues.[24] Intramuscular lipomas are often ill-defined and insinuate into the adjacent muscle fibers. Echogenicity is variable, often isoechoic to hyperechoic, relative to the surrounding muscle **(Fig. 9.5)**. When a deep lipoma is identified on ultrasound, MRI should be recommended to confirm that there are no suspicious features.

Other benign lesions can be considered in the differential diagnosis of superficial lipomas. If a presumed subcutaneous lipoma is hyperechoic and tender, angiolipoma and fat necrosis should be considered (see later discussion).[25,26] Most malignant processes tend to be hypoechoic. Dermatofibrosarcoma protuberans may be hyperechoic,[27] but does not have the other ultrasound features of a superficial lipoma.

Other Benign Lipomatous Masses

Several less common benign lipomatous masses deserve brief comment.[20] Diffuse lipomatosis is diffuse infiltration of an anatomic region with mature fat, usually presenting by the age of 2 years when involving the extremity. Lipomatosis of nerve (also termed fibrolipomatous hamartoma) is fibrofatty infiltration of a peripheral nerve, typically the median nerve at the wrist and associated with

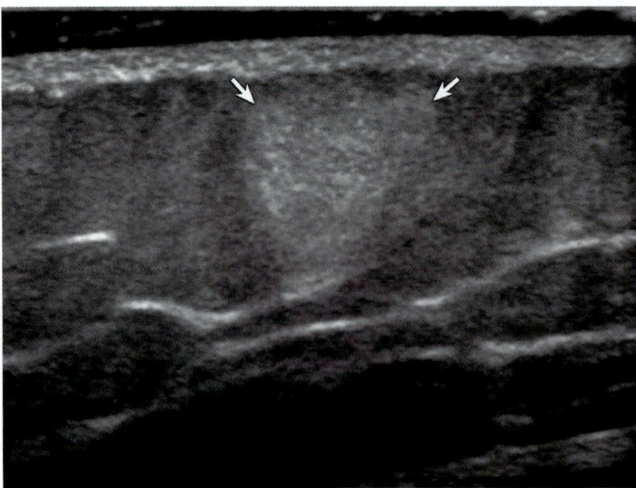

Figure 9.3.   Lipoma. Ultrasound image shows round hyperechoic subcutaneous lipoma (*arrows*) (pathologically proven).

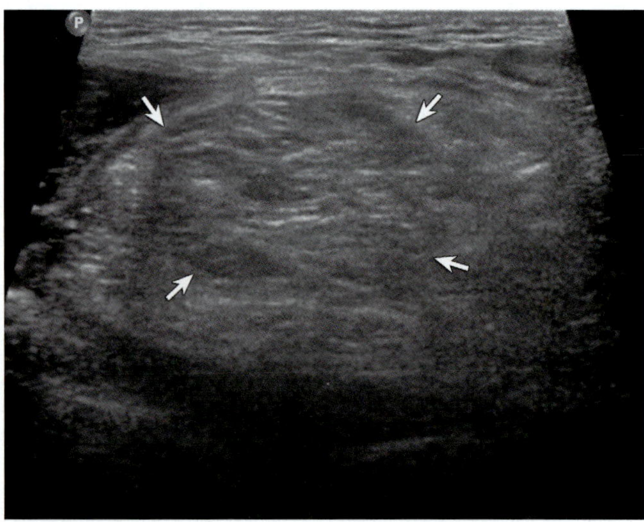

Figure 9.5.   Lipoma: intramuscular. Ultrasound image shows isoechoic intramuscular lipoma (*arrows*) with internal linear hyperechoic fibrous tissue (pathologically proven).

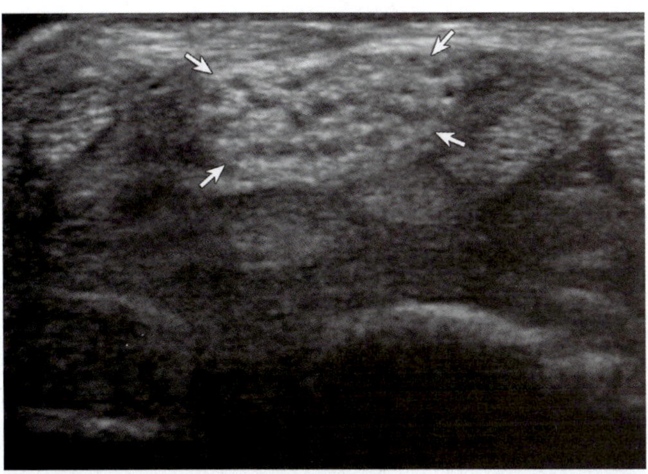

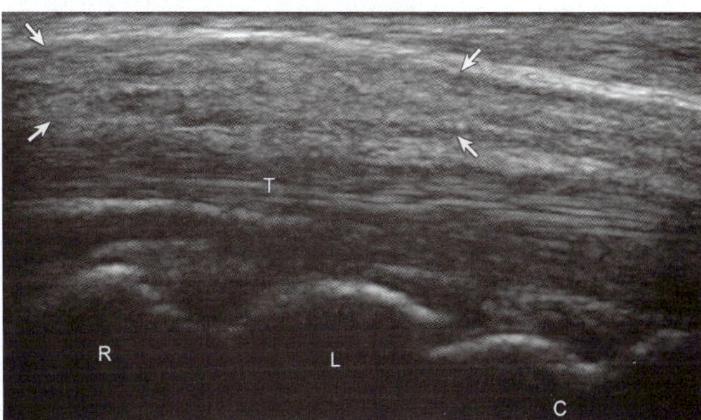

Figure 9.6. Fibrolipomatous hamartoma. Ultrasound images **(A)** short axis and **(B)** long axis to median nerve show increased hyperechoic tissue around the hypoechoic nerve fascicles causing an overall increase in median nerve size (*arrows*) (pathologically proven). R, radius; L, lunate; C, capitate; T, flexor tendon.

macrodystrophia in 67% of cases.[20] Ultrasound shows hyperechoic fibrofatty tissue separating the individual hypoechoic nerve fascicles in the enlarged nerve **(Fig. 9.6)**. Angiolipoma presents as a small (<2 cm), possibly painful circumscribed mass in the subcutaneous tissues. It is typically hyperechoic, and there may be increased vascularity **(Fig. 9.7)**.[25] Hibernoma is a benign tumor composed of brown fat **(Fig. 9.8)**. Although somewhat similar in appearance to a lipoma, the increased echogenicity and possible internal vascularity typically raise concern for other pathologies such as well-differentiated liposarcoma.[28]

Liposarcoma

Liposarcoma is a malignant fat-containing tumor, which has several subtypes and can vary in tumor grade. Liposarcoma is the second most common soft tissue sarcoma, accounting for up to 35% of soft tissue sarcomas.[24] The subtypes of liposarcoma include well-differentiated, dedifferentiated, myxoid, pleomorphic, and mixed liposarcomas.[24] At one end of the spectrum is a well-differentiated, low-grade liposarcoma (previously termed atypical lipoma), while at the other end is a poorly differentiated, high-grade pleomorphic liposarcoma. The imaging appearances of liposarcomas relate to their subtypes and grades of malignancy.

The ultrasound appearances of liposarcomas tend to fall into three categories. The first is the well-differentiated liposarcoma, the most common type of liposarcoma, most frequently located in the deep tissues when involving an extremity.[24] A well-differentiated liposarcoma is predominantly composed of fat (>75%), but may also be characterized by thick septations and/or nodules. At CT or MR imaging, thick septations (>2 mm) or nodules in a fatty tumor, especially if enhancing, indicate well-differentiated low-grade liposarcoma until proven otherwise.[24,29] Although such features may be identified, the septations or nodules are often not well seen at ultrasound, and therefore a well-differentiated liposarcoma may be misdiagnosed as a lipoma **(Fig. 9.9)**. Given the higher prevalence of liposarcomas in deeper soft tissues and the difficulty in providing an accurate diagnosis with ultrasound, any fatty tumor deeper than the subcutaneous tissues warrants MR. Well-differentiated liposarcomas calcify or ossify in 10% to 32% of cases.[24]

Tip:
- Any fatty tumor deeper than the subcutaneous tissues may be a liposarcoma and warrants MRI evaluation.

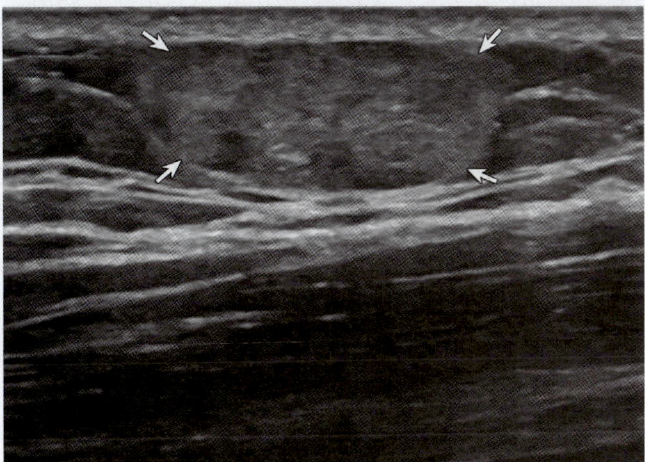

Figure 9.7.   Angiolipoma. Ultrasound image shows well-defined hyperechoic angiolipoma (*arrows*) within the subcutaneous tissues (pathologically proven).

The second ultrasound appearance relates to the myxoid subtype, which is the second most common type of liposarcoma.[24] Myxoid liposarcomas are heterogeneous and contain myxoid, round cell, and fat components,

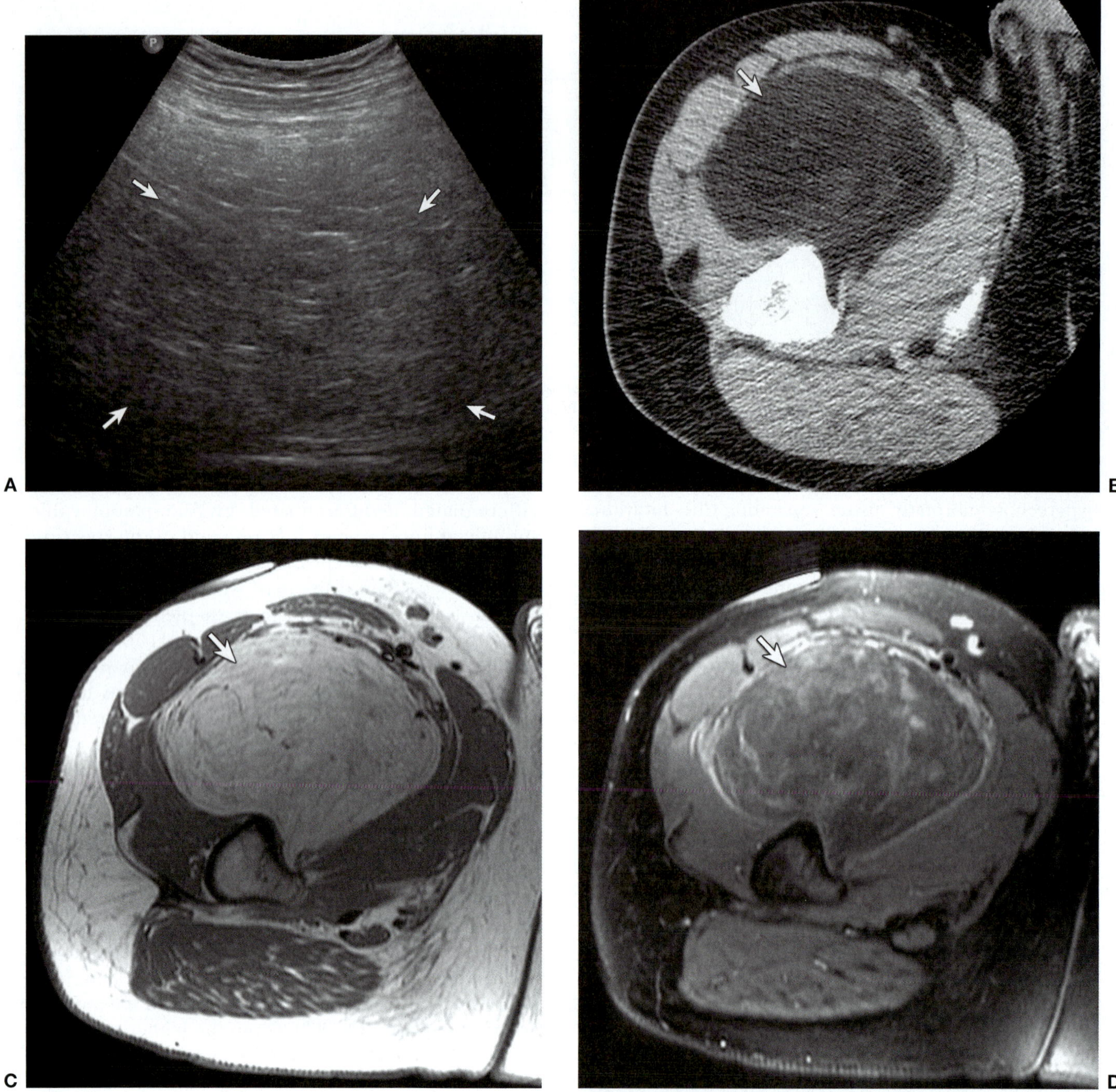

Figure 9.8.   Hibernoma. Ultrasound image **(A)** shows the hibernoma as a homogeneous area of low-level echoes (*arrows*). CT image without contrast **(B)** shows predominantly fatty mass (*arrows*) with internal areas of soft tissue attenuation. Axial T1-weighted **(C)** and fluid-sensitive **(D)** MR images show a fat-containing mass (*arrows*) with internal fluid signal areas (pathologically proven).

although fat may comprise <10% of the tumor volume.[24] The ultrasound appearances depend on the amount of each component. If a myxoid component is predominant, the mass may appear hypoechoic and potentially simulate a complex cyst **(Fig. 9.10)**. To avoid misdiagnosis of a myxoid liposarcoma as a complex cyst, any "cyst-appearing" mass, which does not correspond to a bursa, especially when large, can be biopsied for confirmation.

Tip:
- Consider biopsy of any round "cyst-appearing" mass that does not correspond to a bursa, especially if large, for confirmation of the diagnosis.

A myxoid liposarcoma **(Fig. 9.11)** should not be mistaken for a ganglion cyst, which is usually multilocular

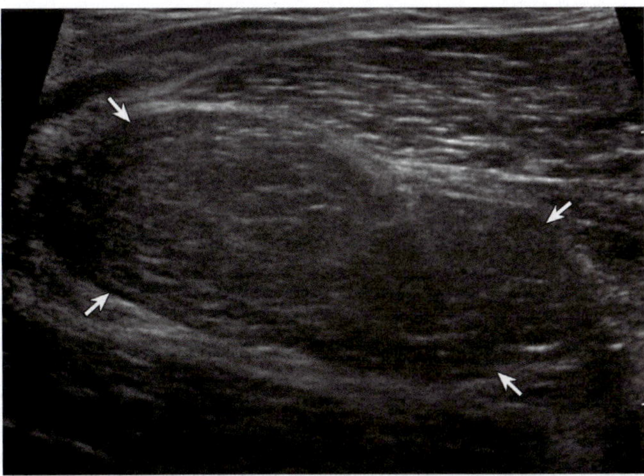

Figure 9.9. Liposarcoma: low-grade well-differentiated. Ultrasound image shows liposarcoma as a well-defined area of low-level echoes (*arrows*) (pathologically proven). Note similar echotexture to lipoma.

and not typically large, or a Baker's cyst, which has a neck between the medial head of the gastrocnemius muscle and the semimembranosus tendon. Myxoid liposarcoma may appear more heterogeneous if increased round cell components are present and therefore appear more nonspecific at ultrasound.

The third ultrasound appearance of liposarcoma occurs with high-grade or poorly differentiated tumors, and includes dedifferentiated, myxoid (if containing a

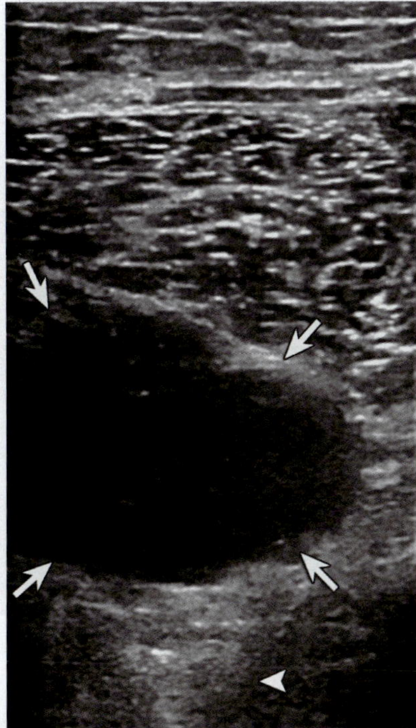

Figure 9.10. Liposarcoma: high-grade myxoid. Ultrasound image shows well-defined hypoechoic liposarcoma (*arrows*) with through-transmission (*arrowhead*) (pathologically proven).

round cell component), pleomorphic, and mixed subtypes. In this situation, the appearance is nonspecific and similar to any high-grade sarcoma. Although predominantly hypoechoic, there are often heterogeneous anechoic areas due to necrosis, heterogeneity, and increased flow on color and power Doppler imaging **(Fig. 9.12)**.

Fibrous Tumors

Soft tissue fibrous proliferation may be categorized as fibromatoses (which includes superficial and deep fibromatoses), benign fibrous proliferations (which includes nodular fasciitis and elastofibroma), fibrosarcomas, and fibrous proliferations of infancy and childhood.[30]

Superficial Fibromatosis

Superficial fibromatosis includes plantar and palmar fibromas.[30] They are benign but, although having no malignant potential, may behave aggressively. Palmar fibromatosis (or Dupuytren disease) is the most common superficial fibromatosis. It occurs typically in men over the age of 30 and is bilateral in approximately 50% of cases.[30] Palmar fibromatosis involves the volar hand and appears as hypoechoic fusiform masses or nodules along the palmar fascia, often associated with flexion deformity of the digits **(Fig. 9.13)**.[31] Plantar fibromatosis (Ledderhose disease) appears as single or multiple discrete fusiform hypoechoic nodules or thickenings along the plantar fascia of the foot **(Fig. 9.14)**. Increased flow on color and power Doppler imaging may be present **(Fig. 9.15)**.[32] Plantar fibromatosis more commonly involves men, is associated with palmar fibromatosis in up to 65% of cases,

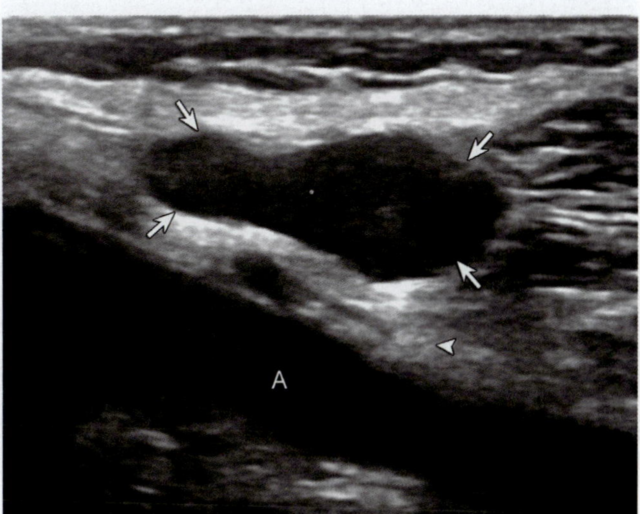

Figure 9.11. Liposarcoma: low-grade myxoid recurrent. Ultrasound image (**A**) shows hypoechoic liposarcoma (*arrows*) with increased through-transmission (*arrowhead*). A, popliteal artery. (pathologically proven).

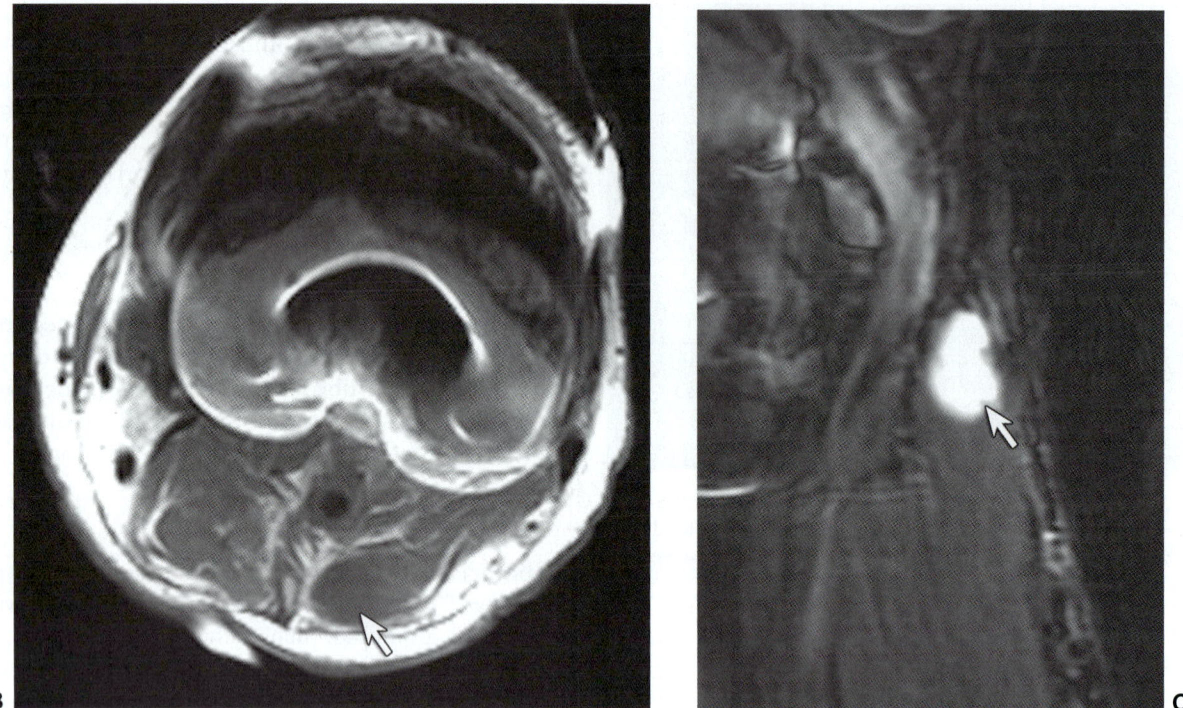

Figure 9.11.   (*continued*) Axial T1-weighted (**B**) and sagittal fluid-sensitive (**C**) MR images show a fluid signal lobular mass (*arrow*). Note artifact related to total knee arthroplasty.

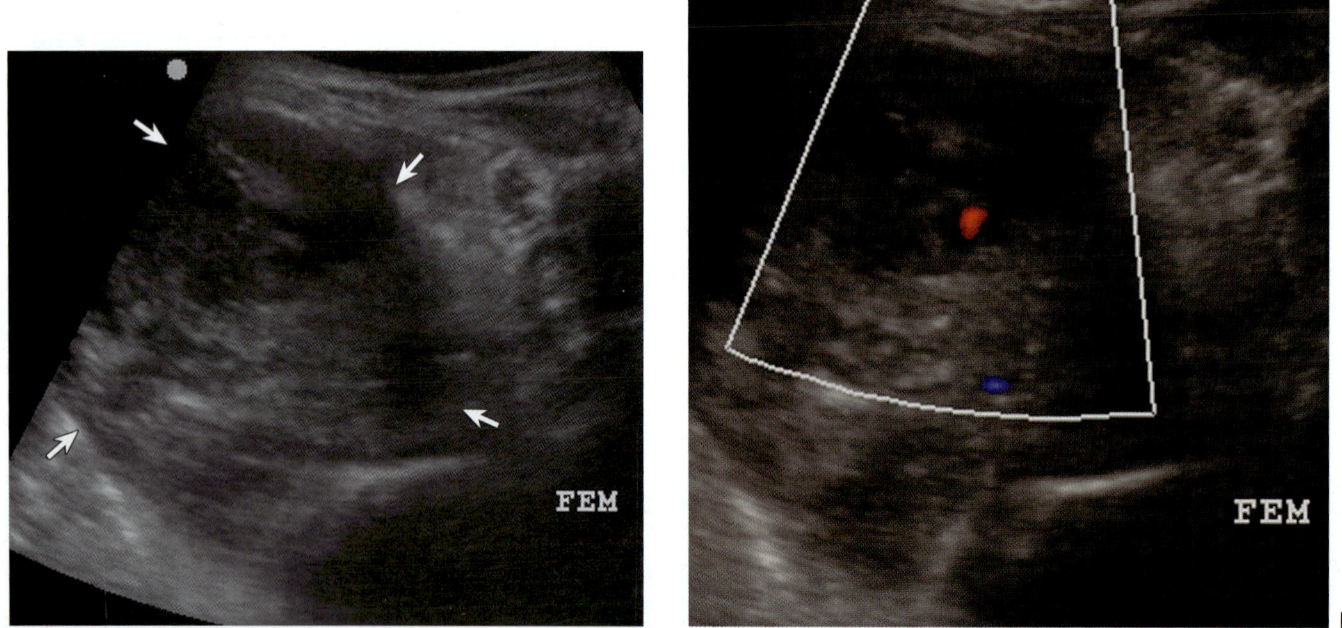

Figure 9.12.   Liposarcoma: high grade undifferentiated. Ultrasound gray scale (**A**) and color Doppler (**B**) images show heterogeneous but predominantly hypoechoic liposarcoma (*arrows* in **A**). FEM, femur (pathologically proven).

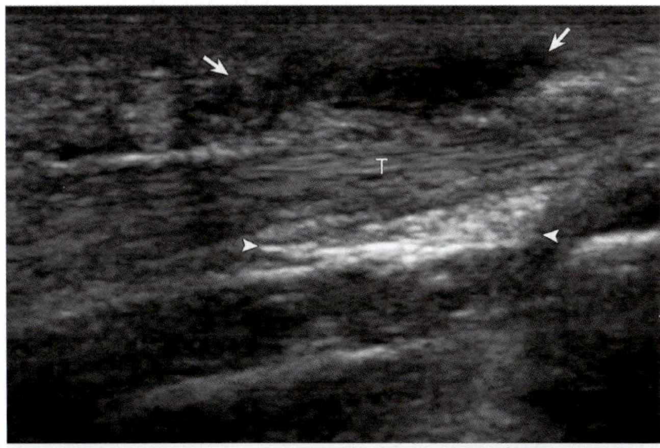

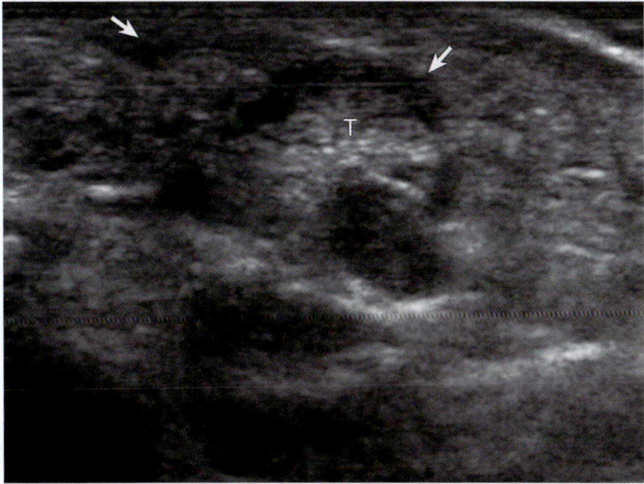

Figure 9.13. Palmar fibromatosis. Ultrasound images long axis (**A**) and short axis (**B**) to flexor tendon (*T*) of hand show a hypoechoic superficial mass-like area (*arrows*) with increased through-transmission (*arrowheads*).

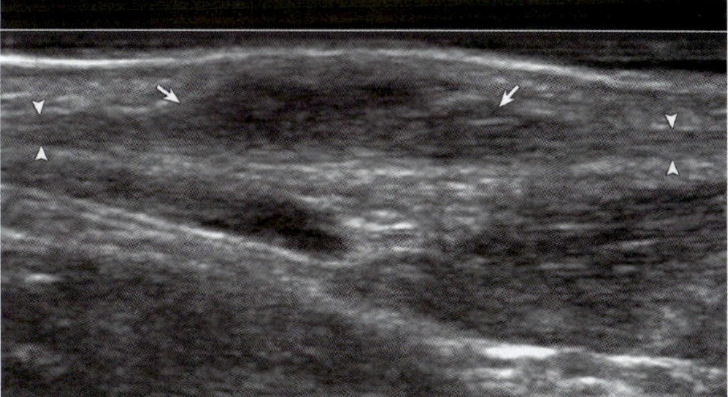

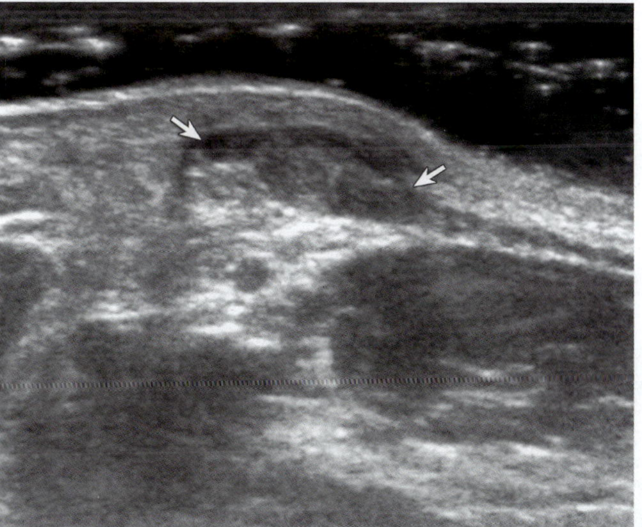

Figure 9.14. Plantar fibromatosis. Ultrasound images long axis (**A**) and short axis (**B**) to plantar aponeurosis (*arrowheads*) of foot show hypoechoic mass-like area (*arrows*).

and is bilateral in 20% to 50% of cases.[30] The presence of multiple plantar aponeurosis nodules, unilateral or bilateral, is diagnostic of plantar fibromatosis.

> **Tip:**
> - Multiple nodules on the plantar fascia are diagnostic of plantar fibromatosis.

Deep Fibromatoses

Deep fibromatoses or desmoid tumors (also termed aggressive fibromatosis) are benign fibrous proliferations at musculoaponeurotic sites, most common in adults between the ages of 25 and 35,[33] and multiple in 15% of cases.[30] Common locations include the shoulder, chest wall, back, thigh, and knee.[30] Similar to superficial fibromatoses, desmoid tumors do not metastasize but may be locally aggressive. Desmoid tumors can be intra-abdominal, within the abdominal wall, or extra-abdominal.[34] They are typically hypoechoic with possible

acoustic shadowing, and flow on color and power Doppler imaging (**Fig. 9.16**).[31] Extra-abdominal desmoids are characterized by an aggressive and infiltrative pattern. A characteristic ultrasound feature is an ill-defined border where it extends through fascial planes, creating a "fascial tail."[33] Patients who have desmoids are at risk of having familial adenomatous polyposis (FAP) and should be screened for FAP.

Nodular Fasciitis

Nodular fasciitis is a benign proliferation of fibroblasts and myofibroblasts, most common between the ages of 20 and 40 years.[30] Two notable features include its propensity to involve the volar aspect of the forearm, and its rapid growth,[30] which often leads to a mistaken diagnosis of soft tissue sarcoma. Ultrasound shows a well-defined soft tissue mass that may be isoechoic to the surrounding tissues or heterogeneous with mixed hypoechoic and isoechoic areas (**Fig. 9.17**).[35] Increased through-transmission has also been described, similar to other soft tissue masses.[35]

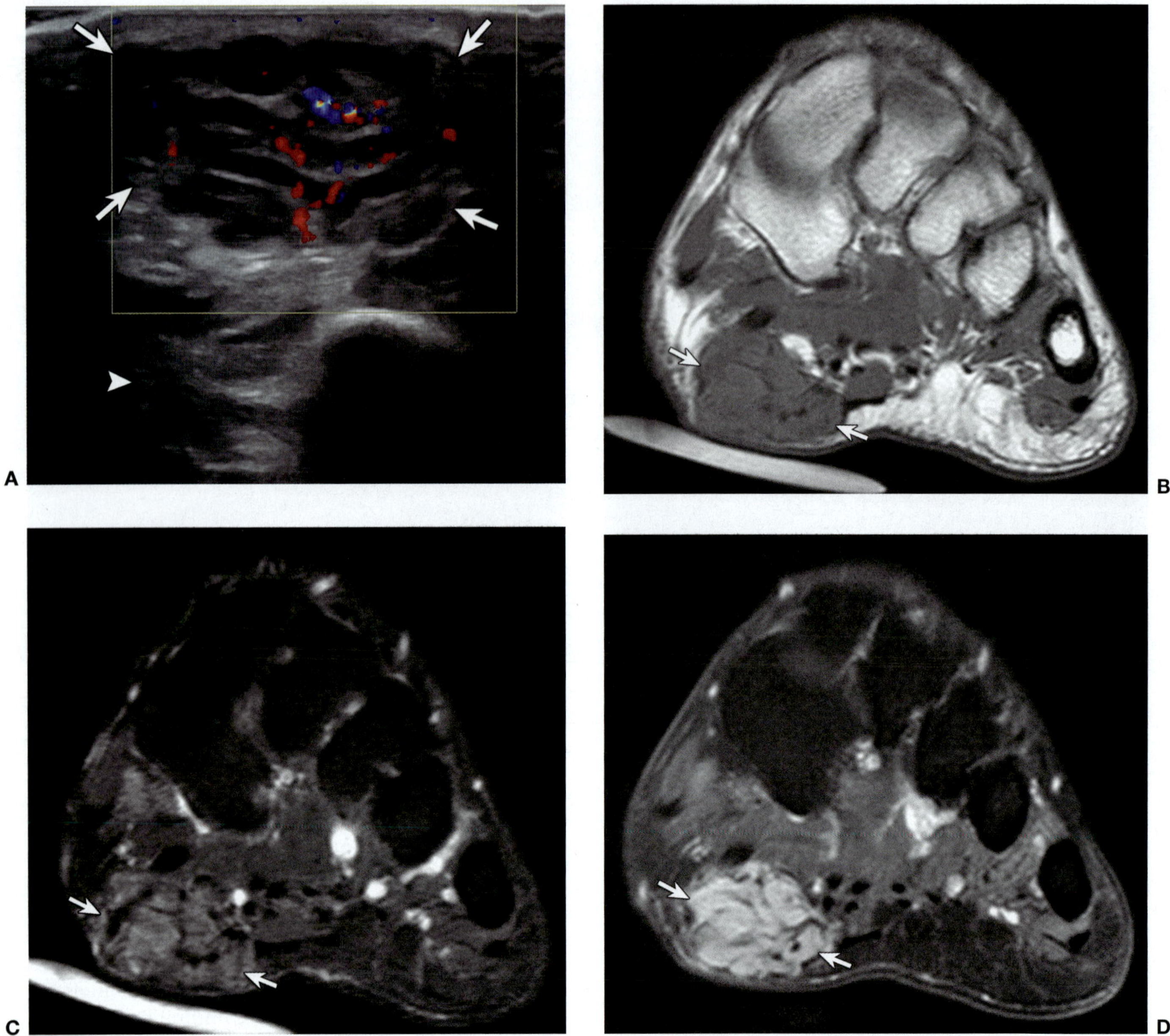

Figure 9.15.   Plantar fibromatosis. Ultrasound color Doppler image **(A)** shows hypoechoic mass (*arrows*) with serpiginous channels, hyperemia, and increased through-transmission (*arrowhead*) (pathologically proven). Axial T1-weighted **(B),** fluid-sensitive **(C),** and T1-weighted fat-saturation post-intravenous gadolinium enhanced **(D)** MR images show an intermediate signal and enhancing heterogeneous mass (*arrows*).

Tip:
- A rapidly growing mass in the volar forearm suggests nodular fasciitis.

Elastofibroma Dorsi

Elastofibroma dorsi is a benign fibroelastic pseudotumor, believed to result from friction between the scapula and chest wall,[36] that almost exclusively occurs at the inferior margin of the scapula, deep to the serratus anterior, rhomboid major and latissimus dorsi muscles. It is usually seen in elderly women, often asymptomatic and bilateral in up to 66% of patients.[36] Elastofibroma contains alternating fatty and fibrous tissue layers, which produce a characteristic heterogeneous and striated appearance with numerous linear and curvilinear hypoechoic fat and hyperechoic fibrous tissue interfaces **(Fig. 9.18).**[36] Dynamic imaging is helpful as the mass may be obscured by the scapula in neutral position.[37] Placing the ipsilateral hand on the opposite shoulder may throw the scapula off the mass.

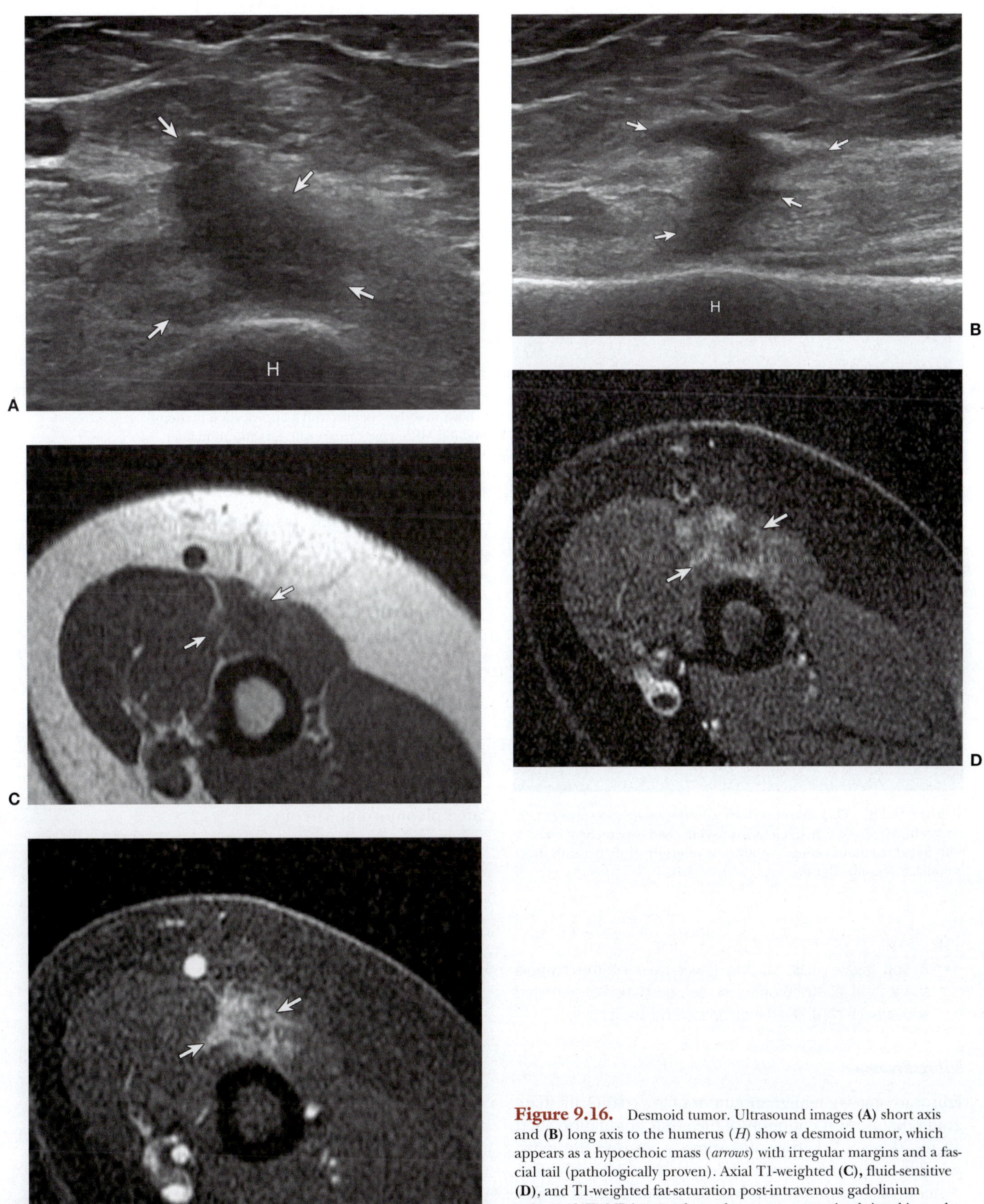

Figure 9.16. Desmoid tumor. Ultrasound images **(A)** short axis and **(B)** long axis to the humerus (*H*) show a desmoid tumor, which appears as a hypoechoic mass (*arrows*) with irregular margins and a fascial tail (pathologically proven). Axial T1-weighted **(C),** fluid-sensitive **(D),** and T1-weighted fat-saturation post-intravenous gadolinium enhanced **(E)** MR images show a heterogeneous mixed signal irregular mass (*arrows*) with moderate enhancement.

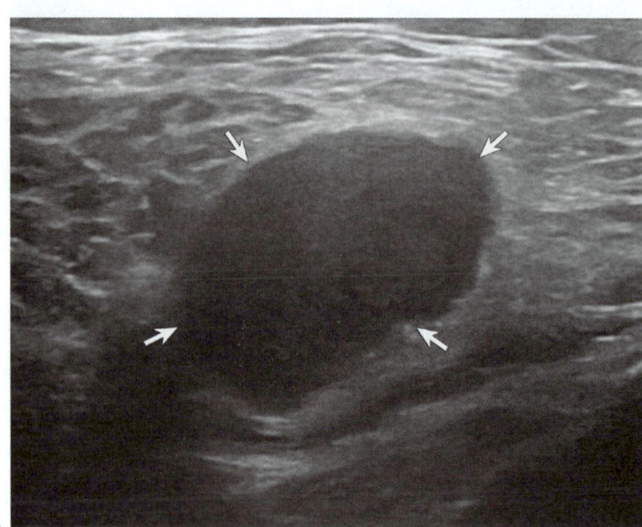

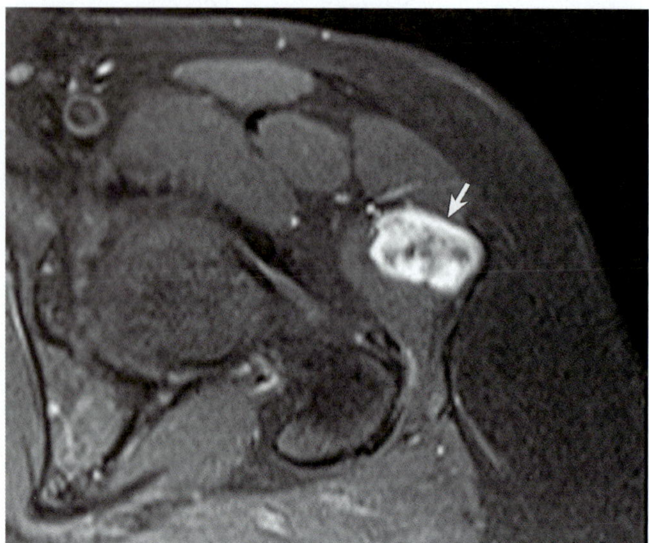

Figure 9.17.   Nodular fasciitis. Ultrasound image **(A)** shows nodular fasciitis, which appears as a predominantly hypoechoic mass (*arrows*), also shown on **(B)** T1-weighted MR image (*arrow*) with fat-saturation after intravenous gadolinium administration (pathologically proven).

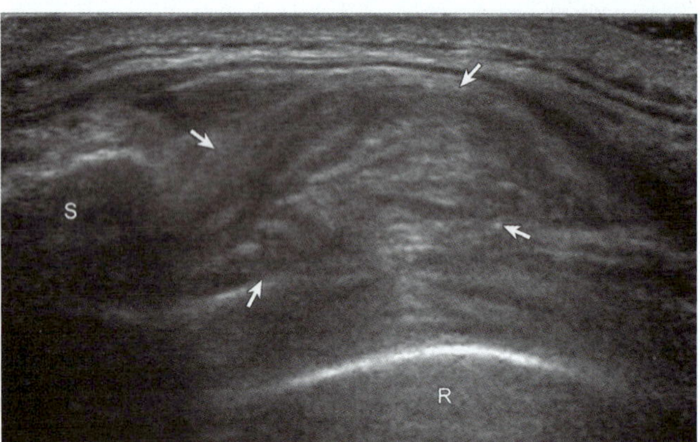

Figure 9.18.   Elastofibroma dorsi. Ultrasound images show a well-defined, mixed echogenicity hypoechoic and hyperechoic mass with linear striations (*arrows*) protruding inferiorly from beneath the scapula. S, scapula; R, rib.

Tip:
- A soft tissue mass at the lower pole of the scapula suggests an elastofibroma, and demonstration of a striated appearance confirms the diagnosis and avoids biopsy.

Fibrosarcoma

Fibrosarcoma is a malignant tumor of low-to-intermediate grade that is most common in the adult population aged 40 to 70 years.[38] Ultrasound shows a nonspecific mass, possibly heterogeneous with calcifications.[1] Myxofibrosarcoma most commonly involves the subcutaneous tissues of the extremities and has a propensity to spread along fascial and vascular planes; recurrent tumor is associated with higher grade and distant metastases **(Fig. 9.19)**.[39]

Malignant fibrous histiocytoma or undifferentiated pleomorphic sarcoma is the most common soft tissue sarcoma. It has a peak incidence in the fifth decade of life, is more common in men, and is the most common radiation-induced soft tissue sarcoma.[38] Most (70%) are intramuscular, usually in the extremities, but 5% to 10% are subcutaneous.[38] Ultrasound demonstrates a nonspecific heterogeneous soft tissue mass with mixed hypoechoic and echogenic regions and increased vascularity **(Fig. 9.20)**.[1] Anechoic regions are due to tumor necrosis. In 2002, the WHO reorganized the classification of soft tissue sarcomas, and the term malignant fibrous histiocytoma has been replaced by undifferentiated pleomorphic sarcoma.[38]

Dermatofibrosarcoma Protuberans

Dermatofibrosarcoma protuberans (DFSP) is one of the more common malignant soft tissue tumors and accounts for 6% of soft tissue sarcomas.[38] It frequently involves males in the third to fifth decades of life and presents as a growing palpable soft tissue nodule.[38] A phase of rapid tumor growth has been described after a quiescent phase of months to years.[40] Because DFSP is dermal and clinically apparent, it is frequently not imaged prior to biopsy or attempted removal. Ultrasound shows a superficial hypoechoic or mixed echogenicity dermal mass with variable flow on color and power Doppler imaging **(Fig. 9.21)**.[27,40] A hyperechoic appearance may be seen due to interfaces between fibrous tissue and tumor cells **(Fig. 9.22)**,[27] and this appearance is associated with irregular margins due to tumor infiltration, unlike other superficial hyperechoic masses such as lipoma, which are well defined.

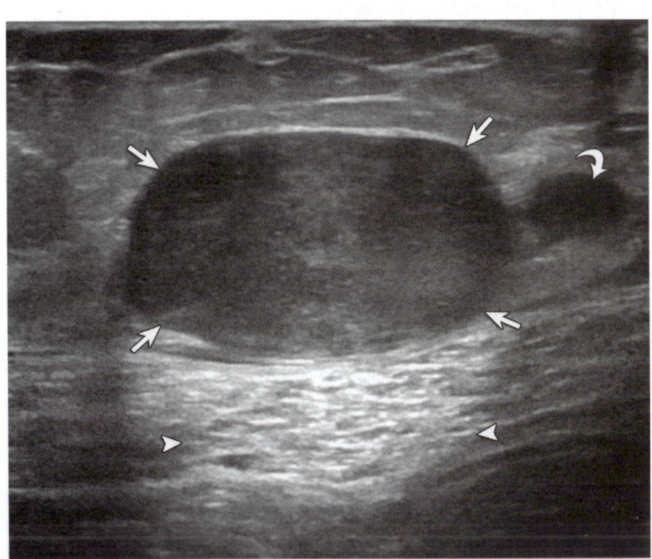
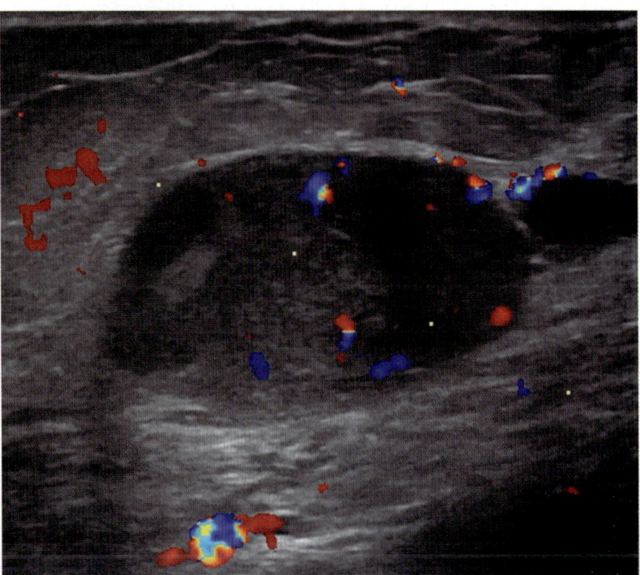

Figure 9.19. Myxofibrosarcoma. Gray scale **(A)** and color Doppler **(B)** ultrasound images show a well-defined hypoechoic mass (*arrows*) with increased through-transmission (*arrowheads*) (pathologically proven). Note adjacent tumor spread (*curved arrow*).

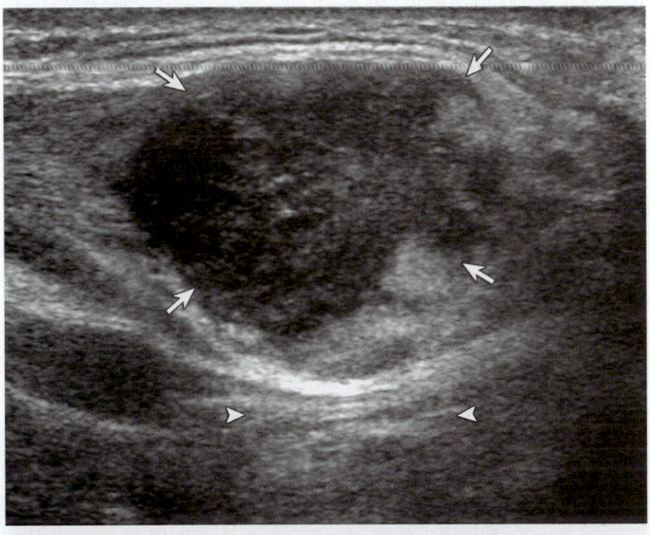

Figure 9.20. Malignant fibrous histiocytoma (undifferentiated pleomorphic sarcoma). Ultrasound image shows a heterogeneous but predominantly hypoechoic mass (*arrows*) with increased through-transmission (*arrowheads*) (pathologically proven).

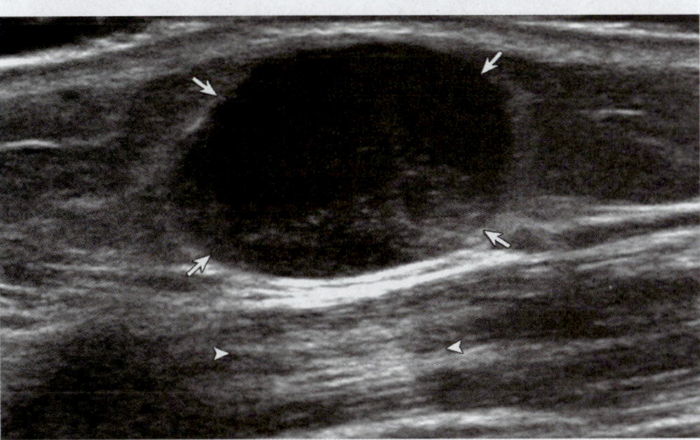
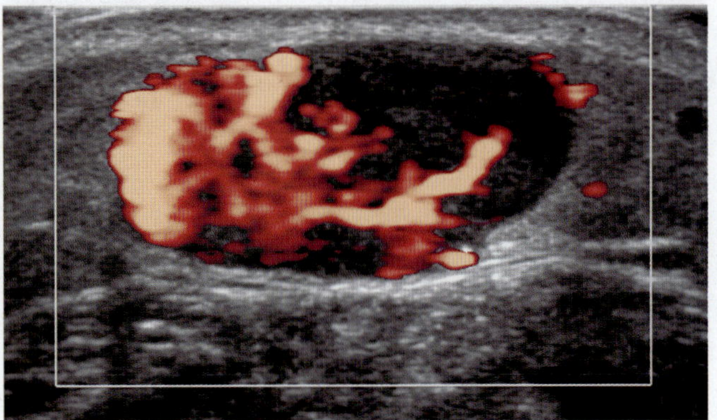

Figure 9.21. Dermatofibrosarcoma protuberans. Gray scale **(A)** and power Doppler **(B)** ultrasound images show a well-defined hypoechoic mass (*arrows*) with hyperemia and increased through-transmission (*arrowheads*) (pathologically proven).

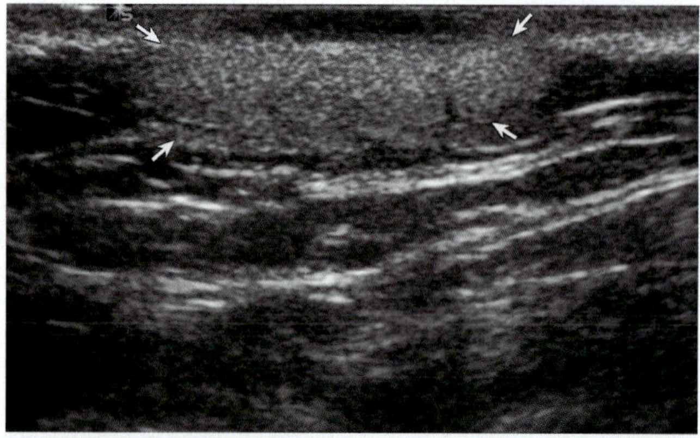

Figure 9.22.   Dermatofibrosarcoma protuberans. Ultrasound image shows a hyperechoic mass (*arrows*) (pathologically proven).

Smooth Muscle Tumors

Tumors that have a predominant smooth muscle differentiation include benign leiomyomas and malignant leiomyosarcomas. Although leiomyomas are uncommon outside the uterus and gastrointestinal tract, they may be found in the extremities and take one of three forms: cutaneous leiomyoma (most common, located in the dermis), angioleiomyoma (located in the subcutaneous tissues), and leiomyoma of deep tissues.[41] Extra-uterine leiomyosarcoma represents the malignant form, and can be divided into four subtypes: cutaneous, subcutaneous, deep soft tissue, and vascular.[42] At ultrasound, a leiomyoma appears as a nonspecific hypoechoic or slightly heterogeneous mass (**Fig. 9.23**), whereas a leiomyosarcoma

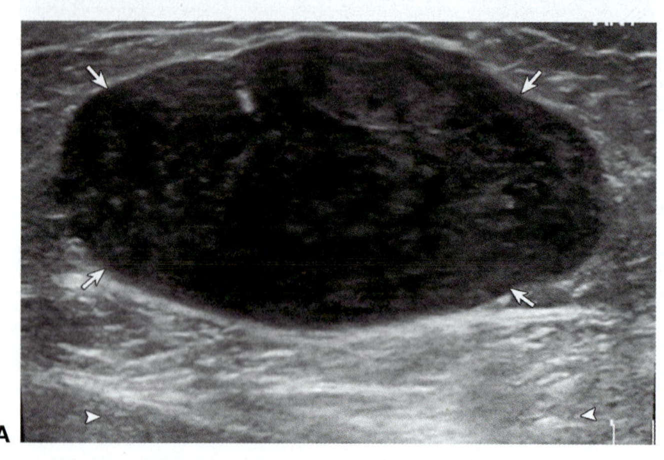

A

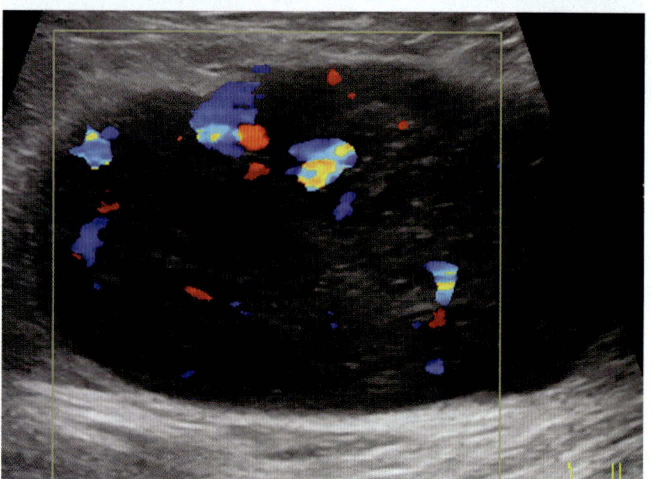

B

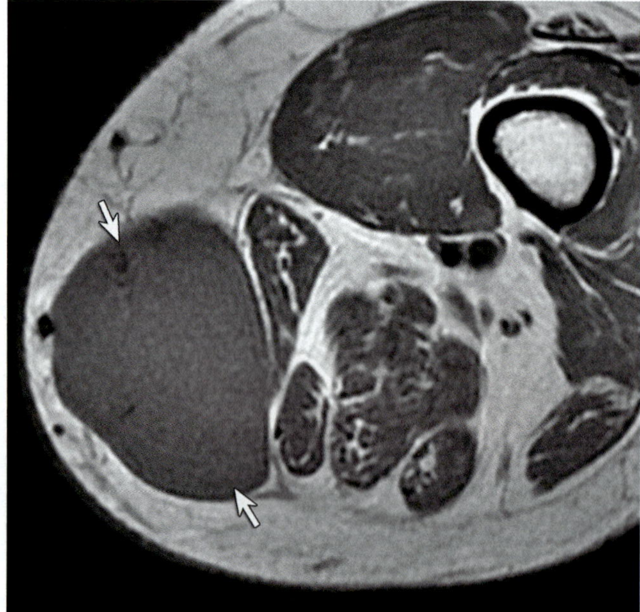

C

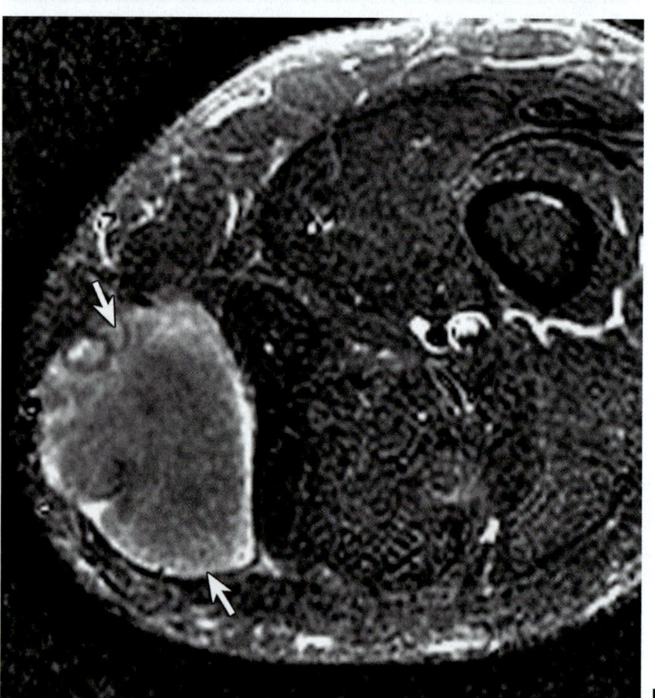

D

Figure 9.23.   Leiomyoma. Gray scale (**A**) and color Doppler (**B**) ultrasound images show a mildly heterogeneous but predominantly hypoechoic mass (*arrows*) with hyperemia and increased through-transmission (*arrowheads*). Axial T1-weighted (**C**), fluid-sensitive (**D**), and T1-weighted fat-saturation post-intravenous gadolinium enhanced (**E**) MR images show a heterogeneous mass (*arrows*) with marked enhancement (pathologically proven).

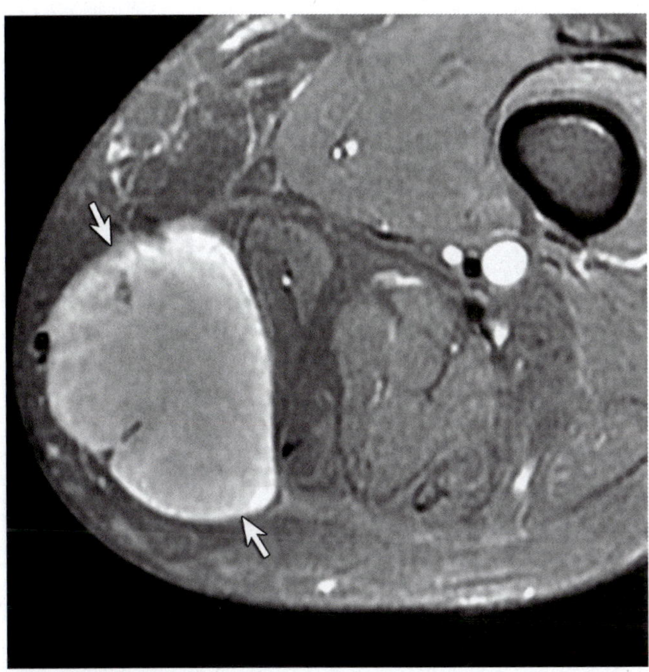

E

Figure 9.23. (*Continued*)

will more likely show heterogeneity **(Fig. 9.24)**, increased vascularity, and possible necrosis.

Lymphoid Tumors

Lymphoma

Lymphoid neoplasms may be categorized as Hodgkin, non-Hodgkin, and plasma cell neoplasms, of which 80% to 85% originate from B cells.[43] The typical presentation is of localized or generalized lymph node enlargement.[44] Extra-nodal involvement, especially involving the soft tissues of the extremities, is rare.[44]

Lymph node involvement in lymphoma has an appearance that it is consistent with malignant infiltration but is otherwise nonspecific, including enlargement, a round rather than oval shape, thickening of the node cortex, and narrowing or obliteration of the echogenic hilum. Malignant nodes often have a peripheral or mixed rather than hilar vascular pattern on color and power Doppler imaging **(Fig. 9.25)**[45] but a hilar pattern is commonly seen in lymphoma and may also be seen with reactive lymph nodes.[46] Although lymph node measurements may be used as guidelines for tumor involvement, it is more critical to assess the morphology of a lymph node than rely on measurements.[47]

Extra-nodal lymphoma of soft tissues most commonly appears as a hypoechoic mass with infiltrative margins and significantly increased vascularity on color and power Doppler imaging.[44] In spite of often large size, necrosis is typically absent.[44] Another characteristic feature is its ability to extend through the soft tissues while preserving the surrounding soft tissues.[43] The characteristic sonographic features of extreme hypervascularity, lack of necrosis, and

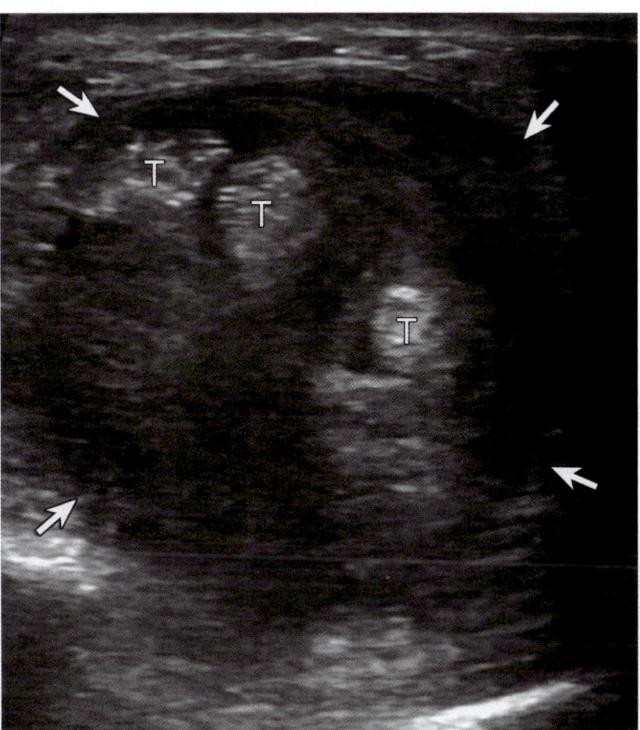

A

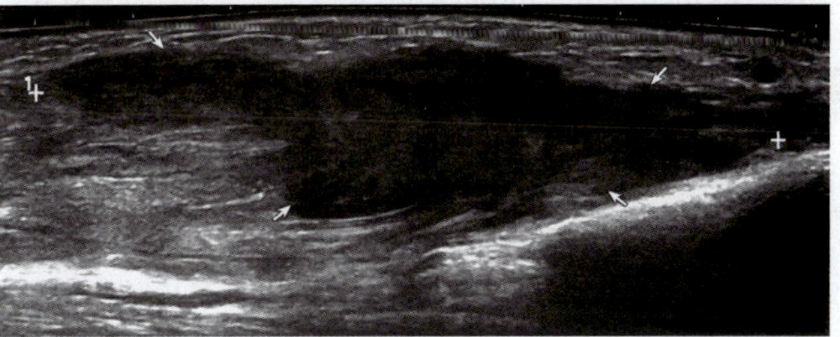

B

Figure 9.24. Leiomyosarcoma. Ultrasound images **(A)** short axis and **(B)** long axis to extensor tendons of forearm (*T*) show hypoechoic mass (*arrows in A and between cursors and arrows* in B) with increased through transmission (pathologically proven).

infiltrative pattern may suggest the diagnosis. Another presentation is of heterogeneous muscle infiltration with preservation of the muscle architecture and plump muscle bundles **(Fig. 9.26)**.[44] Osseous invasion produces discontinuity or destruction of the normally smooth and echogenic bone cortex. Peripheral nerve involvement has also been described.[48] Lymphoma rarely appears as an ill-defined hyperechoic subcutaneous soft tissue mass as seen with subcutaneous T-cell lymphoma.[49]

Tip:
- A hypervascular soft tissue mass with preserved architecture suggests lymphoma.

Neural Tumors

Peripheral Nerve Sheath Tumors

Schwannoma (or neurilemmoma) and neurofibroma represent two forms of benign peripheral nerve sheath

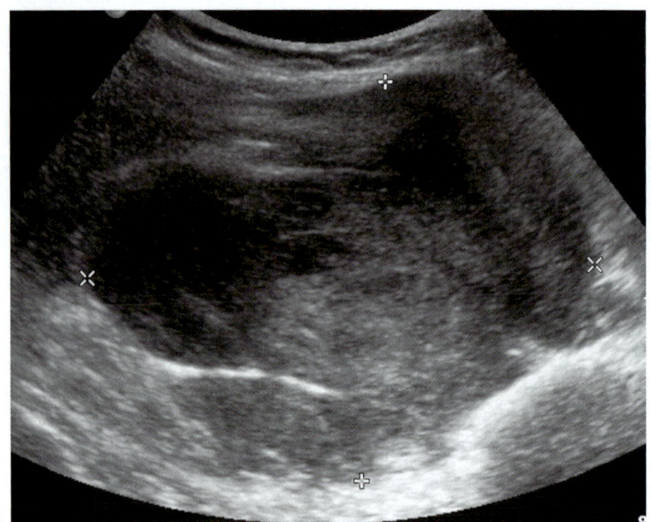
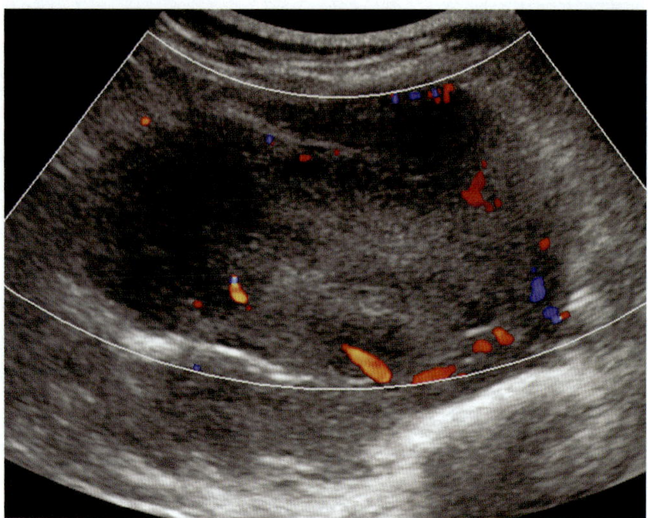

Figure 9.25. Lymphoma: node. Gray scale **(A)** and color Doppler **(B)** ultrasound images show a heterogeneous but predominantly hypoechoic enlarged round-shaped lymph node (*cursors*) with increased through-transmission and irregular blood flow (pathologically proven).

tumors, and commonly present between the ages of 20 and 30 years.[50] Schwannoma tends to be solitary, but can be multiple (termed schwannomatosis) and can be associated with neurofibromatosis type I.[50] The characteristic histologic features of a schwannoma are the presence of Antoni A and B regions.[50] Neurofibromas have three different forms: localized, plexiform, and diffuse.[50] Localized neurofibromas are usually <5 cm in size and painless. Plexiform neurofibromas appear as multiple swellings diffusely involving a nerve trunk or as diffuse enlargement of a nerve. Diffuse neurofibromas cause thickening of the subcutaneous and dermal tissues and envelop tendons, nerves, and vessels. Although

all forms of neurofibromas can be associated with neurofibromatosis I, plexiform neurofibromas are considered pathognomonic.[50] Other hallmarks of neurofibromatosis I include cutaneous neurofibromas (frequently multiple), skin lesions (café au lait spots), skeletal deformities, and mental deficiency.[50] Histologically, in contrast to schwannoma, Antoni A and B regions are not identified. Neurofibromatosis II primarily affects the central nervous system.

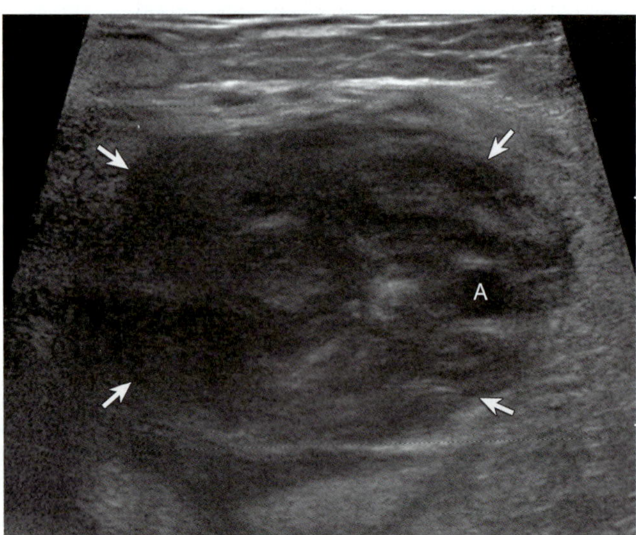
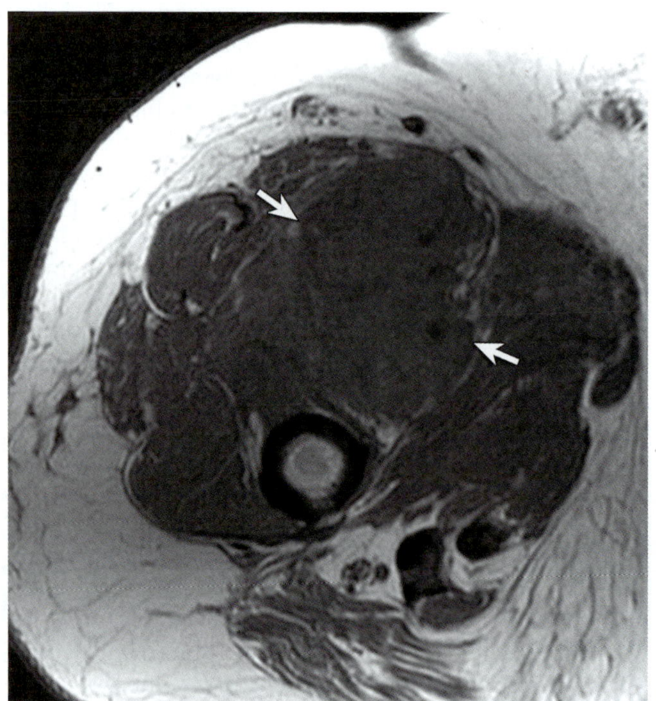

Figure 9.26. Lymphoma: muscle. Ultrasound image **(A)** shows heterogeneous but predominantly hypoechoic infiltrating mass (*arrows*). A, femoral artery. Axial T1-weighted **(B)**, fluid-sensitive **(C)**, and T1-weighted fat-saturation post-intravenous gadolinium enhanced **(D)** MR images show an enhancing heterogeneous mass (*arrows*) (pathologically proven).

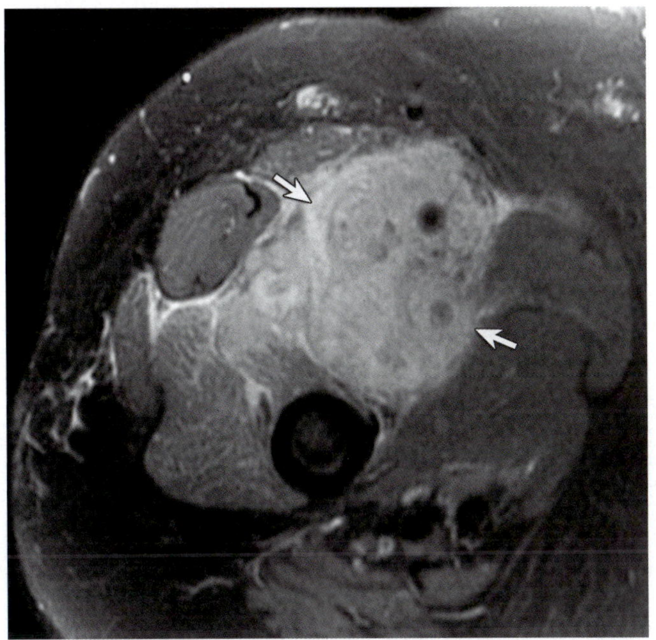

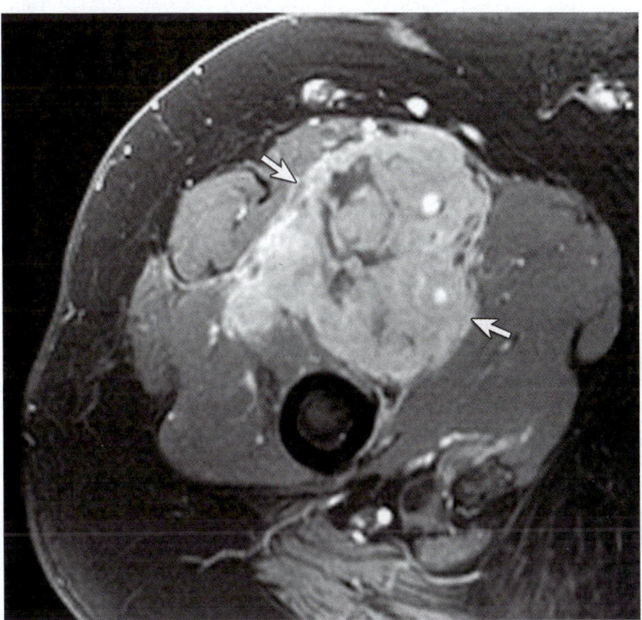

C   D

Figure 9.26. *(Continued)*

At ultrasound, solitary schwannoma **(Fig. 9.27)** and neurofibroma **(Fig. 9.28)** look similar, appearing as well-defined hypoechoic fusiform masses with internal low-level and homogeneous echoes.[51,52] The finding of a peripheral nerve entering and exiting the mass is key to the diagnosis. Often hyperechoic fat is identified around the entering/exiting nerve producing an echogenic, triangular "cap" at the edge of the mass, termed the "split-fat sign."

> **Tip:**
> - The split-fat sign and a nerve entering/exiting a soft tissue mass are characteristic of a nerve tumor.

If the entering or exiting nerve is eccentric to the mass, schwannoma may be suggested, whereas in neurofibroma the nerve tends to be central,[52] but these findings are not invariable.

> **Tip:**
> - Ultrasound cannot reliably distinguish between schwannoma and neurofibroma.

Increased through-transmission deep to a nerve sheath tumor is common[51] and should not lead to a mistaken diagnosis of a complex cyst. Blood flow within neural tumors is typical and is absent in complex cysts. Schwannomas may be heterogeneous due to cyst formation **(Fig. 9.29)**,[52] the so-called "ancient schwannomas." A target appearance has been described due to an echogenic

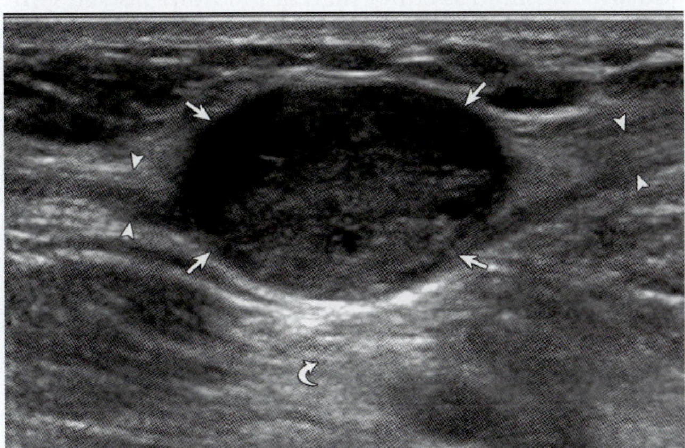

A

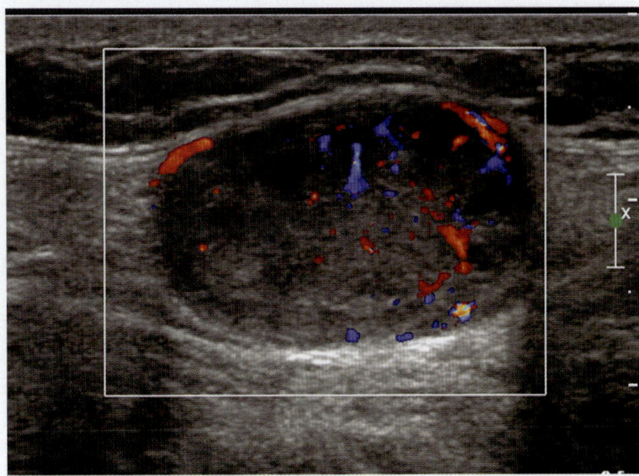

B

Figure 9.27. Schwannoma. Gray scale **(A)** and color Doppler **(B)** ultrasound images show a well-defined mass (*arrows*) with homogeneous low-level echoes that is in continuity with the common peroneal nerve (*arrowheads*). Note hyperemia and increased through-transmission (*curved arrow*) (pathologically proven).

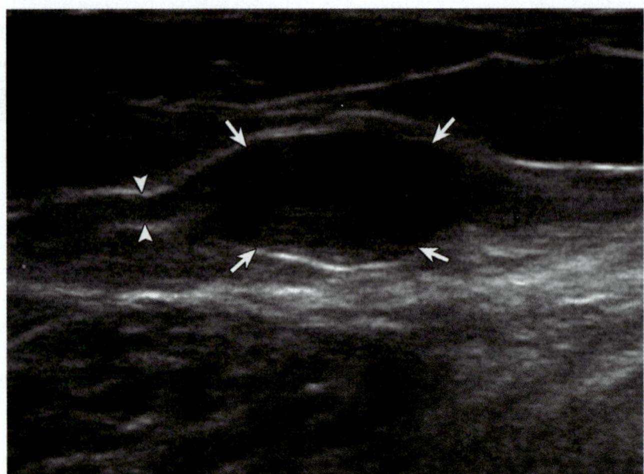

Figure 9.28. Neurofibroma. Ultrasound image shows a well-defined hypoechoic mass (*arrows*) that is in continuity with a peripheral nerve (*arrowheads*) (pathologically proven).

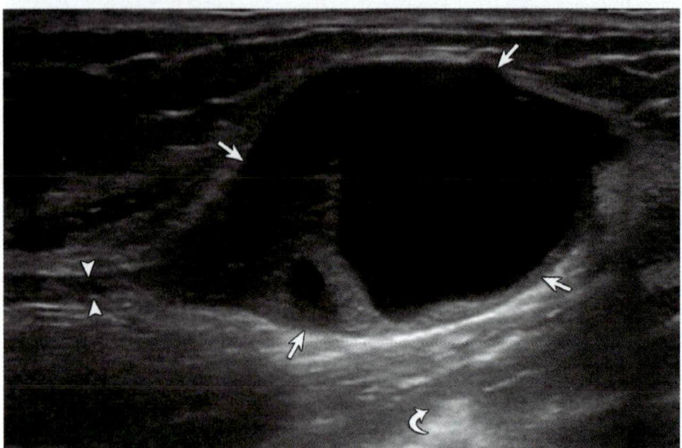

Figure 9.29. Schwannoma: cystic. Ultrasound image shows a well-defined hypoechoic mass (*arrows*), with anechoic cyst formation, that is in continuity with a peripheral nerve (*arrowheads*). Note increased through-transmission (*curved arrow*) (pathologically proven).

fibrocollagenous center and surrounding hypoechoic myxoid area, most notably with benign neurofibromas.[53] Plexiform neurofibromas appear as multiple lobular, predominantly hypoechoic masses with possible target appearances involving a large nerve trunk.[53] Diffuse neurofibroma appears as hyperechoic dermal and subcutaneous tissue thickening with intervening hypoechoic tubular or nodular areas.[54] As they are frequently extensive, plexiform and diffuse neurofibromas are best imaged by MRI.

Malignant peripheral nerve sheath tumors commonly involve large nerve trunks and are associated with neurofibromatosis I in 25% to 70% of cases or prior radiotherapy.[50] The ultrasound appearances are nonspecific. Continuity between the mass and a peripheral nerve may be demonstrated, but often the large size and heterogeneous echotexture of the mass make identification of the nerve difficult. The presence of intra-tumoral cysts or absence of a target sign in a large peripheral nerve sheath

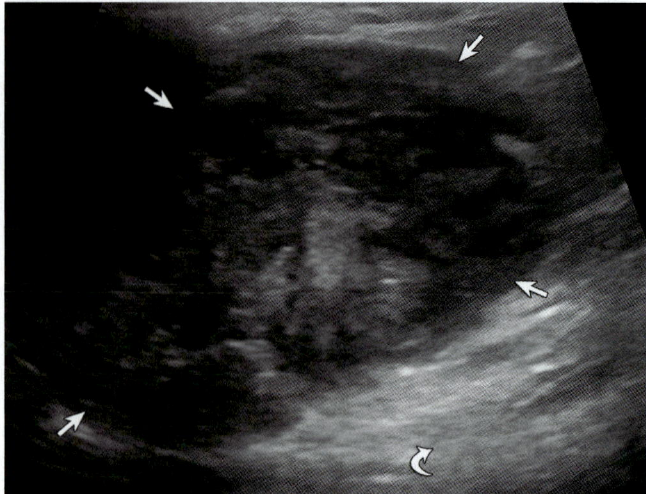

Figure 9.30. Malignant peripheral nerve sheath tumor. Ultrasound image shows a heterogeneous but predominantly hypoechoic mass (*arrows*) with increased through-transmission (*curved arrow*) (pathologically proven).

tumor should raise concern for malignancy **(Fig. 9.30)**. Rapid growth of a previously stable peripheral nerve sheath tumor or clinical findings of pain, motor weakness, or sensory deficits are also worrying.[50]

Vascular Tumors

Vascular Malformations

Categorization of endothelial malformations has been a controversial topic, primarily concerning the use of the term "hemangioma".[55] The classification system proposed in 1982 separates endothelial malformations into two categories: hemangioma and vascular malformation.[56] Hemangioma presents after birth and is characterized by involution. In contrast, vascular malformation is present at birth and grows with the patient. Vascular malformations may be subcategorized histologically as venous, capillary, arteriovenous, lymphatic, and mixed,[57] and also classified as either high or low flow, based on MR imaging or contrast studies.[58] At ultrasound, a high-flow vascular malformation can demonstrate arterial flow.

Vascular malformations typically demonstrate increased flow on color or power Doppler imaging. With a low-flow vascular malformation, the numerous vascular channels tend to be compressible, and flow may only be seen after compression is relieved and the vessels refill.

Tip:
- Vascular malformations may show no Doppler flow until compressed, and blood returns after the compression is released.

High-flow malformations show numerous vessels with prominent arterial flow. The hallmark of a typical

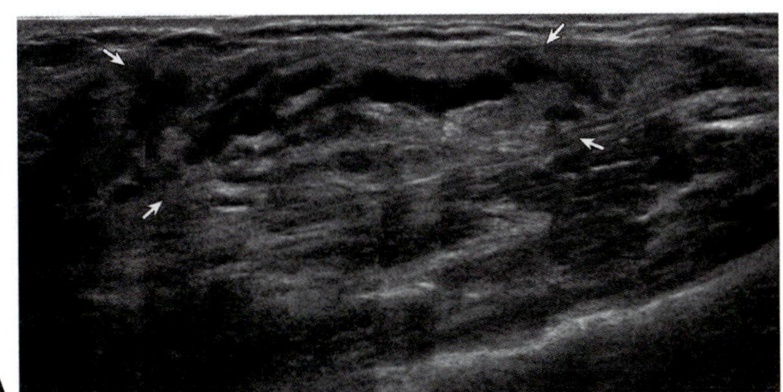

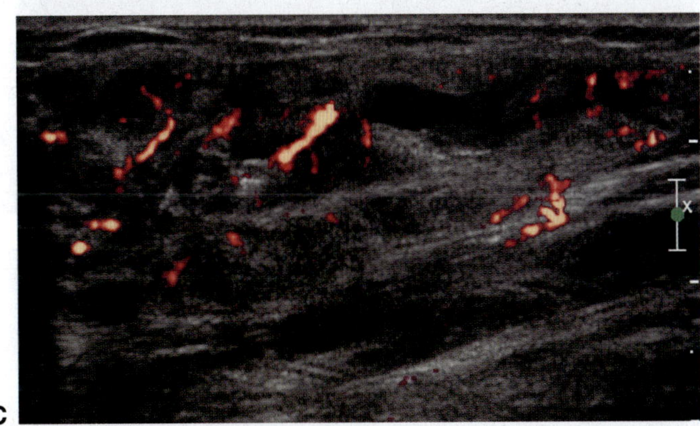

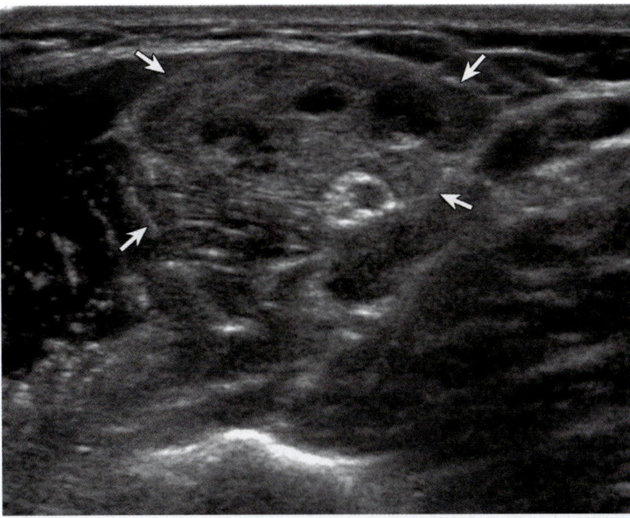

Figure 9.31. Vascular malformation: intramuscular. Ultrasound images (**A** and **B**) show an infiltrating heterogeneous mixed hypoechoic, isoechoic, and hyperechoic area with anechoic channels (*arrows*) and hyperemia on color Doppler imaging (**C**) within triceps brachii muscle (pathologically proven).

intramuscular vascular malformation (also described as an intramuscular hemangioma based on an anatomic approach)[55] is an abnormal heterogeneous area replacing normal muscle with vascular channels, hyperechoic fat (with muscle atrophy), and possible phleboliths (calcified thrombus) that cause shadowing **(Fig. 9.31)**.[59]

Tip:
- Vascular malformation should be suspected if echogenic phleboliths are identified in a soft tissue mass.

There may be no flow on color or power Doppler due to thrombosis or extreme low flow.[60] Although the ultrasound features of an intramuscular vascular malformation are suggestive, confirmation with MR imaging or possibly biopsy may be indicated, especially if clinical findings suggest a more aggressive process. MR imaging more accurately assesses the extent and character of the abnormality than ultrasound.

Angiosarcoma

Several vascular neoplasms usually cannot be distinguished from each other with imaging, including hemangioendothelioma, hemangiopericytoma, and angiosarcoma.[38] Hemangioendothelioma and hemangiopericytoma are of intermediate aggressiveness, although the latter has benign and malignant forms and angiosarcoma is an aggressive malignancy.[38] Angiosarcomas involve the skin in 33% of cases and can be secondary to chronic lymphedema or previous radiotherapy, especially for breast carcinoma.[38] They appear predominantly hypoechoic with increased flow on color and power Doppler imaging, similar to other malignant soft tissue masses **(Fig. 9.32)**. Heterogeneity can in part be due to hemorrhage. Vascular channels are often identified at the periphery of the tumor.[38]

Cartilage Tumors

Chondroma

Soft tissue chondroma is a rare benign cartilage-forming tumor that most commonly presents between the ages of 30 and 60 years[61] as a slow-growing discrete lobular mass, usually <2 cm in size. It most commonly involves the hands and feet[62] and is calcified in 33% to 70% of cases.[61] A characteristic but less frequent site is the infrapatellar fat pad at the knee.[63] There is no malignant potential, although local recurrence has been described. Ultrasound shows a well-defined hypoechoic soft tissue mass usually with echogenic foci and shadowing from mineralized chondroid matrix **(Fig. 9.33)**,[64] and this can be confirmed radiographically. The differential diagnosis includes other masses that may mineralize such as myositis ossificans, synovial sarcoma, extraskeletal chondrosarcoma, and extraskeletal osteosarcoma.

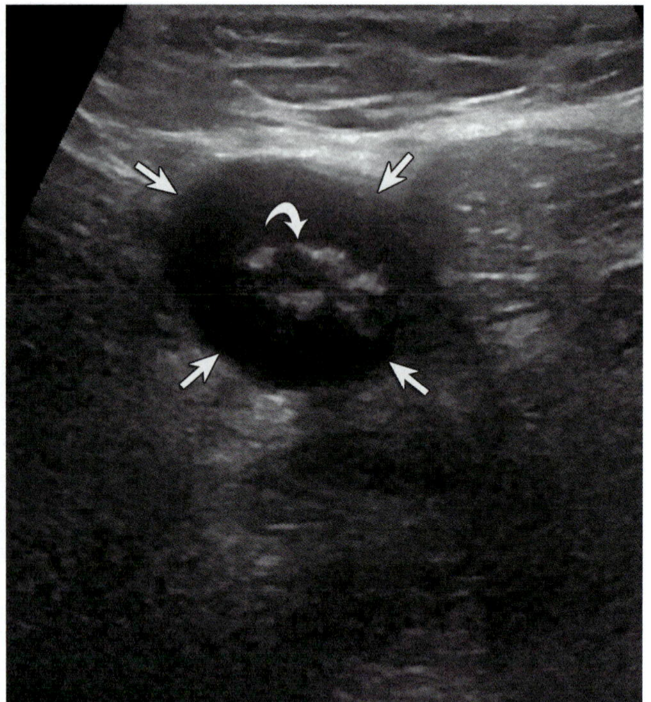

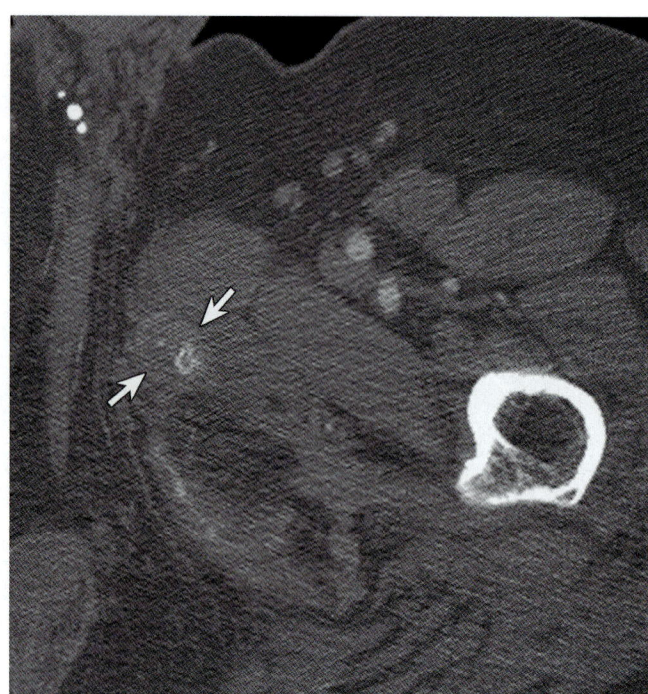

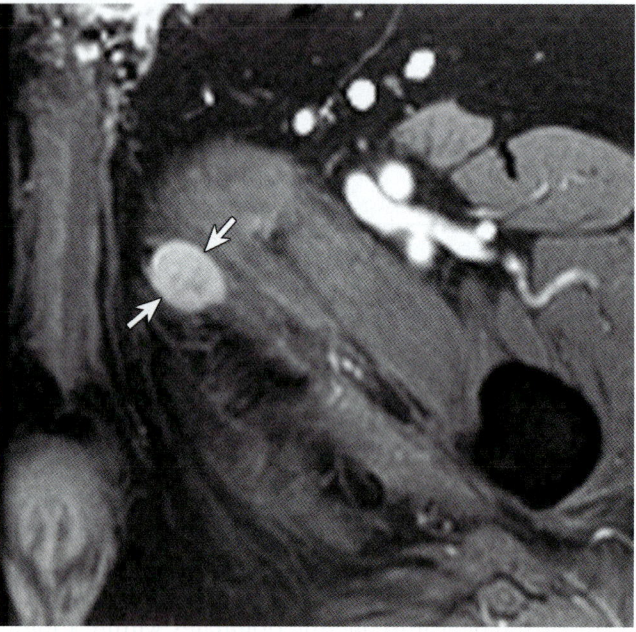

Figure 9.35. Extraskeletal osteosarcoma. Ultrasound image (**A**) shows a hypoechoic mass (*arrows*) with hyperechoic mineralization (*curved arrow* in **A**) and mild increased through-transmission, also shown (arrows) on axial non-contrast CT (**B**) and fluid-sensitive MR image (**C**) (pathologically proven).

margins have also been described.[65] Because synovial sarcoma may demonstrate increased through-transmission, the presence of a round hypoechoic mass with well-defined borders may simulate a complex cyst (**Fig. 9.37**). It is important to consider synovial sarcoma (or a myxomatous neoplasm) when a large unilocular cyst-like mass is identified. At the knee this can be differentiated from a Baker's cyst (which should show a neck between the semimembranosus tendon and the medial head of gastrocnemius),[66,67] more generally from a bursa (which should be located in the expected location of a bursa and often compressible), or a ganglion cyst (which is most commonly multilocular). If there is uncertainty, ultrasound-guided aspiration/biopsy should be considered.

Myeloid Sarcoma (Granulocytic Sarcoma or Chloroma)

Myeloid sarcoma, also called granulocytic sarcoma or chloroma, is a rare form of extra-medullary acute myeloid leukemia, which occurs in 3% to 5% of those with acute myeloid leukemia and presents during remission or relapse.[68] Myeloid sarcoma may also be considered a

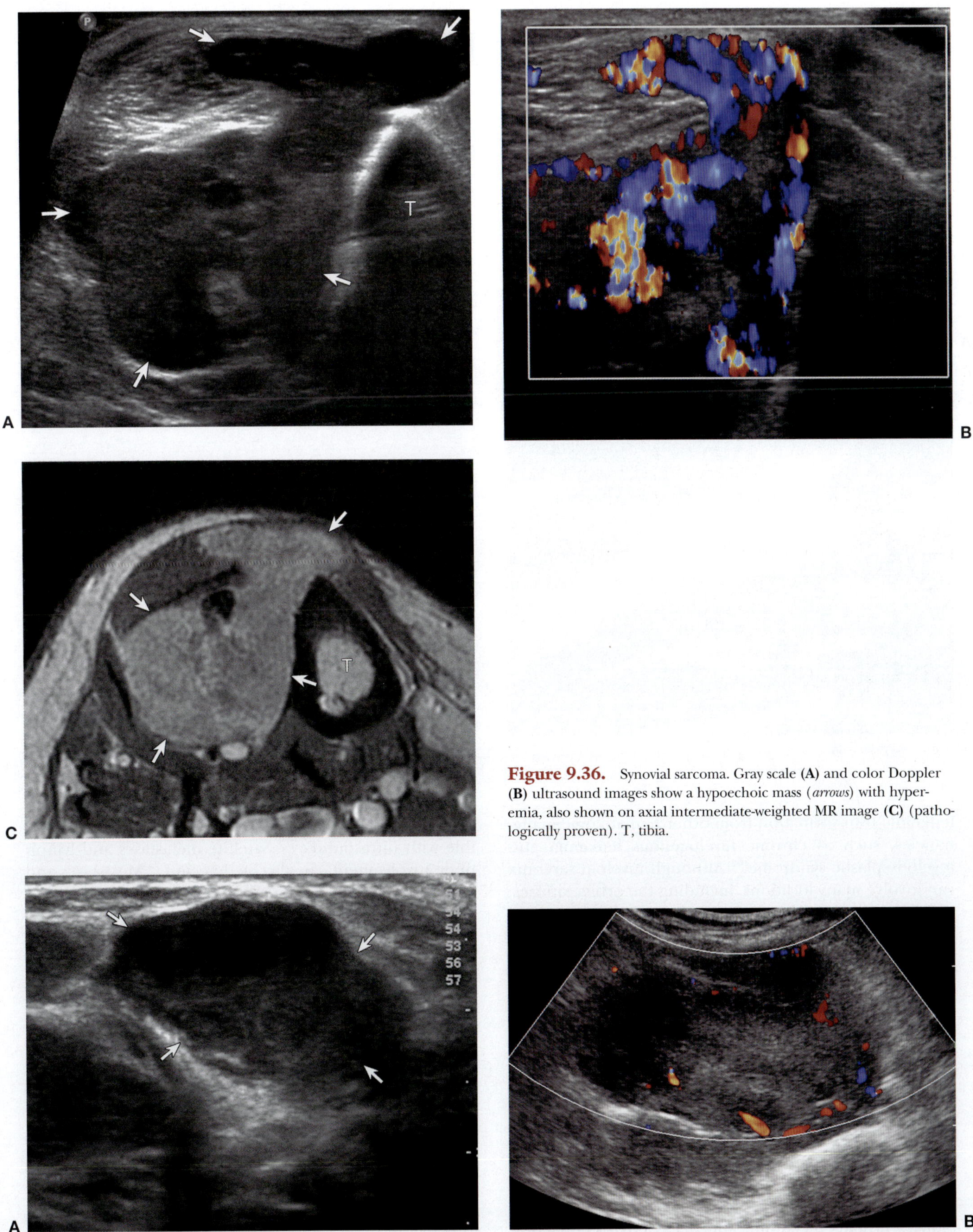

Figure 9.36. Synovial sarcoma. Gray scale **(A)** and color Doppler **(B)** ultrasound images show a hypoechoic mass (*arrows*) with hyperemia, also shown on axial intermediate-weighted MR image **(C)** (pathologically proven). T, tibia.

Figure 9.37. Synovial sarcoma. Gray scale **(A)** and color Doppler **(B)** ultrasound images show a hypoechoic mass (*arrows*) with hyperemia and increased through-transmission (pathologically proven).

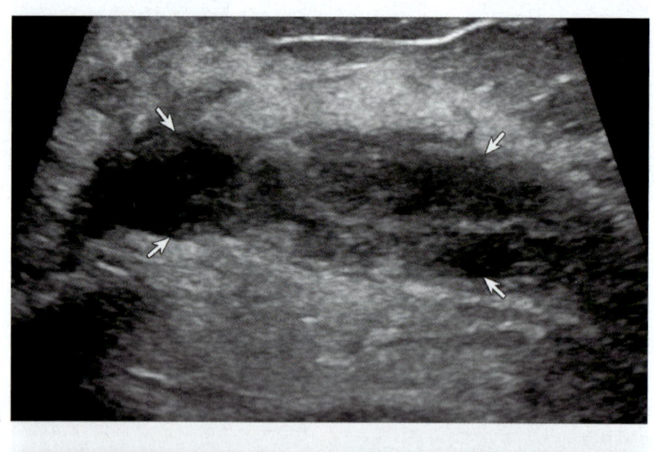

A

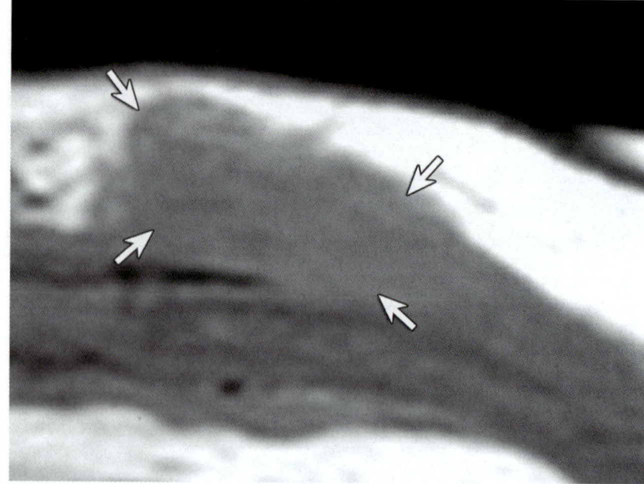

B

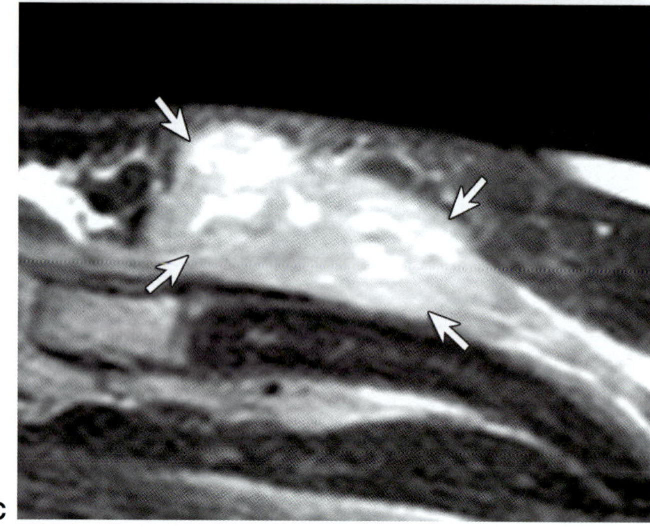

C

Figure 9.38. Myeloid sarcoma (granulocytic sarcoma or chloroma). Ultrasound image (**A**) shows heterogeneous but predominantly hypoechoic mass (*arrows*), also shown on the axial T1-weighted (**B**) and fluid-sensitive (**C**) MR images (pathologically proven).

leukemic transformation from other hematologic malignancies, such as chronic myelogenous leukemia and myelodysplastic syndrome.[68] Although myeloid sarcoma can involve many locations, including the orbits, sinuses, lymph nodes, and bone, 24% of cases have reported subcutaneous involvement (**Fig. 9.38**).[69] Little has been written about the ultrasound appearance of myeloid sarcoma, although a hyperechoic appearance (**Fig. 9.39**),[69] mixed echogenicity in a breast mass,[70] and necrotic lymph nodes[71] have been described.

Melanoma

Cutaneous malignant melanoma accounts for 4% to 11% of all skin cancers.[72] Ultrasound has been used to characterize primary melanoma and evaluate tumor spread or recurrence after treatment.[7,72,73] Ultrasound can detect non-palpable sites of melanoma and guide biopsy.[7] Primary melanoma appears as a hypoechoic oval or fusiform mass, which may have increased color flow

and invade the dermis, but small lesions may not be visible with ultrasound.[72,73] Satellite metastases and lymph node involvement can also be detected.[74] Metastases and recurrence appear hypoechoic (**Fig. 9.40**). Early lymph node involvement shows focal thickening of the node

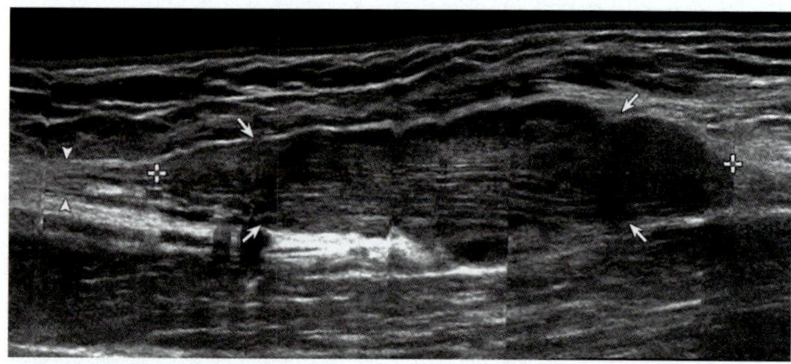

Figure 9.39. Myeloid sarcoma (granulocytic sarcoma or chloroma). Ultrasound image long axis to the median nerve (*arrowheads*) shows hypoechoic mass (*between cursors and arrows*), which infiltrates the median nerve (pathologically proven).

as MR in evaluating sarcoma recurrence **(Fig. 9.42)**.[6] It can show superficial soft tissue recurrence or metastasis in the absence of abnormality on physical examination.[75] Detection and subsequent ultrasound-guided biopsy of recurrence can have a significant effect on patient management.[7] Residual or recurrent tumor or metastasis commonly appears as a well-defined round or lobular hypoechoic mass **(Fig. 9.43)**.[5,76] Flow on color or power Doppler imaging is variable but usually present in superficial metastases.[5] Calcification or ossification may occur depending on the histology of the original tumor. A high-grade tumor may demonstrate

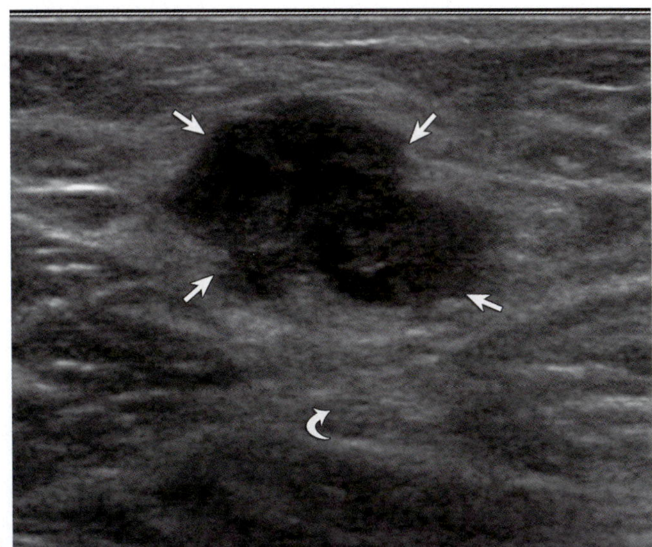

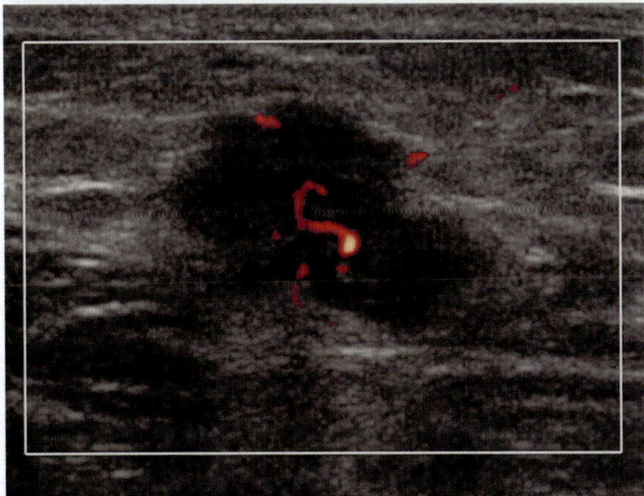

Figure 9.40. Melanoma: metastasis. Gray scale **(A)** and power Doppler **(B)** ultrasound images show a hypoechoic mass (*arrows*) with hyperemia and increased through-transmission (*curved arrow*) (pathologically proven).

cortex and possibly increased flow. Later, involved nodes show enlargement, focal or diffuse thickening of the cortex, narrowing of the echogenic hilum, and a mixed or peripheral vascular pattern.[45]

Plasma Cell Myeloma

Uncommonly, plasmacytoma **(Fig. 9.41)** and multiple myeloma may present as soft tissue masses that are nonspecific at ultrasound and appear hypoechoic with variable flow on color and power Doppler imaging. Bone destruction may also be seen.

Tumor Recurrence and Metastasis

Ultrasound is effective in evaluating residual or recurrent tumor or soft tissue metastasis and is as effective

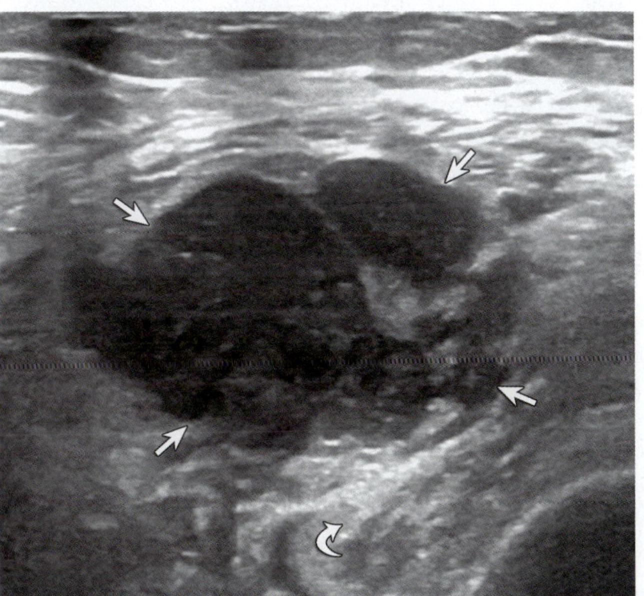

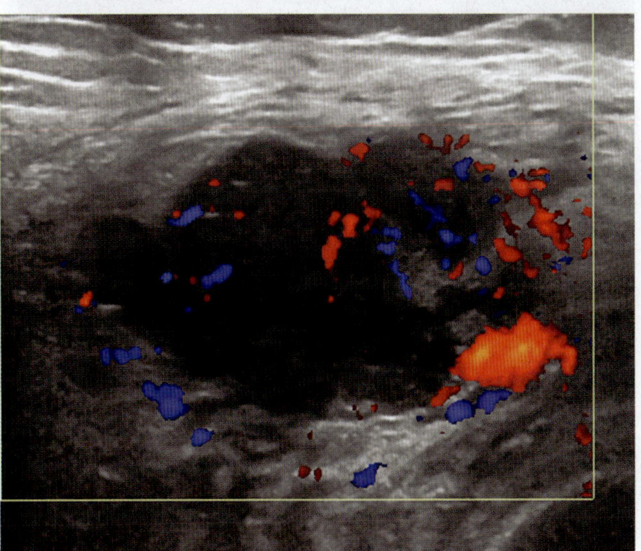

Figure 9.41. Plasmacytoma. Gray scale **(A)** and color Doppler **(B)** ultrasound images show a heterogeneous but predominantly hypoechoic mass (*arrows*) with increased through-transmission (*curved arrow*) and hyperemia, also shown on axial T1-weighted **(C)**, fluid-sensitive **(D)**, and T1-weighted fat-saturation post-intravenous gadolinium enhanced **(E)** MR images (pathologically proven).

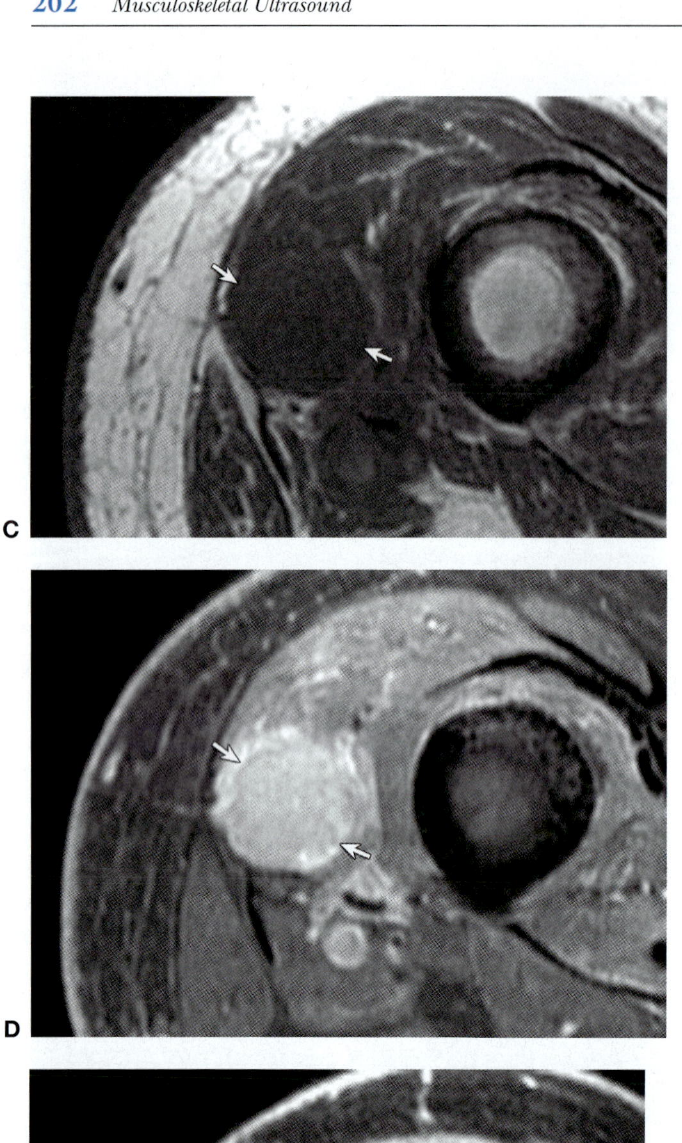

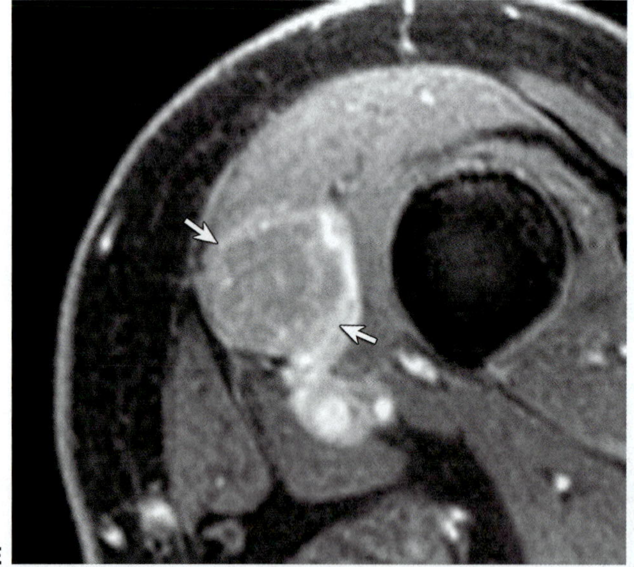

Figure 9.41.   (*Continued*)

heterogeneity and necrosis and be associated with hemorrhage **(Fig. 9.44)**. In contrast, a seroma appears as a well-defined, often lenticular, anechoic fluid collection that lacks internal blood flow on color or power Doppler imaging and is often compressible. Nonspecific

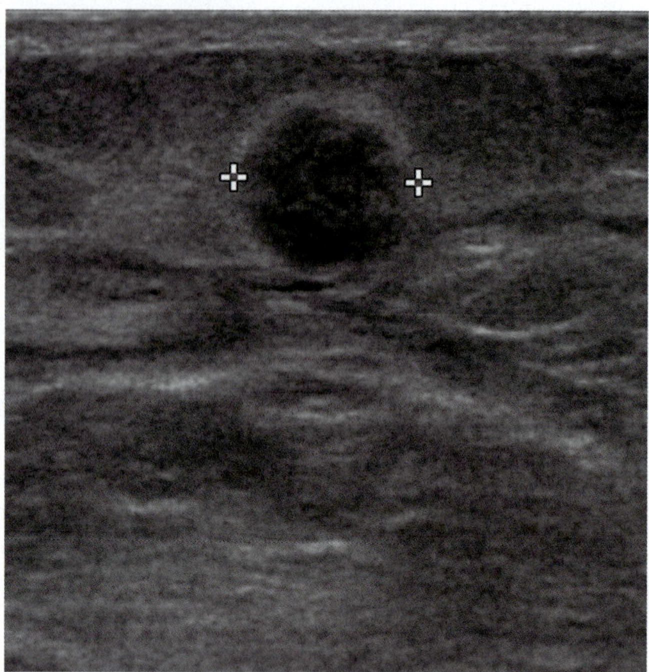

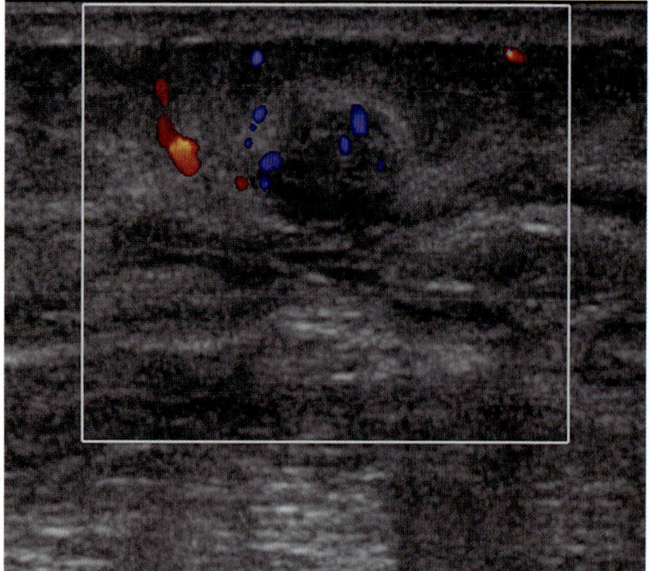

Figure 9.42.   Recurrence: high-grade myxofibrosarcoma. Gray scale **(A)** and color Doppler **(B)** ultrasound images show a hypoechoic mass (*between cursors*) with hyperemia and subtle increased through-transmission (pathologically proven).

postoperative or radiation changes may appear somewhat heterogeneous and perhaps hypoechoic, but are not typically well-defined or mass-like. If differentiation between posttreatment changes and tumor recurrence is difficult, follow-up ultrasound, evaluation with MR imaging including intravenous gadolinium contrast administration, or ultrasound-guided percutaneous biopsy should be considered. An increased incidence of metastases to skeletal muscle has been described at sites of prior trauma.[77]

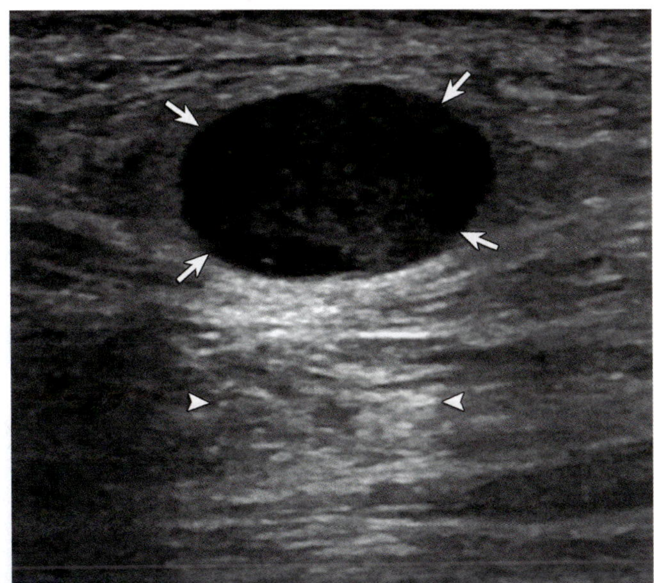

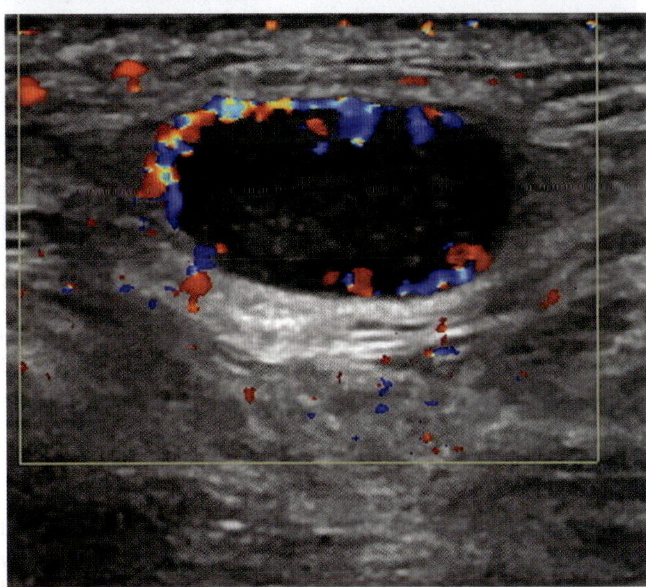

Figure 9.43. Metastasis: squamous cell carcinoma. Gray scale (**A**) and color Doppler (**B**) ultrasound images show a hypoechoic mass (*arrows*) with hyperemia and marked increased through-transmission (*arrowheads*) (pathologically proven).

Other Benign Tumors

Intramuscular Myxoma

Myxoma is a mesenchymal neoplasm composed of undifferentiated stellate cells in a myxoid stroma.[78] While the most common site of a myxoma is the heart, the most common extremity location is intramuscular (82%), especially the thigh (51%).[78] The average age at presentation is 64 (range 15 to 85 years).[79] The combination of intramuscular myxoma and polyostotic fibrous dysplasia (usually involving an adjacent bone) occurs in Mazabraud syndrome.[78]

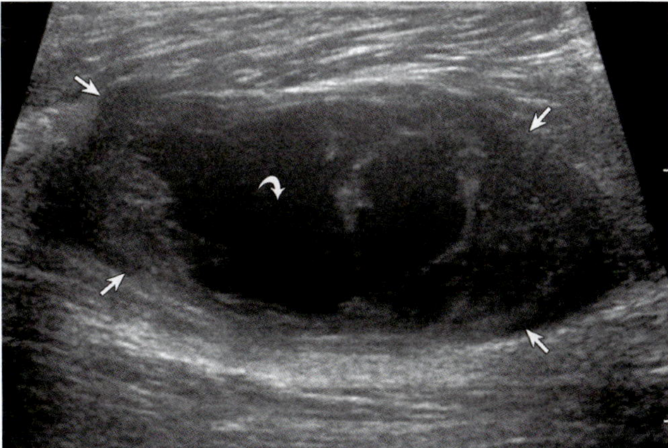

Figure 9.44. Metastasis with hemorrhage: urothelial carcinoma. Ultrasound image shows a heterogeneous but predominantly hypoechoic calf mass (*arrows*) with anechoic area of acute hemorrhage (*curved arrow*) and increased through-transmission (pathologically proven).

Intramuscular myxoma has a characteristic appearance at ultrasound. It is a well-defined, oval, or round intramuscular mass that is hypoechoic with uniform low-level internal echoes (**Fig. 9.45**)[78,80] and increased through-transmission. Hyperechoic areas surrounding the mass (called the bright rim and bright cap signs) may be seen, related to adjacent muscle atrophy and resulting fat deposition.[78–80] The differential diagnosis includes other myxoid tumors and complex ganglion cyst. Internal flow on color or power Doppler imaging, although not always present, indicates a solid mass rather than a complex cyst.[80,81] The differential diagnosis of a fusiform hypoechoic mass surrounded by a hyperechoic rim includes the split-fat sign of a peripheral nerve sheath tumor, which can be confirmed by finding the nerve entering and exiting the mass.[50]

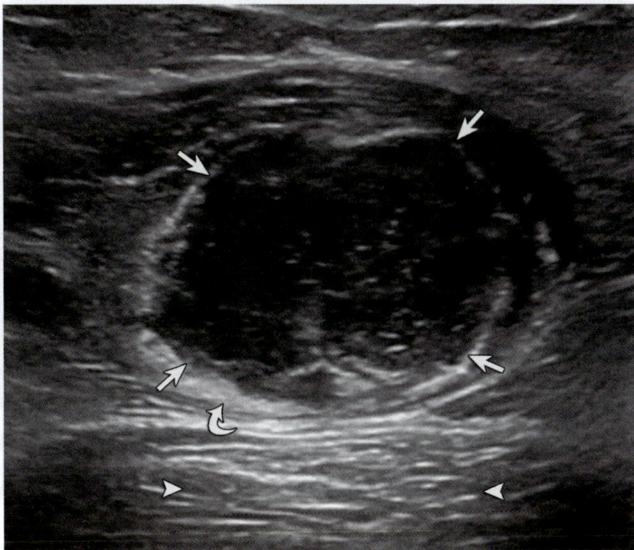

Figure 9.45. Intramuscular myxoma. Ultrasound image shows well-defined hypoechoic mass (*arrows*) with low-level internal echoes and increased through-transmission (*arrowheads*). Note bright rim sign (*curved arrow*) (pathologically proven).

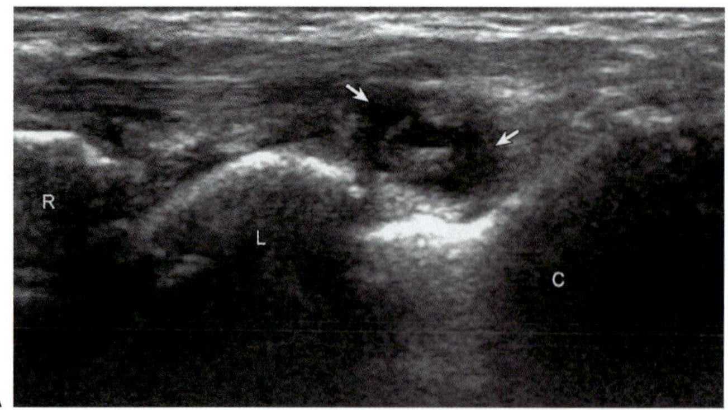

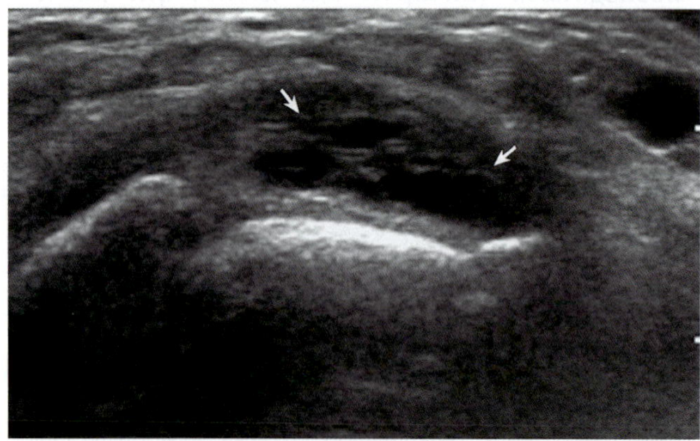

Figure 9.50.   Ganglion cyst: dorsal wrist. Ultrasound images long axis (**A**) and short axis (**B**) to dorsal extensor tendons of wrist show multilobular hypoechoic ganglion cyst (*arrows*) with increased through transmission. R, radius; L, lunate; C, capitate.

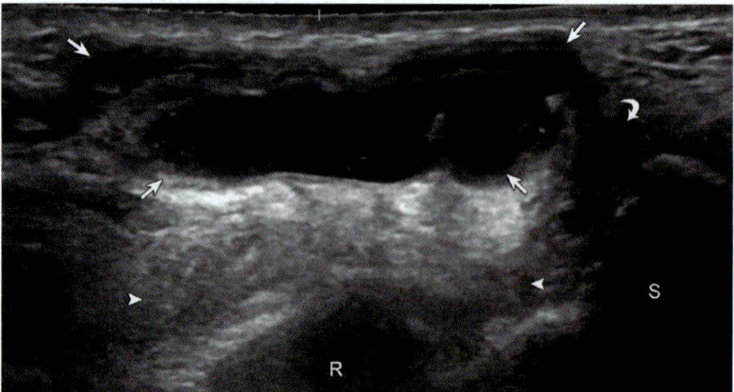

Figure 9.51.   Ganglion cyst: volar wrist. Ultrasound image long axis to radius (*R*) shows multilobular hypoechoic ganglion cyst (*arrows*) with increased through-transmission (*arrowheads*). Note neck of cyst extending from radiocarpal joint (*curved arrow*). S, scaphoid.

diameter[88,90–92] and multilocular, because the multiple septations and internal interfaces create a more hyper-echoic and heterogeneous appearance. Thick mucinous jelly-like contents may be relatively echogenic. Inter-nal echoes from intra-articular gas are also possible. Increased through-transmission may not be obvious if the ganglion is directly adjacent to cortical bone. Ultrasound is effective in the diagnosis of occult dorsal wrist ganglion cysts,[91] which should not be misdiagnosed as distended

dorsal radiocarpal or mid-carpal joint recesses. Ganglion cysts are typically noncompressible in contrast to a dis-tended joint recess.[91]

A unique presentation is an intraneural ganglion cyst of the common peroneal nerve, which is present in up to 18% of patients with foot drop.[93] The ganglion extends from the proximal tibiofibular joint to the common peroneal nerve via the articular branch of the nerve[94,95] and can also extend proximally, into the sciatic nerve or the tibial nerve. The typical clinical presentation of idio-pathic foot drop is of a patient with weight loss, localized trauma, or habitual leg crossing that causes nerve com-pression. Patients with an intraneural ganglion tend to have higher body mass index[93] and may have a higher likelihood of internal derangement of the knee causing joint effusion and increased intra-articular pressure that extends into the proximal tibiofibular joint. Ultrasound shows a multilobular hypoechoic ganglion cyst at the level of the fibular neck in the expected location of the com-mon peroneal nerve and its articular branch (**Fig. 9.52**). The location of the ganglion cyst immediately adjacent to the common peroneal nerve has been termed as the signet ring sign. Ultrasound can identify the extent of the intraneural ganglion cyst, possibly into the sciatic or tibial nerves, and guide percutaneous aspiration.[96] Sec-ondary denervation changes including increased echo-genicity and possibly decreased muscle size (**Fig. 9.52c**) may be identified in the anterior compartment muscles.

Diagnosis of ganglion cyst by ultrasound often relies on the multilocular appearance in a location common to ganglion cysts. If in contact with fibrocartilage at a joint, such as the labrum of the hip or shoulder or the meniscus in the knee, a cyst may represent a paralabral (**Fig. 9.53**) or parameniscal cyst (**Fig. 9.54**) and indicate underlying labral or meniscal damage. When a para-labral cyst at the shoulder is found, the infraspinatus muscle should be evaluated for denervation changes such as atrophy and echogenic fatty infiltration as the cyst may compress the suprascapular nerve in the spino-glenoid notch.

A large unilocular cyst-like abnormality should not be presumed to represent a ganglion cyst, especially if not associated with a tendon. A distended bursa would be in the differential diagnosis especially if the abnormality was in the expected location of a bursa and compress-ible. A large unilocular cyst-like abnormality that is not in the expected location of a bursa should raise concern for a solid lesion such as a myxomatous mass or synovial sarcoma.[66,80] Biopsy may be required.

Epidermal Inclusion Cyst

An epidermal inclusion cyst is a unilocular cyst, lined by squamous cells, encapsulated with fibrous tissue, and located in the epidermis.[97] Etiological theories include congenital, squamous metaplasia, downward growth

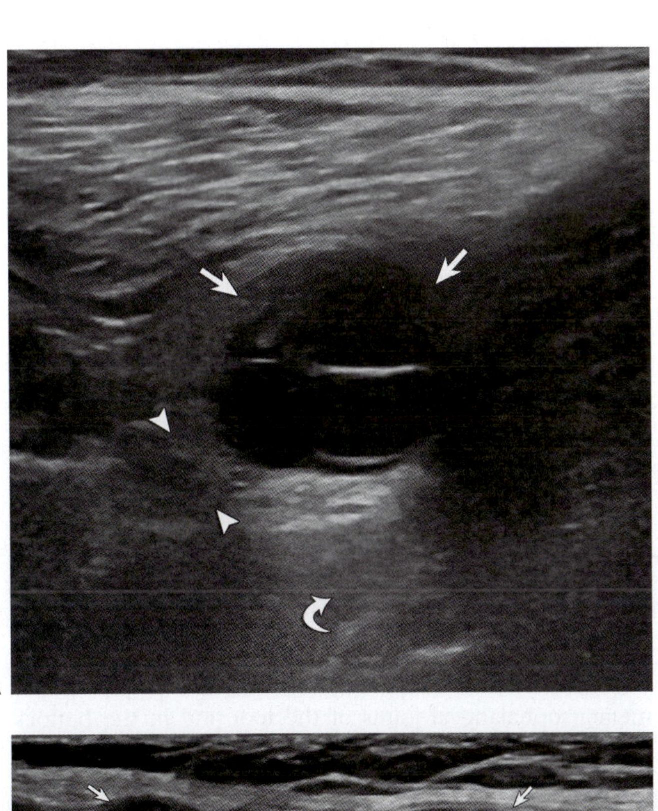

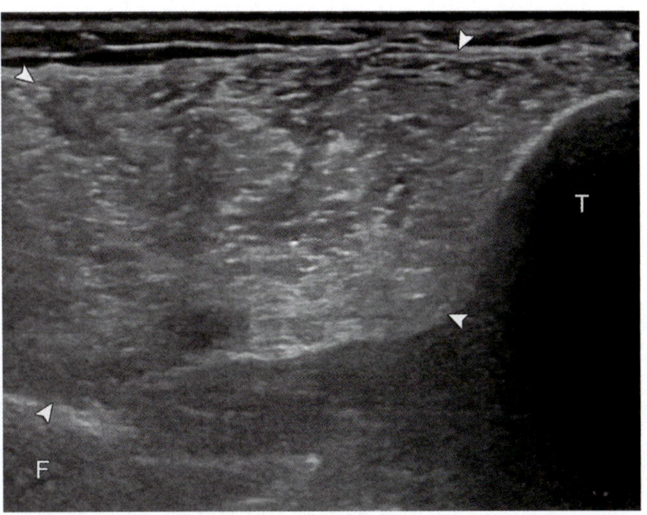

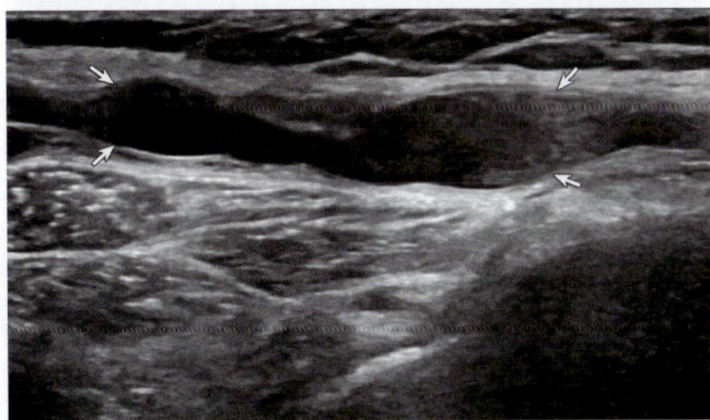

Figure 9.52. Intraneural ganglion cyst. Ultrasound images **(A)** short axis and **(B)** long axis to common peroneal nerve (*arrowheads*) show multilobular hypoechoic ganglion cyst (*arrows*) with increased through-transmission (*curved arrow*). Note **(C)** increased echogenicity of the extensor musculature due to denervation (*arrowheads*). T, tibia; F, fibula.

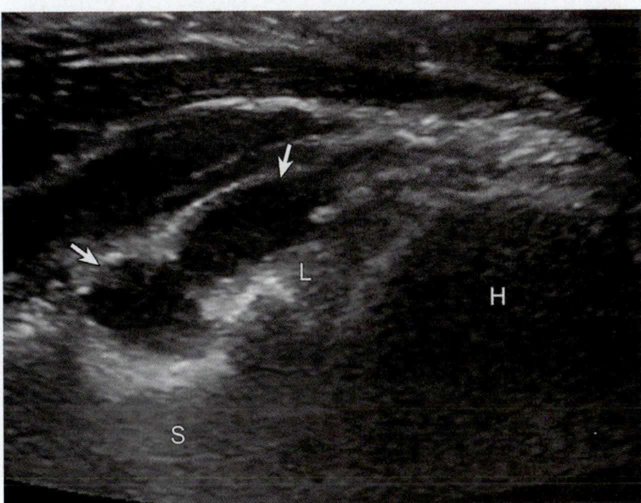

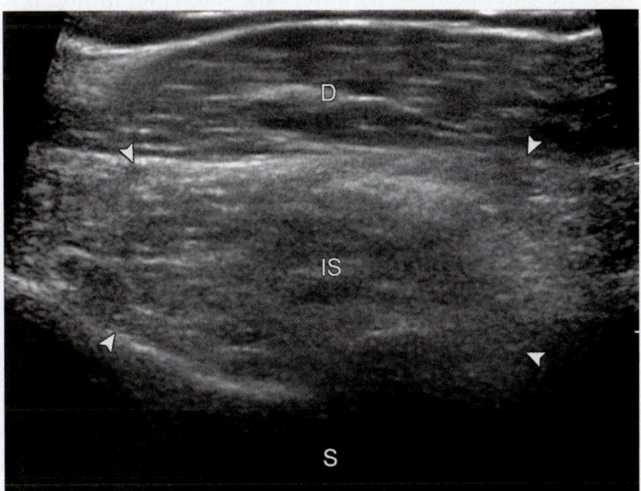

Figure 9.53. Paralabral cyst: shoulder. Ultrasound image **(A)** long axis to infraspinatus shows hypoechoic and lobular paralabral cyst (*arrows*) within the spinoglenoid notch. S, scapula; L, labrum; H, humeral head. Note **(B)** increased echogenicity (*arrowheads*) of the infraspinatus muscle (*IS*) due to denervation. D, deltoid muscle.

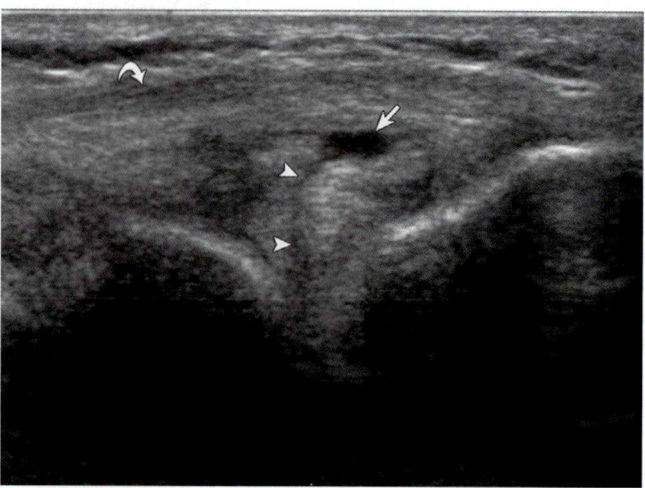

Figure 9.54.   Parameniscal cyst. Ultrasound images over the medial knee in the coronal plane show a heterogeneous and hypoechoic parameniscal cyst (*arrows*) that is located at the base of the medial meniscus (*M*) associated with a meniscal tear (*arrowheads*). F, femur; T, tibia; *curved arrow* in B, tibial collateral ligament.

of epidermal cells from hair follicle obstruction, and growth of implanted dermal tissues from trauma or penetrating injury.[97] Cysts arise anywhere on the body that has hair, although head, neck, trunk, and back are common sites.[98] Cysts contain dermal products, such as keratin, cholesterol, protein, and cell membrane lipids[97] and grow slowly but may become symptomatic after trauma, rupture, or infection.[98]

Ultrasound appearances can be characteristic, although some variability exists depending on the level of maturation, compactness, keratin contents, and whether the cyst has ruptured.[97] Most are round or oval and predominantly hypoechoic, although there are usually scattered internal echoes that may make the cyst nearly isoechoic to muscle (**Fig. 9.55**).[97,98] Increased through-transmission is usually present and internal linear anechoic and echogenic areas may be seen.[97,98] Another characteristic finding is a hypoechoic halo surrounding the cyst.[97,98] Hyperemia is usually absent if the cyst has not ruptured.[97,98]

Rupture is more common when located plantar to the metatarsophalangeal joints of the foot and in the buttock region, and may result in a more variable appearance[99,100] with a lobular shape, ill-defined borders, and an absent hypoechoic halo.[99,100] Hyperemia is usually present and there may be an adjacent abscess.[99,100] Hypoechoic ruptured contents may extend from the cyst along tissue planes (**Fig. 9.56**).

Fat Necrosis

Fat necrosis outside the breast commonly involves the subcutaneous tissues of the lower abdomen and thigh in women and may present as a focal painful palpable area or nodule.[26] Proposed etiologies include trauma, although a history of trauma is often absent, autoimmune disease, vasculitis, cold exposure, and prior injections.[26] Regardless of the inciting event, it is believed that focal fat necrosis is the result of vascular impairment or saponification of fat by lipase from blood.[26]

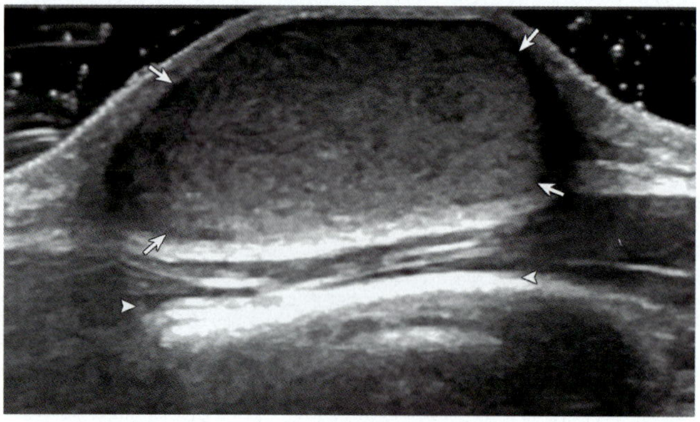

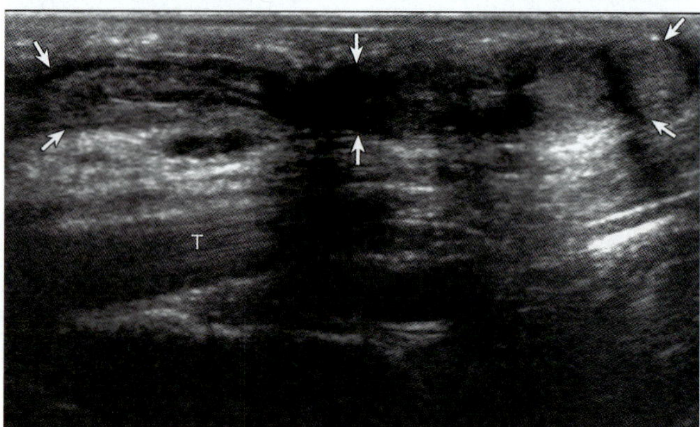

Figure 9.55.   Epidermal inclusion cyst. Ultrasound image shows predominantly hypoechoic epidermal inclusion cyst with low-level homogeneous echoes (*arrows*) and significant increased through-transmission (*arrowheads*).

Figure 9.56.   Epidermal inclusion cyst: ruptured. Ultrasound image long axis to the flexor tendons of the hand (*T*) shows heterogeneous but predominantly hypoechoic ruptured epidermal inclusion (*arrows*) (pathologically proven).

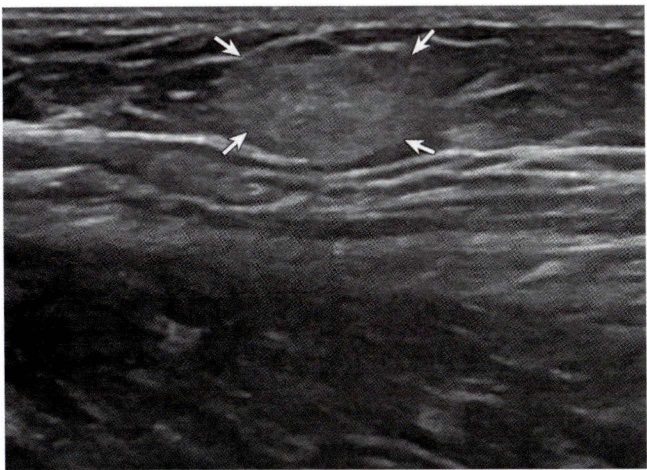

Figure 9.57. Fat necrosis. Ultrasound image shows fat necrosis (*arrows*) as well-defined and hyperechoic within the subcutaneous fat (pathologically proven).

Fat necrosis may be associated with an inflammatory infiltrate, a lipomatous mass, or a Morel-Lavallée lesion (a post-traumatic fluid collection most common in the lateral hip and thigh region at the muscle–subcutaneous fat tissue plane related to separation of the subcutaneous tissues from the underlying fascia), and may appear hypoechoic or hyperechoic.[101] Isolated fat necrosis may appear as a focal, well-defined isoechoic mass with a hypoechoic halo due to a fibrous capsule **(Fig. 9.57)**.[26] The differential diagnosis of this appearance includes lipoma or a variant of lipoma such as angiomyolipoma, epidermal inclusion cyst, or dermatofibrosarcoma protuberans. Alternatively, fat necrosis may appear as an ill-defined area of increased echogenicity due to necrotic adipose tissue and inflammation **(Fig. 9.58)**.

Tip:
- Fat necrosis is not uncommon in obese adolescents and typically presents with minor pain and swelling and ill-defined increased echogenicity in the subcutaneous fat.

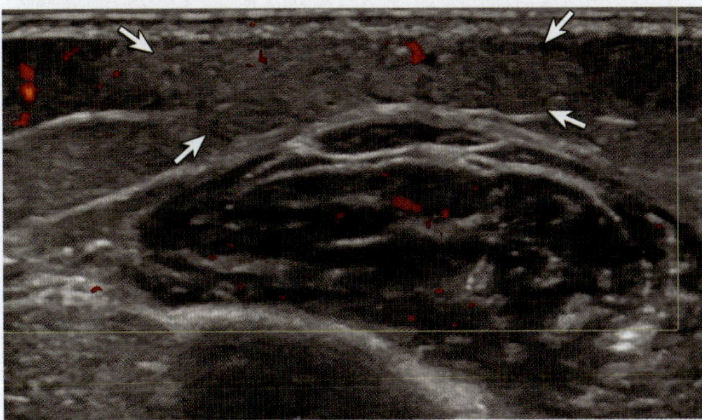

Figure 9.58. Fat necrosis. Color Doppler ultrasound image shows a focal area of increased echogenicity within the subcutaneous fat (*arrows*) with minimal blood flow (pathologically proven).

The differential diagnosis of this appearance primarily includes cellulitis. However, fat necrosis is usually relatively circumscribed and lacks erythema, whereas cellulitis is typically more widespread and is erythematous. Differences between the two forms of isolated fat necrosis may relate to chronicity and extent. Rarely, subcutaneous T-cell lymphoma may appear as an ill-defined hyperechoic soft tissue abnormality.[49]

Soft Tissue Infection

Pyomyositis is a purulent infection of muscle that often presents clinically with a hard swelling and erythema. Ultrasound shows a swollen, echogenic muscle, possibly with small hypoechoic areas due to necrosis and early abscesses.

An abscess may present as a soft tissue mass, although typically clinical signs of infection, such as erythema, warmth, tenderness and fever, and an elevated white blood cell count are present. A focal infected fluid collection may occur in a bursa. Ultrasound is effective in identifying an extremity abscess, especially when superficial. A deep infection in a proximal extremity, especially the thigh, may be more difficult to characterize and MR may be needed to provide a comprehensive evaluation. A soft tissue fluid collection in contact with bone should raise concern for osteomyelitis, especially if the bone cortex is irregular.

At ultrasound, an abscess is most commonly hypoechoic and heterogeneous. A very purulent abscess or bursitis may have numerous internal echoes and may be isoechoic or slightly hyperechoic to surrounding soft tissues, although increased-through transmission is typically present **(Fig. 9.59)**. Numerous punctate hyperechoic foci with short ring-down artifacts are characteristic of

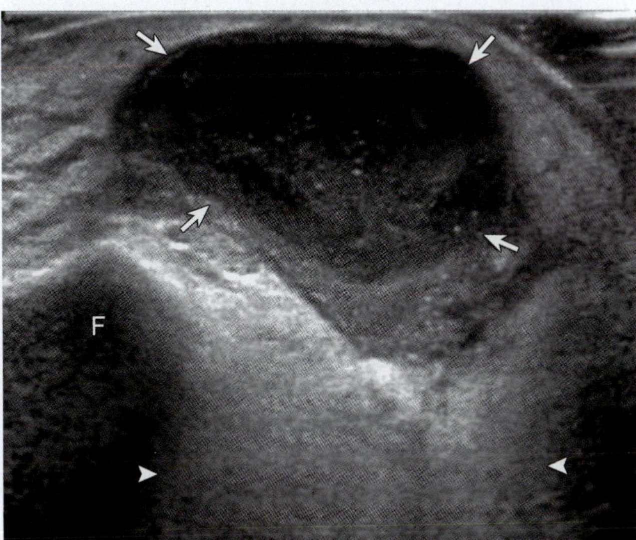

Figure 9.59. Abscess. Ultrasound image shows hypoechoic abscess (*arrows*) with low-level internal echoes that demonstrated swirling motion with transducer pressure (pathologically proven). Note increased through-transmission (*arrowheads*). F, fibula.

soft tissue gas.[102] Some infected fluid collections may be nearly anechoic. Although surrounding increased flow on color or power Doppler imaging supports the diagnosis of inflammation and possible infection, their absence does not exclude infection. Ultrasound-guided aspiration to obtain fluid for microbiology is recommended when there is clinical concern in the presence of a soft tissue fluid collection. An 18G spinal needle is usually adequate, but a wider bore needle is required if the pus is thick, or the abscess may have to be irrigated with saline, and then aspirated.

> **Tip:**
> - Use an 18G (or larger bore) needle to aspirate abscesses.

Chronic infection associated with a retained surgical cotton or gauze swab (called a gossypiboma or textiloma) may present as a soft tissue mass **(Fig. 9.60)**.[103] The retained material may incite an exudative or a sterile fibrotic response.[103] Often the history of prior surgery is not included or is forgotten as the time interval between surgery and presentation may be long. At ultrasound, a gossypiboma has a variable appearance with possible acoustic shadowing. Multiple internal echoes are often seen from the interfaces with the surgical sponge and possible gas.

Muscle Hernia

Muscle hernia, when muscle protrudes through a fascial defect, most commonly involves the lower leg, especially the tibialis anterior muscle.[104] Causes include acute or repetitive trauma, chronic compartment syndrome, and weakening of the fascia from perforating vessels.[104] Dynamic evaluation when the muscle is contracted or the patient erect is often useful. Ultrasound demonstrates that the mass is muscle. It appears hypoechoic with interspersed hyperechoic fibroadipose septations and is in continuity with the muscle of origin **(Fig. 9.61)**.[104,105] Fascial thinning or a defect, sometimes at the site of a perforating arterial vessel, is usually identified. Care must be taken not to press too hard as this may efface the hernia.

> **Tip:**
> - Muscle hernias may become more conspicuous if the patient is examined erect or while contracting the muscle.
> - Use light transducer pressure when examining for a muscle hernia to avoid reducing and missing the hernia.

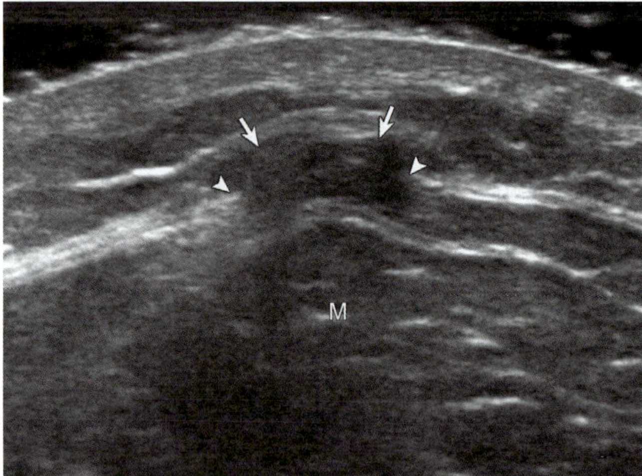

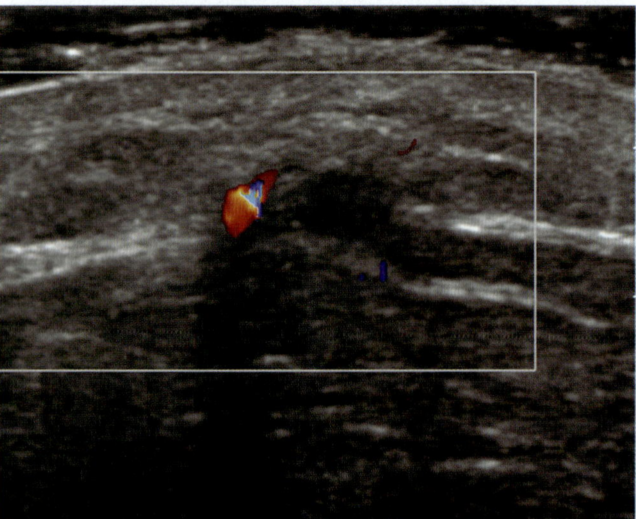

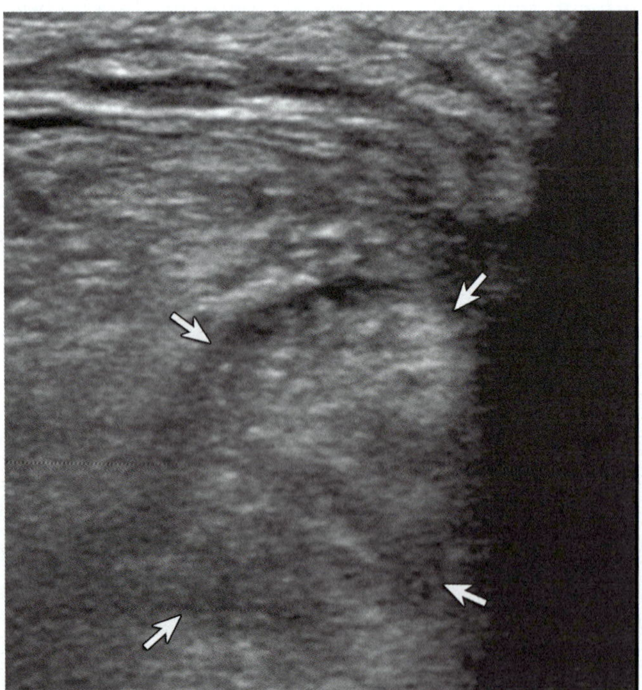

Figure 9.60.   Gossypiboma. Ultrasound image shows heterogeneous but predominantly echogenic infected retained sponge with minimal surrounding hypoechoic halo (*arrows*) (surgically proven).

Figure 9.61.   Muscle hernia. Gray scale **(A)** and color Doppler **(B)** ultrasound images short axis to the tibialis anterior (*M*) show a defect in the overlying fascia (*arrowheads*) with protruding muscle hernia (*arrows*). Note perforating vessel.

Accessory and Anomalous Muscles

Most accessory or anomalous muscles are asymptomatic but they may produce symptoms by compressing neurovascular structures or present as palpable masses.[106] Accessory muscles are diagnosed on ultrasound by demonstrating that a swelling has normal muscle echotexture, often in a characteristic site. Of the many accessory muscles, two that warrant discussion are the extensor digitorum brevis manus at the wrist and the accessory soleus in the ankle and calf. Other accessory muscles are discussed in Chapters 5, 8, and 11.

The extensor digitorum brevis manus occurs in approximately 2% to 3% of the population and is bilateral in 54% of cases.[107] It is located at the dorsum of the wrist, may originate from the distal radius, wrist joint capsule, or fascia and most commonly inserts on the dorsal hood of the index or middle fingers.[106] Ultrasound shows muscle tissue over the dorsum of the wrist that extends distally with the extensor tendons of the index and middle fingers **(Fig. 9.62)**. A characteristic clinical finding is an increase in size of the mass with active finger extension against resistance (Garcia's maneuver)

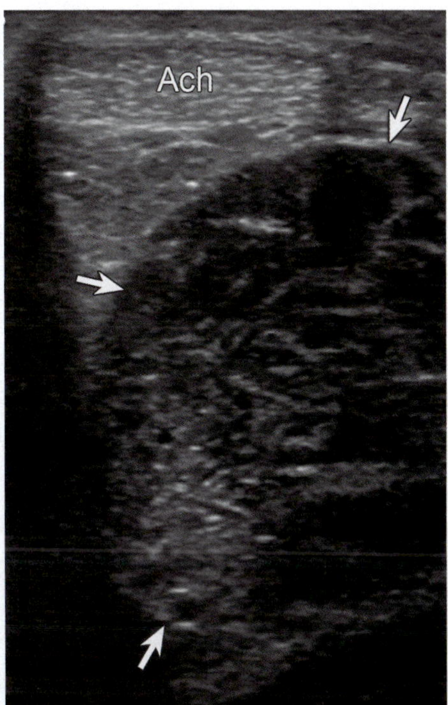

Figure 9.63.   Accessory soleus muscle. Ultrasound image short axis to the Achilles tendon (*Ach*) shows soleus muscle (*arrows*) that extends inferiorly to the level of the distal tibia.

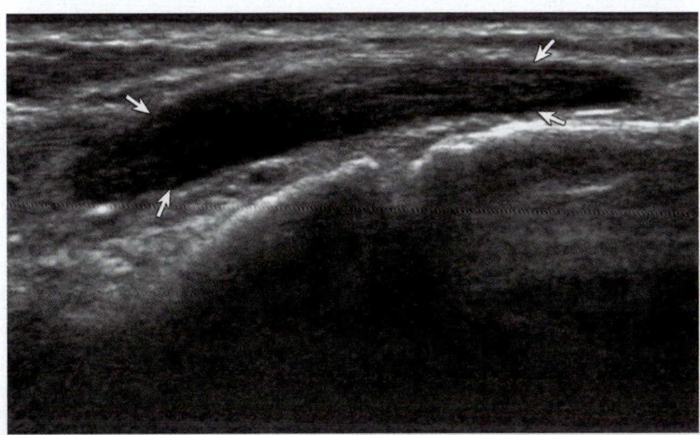

A

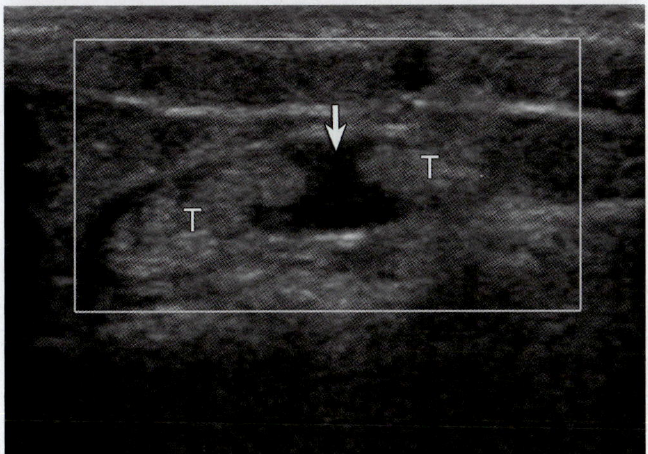

B

Figure 9.62.   Extensor digitorum brevis manus. Ultrasound images long axis **(A)** and short axis **(B)** to the extensor tendons (*T*) of the dorsal wrist at the level of the mid-carpal joint show muscle tissue (*arrows*) between the extensor tendons of the index and middle fingers.

best recognized as increased cross-sectional diameter of the muscle on ultrasound.[107]

The accessory soleus muscle is present in up to 5.5% of the population and is usually unilateral.[106] It originates from the soleus muscle or distal tibia and fibula, lies anterior or anteromedial to the Achilles tendon, and inserts on the Achilles tendon or separately from the Achilles on the calcaneus.[106,108] Ultrasound shows that the mass is muscle **(Fig. 9.63)** in the characteristic location, and a small tendon inserting on the calcaneus may be identified.[109]

Myositis Ossificans

Myositis ossificans is heterotopic ossification in muscle and most commonly involves the thigh and arm.[110] Post-traumatic myositis ossificans is the most common form and is due to degeneration and necrosis of damaged muscle, which mineralizes and forms bone.[111] Peripheral ossification is characteristic.

Early or immature post-traumatic myositis ossificans results in a focal hypoechoic mass, possibly with internal echoes due to early mineralization **(Fig. 9.64)**.[110,111] As the abnormal area matures, foci of echogenic ossification appear at the periphery of the mass, then become continuous and cause acoustic shadowing similar to other forms of heterotopic ossification **(Fig. 9.65)**.[110,111] When myositis ossificans is suspected at ultrasound, radiography is indicated to characterize the ossification. Well-defined circumferential ossification within muscle indicates myositis ossificans.[110] If the radiographic appearance is not diagnostic,

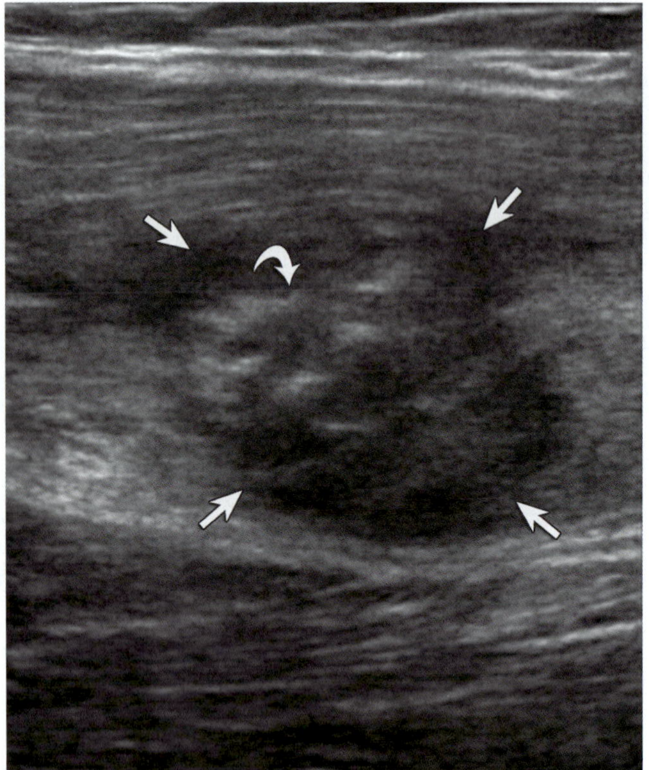

Figure 9.64. Myositis ossificans: early. Ultrasound image shows early myositis ossificans as a hypoechoic area (*arrows*) with internal echogenic mineralization (*curved arrow*) (pathologically proven).

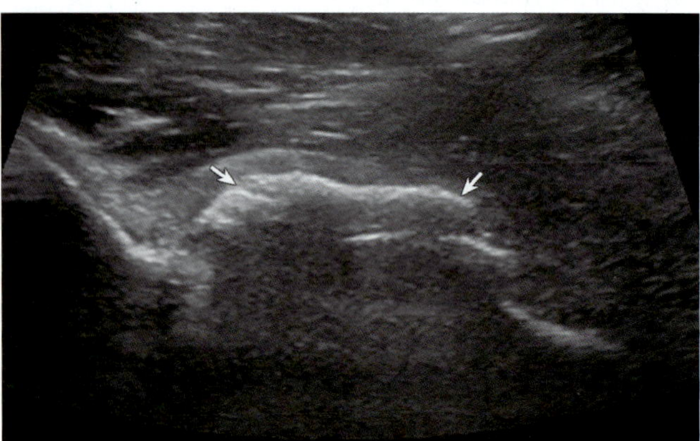

Figure 9.65. Heterotopic ossification: mature. Ultrasound image shows hyperechoic surface of the soft tissue ossification (*arrows*) with acoustic shadowing.

CT can be employed to demonstrate the peripheral nature of the ossification.[110] If ossification is not peripheral or is incomplete, short-term follow-up with radiography or CT is recommended to ensure continued organization and ossification. If the diagnosis of myositis ossificans remains in question, percutaneous biopsy is indicated to exclude soft tissue chondroma, synovial sarcoma, extraskeletal chondrosarcoma, or extraskeletal osteosarcoma, although a skilled histopathologist is required as the immature bone of myositis ossificans may simulate a tumor.

Rheumatoid Nodule

Rheumatoid nodules present as firm, non-tender, mobile, subcutaneous masses at pressure sites[112] and occasionally in non-subcutaneous sites. Usually associated with severe rheumatoid arthritis, nodules may also occur with other collagen vascular diseases.[112] The etiology is believed to relate to immune complex-mediated vasculitis.[112] Histologically, a rheumatoid nodule has an inner necrotic zone, a surrounding layer of granulomas and macrophages, and an outer perivascular layer of chronic inflammatory cells.[112]

Nodules appear as oval homogeneous hypoechoic masses **(Fig. 9.66)**.[113] Hyperemia may be present. A nodule may be adjacent to bone but erosions are not typically seen. In contrast, a gouty tophus typically has a hypoechoic to hyperechoic appearance with multiple internal echoes and is often associated with adjacent cortical erosion.

Gouty Tophus

Gout is due to deposition of monosodium urate crystals that may form organized tophi, commonly in joints, bursae, and the medial aspect of the distal first metatarsal. Tophi may be deposited in and around tendons and present as soft tissue masses. They tend to occur at the extensor aspect of a joint (e.g., in the patellar tendon) and present as a soft tissue mass. Any soft tissue mass that originates in and is isolated to a tendon should raise concern for gout.

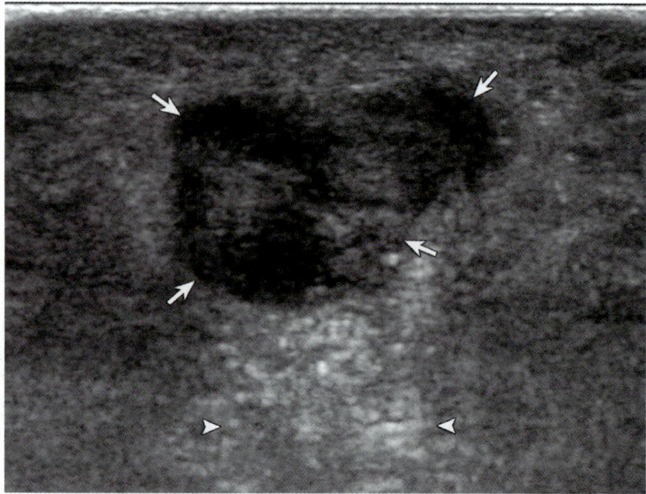

Figure 9.66. Rheumatoid nodule. Ultrasound image shows hypoechoic rheumatoid nodule (*arrows*) with increased through-transmission (*arrowheads*).

At ultrasound, a tophus appears as a focal area of scattered internal echoes **(Fig. 9.67)**[114] and depending on the echogenicity of surrounding tissues, can vary from hypoechoic to hyperechoic. Typical echogenic tophi with multiple internal reflections are best appreciated during real-time scanning. A hypoechoic halo and variable increased flow on color and power Doppler imaging[114] may be present. If a cortical erosion is present, a tophus usually extends into the erosion. Other findings of gout related to joint involvement include joint effusion, synovial proliferation, intra-articular crystals, and "icing" of hyaline cartilage due to crystals on the surface of the cartilage (double contour sign).[114]

Tumoral Calcinosis

Tumoral calcinosis is a hereditary metabolic dysfunction of phosphate regulation that is associated with mass-like peri-articular calcification.[115] Patients often present in the first or second decades of life with a painless soft tissue mass.[115] Laboratory results typically show hyperphosphatemia and normocalcemia. Ultrasound can demonstrate idiopathic calcinosis as a soft tissue mass with a hyperechoic surface and distal shadowing. The differential diagnosis includes soft tissue calcification

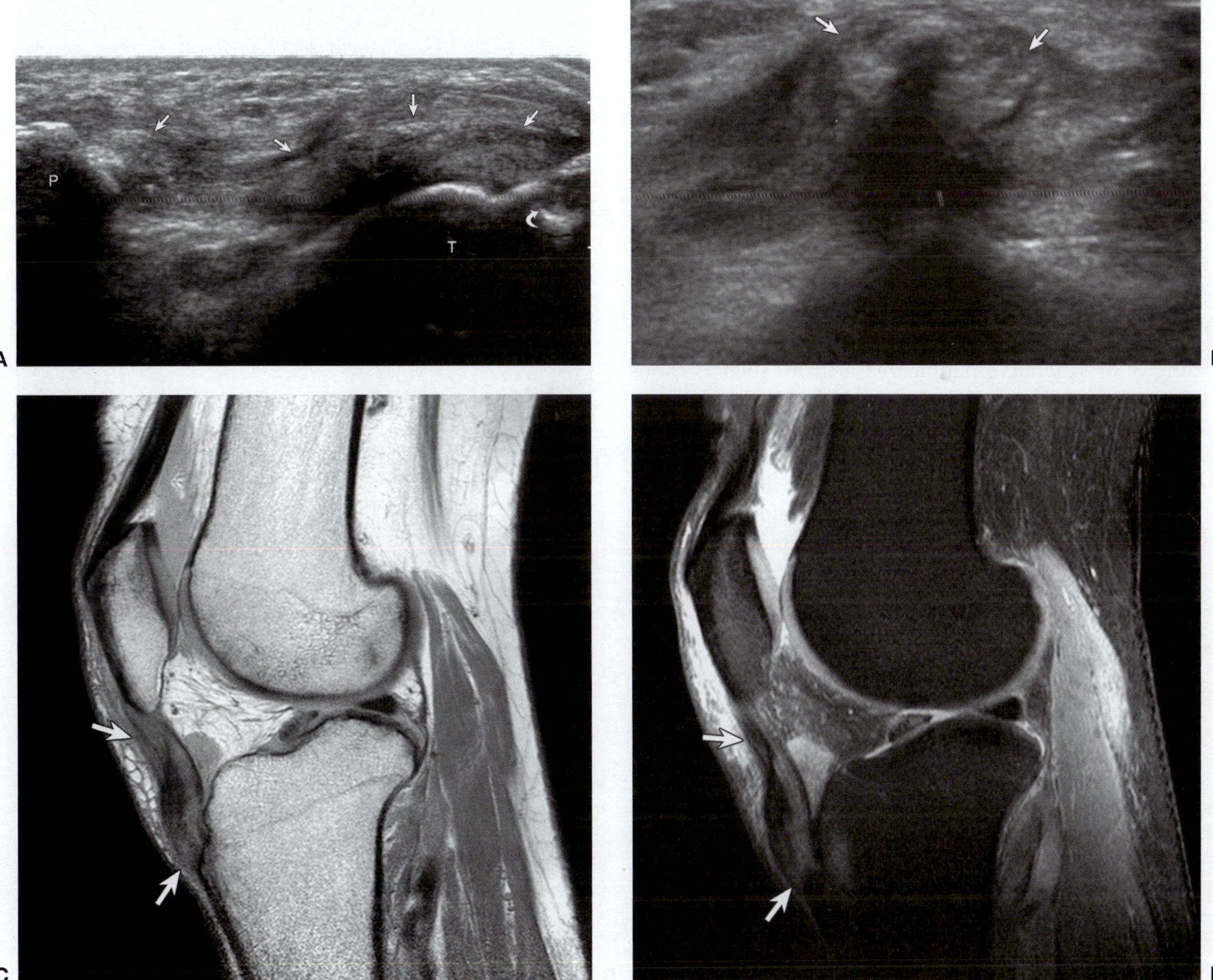

Figure 9.67. Tophus. Ultrasound images long axis **(A)** and short axis **(B)** to patellar tendon show heterogeneous appearance of the patellar tendon with hyperechoic tophi (*arrows*) and variable shadowing, also shown on sagittal proton-density **(C)** and fluid-sensitive fat-saturated **(D)** MR images. Note tibial erosion (*curved arrow* in **A**).

from metabolic disease such as chronic renal failure, although laboratory results and history assist in providing the proper diagnosis.[115] Other causes of soft tissue calcification discussed elsewhere include dystrophic calcification, connective tissue disease, neoplasm, and degenerative conditions.[115]

Other Masses

Several other benign soft tissue pathologies may present clinically as masses. A chronic and retracted tendon or muscle tear may present as a palpable soft tissue mass, such as a tear of the distal rectus femoris.[116,117] Inflammatory lymph nodes may present as masses, for example, the epitrochlear lymph nodes in the medial elbow or axillary lymph nodes.[118] An aneurysm or pseudoaneurysm can cause a soft tissue mass that is ideally evaluated with color or power Doppler ultrasound, which shows typical swirling flow. A thrombosed superficial vein or varix in the leg has no or minimal flow on Doppler and is in continuity with an adjacent vein. Other normal structures, such as the xiphoid process, may present as palpable soft tissue masses.

JOINT AND SYNOVIAL PROCESSES

If a soft tissue mass corresponds to a synovial space such as a joint recess, bursa, or tendon sheath, a benign synovial process is likely. Considerations include chronic inflammation (atypical infection such as tuberculosis or fungus, or systemic inflammatory arthritis such as rheumatoid arthritis), chronic hemorrhage (hemophilia or other causes of hemorrhage), or other synovial process such as amyloidosis, pigmented villonodular synovitis, localized nodular synovitis, intra-articular fibroma, intracapsular chondroma (see earlier discussion), or synovial (osteo) chondromatosis. Most synovial processes

appear nonspecific and are predominantly hypoechoic to isoechoic with variable associated joint fluid and variable flow on color and power Doppler. Patient history is helpful in the diagnosis of atypical infection, systemic inflammatory arthritis, or hemophilia. Amyloid deposition may occur in patients with a history of long-term dialysis, plasma cell myeloma, or chronic inflammation.

At ultrasound, pigmented villonodular synovitis produces significant distention of joint recesses by hypoechoic to isoechoic synovial proliferation and joint effusion (**Figs. 9.68 and 9.69**).[82,119] Localized nodular synovitis

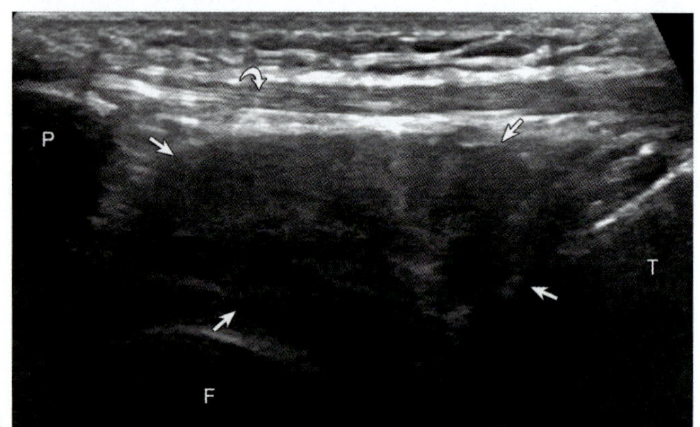

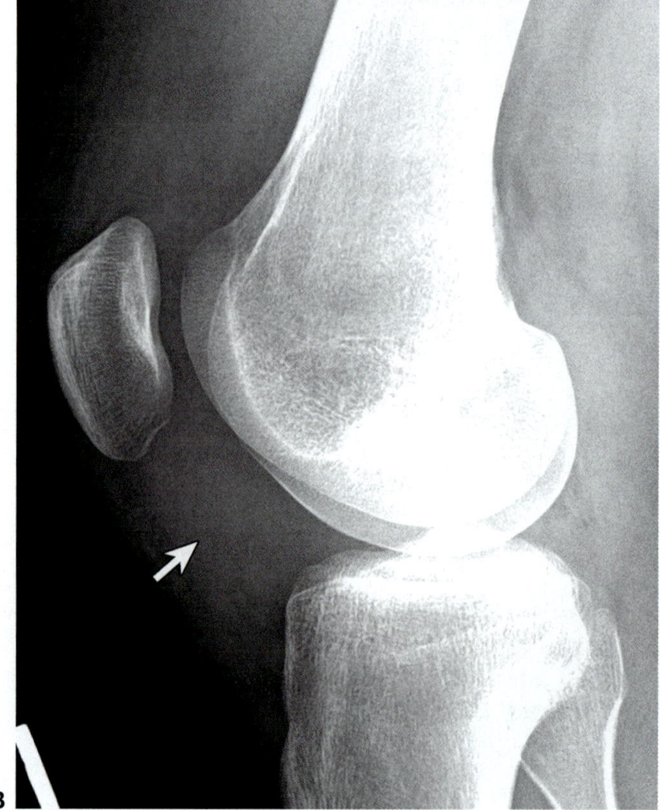

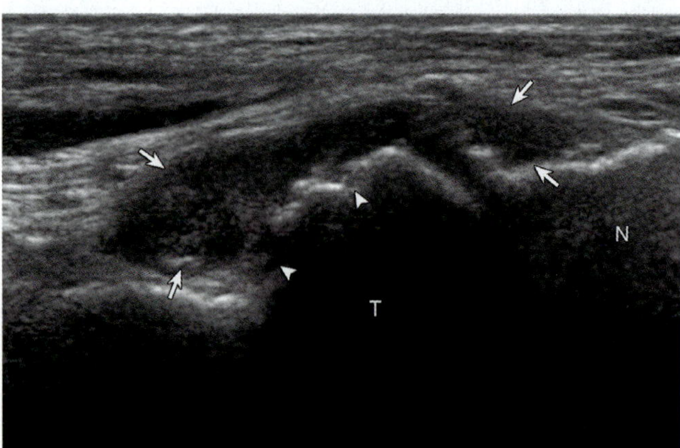

Figure 9.68. Pigmented villonodular synovitis. Ultrasound image in the sagittal plane over the dorsal ankle shows hypoechoic distention of the talonavicular joint (*arrows*) with bone erosions (*arrowheads*) (pathologically proven). T, talus; N, navicular.

Figure 9.69. Pigmented villonodular synovitis. Ultrasound image (**A**) long axis to patellar tendon (*curved arrow*) shows hypoechoic mass (*arrows*), also shown on radiography (**B**), and sagittal T1-weighted (**C**) MR image (pathologically proven). P, patella; F, femur; T, tibia.

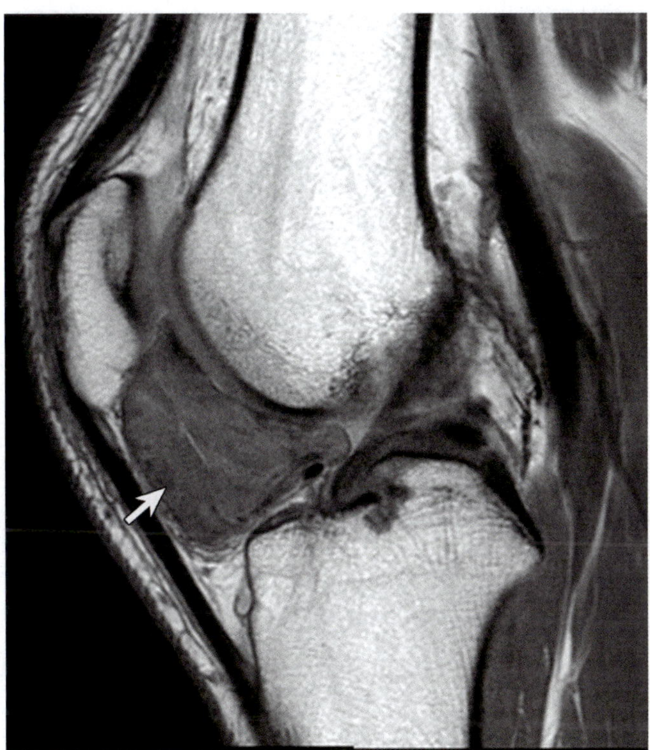

Figure 9.69. (*Continued*)

represents a more focal presentation and typically appears hypoechoic. Uncommonly, a focal hypoechoic to isoechoic intra-articular mass is due to a fibroma (**Fig. 9.70**). Synovial chondromatosis less commonly presents as a mass but produces synovial proliferation with possible hyperechoic calcification and shadowing (**Fig. 9.71**).[120,121] Lipoma arborescens may be primary or secondary to arthritis and usually involves the knee. It represents subsynovial fat

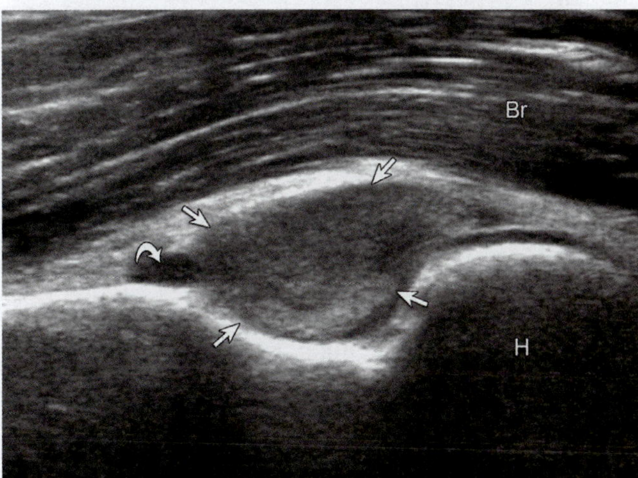

Figure 9.70. Fibroma. Ultrasound image in the sagittal plane over the anterior elbow shows hypoechoic to isoechoic intra-articular fibroma within the anterior elbow joint recess (pathologically proven). H, humerus; Br, brachialis; *curved arrow* = joint fluid.

proliferation and appears as hyperechoic frond-like synovial proliferation (**Fig. 9.72**).[122]

BONE TUMORS

Ultrasound evaluation of bone is relatively limited when compared with radiography, CT, and MR, and is restricted to the extra-osseous soft tissue component of a bone lesion, the integrity of the bone cortex, and assessment for periostitis. Further evaluation with radiography and/or cross-sectional imaging is indicated if a bone abnormality is identified with ultrasound.

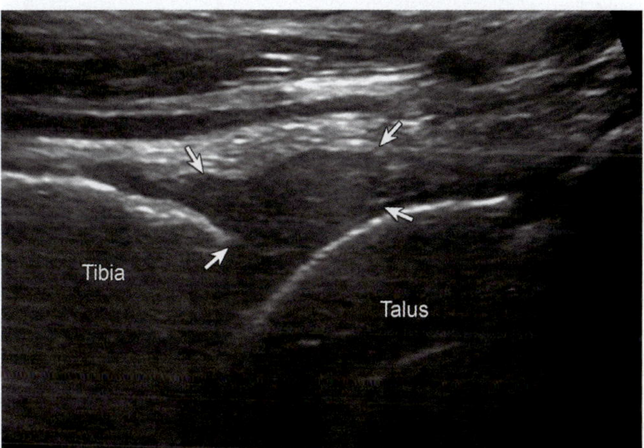

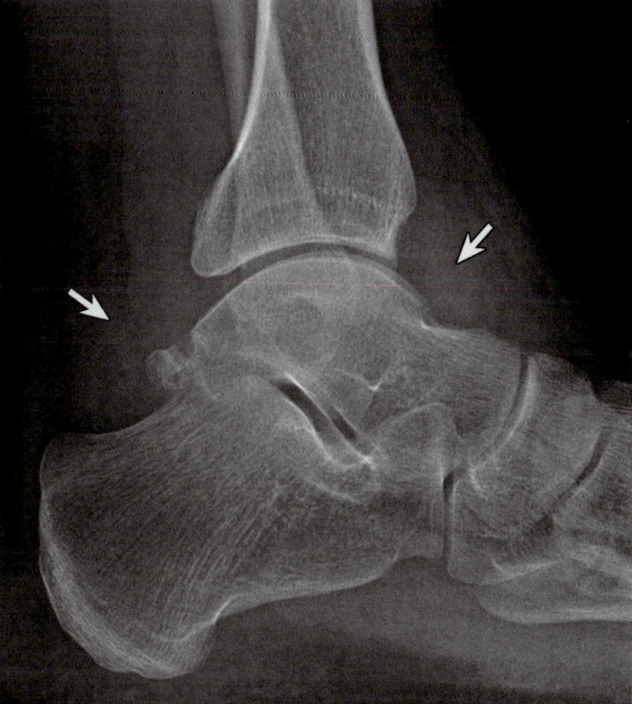

Figure 9.71. Synovial chondromatosis. Ultrasound image (**A**) in the sagittal plane over the dorsal ankle shows hypoechoic distention of the anterior ankle joint recess (*arrows*). Involvement of the both the anterior and posterior ankle joint recesses (*arrows*) are shown on radiography (**B**) and sagittal fluid-sensitive MR image (**C**) (pathologically proven).

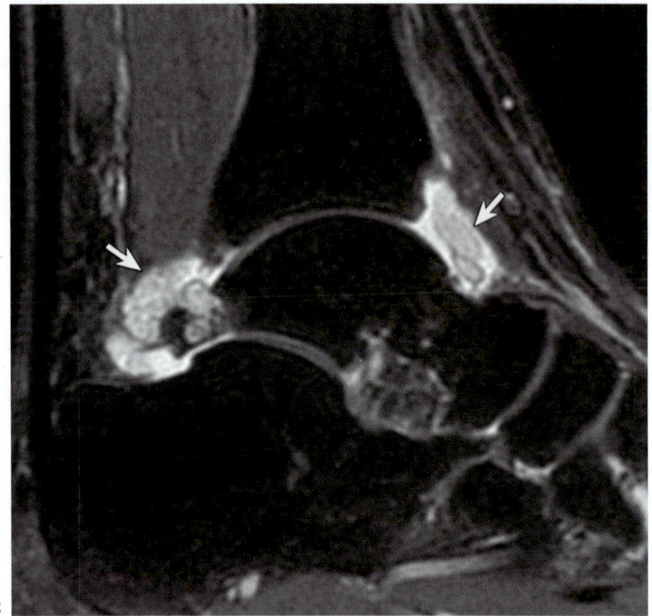

C

Figure 9.71. (*Continued*)

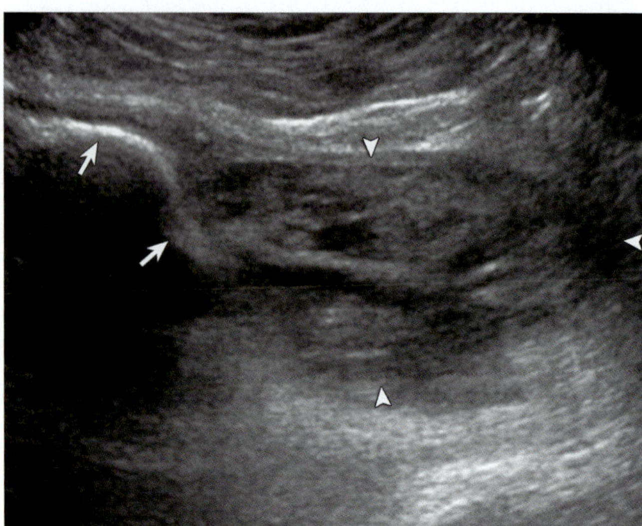

Figure 9.73. Osteochondroma (exostosis). Ultrasound image shows echogenic surface of the osteochondroma (*arrows*) with overlying heterogeneous bursa (*arrowheads*).

tumors, notably Ewing sarcoma and lymphoma, often present as soft tissue masses as the tumor extends beyond the confines of the bone without gross destruction of the cortex **(Fig. 9.74)**.[125,126] Bone destruction with or without a soft tissue mass should raise concern for an aggressive process such as high-grade primary bone tumor **(Fig. 9.75)**, metastasis **(Fig. 9.76)**, or plasmacytoma.

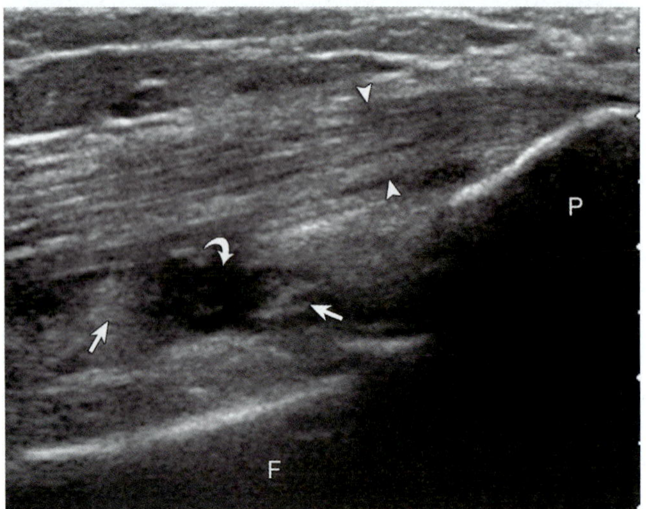

Figure 9.72. Lipoma arborescens. Ultrasound image long axis to quadriceps tendon (*arrowheads*) show frond-like echogenic tissue (*arrows*) within the suprapatellar recess. F, femur; P, patellar; *curved arrow*, joint fluid.

An exostosis or osteochondroma is a benign bone excrescence. If pedunculated, it may extend into the soft tissues, pointing away from a joint **(Fig. 9.73)**.[123] The cartilage cap of an osteochondroma can be assessed with ultrasound.[123] A cartilage cap ≤1 cm thick is benign, whereas a cap >1 to 3 cm or an associated soft tissue mass may indicate malignant degeneration into chondrosarcoma.[124] Ultrasound can show other complications such as an overlying bursa or impingement of an adjacent nerve or vessel.

A bone tumor should be considered when a soft tissue mass is in contact with a bone. Several malignant bone

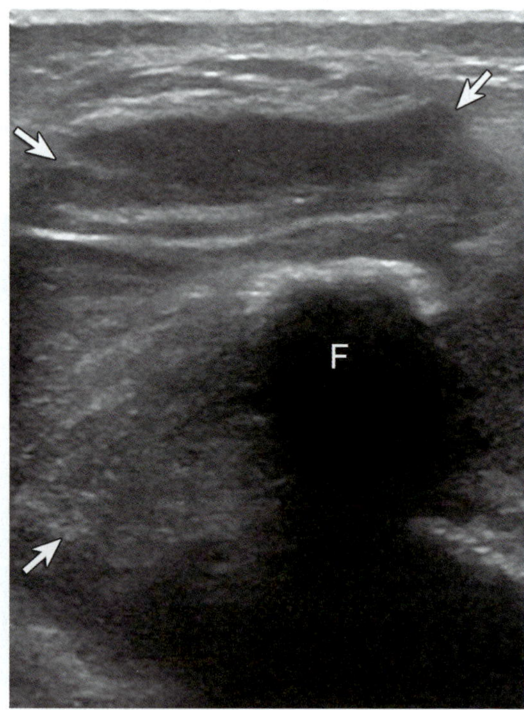

Figure 9.74. Ewing sarcoma. Ultrasound image shows heterogeneous mass (*arrows*) originating from and surrounding the fibula (*F*) (pathologically proven).

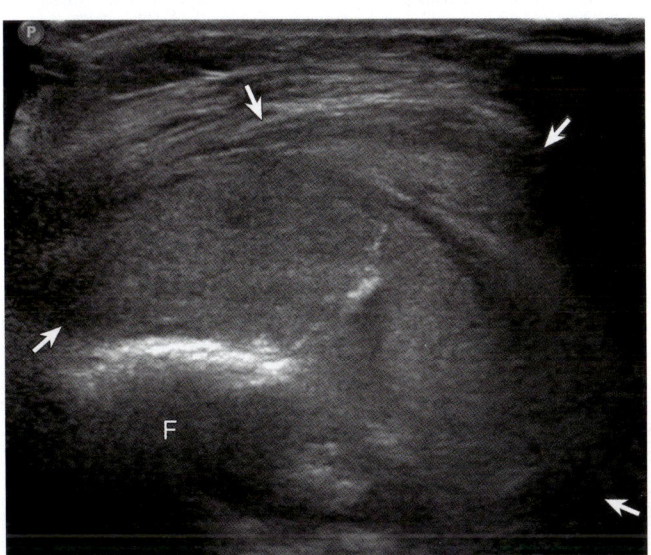 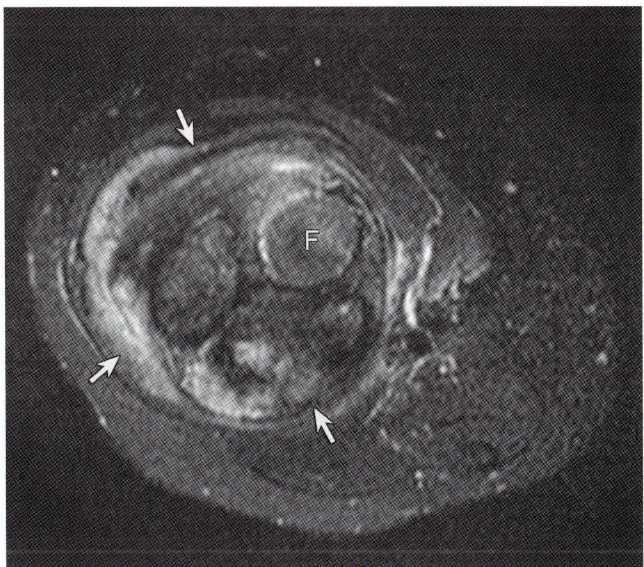

Figure 9.75.   Osteosarcoma. Ultrasound image **(A)** and axial fluid sensitive MR image **(B)** show heterogeneous mass (*arrows*) originating from and surrounding the femur (*F*) (pathologically proven).

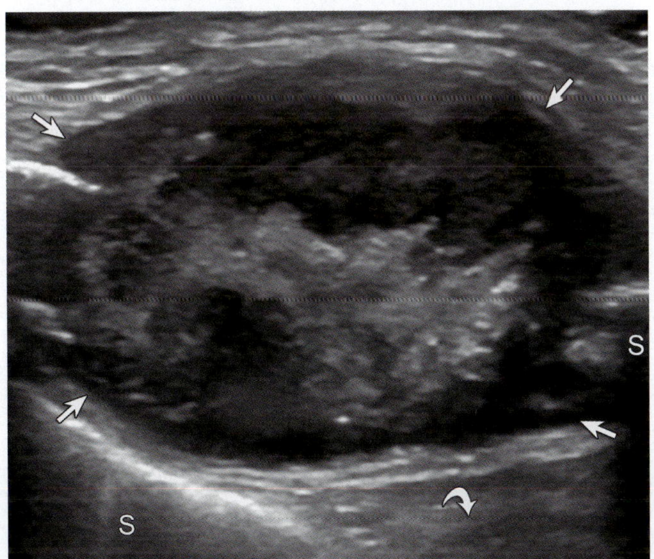 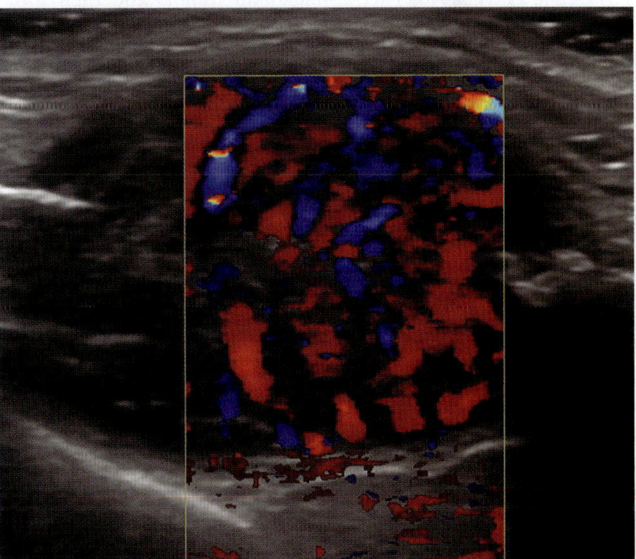

Figure 9.76.   Metastasis: malignant peripheral nerve sheath tumor to sternum. Ultrasound gray scale **(A)** and color Doppler **(B)** images show heterogeneous and hypervascular soft tissue mass (*arrows*) that originates from the sternum (*S*) (pathologically proven). Note destruction of the sternum (*curved arrow*).

CONCLUSION

Ultrasound is an effective imaging method of evaluating soft tissue masses. Initial evaluation distinguishes cystic from solid masses, and characteristic features may allow further differentiation. Several benign and common soft tissue masses can often be diagnosed with ultrasound such as superficial lipoma or ganglion cyst. A soft tissue mass that originates from a synovial space such as a joint limits the differential diagnosis to a likely benign synovial process. Identification of a mass that originates from or involves bone requires further evaluation with cross-sectional imaging and radiographs. Once a mass is identified and characterized, a tissue diagnosis may be needed. Ultrasound-guided biopsy is an ideal method to obtain histologic material in many cases. Ultrasound can also be helpful in evaluating tumor recurrence, particularly if a prosthesis is present.

REFERENCES

1. Widmann G, Riedl A, Schoepf D, et al. State-of-the-art HR-Ultrasound imaging findings of the most frequent musculoskeletal soft-tissue tumors. *Skeletal Radiol.* 2009;38(7):637–649.
2. Kuwano Y, Ishizaki K, Watanabe R, et al. Efficacy of diagnostic ultrasonography of lipomas, epidermal cysts, and ganglions. *Arch Dermatol.* 2009;145(7):761–764.

3. Briccoli A, Galletti S, Salone M, et al. Ultrasonography is superior to computed tomography and magnetic resonance imaging in determining superficial resection margins of malignant chest wall tumors. *J Ultrasound Med.* 2007;26(2):157–162.

4. Lee MH, Kim NR, Ryu JA. Cyst-like solid tumors of the musculoskeletal system: an analysis of ultrasound findings. *Skeletal Radiol.* 2010;39(10):981–986.

5. Arya S, Nagarkatti DG, Dudhat SB, et al. Soft tissue sarcomas: ultrasonographic evaluation of local recurrences. *Clin Radiol.* 2000;55(3):193–197.

6. Choi H, Varma DG, Fornage BD, et al. Soft-tissue sarcoma: MR imaging vs. sonography for detection of local recurrence after surgery. *AJR Am J Roentgenol.* 1991;157(2):353–358.

7. Nazarian LN, Alexander AA, Rawool NM, et al. Malignant melanoma: impact of superficial ultrasound on management. *Radiology.* 1996;199(1):273–277.

8. Fleischer AC. Sonographic depiction of tumor vascularity and flow: from in vivo models to clinical applications. *J Ultrasound Med.* 2000;19(1):55–61.

9. Jin W, Kim GY, Park SY, et al. The spectrum of vascularized superficial soft-tissue tumors on sonography with a histopathologic correlation: Part 1, benign tumors. *AJR Am J Roentgenol.* 2010;195(2):439–445.

10. Jin W, Kim GY, Park SY, et al. The spectrum of vascularized superficial soft-tissue tumors on sonography with a histopathologic correlation: Part 2, malignant tumors and their lookalikes. *AJR Am J Roentgenol.* 2010;195(2):446–453.

11. Kaushik S, Miller TT, Nazarian LN, et al. Spectral Doppler sonography of musculoskeletal soft tissue masses. *J Ultrasound Med.* 2003;22(12):1333–1336.

12. Ferrara KW, Merritt CR, Burns PN, et al. Evaluation of tumor angiogenesis with US: imaging, Doppler, and contrast agents. *Acad Radiol.* 2000;7(10):824–839.

13. Kransdorf MJ. Malignant soft-tissue tumors in a large referral population: distribution of diagnoses by age, sex, and location. *AJR Am J Roentgenol.* 1995;164(1):129–134.

14. Kransdorf MJ. Benign soft-tissue tumors in a large referral population: distribution of specific diagnoses by age, sex, and location. *AJR Am J Roentgenol.* 1995;164(2):395–402.

15. Murphey MD. World Health Organization classification of bone and soft tissue tumors: modifications and implications for radiologists. *Semin Musculoskelet Radiol.* 2007;11(3):201–214.

16. Razek AA, Huang BY. Soft tissue tumors of the head and neck: imaging-based review of the WHO classification. *Radiographics.* 2011;31(7):1923–1954.

17. Konermann W, Wuisman P, Ellermann A, et al. Ultrasonographically guided needle biopsy of benign and malignant soft tissue and bone tumors. *J Ultrasound Med.* 2000;19(7):465–471.

18. Sofka CM, Collins AJ, Adler RS. Use of ultrasonographic guidance in interventional musculoskeletal procedures: a review from a single institution. *J Ultrasound Med.* 2001;20(1):21–26.

19. Yeow KM, Tan CF, Chen JS, et al. Diagnostic sensitivity of ultrasound-guided needle biopsy in soft tissue masses about superficial bone lesions. *J Ultrasound Med.* 2000;19(12):849–855.

20. Murphey MD, Carroll JF, Flemming DJ, et al. From the archives of the AFIP: benign musculoskeletal lipomatous lesions. *Radiographics.* 2004;24(5):1433–1466.

21. Fornage BD, Tassin GB. Sonographic appearances of superficial soft tissue lipomas. *J Clin Ultrasound.* 1991;19(4):215–220.

22. Inampudi P, Jacobson JA, Fessell DP, et al. Soft-tissue lipomas: accuracy of sonography in diagnosis with pathologic correlation. *Radiology.* 2004;233(3):763–767.

23. Paunipagar BK, Griffith JF, Rasalkar DD, et al. Ultrasound features of deep-seated lipomas. *Insights Imaging.* 2010;1(3):149–153.

24. Murphey MD, Arcara LK, Fanburg-Smith J. From the archives of the AFIP: imaging of musculoskeletal liposarcoma with radiologic–pathologic correlation. *Radiographics.* 2005;25(5):1371–1395.

25. Bang M, Kang BS, Hwang JC, et al. Ultrasonographic analysis of subcutaneous angiolipoma. *Skeletal Radiol.* 2011;41(9):1055–1059.

26. Walsh M, Jacobson JA, Kim SM, et al. Sonography of fat necrosis involving the extremity and torso with magnetic resonance imaging and histologic correlation. *J Ultrasound Med.* 2008;27(12):1751–1757.

27. Shin YR, Kim JY, Sung MS, et al. Sonographic findings of dermatofibrosarcoma protuberans with pathologic correlation. *J Ultrasound Med.* 2008;27(2):269–274.

28. Hardes J, Scheil-Bertram S, Hartwig E, et al. Sonographic findings of hibernoma. A report of two cases. *J Clin Ultrasound.* 2005;33(6):298–301.

29. Kransdorf MJ, Bancroft LW, Peterson JJ, et al. Imaging of fatty tumors: distinction of lipoma and well-differentiated liposarcoma. *Radiology.* 2002;224(1):99–104.

30. Dinauer PA, Brixey CJ, Moncur JT, et al. Pathologic and MR imaging features of benign fibrous soft-tissue tumors in adults. *Radiographics.* 2007;27(1):173–187.

31. Murphey MD, Ruble CM, Tyszko SM, et al. From the archives of the AFIP: musculoskeletal fibromatoses: radiologic–pathologic correlation. *Radiographics.* 2009;29(7):2143–2173.

32. Griffith JF, Wong TY, Wong SM, et al. Sonography of plantar fibromatosis. *AJR Am J Roentgenol.* 2002;179(5):1167–1172.

33. Huang CC, Ko SF, Yeh MC, et al. Aggressive fibromatosis of the chest wall: sonographic appearance of the fascial tail and staghorn patterns. *J Ultrasound Med.* 2009;28(3):393–396.

34. Shinagare AB, Ramaiya NH, Jagannathan JP, et al. A to Z of desmoid tumors. *AJR Am J Roentgenol.* 2011;197(6):W1008–W1014.

35. Nikolaidis P, Gabriel HA, Lamba AR, et al. Sonographic appearance of nodular fasciitis. *J Ultrasound Med.* 2006;25(2):281–285.

36. Bianchi S, Martinoli C, Abdelwahab IF, et al. Elastofibroma dorsi: sonographic findings. *AJR Am J Roentgenol.* 1997;169(4):1113–1115.

37. Dalal A, Miller TT, Kenan S. Sonographic detection of elastofibroma dorsi. *J Clin Ultrasound.* 2003;31(7):375–378.

38. Walker EA, Song AJ, Murphey MD. Magnetic resonance imaging of soft-tissue masses. *Semin Roentgenol.* 2010;45(4):277–297.

39. Waters B, Panicek DM, Lefkowitz RA, et al. Low-grade myxofibrosarcoma: CT and MRI patterns in recurrent disease. *AJR Am J Roentgenol.* 2007;188(2):W193–W198.

40. Kau T, Lesnik G, Arnold G, et al. Sonography of dermatofibrosarcoma protuberans of the groin. *J Clin Ultrasound.* 2008;36(8):520–522.

41. Stock H, Perino G, Athanasian E, et al. Leiomyoma of the foot: sonographic features with pathologic correlation. *HSS J.* 2011;7(1):9498.

42. Davies CE, Davies AM, Kindblom LG, et al. Soft tissue tumors with muscle differentiation. *Semin Musculoskelet Radiol.* 2010;14(2):245–256.

43. ter Braak BP, Guit GL, Bloem JL. Case 111: soft-tissue lymphoma. *Radiology.* 2007;243(1):293–296.

44. Chiou HJ, Chou YH, Chiou SY, et al. High-resolution ultrasonography of primary peripheral soft tissue lymphoma. *J Ultrasound Med.* 2005;24(1):77–86.

45. Vassallo P, Wernecke K, Roos N, et al. Differentiation of benign from malignant superficial lymphadenopathy: the role of high-resolution US. *Radiology.* 1992;183(1):215–220.

46. Giovagnorio F, Galluzzo M, Andreoli C, et al. Color Doppler sonography in the evaluation of superficial lymphomatous lymph nodes. *J Ultrasound Med.* 2002;21(4):403–408.

47. Esen G. Ultrasound of superficial lymph nodes. *Eur J Radiol.* 2006;58(3):345–359.

48. Choi AL, Koh SH, Jun SY, et al. Lymphoma involving the ulnar nerve: sonographic findings. *J Ultrasound Med.* 2008;27(10):1527–1531.

49. Kang BS, Choi SH, Cha HJ, et al. Subcutaneous panniculitis-like T-cell lymphoma: ultrasound and CT findings in three patients. *Skeletal Radiol.* 2007;36(suppl 1):67–71.

50. Murphey MD, Smith WS, Smith SE, et al. From the archives of the AFIP. Imaging of musculoskeletal neurogenic tumors: radiologic–pathologic correlation. *Radiographics.* 1999;19(5):1253–1280.

51. Reynolds DL Jr, Jacobson JA, Inampudi P, et al. Sonographic characteristics of peripheral nerve sheath tumors. *AJR Am J Roentgenol.* 2004;182(3):741–744.

52. Tsai WC, Chiou HJ, Chou YH, et al. Differentiation between schwannomas and neurofibromas in the extremities and superficial body: the role of high-resolution and color Doppler ultrasonography. *J Ultrasound Med.* 2008;27(2):161–166.

53. Lin J, Jacobson JA, Hayes CW. Sonographic target sign in neurofibromas. *J Ultrasound Med.* 1999;18(7):513–517.

54. Chen W, Jia JW, Wang JR. Soft tissue diffuse neurofibromas: sonographic findings. *J Ultrasound Med.* 2007;26(4):513–518.

55. Kransdorf MJ, Murphey MD, Fanburg-Smith JC. Classification of benign vascular lesions: history, current nomenclature, and suggestions for imagers. *AJR Am J Roentgenol.* 2011;197(1):8–11.

56. Donnelly LF, Adams DM, Bisset GS III. Vascular malformations and hemangiomas: a practical approach in a multidisciplinary clinic. *AJR Am J Roentgenol.* 2000;174(3):597–608.

57. Flors L, Leiva-Salinas C, Maged IM, et al. MR imaging of soft-tissue vascular malformations: diagnosis, classification, and therapy follow-up. *Radiographics.* 2011;31(5):1321–1340.

58. Dubois J, Alison M. Vascular anomalies: what a radiologist needs to know. *Pediatr Radiol.* 2010;40(6):895–905.

59. Jin W, Kim GY, Lee JII, et al. Intramuscular hemangioma with ossification: emphasis on sonographic findings. *J Ultrasound Med.* 2008;27(2):281–285.

60. Dubois J, Soulez G, Oliva VL, et al. Soft-tissue venous malformations in adult patients: imaging and therapeutic issues. *Radiographics.* 2001;21(6):1519–1531.

61. Hondar Wu HT, Chen W, Lee O, et al. Imaging and pathological correlation of soft-tissue chondroma: a serial five-case study and literature review. *Clin Imaging.* 2006;30(1):32–36.

62. Kransdorf MJ, Meis JM. From the archives of the AFIP. Extraskeletal osseous and cartilaginous tumors of the extremities. *Radiographics.* 1993;13(4):853–884.

63. Jacobson JA, Lenchik L, Ruhoy MK, et al. MR imaging of the infrapatellar fat pad of Hoffa. *Radiographics.* 1997;17(3):675–691.

64. Bianchi S, Zwass A, Abdelwahab IF, et al. Sonographic evaluation of soft tissue chondroma. *J Clin Ultrasound.* 1996;24(3):148–150.

65. Murphey MD, Gibson MS, Jennings BT, et al. From the archives of the AFIP: imaging of synovial sarcoma with radiologic–pathologic correlation. *Radiographics.* 2006;26(5):1543–1565.

66. Bixby SD, Hettmer S, Taylor GA, et al. Synovial sarcoma in children: imaging features and common benign mimics. *AJR Am J Roentgenol.* 2010;195(4):1026–1032.

67. Ward EE, Jacobson JA, Fessell DP, et al. Sonographic detection of Baker's cysts: comparison with MR imaging. *AJR Am J Roentgenol.* 2001;176(2):373–380.

68. Lee EY, Anthony MP, Leung AY, et al. Utility of FDG PET/CT in the assessment of myeloid sarcoma. *AJR Am J Roentgenol.* 2012;198(5):1175–1179.

69. Pui MH, Fletcher BD, Langston JW. Granulocytic sarcoma in childhood leukemia: imaging features. *Radiology.* 1994;190(3):698–702.

70. Lim HS, Park MH, Heo SH, et al. Myeloid sarcoma of the breast mimicking hamartoma on sonography. *J Ultrasound Med.* 2008;27(12):1777–1780.

71. An SB, Cheon JE, Kim IO, et al. Granulocytic sarcoma presenting with necrotic cervical lymph nodes as an initial manifestation of childhood leukaemia: imaging features. *Pediatr Radiol.* 2008;38(6):685–687.

72. Wortsman X. Sonography of the primary cutaneous melanoma: a review. *Radiol Res Pract.* 2012:814396.

73. Nazarian LN, Alexander AA, Kurtz AB, et al. Superficial melanoma metastases: appearances on gray-scale and color Doppler sonography. *AJR Am J Roentgenol.* 1998;170(2):459–463.

74. Catalano O, Caracò C, Mozzillo N, et al. Locoregional spread of cutaneous melanoma: sonography findings. *AJR Am J Roentgenol.* 2010;194(3):735–745.

75. Alexander AA, Nazarian LN, Feld RI. Superficial soft-tissue masses suggestive of recurrent malignancy: sonographic localization and biopsy. *AJR Am J Roentgenol.* 1997;169(5):1449–1451.

76. Giovagnorio F, Valentini C, Paonessa A. High-resolution and color Doppler sonography in the evaluation of skin metastases. *J Ultrasound Med.* 2003;22(10):1017–1022.

77. Magee T, Rosenthal H. Skeletal muscle metastases at sites of documented trauma. *AJR Am J Roentgenol.* 2002;178(4):985–988.

78. Murphey MD, McRae GA, Fanburg-Smith JC. Imaging of soft-tissue myxoma with emphasis on CT and MR and comparison of radiologic and pathologic findings. *Radiology.* 2002;225(1):215–224.

79. Bancroft LW, Kransdorf MJ, Menke DM, et al. Intramuscular myxoma: characteristic MR imaging features. *AJR Am J Roentgenol.* 2002;178(5):1255–1259.

80. Girish G, Jamadar DA, Landry D, et al. Sonography of intramuscular myxomas: the bright rim and bright cap signs. *J Ultrasound Med.* 2006;25(7):865–869.

81. Fornage BD, Romsdahl MM. Intramuscular myxoma: sonographic appearance and sonographically guided needle biopsy. *J Ultrasound Med.* 1994;13(2):91–94.

82. Murphey MD, Rhee JH, Lewis RB, et al. Pigmented villonodular synovitis: radiologic-pathologic correlation. *Radiographics.* 2008;28(5):1493–1518.

83. Middleton WD, Patel V, Teefey SA, et al. Giant cell tumors of the tendon sheath: analysis of sonographic findings. *AJR Am J Roentgenol.* 2004;183(2):337–339.

84. Wang Y, Tang J, Luo Y. The value of sonography in diagnosing giant cell tumors of the tendon sheath. *J Ultrasound Med.* 2007;26(10):1333–1340.

85. Glazebrook KN, Laundre BJ, Schiefer TK, et al. Imaging features of glomus tumors. *Skeletal Radiol.* 2011;40(7):855–862.

86. Park HJ, Jeon YH, Kim SS, et al. Gray-scale and color Doppler sonographic appearances of nonsubbungual soft-tissue glomus tumors. *J Clin Ultrasound.* 2011;39(6):305–309.

87. Hwang JY, Lee SW, Lee SM. The common ultrasonographic features of pilomatricoma. *J Ultrasound Med.* 2005;24(10):1397–1402.

88. Wang G, Jacobson JA, Feng FY, et al. Sonography of wrist ganglion cysts: variable and noncystic appearances. *J Ultrasound Med.* 2007;26(10):1323–1328.

89. Bui-Mansfield LT, Youngberg RA. Intraarticular ganglia of the knee: prevalence, presentation, etiology, and management. *AJR Am J Roentgenol.* 1997;168(1):123–127.

90. Ortega R, Fessell DP, Jacobson JA, et al. Sonography of ankle ganglia with pathologic correlation in 10 pediatric and adult patients. *AJR Am J Roentgenol.* 2002;178(6):1445–1449.

91. Cardinal E, Buckwalter KA, Braunstein EM, et al. Occult dorsal carpal ganglion: comparison of ultrasound and MR imaging. *Radiology.* 1994;193(1):259–62.

92. Teefey SA, Dahiya N, Middleton WD, et al. Ganglia of the hand and wrist: a sonographic analysis. *AJR Am J Roentgenol.* 2008;191(3):716–720.

93. Young NP, Sorenson EJ, Spinner RJ, et al. Clinical and electrodiagnostic correlates of peroneal intraneural ganglia. *Neurology.* 2009;72(5):447–452.

94. Spinner RJ, Desy NM, Amrami KK. Sequential tibial and peroneal intraneural ganglia arising from the superior tibiofibular joint. *Skeletal Radiol.* 2008;37(1):79–84.

95. Spinner RJ, Luthra G, Desy NM, et al. The clock face guide to peroneal intraneural ganglia: critical "times" and sites for accurate diagnosis. *Skeletal Radiol.* 2008;37(12):1091–1099.

96. Jose J, Fourzali R, Lesniak B, et al. Ultrasound-guided aspiration of symptomatic intraneural ganglion cyst within the tibial nerve. *Skeletal Radiol.* 2011;40(11):1473–1478.

97. Kim HK, Kim SM, Lee SH, et al. Subcutaneous epidermal inclusion cysts: ultrasound (US) and MR imaging findings. *Skeletal Radiol.* 2011;40(11):1415–1419.

98. Lee HS, Joo KB, Song HT, et al. Relationship between sonographic and pathologic findings in epidermal inclusion cysts. *J Clin Ultrasound.* 2001;29(7):374–383.

99. Jin W, Ryu KN, Kim GY, et al. Sonographic findings of ruptured epidermal inclusion cysts in superficial soft tissue: emphasis on shapes, pericystic changes, and pericystic vascularity. *J Ultrasound Med.* 2008;27(2):171–176.

100. Yuan WH, Hsu HC, Lai YC, et al. Differences in sonographic features of ruptured and unruptured epidermal cysts. *J Ultrasound Med.* 2012;31(2):265–272.

101. Robinson P, Farrant JM, Bourke G, et al. Ultrasound and MRI findings in appendicular and truncal fat necrosis. *Skeletal Radiol.* 2008;37(3):217–224.

102. Turecki MB, Taljanovic MS, Stubbs AY, et al. Imaging of musculoskeletal soft tissue infections. *Skeletal Radiol.* 2010;39(10):957–971.

103. Manzella A, Filho PB, Albuquerque E, et al. Imaging of gossypibomas: pictorial review. *AJR Am J Roentgenol.* 2009;193(suppl 6):94–101.

104. Beggs I. Sonography of muscle hernias. *AJR Am J Roentgenol.* 2003;180(2):395–399.

105. Bianchi S, Abdelwahab IF, Mazzola CG, et al. Sonographic examination of muscle herniation. *J Ultrasound Med.* 1995;14(5):357–360.

106. Sookur PA, Naraghi AM, Bleakney RR, et al. Accessory muscles: anatomy, symptoms, and radiologic evaluation. *Radiographics.* 2008;28(2):481–499.

107. Ouellette H, Thomas BJ, Torriani M. Using dynamic sonography to diagnose extensor digitorum brevis manus. *AJR Am J Roentgenol.* 2003;181(5):1224–1226.

108. Yu JS, Resnick D. MR imaging of the accessory soleus muscle appearance in six patients and a review of the literature. *Skeletal Radiol.* 1994;23(7):525–528.

109. Bianchi S, Abdelwahab IF, Oliveri M, et al. Sonographic diagnosis of accessory soleus muscle mimicking a soft tissue tumor. *J Ultrasound Med.* 1995;14(9):707–709.

110. Tyler P, Saifuddin A. The imaging of myositis ossificans. *Semin Musculoskelet Radiol.* 2010;14(2):201–216.

111. Abate M, Salini V, Rimondi E, et al. Post traumatic myositis ossificans: sonographic findings. *J Clin Ultrasound.* 2011;39(3):135–140.

112. Nakamura T, Higashi S, Tomoda K, et al. Cutaneous nodules in patients with rheumatoid arthritis: a case report and review of literatures. *Clin Rheumatol.* 2011;30(5):719–722.

113. Nalbant S, Corominas H, Hsu B, et al. Ultrasonography for assessment of subcutaneous nodules. *J Rheumatol.* 2003;30(6):1191–1195.

114. Thiele RG. Role of ultrasound and other advanced imaging in the diagnosis and management of gout. *Curr Rheumatol Rep.* 2011;13(2):146–153.

115. Olsen KM, Chew FS. Tumoral calcinosis: pearls, polemics, and alternative possibilities. *Radiographics.* 2006;26(3):871–885.

116. Bianchi S, Martinoli C, Waser NP, et al. Central aponeurosis tears of the rectus femoris: sonographic findings. *Skeletal Radiol.* 2002;31(10):581–586.

117. Bianchi S, Zwass A, Abdelwahab IF, et al. Diagnosis of tears of the quadriceps tendon of the knee: value of sonography. *AJR Am J Roentgenol.* 1994;162(5):1137–1140.

118. García CJ, Varela C, Abarca K, et al. Regional lymphadenopathy in cat-scratch disease: ultrasonographic findings. *Pediatr Radiol.* 2000;30(9):640–643.

119. Lin J, Jacobson JA, Jamadar DA, et al. Pigmented villonodular synovitis and related lesions: the spectrum of imaging findings. *AJR Am J Roentgenol.* 1999;172(1):191–197.

120. Murphey MD, Vidal JA, Fanburg-Smith JC, et al. Imaging of synovial chondromatosis with radiologic-pathologic correlation. *Radiographics.* 2007;27(5):1465–1488.

121. Roberts D, Miller TT, Erlanger SM. Sonographic appearance of primary synovial chondromatosis of the knee. *J Ultrasound Med.* 2004;23(5):707–709.

122. Learch TJ, Braaton M. Lipoma arborescens: high-resolution ultrasonographic findings. *J Ultrasound Med.* 2000;19(6):385–389.

123. Murphey MD, Choi JJ, Kransdorf MJ, et al. Imaging of osteochondroma: variants and complications with radiologic–pathologic correlation. *Radiographics.* 2000;20(5):1407–1434.

124. Bernard SA, Murphey MD, Flemming DJ, et al. Improved differentiation of benign osteochondromas from secondary chondrosarcomas with standardized measurement of cartilage cap at CT and MR imaging. *Radiology.* 2010;255(3):857–865.

125. Peersman B, Vanhoenacker FM, Heyman S, et al. Ewing's sarcoma: imaging features. *JBR-BTR.* 2007;90(5):368–376.

126. Mulligan ME, McRae GA, Murphey MD. Imaging features of primary lymphoma of bone. *AJR Am J Roentgenol.* 1999;173(6):1691–1697.

CHAPTER

10

Michel Court-Payen
Marcin Szkudlarek
Ian Beggs

Inflammatory Joint Diseases

INTRODUCTION

Ultrasound is increasingly used as a diagnostic modality in joint imaging by radiologists and rheumatologists. Several factors explain this development. Technical advances have improved image quality, simplified equipment, reduced cost, and improved diagnostic capability. New, highly effective treatments have become available that control joint inflammation and prevent or retard long-term joint damage, but early diagnosis of pre-destructive soft tissue changes is critical and best achieved by magnetic resonance imaging (MRI) or ultrasound. With the exception of pre-erosions (subcortical bone edema) and assessment of articular cartilage, MRI and ultrasound are equally effective in the diagnosis of inflammatory arthropathy.[1] Ultrasound is more operator-dependent than MRI and cannot always access all parts of a joint (e.g., between metacarpal heads). However, ultrasound has better spatial resolution than MRI in superficial areas, can be used to scan multiple joints and sites quickly, and readily distinguishes effusion from synovitis without needing intravenous contrast. Ultrasound is now viable as a diagnostic tool for office-based practice and for this reason has been adopted by many rheumatologists in their routine practice.

In this chapter we will present the ultrasound technique and criteria for examining patients with arthropathies, and discuss initial diagnosis and follow-up. We will discuss the ultrasound findings in conditions that target the synovial membrane (e.g., rheumatoid arthritis, juvenile idiopathic arthritis, and crystal arthropathies); inflammatory arthropathies that target both entheses and synovial membrane (spondyloarthopathies); and other arthropathies (osteoarthritis, pigmented villonodular synovitis, synovial osteochondromatosis, amyloid, septic arthritis, and hemophiliac arthropathy). Finally, we will describe ultrasound-guided interventions.

Although the cost of ultrasound equipment has reduced considerably in real terms, high-quality equipment remains essential. High-frequency (>10 MHz) linear array transducers are essential, although larger joints may need curvilinear transducers and lower frequencies.

Small footprint transducers are useful for the small joints of the hands and feet. A standoff is not required, but copious jelly helps. Beam steering and compound imaging are also useful. Joints should be relaxed when examined, and transducer pressure should be light or fluid may be displaced and missed or vascularity effaced.

> **Tip:**
> Use light transducer pressure or fluid or hyperemia may be missed.

New developments are being assessed for possible roles in joint disease: 3D imaging (possible quantification of the volume of inflamed synovium, regional vessels, or erosions); intravenous contrast agents (improved visualization of vascularity); elastography (compressibility of soft tissues); and fusion imaging (direct correlation of ultrasound to computed tomography [CT] and/or MRI). As yet, no practical applications for these techniques have been established in routine rheumatological practices.

Standardization of technique and diagnoses has been facilitated by the adoption of a number of consensus definitions[2]:

Synovial fluid: Intra-articular material that is displaceable and compressible and does not exhibit Doppler signal. It is usually anechoic **(Fig. 10.1)** or hypoechoic but may be hyperechoic.

Synovial hypertrophy: Abnormal intra-articular tissue that is not displaceable and is poorly compressible. It may/may not exhibit Doppler signal and is usually hypoechoic **(Figs. 10.2 and 10.3)**.

Tenosynovitis: Thickened tissue (+/− fluid) within a tendon sheath seen in two perpendicular planes. It may/may not exhibit Doppler signal and is usually hypoechoic **(Figs. 10.4 and 10.5)**.

Bone erosion: An intra-articular discontinuity in the bone surface that is visible in two perpendicular planes **(Fig. 10.6)**.

Enthesopathy: Abnormally hypoechoic and/or thickened tendon or ligament at its bony attachment with loss

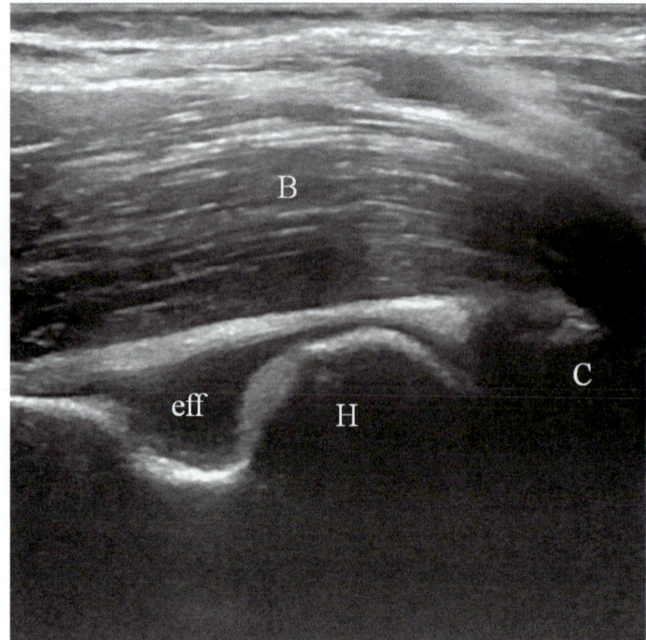

Figure 10.1. Longitudinal scan of anterior elbow. Anechoic effusion (*eff*) in anterior recess. B, brachialis muscle; C, coronoid process of ulna; H, humerus.

of the normal fibrillar pattern seen in two perpendicular planes. Echogenic foci due to calcification, Doppler signal, and bony changes (due to enthesophytes, erosions, or irregularity) may be present.

In clinical practice, the diagnosis of "active arthritis" (or clinical synovitis) is based primarily on clinical evaluation, but it is often difficult to determine whether

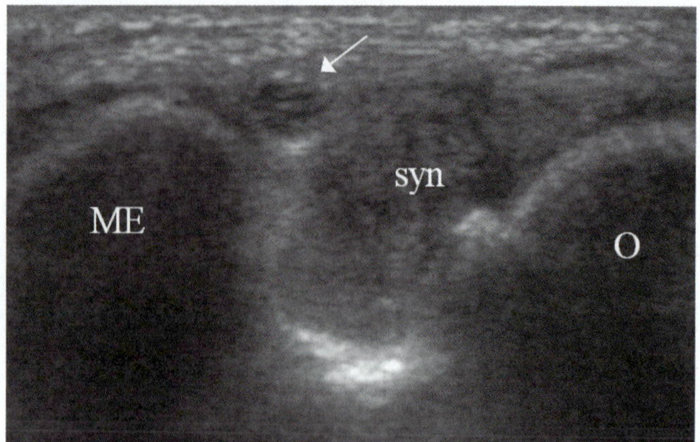

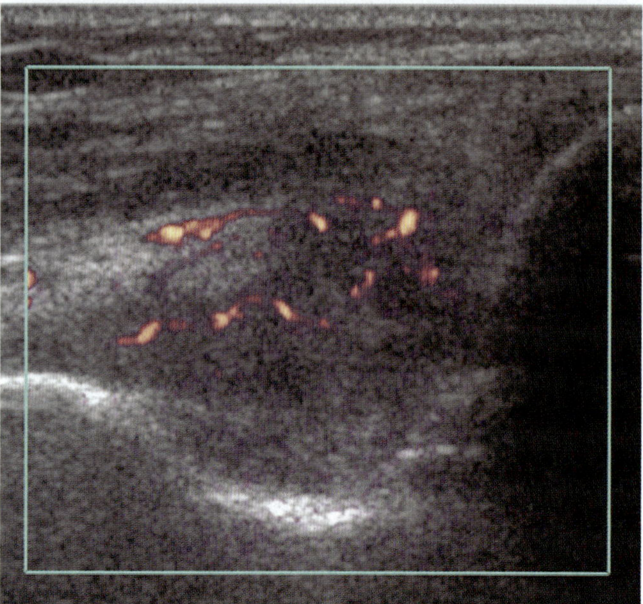

Figure 10.2. Patient with synovial hypertrophy (*syn*) in elbow. **A:** Transverse posteromedial ultrasound scan showing displacement of ulnar nerve (*arrow*). O, olecranon; ME, medial epicondyle of humerus. **B:** Power Doppler examination shows synovial hyperemia.

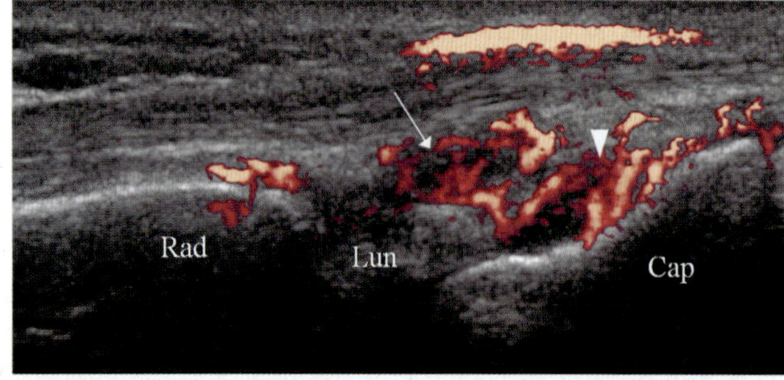

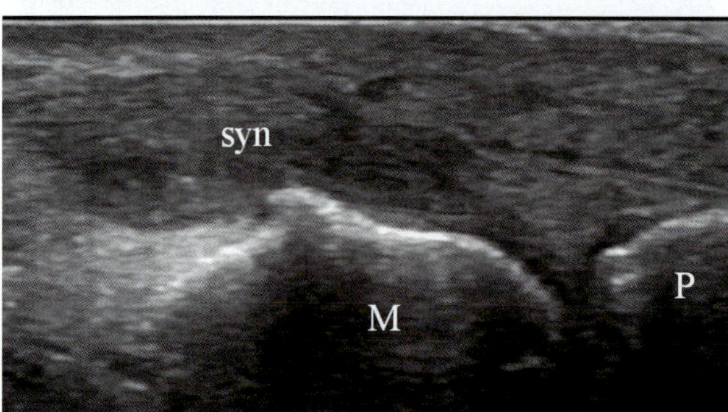

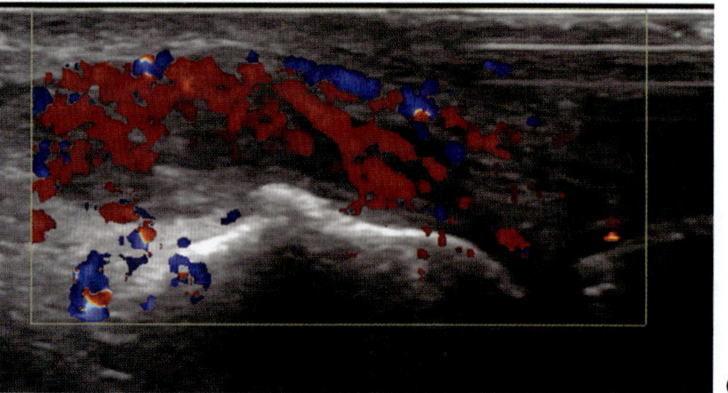

Figure 10.3. Rheumatoid arthritis patients. **A:** Dorsal longitudinal ultrasound scan of the wrist shows synovial thickening in the recesses of the radiocarpal (*arrow*) and midcarpal (*arrowhead*) joints. Synovial hyperemia on power Doppler examination confirms active synovitis. Rad, radius; Lun, lunate; Cap, capitate **B:** Dorsal longitudinal ultrasound scan of the third MCP joint shows synovial thickening (*syn*) extending from the joint line and along the metacarpal head (*M*). P, proximal phalanx. **C:** Synovial hyperemia on color Doppler examination confirms active synovitis.

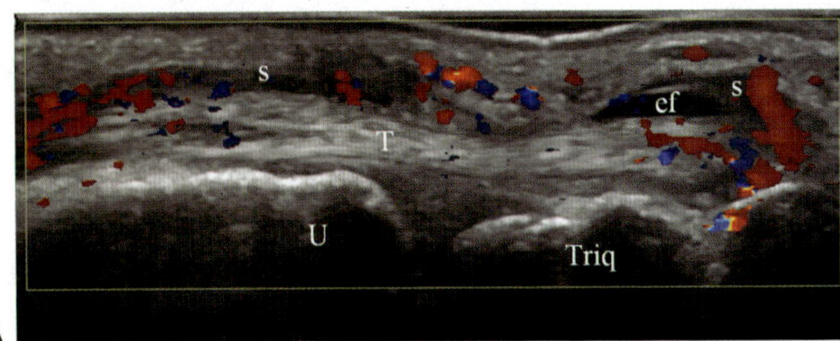

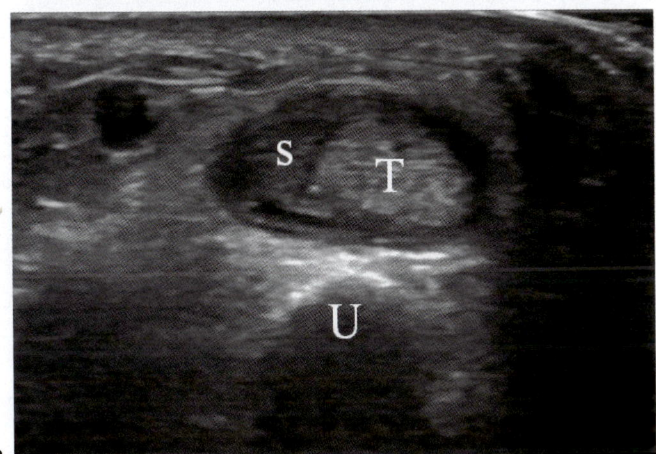

Figure 10.4. Longitudinal (**A**) and transverse (**B**) scans of the extensor carpi ulnaris tendon (*T*) at the wrist of a patient with RA and tenosynovitis. The tendon is slightly enlarged. Effusion (*ef*) and synovial thickening (*S*) in the tendon sheath. Color Doppler (*A*) shows tendon and synovial hyperemia. U, ulna; Triq, triquetrum.

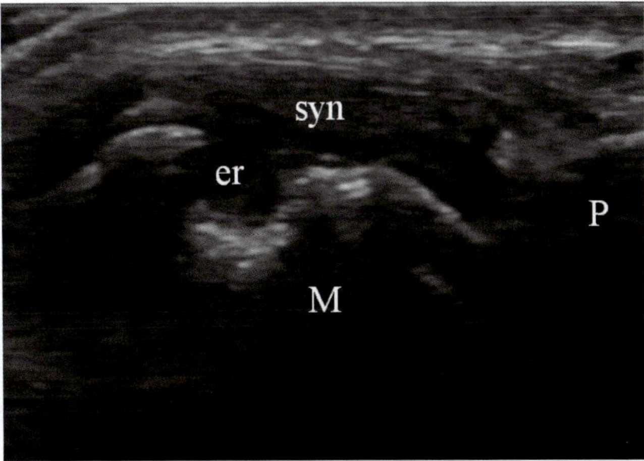

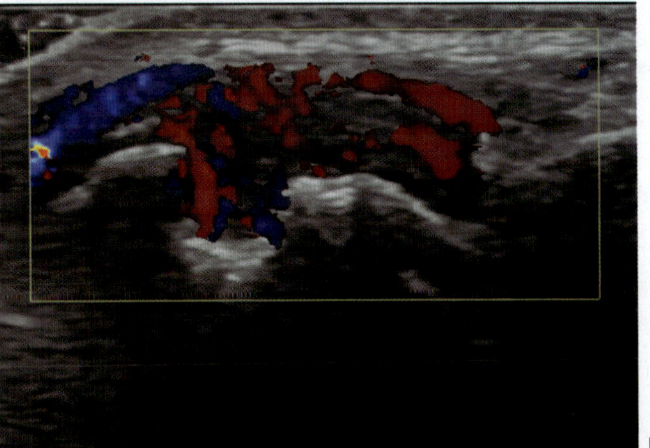

Figure 10.6. Dorsal longitudinal scans of second MTP joint in patient with RA. **A:** Synovial hypertrophy (*syn*) with erosion of metatarsal head (*er*). M, metatarsal head; P, proximal phalanx. **B:** Synovial hyperemia on color Doppler examination confirms active synovitis.

joint pain, swelling, and/or limitation of mobility are caused by synovitis, tenosynovitis, enthesitis, or peri-articular edema. Ultrasound has become a valuable adjunct in rheumatology. Ultrasound examination of joints demonstrates with high accuracy most of the ana-tomical structures involved: synovial recesses, articular/periarticular bone contours, ligaments, tendons, and tendon sheaths (including the bony insertions or enthe-ses of ligaments and tendons), and bursae. Ultrasound can demonstrate inflammatory changes (hyperemia, synovial thickening, or effusion in joint recesses, bur-sae, or tendon sheaths) and destructive changes (bone erosions, joint destruction or ankylosis, cartilage loss, and tendon tears).

Most of the early studies that described the ultrasound findings in inflammatory arthropathy were performed on patients with rheumatoid arthritis (RA), but these findings are not specific and can be found in most types of joint diseases.

EXAMINATION TECHNIQUE

In general, joints are best examined with long-axis scans to show the joint recesses. Tendon sheaths are best stud-ied in short axis when the transducer can be moved proximally and distally, employing an "elevator" tech-nique. Bursae and Baker cysts are shown in two planes. Typical sites of synovitis include the ulnar aspect of the

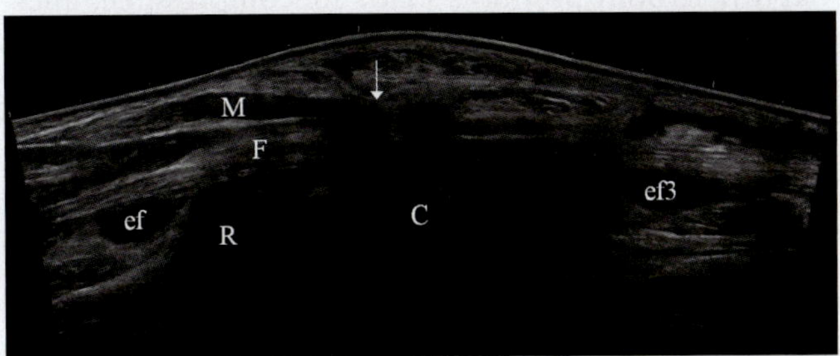

Figure 10.5. Tenosynovitis of the flexor digitorum tendons of the long finger (*F*). Longitudinal ultrasound scan shows effusion in the flexor tendon sheath proximal (*ef*) and distal (*ef3*) to the carpal tun-nel. Median nerve is enlarged proximal to the carpal tunnel (*M*) and compressed under the flexor retinaculum (*arrow*). R, radius; C, carpus.

wrist, the metacarpophalangeal joints (MCPJs) especially the dorsal margins, and the suprapatellar recess of the knee.

Hand and Wrist

The hand/wrist is the area most frequently examined for inflammatory arthropathy. Ultrasound anatomy and technique have been described in Chapter 5 and will not be repeated in detail here, but a systematic approach to the examination is essential. The thumb and interphalangeal joints are not usually included unless there is a specific indication. By moving the transducer slowly, the entire examination can be performed as a combined grayscale and Doppler procedure.

Start by examining the dorsal aspects of the second to fifth MCPJs with the hand pronated, fingers extended, and the transducer placed longitudinally (**Fig. 10.7**). Flexion at the wrist or MCPJs reduces the conspicuity of both grayscale and Doppler evidence of synovitis.[3] With grayscale and Doppler gain and focal zone suitably adjusted, examine each joint in turn by moving the transducer slowly backward and forward from medial to lateral. At the second and fifth MCPJs, respectively, continue the movement to examine the radial and ulnar aspects of the joints.

Now place the transducer transversely on Lister tubercle to examine the second to fifth extensor compartments before internally and externally rotating the wrist to examine the sixth and first extensor compartments, respectively. In each position, an "elevator" technique is employed by moving the transducer to and fro, proximally and distally. The transducer is then rotated through 90 degrees on the dorsal aspect of the carpals and again moved backward and forward, from radial to ulnar, to examine the wrist and midcarpal joints. The hand is then supinated and the transducer placed transversely across the carpal tunnel and moved proximally and distally looking for evidence of flexor tenosynovitis. Finally, the volar aspects of the second to fifth MCPJs are examined in similar fashion to the dorsal aspects.

Foot and Ankle

A similar approach to the hand/wrist is used. The dorsal and plantar aspects of the metatarsophalangeal (MTP) joints and the dorsal midfoot are examined with the transducer placed longitudinally. The medial, peroneal, and anterior tendons at the ankle are examined transversely using a proximal and distal elevator technique, and the anteromedial and lateral gutters are also examined transversely.

Other Joints

Although long-axis scans of joints are usually preferred, short-axis scans can be useful, for example, in looking for fluid or synovitis in the medial and lateral pouches of the suprapatellar recess of the knee.

ULTRASOUND FINDINGS IN INFLAMMATORY JOINT DISEASES

Synovitis

Detection of synovitis is important because synovitis precedes bone erosions. Ultrasound is better than clinical examination and radiographs, and comparable to MRI in detecting synovitis.[1] Synovial hypertrophy and joint fluid are both frequently present (**Fig. 10.8**). Normal synovium is so thin it is not seen with ultrasound. Synovial hypertrophy produces solid, noncompressible, thickened hypoechoic tissue in joints and tendon sheaths.[2,4,5] The echogenicity of the thickened synovium is inversely proportional to its water content: the more fluid that is present, the less echogenic the synovium. A semiquantitative grading system (normal/mild/moderate/large) for synovial hypertrophy may be employed.[6] Joint or tendon sheath fluid is usually anechoic or hypoechoic, and compressible. A complex or echogenic appearance is due to proteinaceous fluid, crystals, or debris. Even in large and easily palpable joints such as the knee, ultrasound is more sensitive in detecting fluid than clinical examination or radiographs.[7,8] Volumes as small as 1 mL

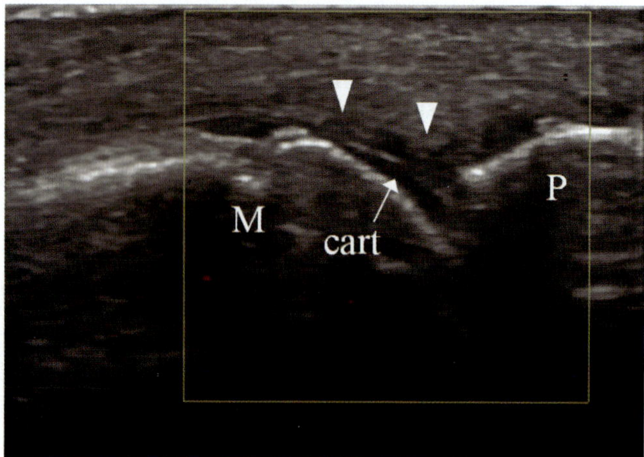

Figure 10.7. Dorsal longitudinal scan of normal second MCP joint showing normal capsule (*arrowheads*) and no synovial thickening. M, metacarpal head with anechoic cartilage (*cart*); P, proximal phalanx.

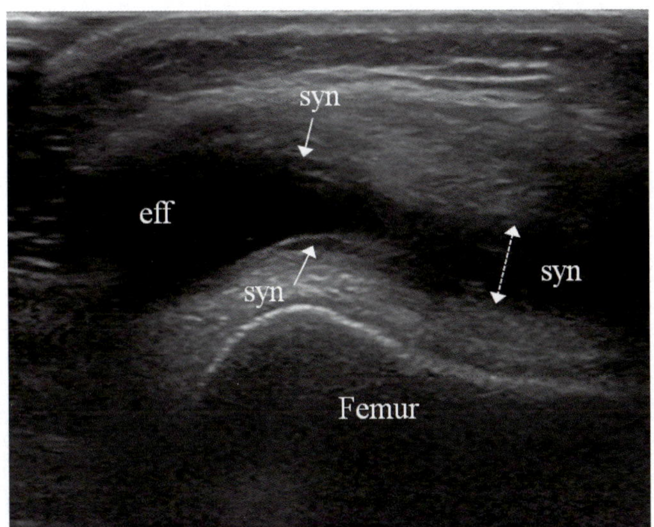

Figure 10.8.   Transverse scan of suprapatellar recess of knee. Transducer pressure on right of image displaces fluid to left and distinguishes effusion (*eff*) from synovial hypertrophy (*syn*).

and interobserver agreement of 79% can be found in small joints of the hands and feet.[8]

In patients with doubtful hypoechoic or anechoic areas in superficial joints, compression with the transducer[9] distinguishes between synovial hypertrophy (poorly compressible, non-displaceable) and effusion (compressible, displaceable) **(Fig. 10.8)**. This does not work for deep joints like the hip.

> **Tip:**
> Joint fluid is compressible and displaceable. Synovial thickening is poorly compressible and non-displaceable.

Synovial hypertrophy occurs in both acute (inflammation) and chronic (fibrosis) stages of inflammatory joint disease, and it is not possible to distinguish between them using grayscale ultrasound. Doppler techniques (color or power Doppler) are therefore widely employed for diagnosis and follow-up of arthritic joints.

> **Tip:**
> Use Doppler to distinguish between active and chronic (inactive) synovitis.

Doppler techniques detect tissue hyperemia, which is associated with disease activity **(Figs. 10.2 and 10.3)**. Some authors use power Doppler. Depending on the sensitivity of the ultrasound equipment, others prefer color Doppler. Synovial hyperemia on Doppler ultrasound correlates well with contrast enhancement on MRI[10,11] and microvascular density on histology.[12] Synovial tissue may be seen extending into erosions **(Fig. 10.6)**, sometimes with vascular signal,[13] probably related to erosion

activity **(Fig. 10.6)**. Fluid does not show Doppler signal and this helps to distinguish active synovitis from fluid. Light transducer pressure is essential as even moderate pressure may efface vessels and flow.

Intravenous injection of ultrasound contrast has been used to increase the sensitivity of Doppler examinations.[10,14,15] However, the sensitivity of current generation ultrasound machines has improved dramatically, even without contrast enhancement, and with high-end units it is now possible to display physiological joint flow.[16] The use of intravenous ultrasound contrast increases the cost and time of the examination, and is invasive. Contrast is not used in routine clinical practice although it has been shown to improve the diagnosis of sacroiliitis.[17]

Doppler findings[5] can be reported in three different ways: qualitative assessment, semiquantitative grading, and quantitative assessment. Qualitative assessment is a simple report of the presence or absence of synovial flow. Semiquantitative scoring is the most often used technique in daily practice[10,13] and employs a grading scale depending on the severity of findings.[1] Quantitative assessment[18,19] is time-consuming but is more precise and is used for trials. It is performed by calculating the number of pixels showing power Doppler signal or by calculating the resistive index from spectral Doppler measurements. Future ultrasound systems may provide automatic measurements.

Bony Changes

Ultrasound of articular and periarticular bone surfaces can display erosions **(Fig. 10.3)**, which are important signs in aggressive arthritis such as RA. Erosions are not disease-specific and can occur in other types of inflammatory joint disease. Small bone defects resembling erosions can be found in healthy controls.[20] Erosions typically occur in the bare area of a joint (i.e., the intracapsular cortex that is not covered by hyaline cartilage) and are seen as focal cortical defects identified in two perpendicular planes. Active erosions may show Doppler signal **(Fig. 10.6)**.

> **Tip:**
> Erosions usually occur at the bare area of a joint.

Ultrasound is more sensitive than radiographs and comparable to MRI in detecting erosions in fingers[21,22] or toes.[1] The specificity of ultrasound is lower than that of CT, probably because small cortical defects occur as normal findings. Some studies have found ultrasound to be less sensitive in detecting erosions than MRI,[23] possibly because of inaccessibility (e.g., on the lateral and medial margins of metacarpal and metatarsal heads or at the wrist joint).[1,22] A drawback of ultrasound is that it cannot detect bone marrow edema, which has been shown to be an important prognostic factor on MRI. Bone erosions in early undifferentiated arthritis increase the risk of developing persistent arthritis.[23]

Cartilage Changes

Normal hyaline or articular cartilage forms a hypoechoic layer that covers the bright surface of the subchondral bone plate. Its thickness can be measured by ultrasound.[9] The superficial surface of normal cartilage is seen as a smooth, thin echogenic line. In inflammatory and degenerative joint diseases, nonspecific destructive cartilaginous changes can be detected with diffuse or focal thinning **(Fig. 10.9)**, irregularity of the surface, or defects.

Tenosynovitis

In tenosynovitis, hypoechoic or anechoic fluid and/or synovial proliferation are seen around the tendon in the tendon sheath. Synovial hypertrophy may be nodular and show abnormal Doppler signal. Tendinopathy (with or without tenosynovitis) is defined by intratendinous changes: hypoechoic thickening best demonstrated on transverse scans, and disorganization of the fibrillar tendon structure best seen on longitudinal scans. Paratendinitis is an inflammatory thickening of the para-tendon, which can be pronounced in some arthritides (RA, crystal or infectious arthritides, and juvenile idiopathic arthritis). Tendon tears are defined by areas of interruption of tendon fibers and may be partial (transverse or longitudinal with tendon split) or complete (transverse tears). In aggressive inflammatory joint diseases such as RA, synovial tissue can enter tendon erosions, similarly to bony erosions.

Enthesitis

Enthesopathy refers to a pathological condition at the bony attachment of tendons, ligaments, capsule, or fascia, and can be mechanical or secondary to an inflammatory process (enthesitis). Enthesitis is characteristic of sero-negative spondyloarthropathies such as ankylosing spondylitis and psoriasis. Signs of inflammation in the spondyloarthropathies are more frequent at insertion sites than in the synovial membrane of joints or tendon sheaths. This is the opposite of RA[24] and is useful when considering the differential diagnosis, although a specific diagnosis cannot be achieved with ultrasound alone.

The presence of inflammation at insertion sites is difficult to assess clinically. Radiographs show bony changes (enthesophytes, bony irregularity, and erosions) and tendon calcification at a late stage, often only after many years of symptoms.[25] Ultrasound and MRI can demonstrate the early soft tissue signs of inflammation. Ultrasound shows the soft tissue part of insertion sites in greater detail than MRI, especially at small structures, and is a helpful adjunct to clinical examination. Ultrasound shows focal hypoechoic thickening of the tendon insertion in two orthogonal planes, sometimes with hyperemia, calcifications, or bony changes.[2] Adjacent bursae may also be inflamed (e.g., enthesitis of the Achilles tendon and retrocalcaneal bursitis). As ultrasound can show only the surface of bone at an enthesis, local bone edema is not detectable, and this is a disadvantage compared with water-sensitive MRI sequences (STIR, fat-suppressed T2-weighted) or fat-suppressed contrast-enhanced T1-weighted sequences.[26] However, only large calcifications or spurs can be seen on MRI, whereas ultrasound shows even small enthesophytes.

Bursitis

Most peripheral bursae are accessible to ultrasound. Bursitis is diagnosed when a bursa is enlarged with fluid and synovial thickening or completely filled with synovial tissue **(Fig. 10.10)**. Doppler signal may be present. Bursal fluid is often anechoic but inflammation, infection, blood, and crystals may result in echogenic fluid.

Bursae occur at many sites, for example, the olecranon bursa at the elbow, the retrocalcaneal bursa at the ankle, the subacromial bursa of the shoulder and around the knee.

In patients with swelling and/or pain of the knee and/or popliteal fossa, a Baker cyst is easily diagnosed at ultrasound by demonstrating a comma-shaped cyst with its characteristic neck between the medial head of

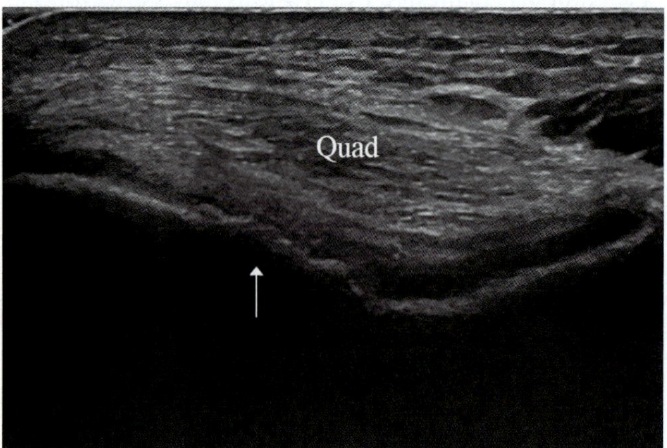

Figure 10.9. Transverse scan of femoral trochlea with knee in full flexion. Cartilage thinning and irregular hyperostosis are present on lateral aspect of trochlea (*arrow*). Quad, Quadriceps tendon.

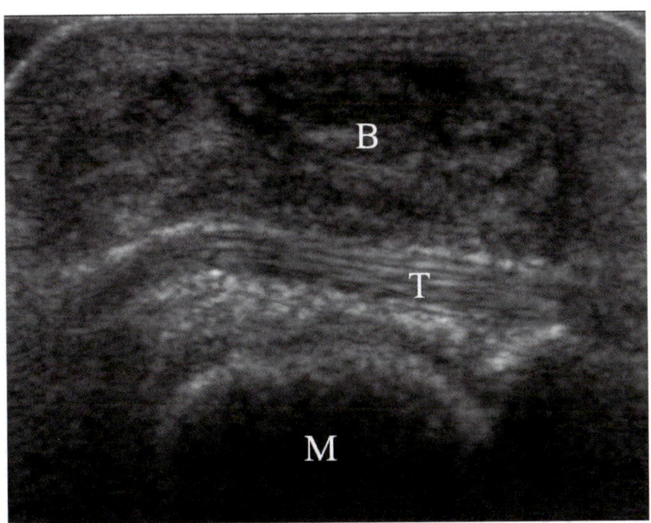

Figure 10.10.   Rheumatoid bursitis superficial to first metatarsophalangeal joint. Longitudinal ultrasound scan shows enlarged hypoechoic bursa (*B*) superficial to flexor hallucis longus tendon (*T*) and first metatarsal head (*M*).

gastrocnemius and the semimembranosus tendon. The cyst may be filled with solid synovial tissue in inflammatory joint disease. Ultrasound identifies other causes of popliteal masses (tumor, aneurysm, ganglion cyst, hematoma, and abscess) and distinguishes between ruptured Baker cyst, when fluid is seen tracking along fascial planes, and deep venous thrombosis in patients with acute leg swelling.

Adventitial bursae occur at sites of mechanical friction, often related to sports or occupation. They fill with fluid and do not have a synovial lining.

INFLAMMATORY JOINT DISEASES

Rheumatoid Arthritis

RA is a chronic, symmetric autoimmune disease characterized by joint inflammation, destruction of small and large joints, and extra-articular manifestations. Until 2010 it was diagnosed according to the American College of Rheumatology (ACR) 1987 Classification Criteria[27] based on clinical assessment, immunological markers (presence of rheumatoid factor), and conventional radiography.

The new 2010 European League Against Rheumatism (EULAR)/ACR Classification Criteria for RA[28] allows ultrasound to supplement the clinical examination. By showing the extent of joint involvement, the status of the disease may change from a mono- or oligoarthritis to polyarthritis,[29] thus potentially changing the diagnosis and instigating potent treatments. Only ultrasound signs of inflammation/synovitis play a role. No place is given to evidence of joint destruction although ultrasound has high sensitivity for the detection of bone erosions in small joints,[1,21,30] particularly in early disease.[22]

Typical symmetrical involvement of the wrist joints (most often around the styloid process of the ulna) **(Fig. 10.11)** and the small joints of the extremities can be easily detected with ultrasound (MCP-, MTP- and proximal interphalangeal [PIP]-joints). Tenosynovitis and possible tendon ruptures can also be detected (extensor carpi ulnaris and other extensor tendons, flexor digitorum tendons with carpal tunnel syndrome) **(Fig. 10.12)**. Ultrasound shows all changes in joints affected by RA with the exception of bone edema and bone/cartilage damages in areas not accessible by ultrasound. Detection of joint effusion, synovial thickening, synovial hyperemia/inflammation with Doppler techniques, tendon pathology such as inflammation, fluid in tendon sheaths and bursae, tendon rupture, cartilage thinning, and bone erosions are all possible with ultrasound.

Rheumatoid Nodules

Rheumatoid nodules are areas of fibrinoid necrosis surrounded by fibrous tissue seen in up to 25% of patients with RA, usually with active disease and high levels of rheumatoid factor. Nodules are usually subcutaneous

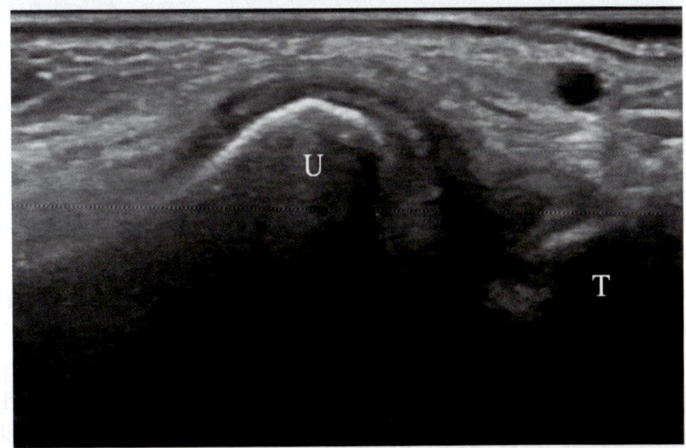

A

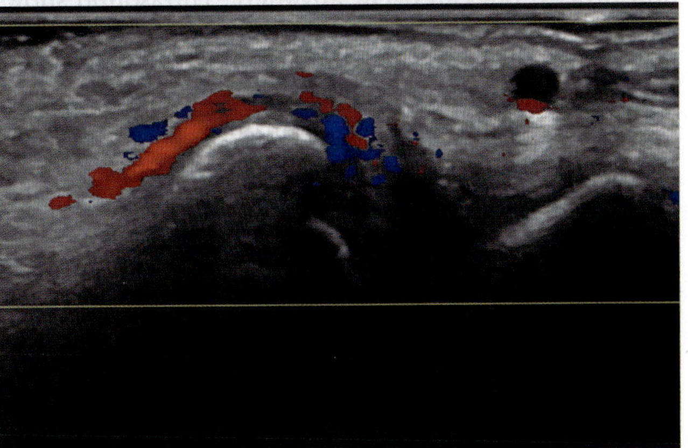

B

Figure 10.11.   Rheumatoid arthritis patient. **A:** Hypoechoic synovial hypertrophy on ulnar aspect of wrist and around ulnar head (*U*). T, triquetrum. **B:** Synovial hyperemia around ulnar head on color Doppler examination is a sign of disease activity.

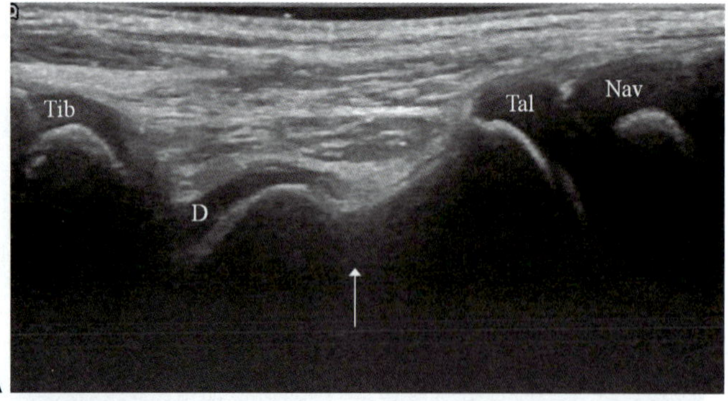

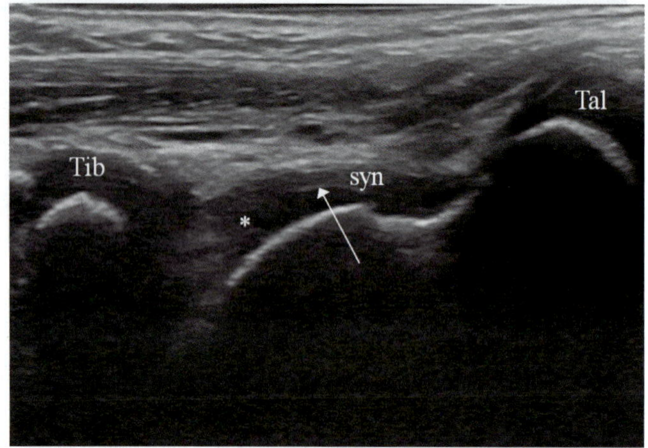

Figure 10.15.   Dorsal longitudinal ultrasound scans of ankles of 4-year-old children. **A:** Normal ankle with thick hypoechoic cartilage on talar dome (*D*) and in growing epiphyses of distal tibia (*Tib*), distal talus (*Tal*), and navicular (*Nav*). No sign of synovitis. **B:** Juvenile idiopathic arthritis with hypoechoic synovial hypertrophy in anterior ankle joint recess. The interface between cartilage and synovium (*syn*) is seen when the ultrasound beam is perpendicular to the cartilage surface (*arrow*), but not identified when the ultrasound beam is angled due to anisotropy (*asterisk*).

Diagnosis with Ultrasound

MRI provides a more complete joint examination than ultrasound, but requires sedation of young children, an age group with a high prevalence of JIA. Consequently, ultrasound has a significant role in the assessment of disease activity. Young children can be seated on a parent's lap or play while being examined. The way a child communicates joint discomfort varies. Ultrasound is particularly useful if there are few verbal complaints, for example, in infants. Ultrasound is also more informative than clinical examination,[49] and subclinical synovitis is frequently detected by ultrasound, particularly in the hands and feet. There are no validated MRI- or ultrasound-scoring systems for evaluating inflammatory and destructive joint abnormalities in JIA.

Follow-up with Ultrasound

Ultrasound may detect decreases in joint effusion and synovial hypertrophy in patients treated systemically or with intra-articular steroid injections.[46,47] Confirmation of remission cannot rely solely on clinical examination, but must include repeated imaging to confirm the absence of subclinical inflammation,[50] although further studies are needed to evaluate the reliability of ultrasound assessment of treatment response.

A proportion of JIA patients who do not receive treatment will develop progressive joint destruction, growth disturbances, and serious functional disability, but the course of the disease is difficult to predict. One important prognostic factor is the JIA subtype. Early use of new highly efficacious treatments has improved the outcome in many patients with JIA. Ultrasound has the potential to detect subclinical synovitis or enthesitis, which might lead to change in disease categorization (e.g., from oligoarthritis to polyarthritis or enthesitis-related arthritis) and early change of therapy. Ultrasound detection of bone erosions early in the course of JIA is also an indicator of poor long-term outcome.

Crystal Deposition Diseases

In crystal deposition diseases, crystals are deposited in joints and periarticular soft tissues. The main crystals are monosodium urate, calcium pyrophosphate (CPPD), and calcium hydroxyapatite (HADD), although mixed crystal deposition may occur. Crystal deposition can cause inflammation or articular damage, although many patients are asymptomatic. Aspiration of joint fluid is needed for definitive diagnosis and may be facilitated by ultrasound-guided aspiration. Examination under polarized light microscopy distinguishes urate from pyrophosphate crystals. However, characteristic patterns of deposition may allow ultrasound differentiation between urate and pyrophosphate deposition.[51] Ultrasound can also show erosions and synovitis in established joint disease.

Gout

Gout results from deposition of monosodium urate crystals. Acute gout can occur at any joint, but preferentially involves the lower limb. Classically it involves the first MTP joint (podagra) and presents with severe pain, erythema, and swelling. Ultrasound shows synovial thickening, Doppler signal, and periarticular edema. Joint fluid during an acute attack may be anechoic, but pressure with the transducer may elicit a "snowstorm" appearance due to displacement of crystals, which are typically heterogeneous in size and shape.

Monosodium urate crystals are characteristically deposited on the surface of articular cartilage. The crystals are strongly reflective, even with low gain settings, and produce echogenic foci on the surface of the cartilage, resulting in a "double contour" appearance **(Fig. 10.16)**.

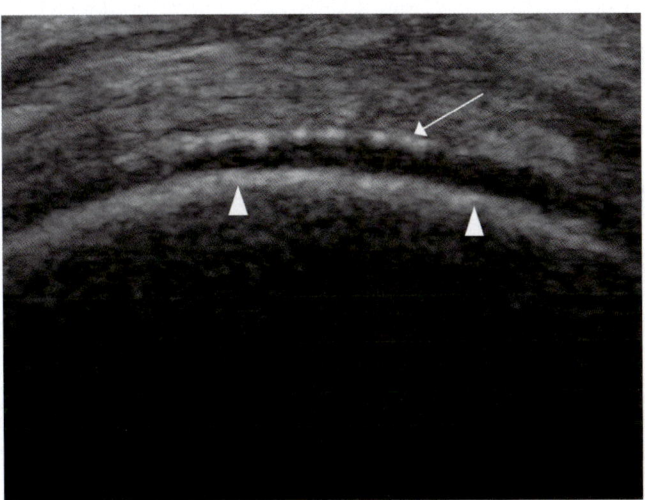

Figure 10.16.   Ultrasound examination of the femoral articular cartilage of the knee of a patient with gout. The double contour appearance due to echogenic crystal deposition on the surface of the cartilage (*arrow*) is characteristic of gout. Note the subchondral bone (*arrowheads*).

> **Tip:**
> A "double contour" appearance due to deposition of echogenic crystals on the surface of articular cartilage is pathognomonic of gout.

Tophi are larger aggregations of monosodium urate crystals, most often seen in fingers, toes, and at the olecranon bursa at the elbow. They may be intra-articular or extra-articular and extend into tendons. Tophi may be soft, hard, or mixed. Soft tophi contain multiple small echogenic foci without distal acoustic shadowing. Hard tophi are echogenic and have distal acoustic shadowing (**Fig. 10.17**). Doppler signal may be prominent. Ultrasound may show intra-articular erosions and synovial thickening. The synovial thickening is uniform, whereas intra-articular tophi are nodular. Erosions in association with tophi are more common in the feet than hands.[52,53]

Calcium Pyrophosphate Deposition Disease

Calcium pyrophosphate deposition in hyaline cartilage and fibrocartilage is often an asymptomatic incidental finding on radiographs. Pseudogout is an acute arthritis due to pyrophosphate deposition and usually affects large joints, typically the knee (**Fig. 10.18**). Pyrophosphate crystals are deposited within articular cartilage. This distinguishes CPPD from gout, in which the crystals are on the surface of the cartilage.

> **Tip:**
> Echogenic crystal deposition deep to the surface of articular cartilage is typical of CPPD.

Pyrophosphate crystals in fibrocartilage, such as the menisci of the knee, result in punctate, echogenic calcifications with or without posterior acoustic shadowing. Streaky calcification may be seen in tendons, synovium, and joint capsules.

Hydroxyapatite Deposition Disease

Hydroxyapatite crystals are characteristic of calcific tendinitis and may be seen in destructive arthropathies such as cuff tear arthropathy. Tendon deposits are frequently densely echogenic and have posterior acoustic shadowing. In acute calcific tendinitis, when the calcium softens and the patient presents with acute, severe pain, the calcium may be only faintly echogenic, difficult to distinguish from adjacent tendon, lack acoustic shadowing, and be surrounded by Doppler signal.

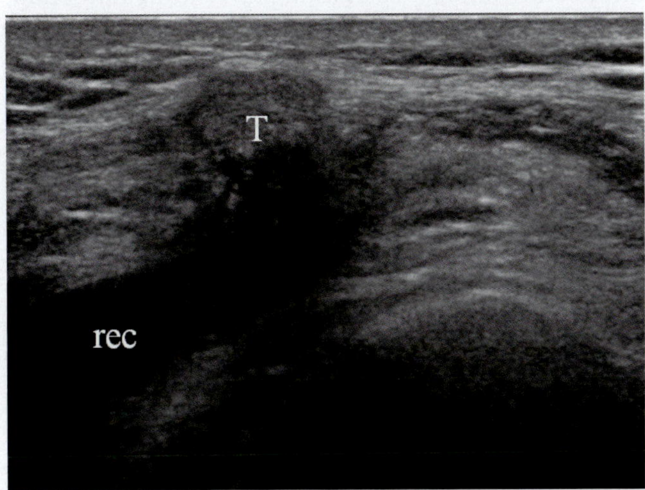

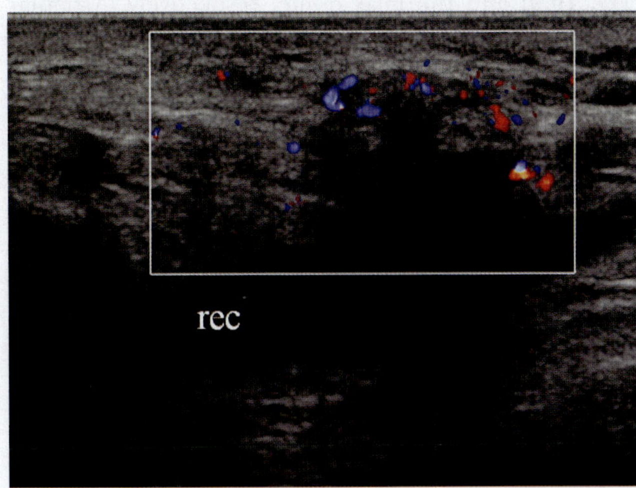

Figure 10.17.   Transverse scan of the parapatellar recess (*rec*) of a patient with gout. **A:** A palpable tophus close to the parapatellar recess is inhomogeneous, hyperechoic, and casts strong acoustic shadowing (*T*). **B:** Peripheral hyperemia on color Doppler confirms the presence of inflammation.

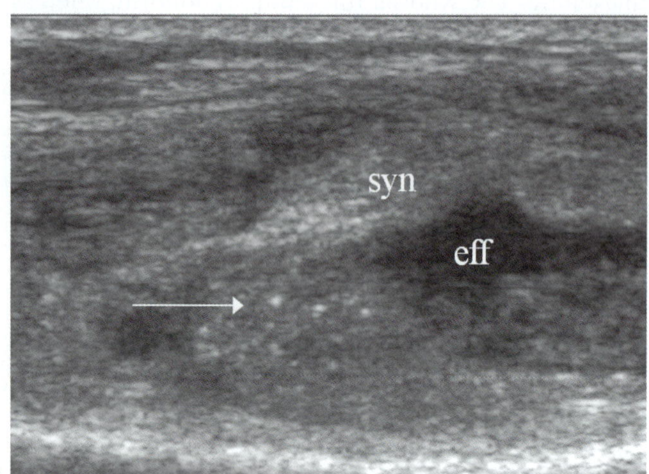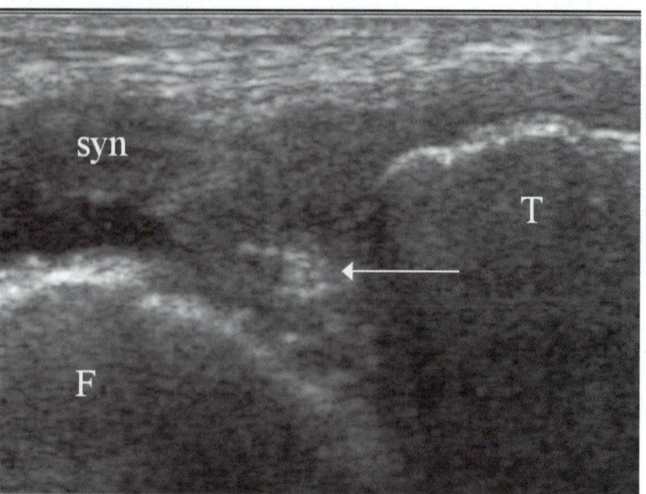

Figure 10.18.   Patient with CPPD disease. **A:** Effusion (*eff*) and synovial thickening (*syn*) in the knee, with tiny echogenic foci of micro-calcification in synovium (*arrow*). **B:** Calcific deposits in the medial meniscus (*arrow*). F, femur; T, tibia.

OTHER JOINT DISEASES

Osteoarthritis

Nonspecific changes in osteoarthritis include joint fluid, synovial thickening, and thickening and bulging of the joint capsule.[54,55] Enthesopathic changes, such as thickening and loss of fibrillar architecture, may be seen at tendon and ligament insertions. Abnormal Doppler signal in joints or at entheses and intra-articular erosions may be present and are not exclusive to inflammatory arthropathy. Articular surface changes tend to be central, and this can be a problem because of limited ultrasound access. Improved visualization of articular surfaces can be obtained by examining some joints in flexion, for example, the MCP/MTP and interphalangeal joints. Knee flexion and plantar flexion at the ankle improve access to the trochlea of the knee **(Fig. 10.9)** and the talar dome, respectively. Articular cartilage may become ill-defined, heterogeneous, and thinned, and the articular cortex irregular. Osteophytes and enthesophytes appear as small bony prominences at the joint margin **(Fig. 10.19)**, for example, Heberden and Bouchard nodes at the distal and PIP joints, respectively.

Pigmented Villonodular Synovitis, Synovial Osteochondromatosis, Amyloid

In addition to systemic arthropathies such as RA or gout, synovial proliferative conditions such as pigmented villonodular synovitis (PVNS), synovial osteochondromatosis, and amyloid[56–58] may cause intra-articular masses and large erosions. The synovial masses may be localized or diffusely involve a joint. PVNS is a benign neoplastic process that results in villous/nodular synovial hypertrophy. Repeated bleeding causes hemosiderin deposition.

Localized intra-articular PVNS usually occurs at the knee. Another localized form of PVNS occurs in relation to tendon sheaths, particularly in the hand, and is also known as giant cell tumor of tendon sheath (GCTTS). Synovial osteochondromatosis occurs in joints, bursae, and tendon sheaths. It is thought to be a benign neoplastic process rather than a metaplastic process and results in synovial hyperplasia and cartilaginous nodules that may calcify or ossify and form loose bodies. Amyloid arthropathy occurs in patients on long-term hemodialysis, which results in the deposition of $\beta 2$ microglobulin in synovium. Deposits also occur in tendons, bursae, and periarticular soft tissues including the carpal tunnel.

Ultrasound in all three conditions shows joint fluid and hypoechoic synovial masses that may be extensive or localized, nodular, or causing diffuse synovial thickening **(Fig. 10.20)**. Large bony erosions may be present. The three conditions may be indistinguishable on ultrasound, and biopsy is usually required to confirm the diagnosis.

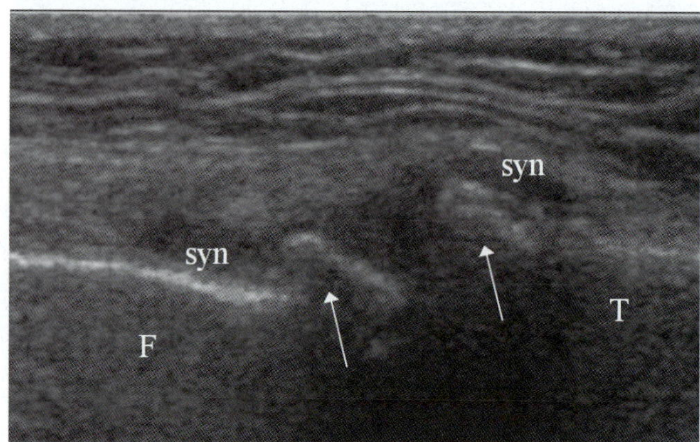

Figure 10.19.   Osteoarthritis of the knee. Longitudinal scan of medial joint line shows osteophytes (*arrows*) and synovial thickening (*syn*). F, femur; T, tibia.

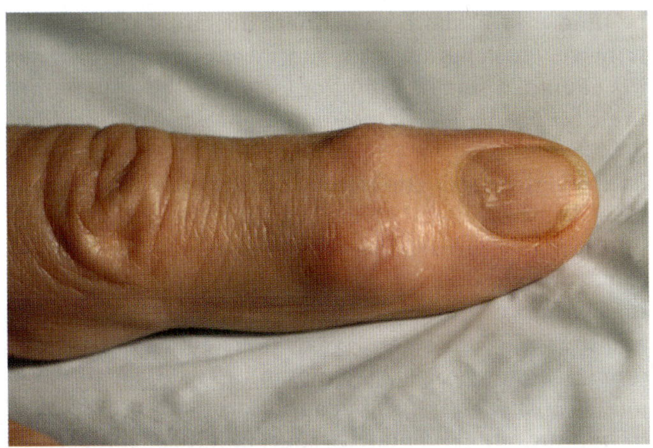

A

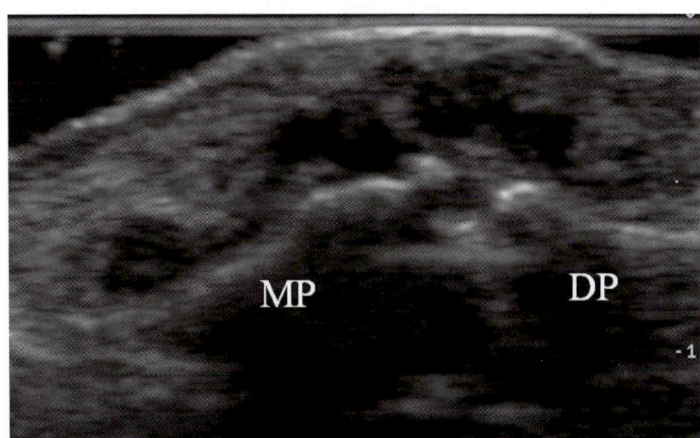

B

Figure 10.20.   Patient with PVNS. **A:** Clinical photograph shows focal soft tissue swelling on ulnar aspect of distal interphalangeal joint of index finger. **B:** Longitudinal ultrasound on dorso-ulnar aspect of the distal interphalangeal joint shows a hypoechoic synovial mass communicating with the joint line. MP, middle phalanx; DP, distal phalanx.

PVNS tends to be hypervascular on ultrasound and is diagnosed on MRI if blooming artifact due to hemosiderin deposition is present on gradient echo images. GCTTS results in a hypoechoic mass that is intimately related to a tendon sheath (see Chapter 9). Synovial osteochondromatosis is hypovascular. Calcification or ossification of cartilage nodules results in echogenic foci **(Fig. 10.21)**. Amyloid has no specific diagnostic ultrasound features, but the history of chronic hemodialysis is characteristic. Amyloid deposits cause tendon thickening, slightly hyperechoic masses in bursae and between muscles, and periarticular fluid collections.

Tip:
PVNS, synovial osteochondromatosis, and amyloid cause larger erosions than inflammatory joint disease.

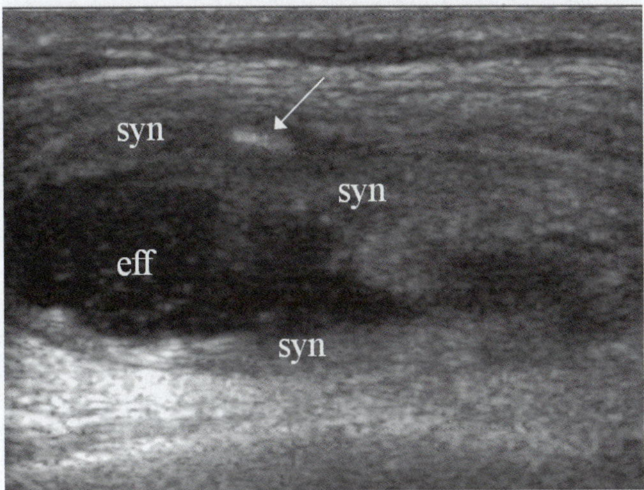

Figure 10.21.   Osteochondromatosis of the knee. Ultrasound shows effusion (*eff*) and synovial hypertrophy (*syn*) in the knee recess. Calcification in the thickened synovial wall is seen (*arrow*).

Septic Arthritis

Joint infection rapidly destroys articular cartilage; therefore, urgent diagnosis and treatment are essential. Patients typically present with a painful, swollen joint, but a more indolent presentation may occur with less aggressive organisms or in immunocompromised patients. Inflammatory markers are not always elevated. To further confuse matters, inflammatory markers may be elevated in acute calcific tendinitis, which has a similar clinical presentation to septic arthritis at the shoulder. Radiographic changes in septic arthritis are delayed. Septic arthritis in children is discussed in Chapter 13.

The key ultrasound feature of septic arthritis is joint fluid, although synovial thickening and synovial and periarticular Doppler signal are also seen. Joint fluid is rarely anechoic and often contains low-level echoes. Echogenic fluid, debris, septations, and even intra-articular gas bubbles may be present. Echogenic fluid may simulate synovial thickening, but fluid can be distinguished from synovial thickening by using the transducer to compress the joint and show typical fluid movement.[59] If fluid is demonstrated, ultrasound-guided joint aspiration should be performed to obtain fluid for an urgent Gram stain and culture, including for TB. Septic bursitis and tenosynovitis are also diagnosed by the presence of fluid in the appropriate clinical setting, and aspiration should be performed. Ultrasound is widely used to look for joint fluid in suspected septic arthritis. However, poor results have been recorded at the hip.[60] Some joints (e.g., the sacroiliac, sternoclavicular, and acromioclavicular joints) have non-distensible capsules, and the absence of fluid does not exclude infection. MRI should be performed if infection is not confirmed.[59] Ultrasound aspiration of prosthetic hips is often employed, although disappointing results have been reported.[61]

Hemophilic Arthropathy

Hemophilic arthropathy is the result of repeated hemarthroses that often start within a few years of birth. The effect of intra-articular blood on the joint may be cartilage-mediated or synovial-mediated.[62] Synovial hypertrophy, inflammation, and hemosiderin deposition predispose to further bleeds. Chronic disease leads to cartilage and subchondral bone destruction with superimposed degenerative changes, and may finally result in ankylosis. Ultrasound can show very small hemarthroses in early disease and nonspecific effusions and synovial hypertrophy in later disease. Problems with standardization and interobserver variability mean that ultrasound is less suited than MRI to monitor disease progression.[63]

ULTRASOUND-GUIDED THERAPEUTIC TECHNIQUES

Local steroid injection is an important element in the treatment of arthritis and osteoarthritis. The clinical effect depends on placing the needle accurately. Ultrasound is increasingly used to guide aspiration or injection of joints, tendon sheaths, bursae, cysts, and around tendon insertions. It ensures accurate and safe needle placement, especially in anatomically complex areas such as the hip, ankle, and wrist. Aseptic technique is essential. The skin should be cleaned and sterile gloves and a transducer cover used. The needle (21G to 23G) should be inserted using a "free hand" technique with the needle inclined obliquely along the scan plane while scanning in real time. When the scan plane is longitudinal, the needle is inserted distal to the transducer and directed obliquely toward the target. Needle puncture of a joint recess or a tendon sheath is easier if it is distended by fluid or synovial hypertrophy. Injection of dry joints is more challenging, and may necessitate preliminary injection of a small amount of local anesthetic to ensure the needle is correctly positioned. Most joint injections are performed with a scan plane that crosses the joint line, and the needle tip is inserted into the joint recess or placed against articular cartilage. For injections in small joints or tendon sheaths of the wrist/hand and ankle/foot, a small "hockey stick" transducer is useful. The injected dose of steroid depends on the type of steroid and the size of the joint, for example, 20 mg of triamcinolone acetonide for small joints and 40 to 80 mg for large joints, usually with an appropriate volume of lidocaine or bupivacaine. The puncture site should be compressed after the procedure so as to minimize the risk of subcutaneous atrophy due to steroid leaking from the joint.

We will here describe injection techniques in two difficult anatomical areas with frequent involvement in rheumatology; the wrist and hand, and the ankle and foot.

Ultrasound-Guided Injections in the Wrist and Hand

Puncture of the dorsal radiocarpal recess is performed with a longitudinal scan plane at the level of the Lister tubercle (**Fig. 10.22**). The dorsal midcarpal recess is punctured in a similar way, slightly distally, generally in a more ulnar longitudinal scan plane, avoiding the ulnar extensor tendons (**Fig. 10.23**). Puncture of the distal radioulnar joint is less frequently performed. A dorsal transverse scan plane and ulnar skin puncture avoid the extensor digiti minimi tendon. The needle is placed either just proximal to the joint in an enlarged superior recess or at the level of the joint line in contact with the cartilage of the ulnar head. Osteoarthritis of the first carpometacarpal

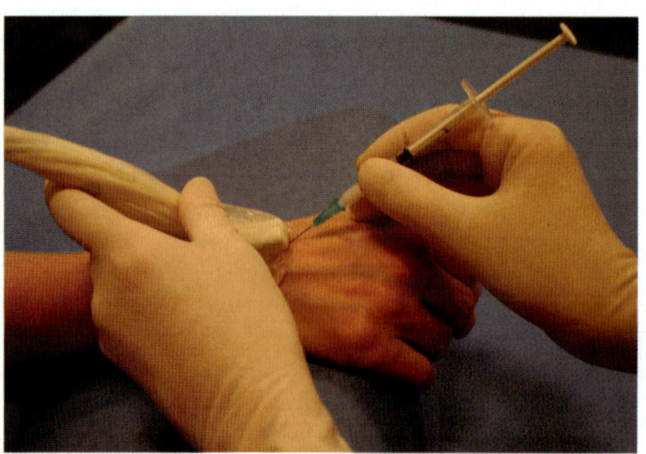

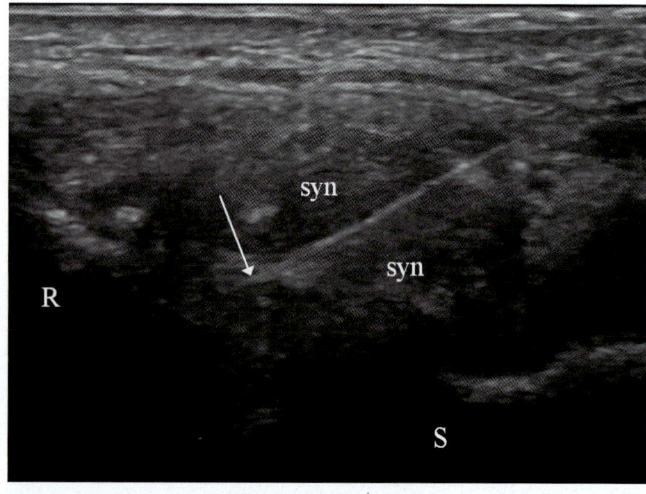

Figure 10.22. Ultrasound-guided injection in the dorsal recess of the radiocarpal joint with a longitudinal scan just distal to the Lister tubercle on the radius. **A:** Position of the transducer. **B:** Needle tip (*arrow*) in the radiocarpal recess enlarged by synovial hypertrophy (*syn*) in a patient with osteoarthrosis. R, radius; S, scaphoid.

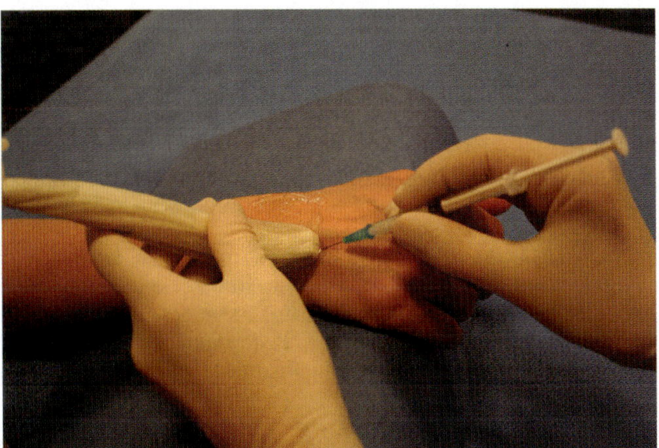

Figure 10.23.   Ultrasound-guided injection in the dorsal recess of the midcarpal joint with a longitudinal scan just distal to the ulna.

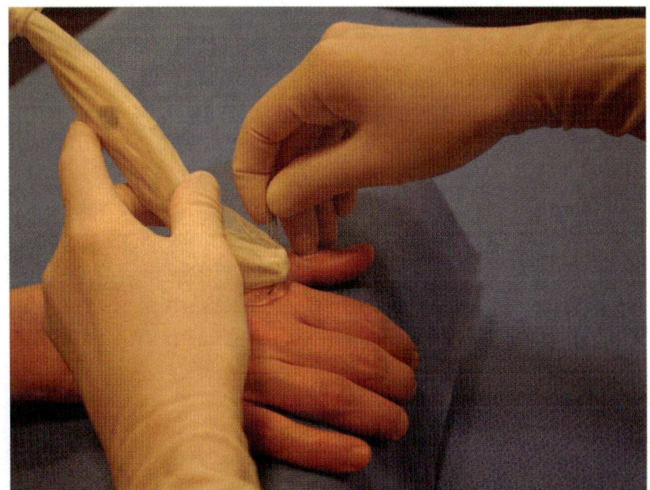

A

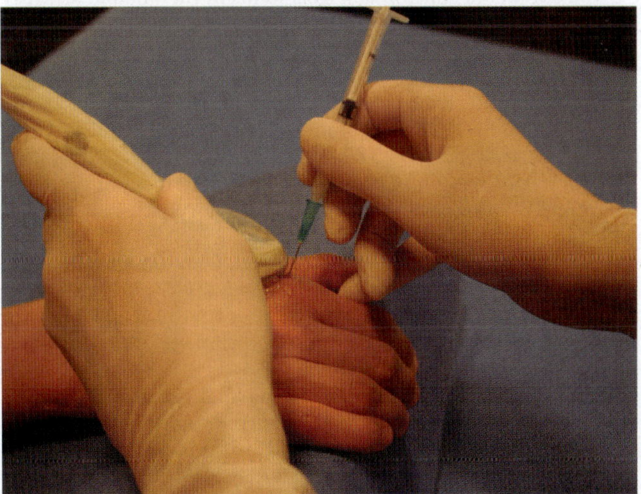

B

Figure 10.24.   Steroid injection in the second MCP joint. **A:** Marking the skin over the joint line with a paperclip. **B:** Ultrasound-guided puncture.

joint is often treated by local steroid injection. Two puncture routes are possible: A dorsal longitudinal route with the needle inclined relatively perpendicular to access the joint while avoiding the branches of the radial nerves, or a palmar longitudinal route through the thenar muscles, with a more oblique approach.

The finger joints are injected dorsomedially or dorsolaterally, avoiding the extensor tendon and the digital arteries and nerves. If the joint recess is distended, a longitudinal scan plane with a distal oblique approach is possible. If the recess is not prominent, it may be easier to visualize and mark the joint line with the help of a needle or paperclip placed between the skin and the transducer (**Fig. 10.24**). It is then generally easy to penetrate the joint line with a single perpendicular puncture using a hockey stick transducer only if the placement is doubtful (**Fig. 10.24**). Tendon sheaths can be injected in a longitudinal plane with a puncture route as tangential as possible and inserting the needle tip as far as possible into the sheath. If the sheath is minimally enlarged, a transverse scan plane may be easier.

Ultrasound-Guided Injections in the Ankle and Foot

The ankle joint is punctured with a longitudinal, anteromedial or anterolateral scan plane, avoiding the extensor tendons and the anterior tibial vessels. The needle tip is inserted into the anterior recess or placed against the cartilage of the talar dome. In osteoarthritis or JIA, injection of the posterior subtalar joint may be needed but can be difficult to perform, especially if the recesses are not bulging. An anterolateral oblique plane, anterior to the peroneal tendons, can be used by moving the transducer posteriorly from a coronal image of the tarsal sinus (**Fig. 10.25**). The anterior subtalar joint (talocalcaneonavicular) or other tarsal joints are punctured dorsally, with an appropriate scanning plane to avoid the tendons and

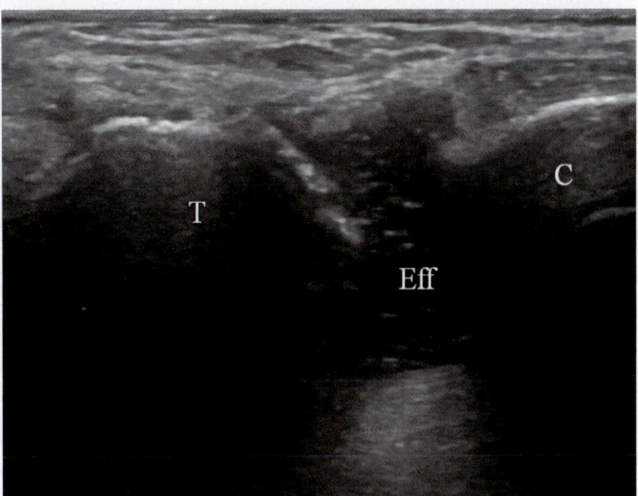

Figure 10.25.   Osteoarthrosis of the posterior talocalcaneal joint. Lateral coronal ultrasound scan showing effusion (*Eff*) in the anterolateral recess.

the vessels. Injections of periarticular tendons and toe joints are similar to the wrist and hand. The flexor hallucis longus tendon is deeply situated and is best accessed with an oblique approach, just proximal to the calcaneus, using a hockey stick transducer and avoiding the posterior tibial artery and the tibial nerve.

CONCLUSION

Ultrasound is now established as an essential tool in the initial assessment, monitoring, and treatment of inflammatory arthropathy.

REFERENCES

1. Szkudlarek M, Narvestad A, Klarlund M, et al. Ultrasonography of the metatarsophalangeal joints in rheumatoid arthritis: comparison with magnetic resonance imaging, conventional radiography, and clinical examination. *Arthritis Rheum.* 2004;50:2103–2112.
2. Wakefield RJ, Balint PV, Szkudlarek M, et al. Musculoskeletal ultrasound including definitions for ultrasonographic pathology. *J Rheumatol.* 2005;32:2485–2487.
3. Zayat AS, Freeston JE, Conaghan PG, et al. Does joint position affect ultrasound findings in inflammatory arthritis? *Rheumatology (Oxford).* 2012;51:921–925.
4. De Flaviis L, Scaglione P, Nessi R, et al. Ultrasonography of the hand in rheumatoid arthritis. *Acta Radiol.* 1988;29(4):457–460.
5. Backhaus M, Burmester GR, Gerber T, et al. Guidelines for musculoskeletal ultrasound in rheumatology. *Ann Rheum Dis.* 2001;60:641–649.
6. Mandl P, Naredo E, Wakefield RJ, et al. A systematic literature review analysis of ultrasound joint count and scoring systems to assess synovitis in rheumatoid arthritis according to the OMERACT filter. *J Rheumatol.* 2011;38:2055–2062.
7. El-Miedany YM, Housny IH, Mansour HM, et al. Ultrasound versus MRI in the evaluation of juvenile idiopathic arthritis of the knee. *Jt Bone Spine.* 2001;68:222–230.
8. Kane D, Balint PV, Sturrock RD. Ultrasonography is superior to clinical examination in the detection and localization of knee joint effusion in rheumatoid arthritis. *J Rheumatol.* 2003;30:966–971.
9. Ostergaard M, Court-Payen M, Gideon P, et al. Ultrasonography in arthritis of the knee. A comparison with MR imaging. *Acta Radiol.* 1995;36(1):19–26.
10. Szkudlarek M, Court-Payen M, Strandberg C, et al. Power Doppler ultrasonography for assessment of synovitis in the metacarpophalangeal joints of patients with rheumatoid arthritis: a comparison with dynamic magnetic resonance imaging. *Arthritis Rheum.* 2001;44(9):2018–2023.
11. Terslev L, Torp-Pedersen S, Savnik A, et al. Doppler ultrasound and magnetic resonance imaging of synovial inflammation of the hand in rheumatoid arthritis: a comparative study. *Arthritis Rheum.* 2003;48(9):2434–2441.
12. Walther M, Harms H, Krenn V, et al. Synovial tissue of the hip at power Doppler US: correlation between vascularity and power Doppler ultrasound signal. *Radiology.* 2002;225(1):225–231.
13. Hau M, Schultz H, Tony HP, et al. Evaluation of pannus and vascularization of the metacarpophalangeal and proximal interphalangeal joints in rheumatoid arthritis by high-resolution ultrasound (multidimensional linear array). *Arthritis Rheum.* 1999;42(11):2303–2308.
14. Terslev L, Torp-Pedersen S, Bang N, et al. Doppler ultrasound findings in healthy wrists and finger joints before and after use of two different contrast agents. *Ann Rheum Dis.* 2005;64(6):824–827.
15. Klauser AS, Franz M, Arora R, et al. Detection of vascularity in wrist tenosynovitis: power Doppler ultrasound compared with contrast-enhanced grey-scale ultrasound. *Arthritis Res Ther.* 2010;12(6):R209.
16. Terslev L, Torp-Pedersen S, Qvistgaard E, et al. Doppler ultrasound findings in healthy wrists and finger joints. *Ann Rheum Dis.* 2004;63(6):644–648.
17. Klauser AS, De Zordo T, Bellmann-Weiler R, et al. Feasibility of second-generation ultrasound contrast media in the detection of active sacroiliitis. *Arthritis Rheum.* 2009;61(7):909–916.
18. Qvistgaard E, Røgind H, Torp-Pedersen S, et al. Quantitative ultrasonography in rheumatoid arthritis: evaluation of inflammation by Doppler technique. *Ann Rheum Dis.* 2001;60(7):690–693.
19. Terslev L, Torp-Pedersen S, Qvistgaard E, et al. Estimation of inflammation by Doppler ultrasound: quantitative changes after intra-articular treatment in rheumatoid arthritis. *Ann Rheum Dis.* 2003;62(11):1049–1053.
20. Ejbjerg B, Narvestad E, Rostrup E, et al. Magnetic resonance imaging of wrist and finger joints in healthy subjects occasionally shows changes resembling erosions and synovitis as seen in rheumatoid arthritis. *Arthritis Rheum.* 2004;50(4):1097–1106.
21. Backhaus M, Kamradt T, Sandrock D, et al. Arthritis of the finger joints: a comprehensive approach comparing conventional radiography, scintigraphy, ultrasound, and contrast-enhanced magnetic resonance imaging. *Arthritis Rheum.* 1999;42(6):1232–1245.
22. Wakefield RJ, Gibbon WW, Conaghan PG, et al. The value of sonography in the detection of bone erosions in patients with rheumatoid arthritis: a comparison with conventional radiography. *Arthritis Rheum.* 2000;43(12):2762–2770.
23. Visser H, le Cessie S, Vos K, et al. How to diagnose rheumatoid arthritis early: a prediction model for persistent (erosive) arthritis. *Arthritis Rheum.* 2002;46(2):357–365.
24. McGonagle D, Gibbon W, Emery P. Classification of inflammatory arthritis by enthesitis. *Lancet.* 1998;352(9134):1137–1140.
25. Resnick D, Niwayama G. Entheses and enthesopathy. Anatomical, pathological, and radiological correlation. *Radiology.* 1983;146(1):1–9.
26. McGonagle D, Gibbon W, O'Connor P, et al. Characteristic magnetic resonance imaging entheseal changes of knee synovitis in spondyloarthropathy. *Arthritis Rheum.* 1998;41(4):694–700.
27. Arnett FC, Edworthy SM, Bloch DA, et al. The American Rheumatism Association 1987 revised criteria for the classification of rheumatoid arthritis. *Arthritis Rheum.* 1988;31(3):315–324.
28. Aletaha D, Neogi T, Silman AJ, et al. 2010 rheumatoid arthritis classification criteria: an American College of Rheumatology/European League Against Rheumatism collaborative initiative. *Ann Rheum Dis.* 2010;69(9):1580–1588.
29. Wakefield RJ, Green MJ, Marzo-Ortega H, et al. Should oligoarthritis be reclassified? Ultrasound reveals a high prevalence of subclinical disease. *Ann Rheum Dis.* 2004;63(4):382–385.
30. Szkudlarek M, Klarlund M, Narvestad E, et al. Ultrasonography of the metacarpophalangeal and proximal interphalangeal joints in rheumatoid arthritis: a comparison with magnetic resonance imaging, conventional radiography and clinical examination. *Arthritis Res Ther.* 2006;8(2):R52.
31. Nalbant S, Corominas H, Hsu B, et al. Ultrasonography for assessment of subcutaneous nodules. *J Rheumatol.* 2003;30(6):1191–1195.
32. Saleem B, Brown AK, Keen H, et al. Should imaging be a component of rheumatoid arthritis remission criteria? A comparison between traditional and modified composite remission scores and imaging assessments. *Ann Rheum Dis.* 2011;70(5):792–798.

33. Brown AK, Conaghan PG, Karim Z, et al. An explanation for the apparent dissociation between clinical remission and continued structural deterioration in rheumatoid arthritis. *Arthritis Rheum.* 2008;58(10):2958–2967.

34. Filippucci E, Farina A, Carotti M, et al. Grey scale and power Doppler sonographic changes induced by intra-articular steroid injection treatment. *Ann Rheum Dis.* 2004;63(6):740–743.

35. Ribbens C, André B, Marcelis S, et al. Rheumatoid hand joint synovitis: gray-scale and power Doppler ultrasound quantifications following anti-tumor necrosis factor-alpha treatment: pilot study. *Radiology.* 2003;229(2):562–569.

36. Newman JS, Laing TJ, McCarthy CJ, et al. Power Doppler sonography of synovitis: assessment of therapeutic response—preliminary observations. *Radiology.* 1996;198(2):582–584.

37. Hau M, Kneitz C, Tony HP, et al. High resolution ultrasound detects a decrease in pannus vascularisation of small finger joints in patients with rheumatoid arthritis receiving treatment with soluble tumour necrosis factor alpha receptor (etanercept). *Ann Rheum Dis.* 2002;61(1):55–58.

38. Terslev L, Torp-Pedersen S, Qvistgaard E, et al. Effects of treatment with etanercept (Enbrel, TNRF:Fc) on rheumatoid arthritis evaluated by Doppler ultrasonography. *Ann Rheum Dis.* 2003;62(2):178–181.

39. Scheel AK, Hermann KG, Ohrndorf S, et al. Prospective 7 year follow up imaging study comparing radiography, ultrasonography, and magnetic resonance imaging in rheumatoid arthritis finger joints. *Ann Rheum Dis.* 2006;65(5):595–600.

40. Taylor PC, Steuer A, Gruber J, et al. Comparison of ultrasonographic assessment of synovitis and joint vascularity with radiographic evaluation in a randomized, placebo-controlled study of infliximab therapy in early rheumatoid arthritis. *Arthritis Rheum.* 2004;50(4):1107–1116.

41. Naredo E, Möller I, Cruz A, et al. Power Doppler ultrasonographic monitoring of response to anti-tumor necrosis factor therapy in patients with rheumatoid arthritis. *Arthritis Rheum.* 2008;58(8):2248–2256.

42. Dougados M, van der Linden S, Juhlin R, et al. The European Spondyloarthropathy Study Group preliminary criteria for the classification of spondyloarthropathy. *Arthritis Rheum.* 1991;34(10):1218–1827.

43. Naredo E, Batlle-Gualda E, Garcia-Vivar ML, et al. Power Doppler ultrasonography assessment of entheses in spondyloarthropathies: response to therapy of entheseal abnormalities. *J Rheumatol.* 2010;37(10):2110–2117.

44. Petty RE, Southwood TR, Manners P, et al. International League of Associations for Rheumatology classification of juvenile idiopathic arthritis: second revision, Edmonton, 2001. *J Rheumatol.* 2004;31(2):390–392.

45. Ravelli A, Martini A. Juvenile idiopathic arthritis. *Lancet.* 2007;369(9563):767–778.

46. Laurell L, Court-Payen M, Nielsen S, et al. Ultrasonography and color Doppler in juvenile idiopathic arthritis: diagnosis and follow-up of ultrasound-guided steroid injection in the ankle region. A descriptive interventional study. *Pediatr Rheumatol. Online J.* 2011;9(1):4.

47. Laurell L, Court-Payen M, Nielsen S, et al. Ultrasonography and color Doppler in juvenile idiopathic arthritis: diagnosis and follow-up of ultrasound- guided steroid injection in the wrist region. A descriptive interventional study. *Pediatr Rheumatol Online J.* 2012;10:11.

48. Breton S, Jousse-Joulin S, Cangemi C, et al. Comparison of clinical and ultrasonographic evaluations for peripheral synovitis in juvenile idiopathic arthritis. *Semin Arthritis Rheum.* 2011;41(2):272–278.

49. Janow GL, Panghaal V, Trinh A, et al. Detection of active disease in juvenile idiopathic arthritis: sensitivity and specificity of the physical examination vs. ultrasound. *J Rheumatol.* 2011;38(12):2671–2674.

50. Rebollo-Polo M, Koujok K, Weisser C, et al. Ultrasound findings on patients with juvenile idiopathic arthritis in clinical remission. *Arthritis Care Res (Hoboken).* 2011;63(7):1013–1019.

51. Delle Sedie A, Riente L, Iagnocco A, et al. Ultrasound imaging for the rheumatologist X. Ultrasound imaging in crystal-related arthropathies. *Clin Exp Rheumatol.* 2007;25(4):513–517.

52. Wright SA, Filippucci E, McVeigh C, et al. High-resolution ultrasonography of the first metatarsal phalangeal joint in gout: a controlled study. *Ann Rheum Dis.* 2007;66(7):859–864.

53. Thiele RG, Schlesinger N. Diagnosis of gout by ultrasound. *Rheumatology (Oxford).* 2007;46(7):1116–1121.

54. Grassi W, Filippucci E, Farina A. Ultrasonography in osteoarthritis. *Semin Arthritis Rheum.* 2005;34(6)(suppl 2):19–23.

55. Keen III, Conaghan PG. Usefulness of ultrasound in osteoarthritis. *Rheum Dis Clin North Am.* 2009;35(3):503–519.

56. Murphey MD, Rhee JH, Lewis RB, et al. Pigmented villonodular synovitis: radiologic-pathologic correlation. *Radiographics.* 2008;28(5):1493–1518.

57. McKenzie G, Raby N, Ritchie D. A pictorial review of primary synovial osteochondromatosis. *Eur Radiol.* 2008;18(11):2662–2669.

58. Kiss E, Keusch G, Zanetti M, et al. Dialysis-related amyloidosis revisited. *AJR Am J Roentgenol.* 2005;185(6):1460–1467.

59. Chau CL, Griffith JF. Musculoskeletal infections: ultrasound appearances. *Clin Radiol.* 2005;60(2):149–159.

60. Weybright PN, Jacobson JA, Murry KH, et al. Limited effectiveness of sonography in revealing hip joint effusion: preliminary results in 21 adult patients with native and postoperative hips. *AJR Am J Roentgenol.* 2003;181(1):215–218.

61. Eisler T, Svensson O, Engström CF, et al. Ultrasound for diagnosis of infection in revision total hip arthroplasty. *J Arthroplasty.* 2001;16(8):1010–1017.

62. Roosendaal G, Lafeber FP. Pathogenesis of haemophilic arthropathy. *Haemophilia.* 2006;12(suppl 3):117–121.

63. Zukotynski K, Jarrin J, Babyn PS, et al. Sonography for assessment of haemophilic arthropathy in children: a systematic protocol. *Haemophilia.* 2007;13(3):293–304.

CHAPTER

11

Muscles

Stefano Bianchi
Jean-Louis Brasseur
Gerard Morvan
Lionel Pesquer
Dien Hung Luong

INTRODUCTION

The elementary structure shared by every skeletal muscle is the *myofiber*, which is enveloped by a thin layer of connective tissue called the endomysium. Muscle fibers are of two types: type I and type II. Type I fibers, the red myofibers, are smaller and more apt to prolonged contractions, while the larger type II fibers are responsible for powerful contractions of short duration. All skeletal muscles contain both types of fibers but the proportions differ depending on functional demands. Myofibers are packed together to form *muscle fascicles* that are surrounded by the perimysium, fibroadipose septa that contain vessels and nerves. Groups of fascicles form *muscles* that are surrounded by a thick epimysium.

When muscles contract, the forces generated by the fascicles are transmitted to fibroadipose septae and then to internal tendons or laminae that converge on the distal tendon or tendon laminae. Muscle fibers parallel to the axis of muscle contraction provide the maximum range of muscle excursion, while oblique fibers have a shorter range but increase the force of contraction. Muscle size, shape, and internal architecture reflect mainly functional requirements.[1–4] Muscles vary in size from a few millimeters to very long muscles such as the sartorius, the longest muscle of the human body.

Ultrasound Technique of Examination and Normal Ultrasound Appearance

A short clinical history and a basic physical examination are always performed before ultrasound (US) examination of muscles.[1] Data concerning the onset and location of symptoms, the presence of a mass, ecchymosis, or local tenderness on palpation or muscle contraction are required to target the zone of interest and aid interpretation of the ultrasound findings.

For the lower limbs, the patient lies supine or prone. For the upper limbs, the patient sits with the arm on the examination couch and the limb positioned according to the region of interest. Special positions, such as squatting for easier detection of herniation of anterolateral leg muscles, can be used when appropriate.

The frequency of the transducer must be adapted to the depth and size of the muscle. For superficial muscles, 10 to 17 MHz transducers are used, whereas 3.5 to 7 MHz transducers are necessary for deeper structures.[3–5] Focus adjustment for depth optimizes spatial resolution. Power or color Doppler allows assessment of vascularity. Power Doppler may be more sensitive than color Doppler, but this seems to depend on the hardware adjustments. Pulsed Doppler, sonoelastography, and three-dimensional or fusion imaging are not used in daily routine. Appropriate annotations are required to allow better understanding of ultrasound images by clinicians,[3] including the name of the region, side, anatomic landmarks, and the scanning plane.

Muscles must be examined in their longitudinal and axial planes (**Fig. 11.1**). The transducer must be perpendicular to the muscle fibers to avoid anisotropy, which can lead to decreased echogenicity of the perimysium, internal septa, aponeuroses, and tendons. In doubtful cases, tilting the transducer can show that the hypoechoic appearance is related to anisotropy. Examination during muscle contraction also reduces artifacts by modifying the orientation of the septa (**Fig. 11.2**). Beam steering can reduce artifactual anisotropy. Harmonic and compound imaging improve the signal-to-noise ratio and tissue contrast.[6] Panoramic scans allow better comprehension of images by clinicians and improve the accuracy of measurements (**Fig. 11.3**).[7]

Local tenderness caused by increasing pressure with the transducer helps to focus the ultrasound examination toward the area of interest. Transducer pressure may reduce the thickness of the subcutaneous tissues and improve the assessment of underlying structures, but pressure can efface fluid collections and muscle hernias. Dynamic ultrasound performed during muscle contraction and relaxation helps to detect subtle muscle injuries and muscle hernias, analyze fibrous scars, and reduce anisotropy.[1,8]

Ultrasound examination must include not only the whole muscle, including its proximal and distal insertions, but also adjacent muscles. Contralateral examination helps in assessing small or doubtful lesions, unilateral muscle agenesis or atrophy/hypertrophy, and allows better evaluation of anatomic variations.

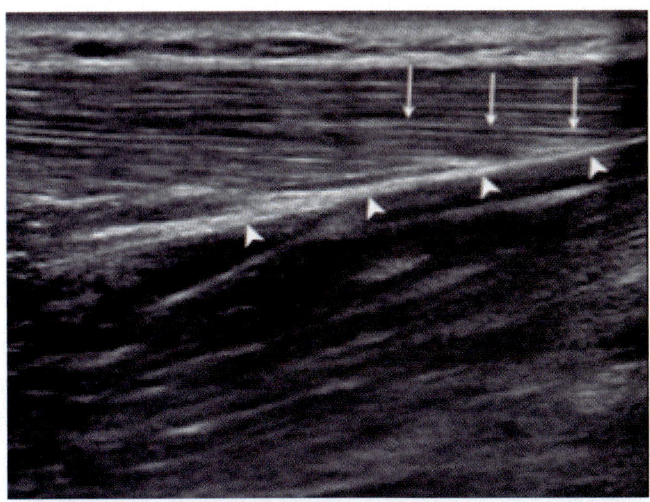 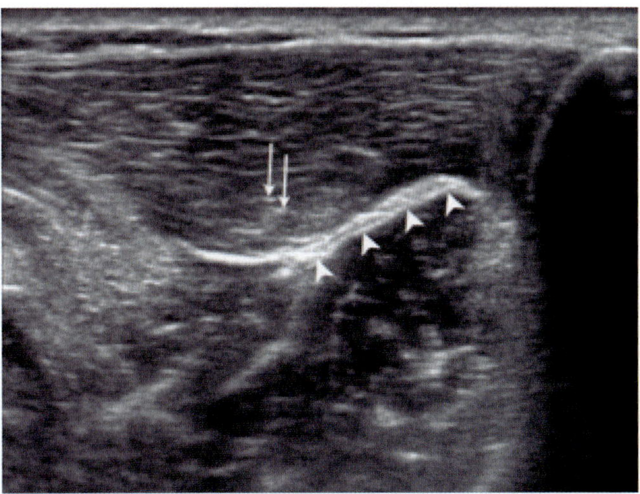

Figure 11.1. Longitudinal ultrasound image (**A**) of tibialis anterior muscle show perimysium (*arrows*) as hyperechoic bands inserting on to a central aponeurosis (*arrowheads*). In short axis (**B**), perimysium appears as dots.

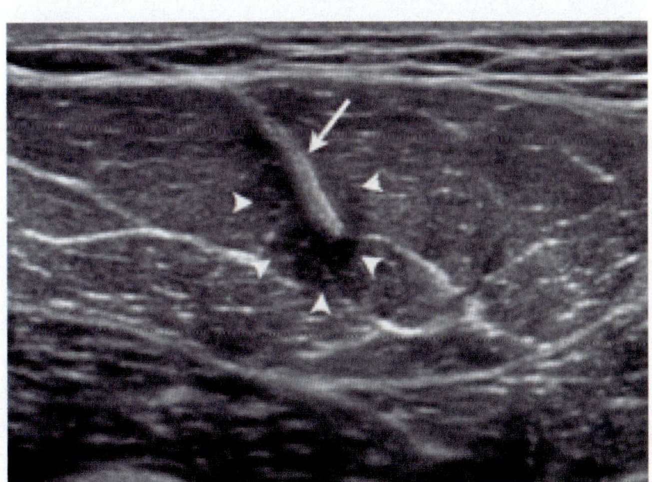 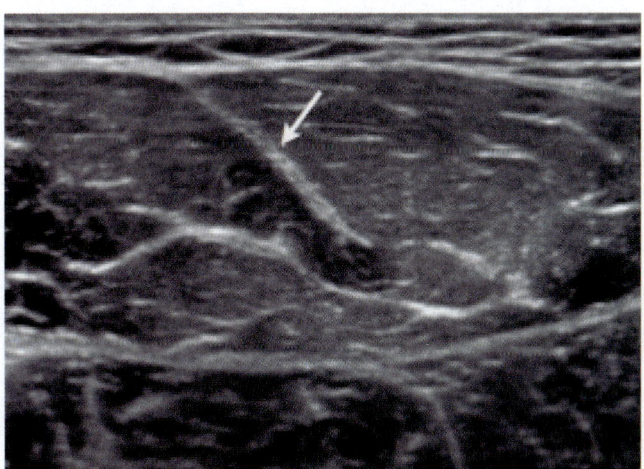

Figure 11.2. Transverse ultrasound images without (**A**) and with (**B**) thigh contraction showing hypoechoic areas due to anisotropy (*arrowheads*) close to the central aponeurosis of the RF (*arrows*). Note the lateral deviation of central aponeurosis during RF muscle contraction.

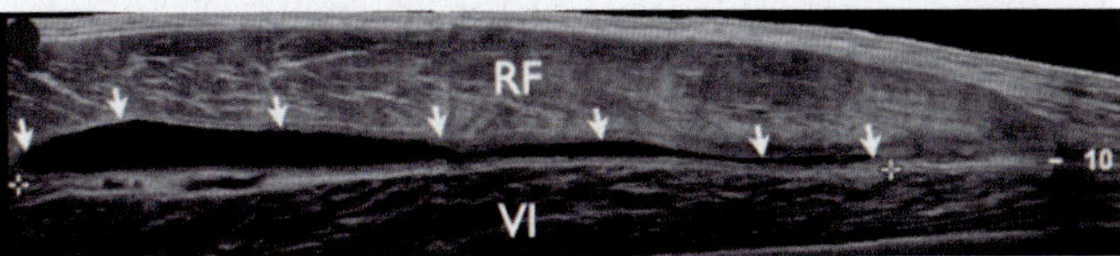

Figure 11.3. Longitudinal extended field-of-view image of anterior thigh. Fluid collection (*arrows*) at the deep margin of the rectus femoris (*RF*) displayed in its full length. VI, vastus intermedialis.

Ultrasound of normal muscles shows regular alternation of myofibers and connective tissue components.[1–5] On *longitudinal* sonograms, myofibers appear as hypoechoic structures separated by hyperechoic thinner bands reflecting the perimysium (fibroadipose septa). The overall appearance is regular alternation of parallel hypo- and hyperechoic bands. *Axial* images of muscles show hypoechoic structures containing short echoic bands or dots due to the perimysium. Peripheral muscle fascia appears as thick hyperechoic bands on both planes. Vessels and nerves run through focal interruptions of the fascia. When correctly examined, internal and terminal aponeuroses and tendons are hyperechoic on both axes but appear hypoechoic if the transducer is not perpendicular.

ACCESSORY MUSCLES

General Considerations

Accessory muscles (AMs) are congenital anomalies[9–16] that are usually asymptomatic and go unnoticed but can be clinically relevant. Frequently they present as asymptomatic masses that can be confused with soft tissue tumors.[17]

If located in fibro-osseous tunnels, they can cause neurologic symptoms due to nerve compression.[18–23] In active patients, they can cause pain during exercise due either to ischemia related to increased intrafascial pressure or to overuse tendinopathy.

The diagnosis of AMs is based mainly on recognition of the typical location and imaging features. Although AMs are congenital, patients often report them as new masses. This can be explained by two mechanisms: hypertrophy due to sports activity, particularly in young patients, and awareness of a swelling after weight loss and thinning of the subcutaneous fat. A clinically evident AM appears as an indolent soft tissue mass covered by normal skin. Signs of inflammation and adhesions to the skin are absent. If the diagnosis is suspected on inspection or palpation, muscle contraction increases firmness, as in normal muscles.

Since AMs are made of normal muscle tissue, they often present at imaging as small, bulky masses with regular internal organization identical to adjacent muscles. When they present as masses, the diagnosis is relatively easy if the possibility of AM is kept in mind and an appropriate imaging modality is used. In other presentations, a high degree of clinical suspicion is necessary to detect smaller AMs. In doubtful cases, bilateral examination can help in demonstrating normal contralateral anatomy, although the rare possibility of bilateral AMs must be kept in mind.

Standard radiographs are of limited value. Computed tomography (CT) shows a mass with density and shape similar to that of adjacent muscles. At magnetic resonance imaging (MRI), anomalous muscles resemble normal muscle morphology and signal/texture on all sequences including after gadolinium injection. Tendons can be detected by ultrasound and MRI, thus confirming the diagnosis.

Knowledge of the appearance and typical locations of AMs is necessary to avoid confusion with pathologic masses and unnecessary biopsy or surgery.

Upper Extremity

Shoulder

AMs found at the anterior aspect of the shoulder include accessory heads of the biceps, coracobrachialis, and subscapularis muscles.[24] The AM located on the anterior surface of the subscapularis muscle has the most clinical importance[24] as it may cause problems at surgery if it covers the anterior circumflex artery, the main nutrient vessel of the humeral head. To avoid damage, it is necessary to locate the artery by splitting the subscapularis AM belly. The muscle inserts into the anterior aspect of the lateral part of the subscapularis tendon and extends inferiorly. Ultrasound shows the muscle position, size, and internal structure **(Fig. 11.4)** and by using color Doppler, defines the precise location of the anterior circumflex artery and its relation to the subscapularis AM. This can be important for presurgical planning.

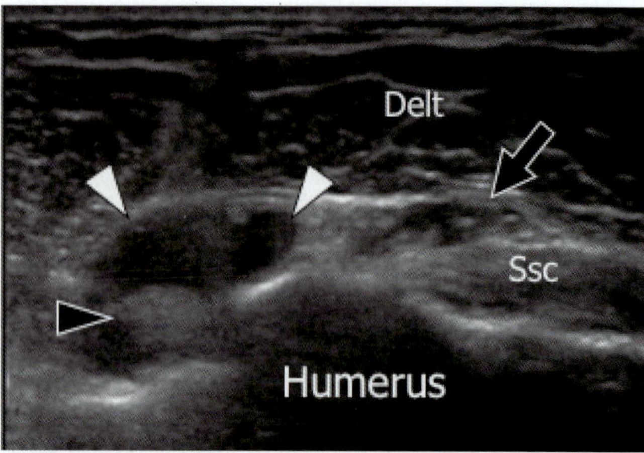

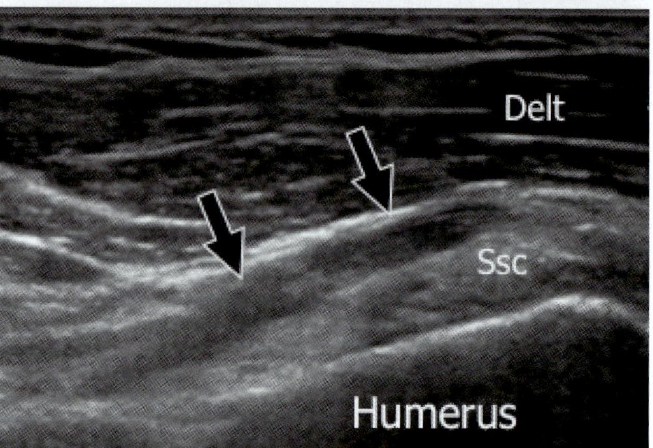

Figure 11.4. Aberrant muscle on the anterior surface of the subscapularis. Axial **(A)** and sagittal **(B)** sonograms obtained over the lateral part of the subscapularis tendon (*Ssc*) show the aberrant muscle (*arrows*) lying between subscapularis and the deltoid muscle (*Delt*). In **(A)**, note the close relationship between the AM and the long head of the biceps tendon (*black arrowhead*), which is surrounded by an effusion (*white arrowheads*).

Elbow

Anconeus epitrochlearis (AE) is a small, often bilateral, AM, and its prevalence is estimated from 1% to 34%. In a recent review of asymptomatic subjects, the AE muscle was seen on MRI in 23% of individuals.[25] It originates from the posterior aspect of the medial condyle of the humerus and inserts into the medial aspect of the olecranon. As it extends into the cubital tunnel, it can compress the ulnar nerve (UN), particularly during full elbow flexion. Chronic intermittent pressure on the nerve occurring during repetitive flexion and extension of the elbow can cause intraneural edema and subsequently internal fibrotic changes responsible for ulnar neuropathy.[26]

Due to its small size, the AE cannot be palpated at physical examination, and imaging is required. Standard radiographs are useful in excluding osteoarthritic changes, the main cause of ulnar neuropathy at the level of the

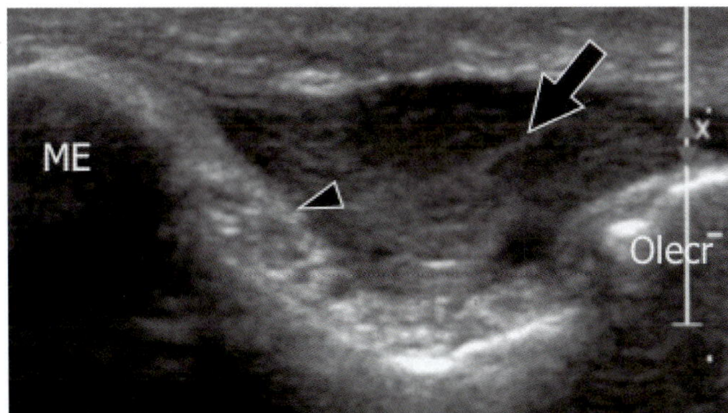

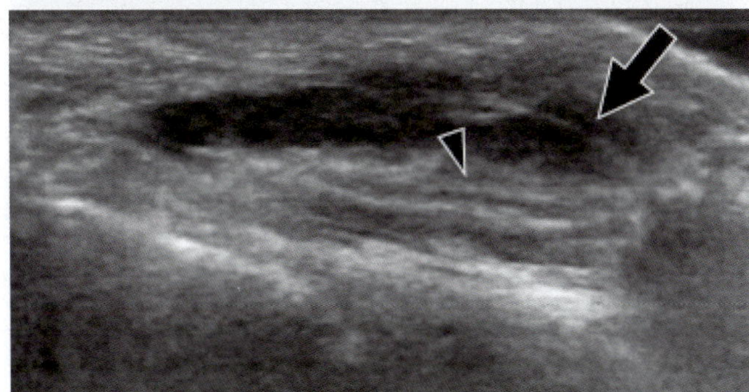

Figure 11.5.   Anconeus epitrochlearis(AE) muscle. Axial **(A)** and sagittal **(B)** sonograms obtained over the cubital tunnel show the AE muscle (*arrow*) and the UN (*arrowhead*). Note the close relations between the two structures inside the cubital tunnel. ME, medial epicondyle; Olecr, olecranon.

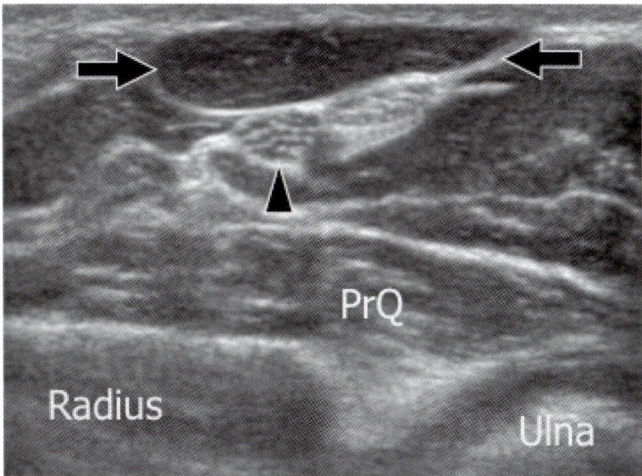

Figure 11.6.   Reversed palmaris longus muscle. Axial sonogram reveals the AM (*arrows*) showing normal muscle internal architecture and well-defined borders. Hyperechoic fascia surrounds the muscle that lies superficial to the median nerve (*arrowhead*). PrQ, pronator quadratus muscle.

cubital tunnel, but are useless in detection of the AE. Ultrasound detects the AE and also evaluates the UN. Due to its superficial location, the AE is easily identified by ultrasound **(Fig. 11.5)**. On axial scans, the AE appears as a hypoechoic structure located superficial to the UN in the cubital tunnel. Scanning during progressive elbow flexion may show anterior displacement of the muscle and impingement on the posterior aspect of the UN. Internal UN changes secondary to long-standing friction include swelling, irregular hypoechoicity, and loss of the normal internal fascicular pattern.

Wrist

Anomalous wrist muscles can be true AMs or anomalous insertions of normal muscles. The most frequent anomalous insertion is proximal extension of the lumbrical muscles. The most common AMs are the accessory abductor digiti minimi (AADM), extensor digitorum brevis manus, and the digastric flexor digitorum superficialis muscle of the index finger,[27] which can be encountered as incidental findings in asymptomatic subjects or present as clinically evident masses or compression of the median or the ulnar nerves in the carpal tunnel or Guyon canal.

Variations of the palmaris longus muscle belly are quite common.[27] Normally, the muscle belly is located proximally and has a very thin tendon that lies in the subcutaneous tissues just superficial to the median nerve and the flexor digitorum tendons, and inserts in the proximal edge of the transverse carpal ligament and the palmar aponeurosis. Occasionally, the muscle belly is in a central or distal position. When located distally, the muscle has a long proximal tendon, giving the appearance of a "reversed" palmaris longus **(Fig. 11.6)**. This variation is mostly asymptomatic and appears as local swelling of the palmar aspect of the distal forearm/wrist, but rarely it has a mass effect on the median nerve and the flexor tendons. Ultrasound easily shows this superficially located anomalous muscle in both axial and sagittal planes.

The AADM is the most common AM of the wrist and is present in approximately 24% of normal individuals.[27] It originates from the palmar carpal ligament and palmaris longus tendon, and inserts on the abductor digiti minimi and the medial aspect of the base of the proximal phalanx of the little finger.[28] The AADM runs inside Guyon canal, a fibro-osseous canal on the ulnar aspect of the palmar wrist that contains the ulnar artery and nerve **(Figs. 11.7, 11.8)**. When present, the AADM is usually located in the anterior part of the canal, but it can also run between the artery and the UN. Although usually asymptomatic, it may cause compression of the nerve against the pisohamate ligament. In this case, a positive Tinel sign can be elicited by gently tapping over the canal. Muscle size may be an important factor. Patel et al.[23] found a difference in the thickness of the AADM muscle between asymptomatic subjects (mean 1.7 mm) and patients (mean 4 mm) with clinical signs of UN entrapment at the wrist. Axial sonograms are best for demonstrating this anomalous muscle inside Guyon canal and show muscle thickness and the shape and size

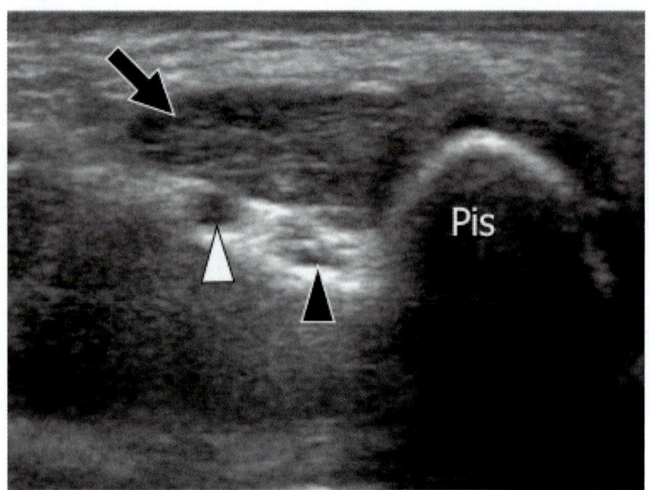

Figure 11.7.   Accessory abductor digiti minimi(AADM) muscle. Axial sonogram shows the accessory muscle (*arrow*) inside the Guyon tunnel. The muscle is superficial to the ulnar artery (*white arrowhead*) and nerve (*black arrowhead*). Pis, pisiform bone.

of the UN. Ultrasound has the advantage over MRI of dynamic examination. Ultrasound performed with active abduction of the little finger can show an increase in the AADM muscle thickness and impingement on the UN. Color and power Doppler allow accurate evaluation of the ulnar artery and its internal flow, thus differentiating nerve compression by the muscle from hypothenar hammer syndrome.

The extensor digitorum brevis manus is present in 1% to 3% of individuals.[28,29] It arises from the distal radius and the distal radiocarpal ligament and inserts into the index or middle finger. It appears clinically as a fusiform lump alongside the extensor tendon of the index finger and is easily mistaken for a dorsal ganglion or tenosynovitis of the extensor tendons. Active resisted extension of the index or middle finger results in increased firmness of the mass and indicates the correct diagnosis. Radiographs are normal. Ultrasound is able to identify the typical echotexture of the muscle and its relationship with the extensor tendons (**Fig. 11.9**).

On the ventral wrist, an unusually situated muscle belly of the flexor digitorum superficialis muscle may cause symptoms related to carpal tunnel syndrome. The anomalous muscle belly can be seen on ultrasound entering the carpal tunnel during extension of the fingers (**Fig. 11.10**). Dynamic scanning during flexion and extension of the fingers shows the muscle entering and exiting the tunnel. An unusual proximal origin of the lumbricals inside the carpal tunnel can also be encountered. These muscles are pulled into the tunnel during flexion of the fingers and may cause median neuropathy. Dynamic scanning with flexion and extension of the fingers is essential for a proper diagnosis of anomalous lumbrical muscles.

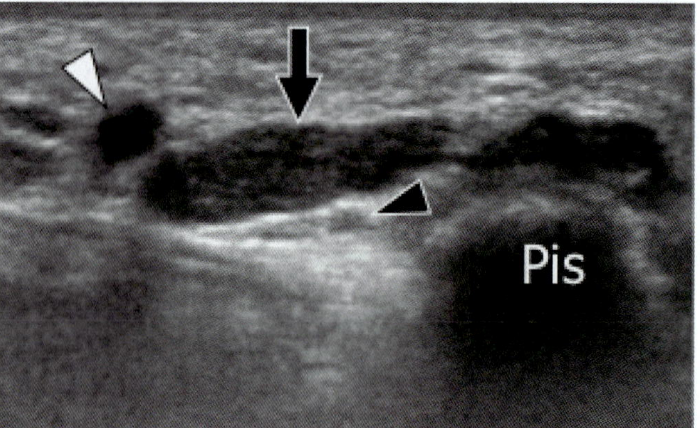

A

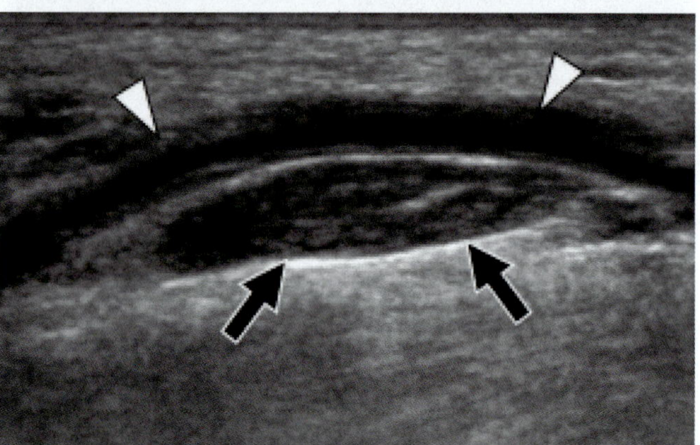

B

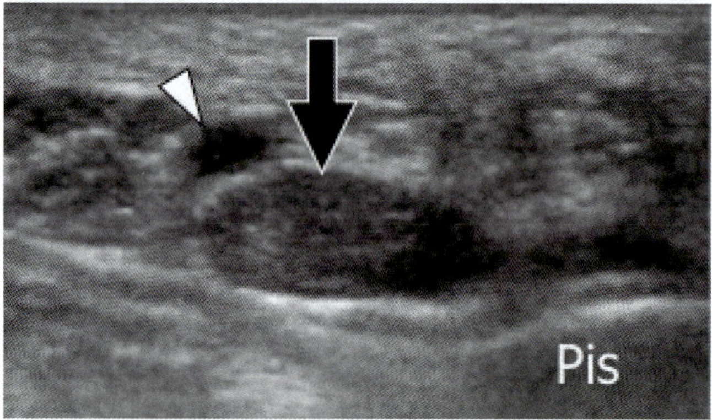

C

Figure 11.8.   Accessory abductor digiti minimi(AADM) muscle. Axial (**A**) and sagittal oblique (**B**) ultrasound images depict the accessory muscle (*black arrows*) inside the Guyon tunnel between the ulnar artery (*white arrowheads*) and nerve (*black arrowhead*). Axial image obtained during active resisted abduction of the little finger (**C**) shows a significant increase in the muscle size (*large arrow*), a possible cause of intermittent compression on the adjacent structures. Pis, pisiform bone.

Lower Extremity

Thigh–knee

The tensor fasciae suralis (TFS) is a rare anomalous muscle in the popliteal region that presents as a popliteal mass. It arises from the semitendinosus muscle, runs superficial to the medial head of the gastrocnemius

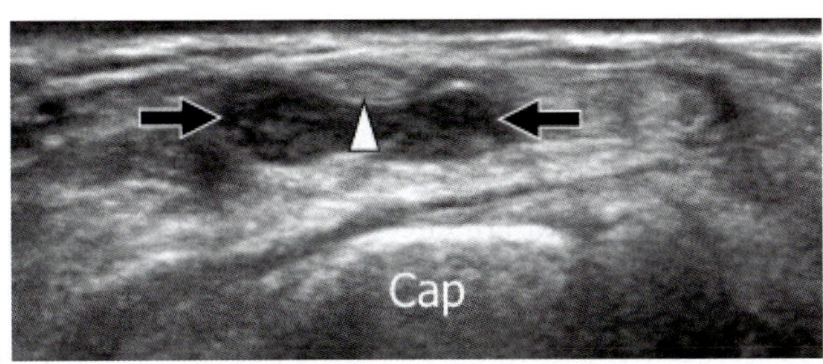
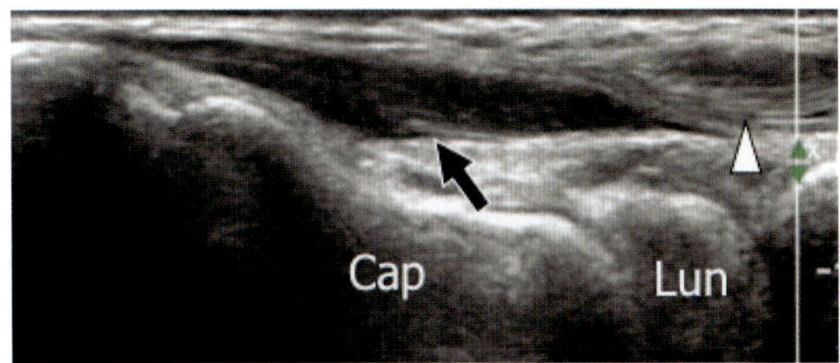

A   **B**

Figure 11.9.   Extensor digitorum brevis manus muscle. Axial **(A)** and sagittal **(B)** sonograms show an extensor digitorum brevis manus muscle (*arrows*) as an hypoechoic well-defined mass overlying the capitate (*Cap*). Note the close relationships of the muscle with the extensor tendon of the long finger (*arrowheads*). Lun, lunate bone.

(MHG), and continues as a thin and long tendon that joins the Achilles tendon.[30,31] In the diagnostic workup of a popliteal mass, ultrasound is commonly used because it differentiates cystic from solid lesions, assesses the popliteal artery, and demonstrates the relation of a mass to the surrounding tendons and nerves.

The actual prevalence of TFS is unknown. Sporadic reports present its ultrasound and MRI appearances.[31,32] Both modalities show the typical internal architecture of fibroadipose septa and muscle fibers inserting into a central tendon (circumpennate muscle). Axial images are particularly helpful in demonstrating the location of the aberrant muscle and its relation to other anatomic structures, whereas sagittal images provide better details of its internal architecture. In evaluating a popliteal solid mass, it is important to be aware of the possibility of a TFS to avoid unnecessary surgical exploration.

Ankle

The largest AM at the ankle is the accessory soleus (AS), which is located between the Achilles tendon and the soleus muscle.[9,11–13,15,16,33–35] Usually it originates from the posterior aspect of the tibia and anterior aspect of the soleus muscle. Depending on the insertion, five types of AS have been described. In type 1, the muscle inserts into the Achilles tendon and ends 1 to 2 cm from the calcaneum. In types 2 to 3, the muscle inserts directly (type 2) or through a short tendon (type 3) anterior to the Achilles tendon on the upper aspect of the calcaneum. In types 4 to 5, the AS inserts directly (type 4) or by its tendon (type 5) into the medial face of the calcaneum.

The AS usually presents on clinical examination as an indolent posteromedial mass that has a soft consistency when the patient is examined in the recumbent position, but becomes tense when the patient is examined standing and tiptoeing actively. The AS can be symptomatic and cause local pain due to ischemia related to overuse in sport. A large AS may compress the tibial nerve. Pain can also come from increased pressure inside the fascia, as indicated by symptom relief following fasciotomy.

Several imaging modalities show the AS **(Fig. 11.11)**. Standard radiographs can suggest the diagnosis by showing a fusiform opacity obliterating the normal triangular fatty space of Kager on the lateral view of the ankle, although this is a nonspecific appearance. Ultrasound shows a muscle located anterior to the Achilles tendon, best evaluated by longitudinal images over the Achilles

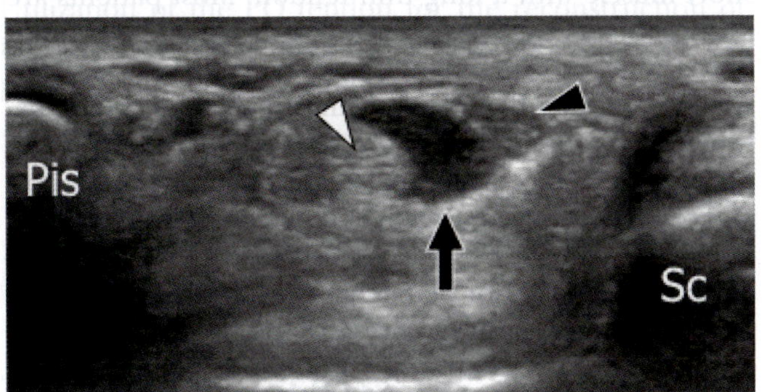
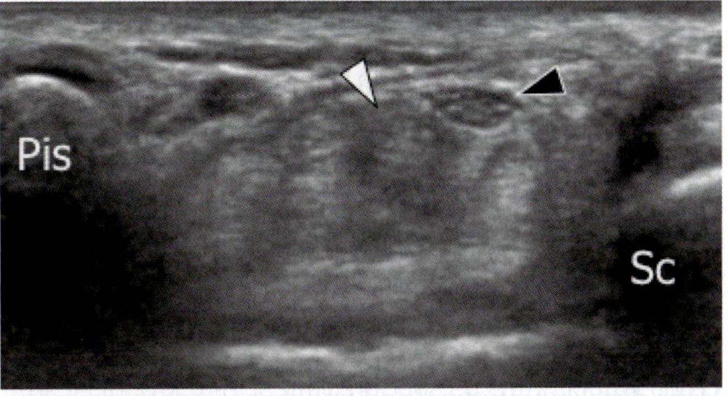

A   **B**

Figure 11.10.   Anomalous muscle belly of the flexor digitorum superficialis. Comparative axial ultrasound images of the proximal carpal tunnel obtained with fingers in extension **(A)** and flexion **(B)**. In extension, ultrasound shows an anomalous muscle (*arrow*) entering the carpal tunnel and displacing the median nerve (*black arrowhead*). The muscle is not located inside the tunnel in finger flexion. Pis, pisiform bone; Sc, scaphoid bone. Note the tendon of the flexor digitorum superficialis of the index finger (*white arrowhead*).

to inadequate treatment and expose patients to complications such as fibrous scar, myositis ossificans, calcific myonecrosis, and compartment syndrome, which increase disability. The role of imaging is to supplement clinical evaluation by describing the type, exact location, and severity of muscle injury. These data are essential since recovery is related to the size of the muscle injury and its location (e.g., injuries of semimembranosus or the central tendon of rectus femoris have a poorer prognosis). Additionally, avulsions may require surgical repair.[46,47]

MRI and ultrasound are widely used in daily routine to assess muscle injuries. Ultrasound is quicker, more available, cheaper, and better tolerated by patients than MRI. High-quality transducers and recent advances in software technologies provide depiction of subtle findings. Nevertheless, accuracy depends also, and even mainly, on the experience of the sonographer. Deep structures such as pelvitrochanteric muscles or adductor or hamstring origins are more difficult to assess with ultrasound, especially in patients with high body mass index,[48] and MRI may be preferable. Comparison of ultrasound and MRI in hamstring injuries shows that sensitivity is equal in acute injuries and suggests that ultrasound should be preferred because of its cheaper cost.[49] Ultrasound has higher sensitivity in the detection of recent fluid collections,[50] whereas MRI allows better analysis of residual abnormalities and remains the modality of choice for healing control and follow-up.

Delayed-onset Muscle Soreness

DOMS is a benign condition that consists of tenderness or stiffness to palpation and/or movement after strenuous muscle activity. Symptoms typically begin 24 to 48 hours after exercise, peak after 2 or 3 days, and disappear after 7 to 10 days. They are located initially at the myotendinous junction and tend to spread to the entire muscle.[51,52] The severity and duration of symptoms depend on the muscle group injured, the level of the athlete, and muscle performance. The pathomechanism of DOMS is still unclear, and various theories (lactic acid accumulation, connective or muscle tissue damage, muscle spasm, local inflammatory changes with enzyme release) have been suggested.[53]

Magnetic resonance shows increased intensity signal on fluid-sensitive sequences without evidence of bleeding, initially located at the myotendinous junction. The edema can progress to the entire muscle and can then be seen and better appreciated on axial images. In severe injuries, edema can even extend into the subcutaneous tissue. MRI changes occur later than the onset of symptoms, about 3 to 5 days after the precipitating exercise and can be observed for up to 80 days after the onset of symptoms.[54,55]

Ultrasound is normal or shows ill-defined focal areas of homogeneously increased echogenicity that can spread to the entire muscle.[56,57] Transverse sonograms are most

helpful in detecting these subtle abnormalities, and comparison with adjacent normal muscles or the opposite limb is frequently necessary to confirm the diagnosis.

Tears

Muscle tears are secondary to two main pathomechanisms: *extrinsic* tears from direct external trauma and *intrinsic* tears caused by forced contraction of an elongated muscle.[58,59]

Extrinsic injuries mainly affect the lower limbs and range from simple disorganization to rupture of muscle fibers and supporting connective tissue associated with a local hematoma. Injuries are more serious if the affected muscle is trapped between the extrinsic compression and the adjacent bone. This explains why in thigh trauma, hamstring injuries are usually less serious than injuries to the quadriceps.[58]

Intrinsic injuries are the result of simultaneous abnormal stretching and forced contraction of a muscle. Lower limb muscles and muscles that cross two joints (e.g., hamstring muscles, rectus femoris) and/or have complex internal architecture are most frequently affected.

Ultrasound Appearance of Acute Traumatic Lesions and Post-traumatic Lesions

Extrinsic Injuries

Ultrasound examination of extrinsic injuries must first assess possible damage to the subcutaneous tissues such as hematoma, fat fracture, or fascial tear. Ultrasound examination of the fascia in the axial plane is important since fascial injuries can be painful and easily overlooked when there are no associated deep muscle injuries. Small injuries can be more painful and more likely to lead to chronic disability than larger lesions. Next, the ultrasound examination assesses the internal muscle architecture. The degree of muscle damage is usually better assessed on axial sonograms. In minor injuries, ultrasound shows only swelling and disorganization of the muscle architecture with loss of parallelism between muscle fascicles. Moderate tears affect <50% of the muscle on axial images, whereas serious ruptures affect >50% of the muscle. Local hematomas are usually absent in minor injuries. In moderate tears, bleeding is often seen as hemorrhagic infiltration of the muscle without a collection. In serious ruptures, well-defined hematomas are frequently seen, and they can lead to enlargement of the muscle. Recent hematomas appear as echoic collections that change shape during compression with the transducer. A recent hematoma can be drained under ultrasound guidance, usually 10 to 14 days after injury, to lower internal pressure within the muscle compartment, help healing, and possibly reduce the chance of secondary ossification, although evidence for these benefits does not exist. Organized hematomas are unsuitable for needle puncture. They are

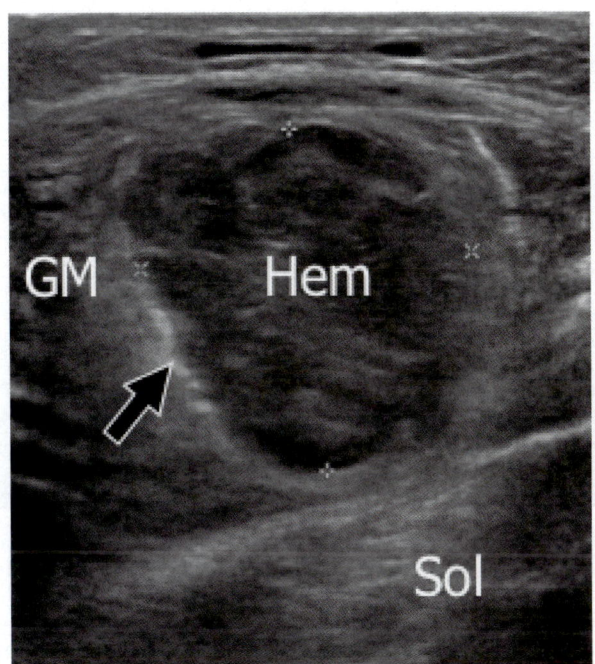

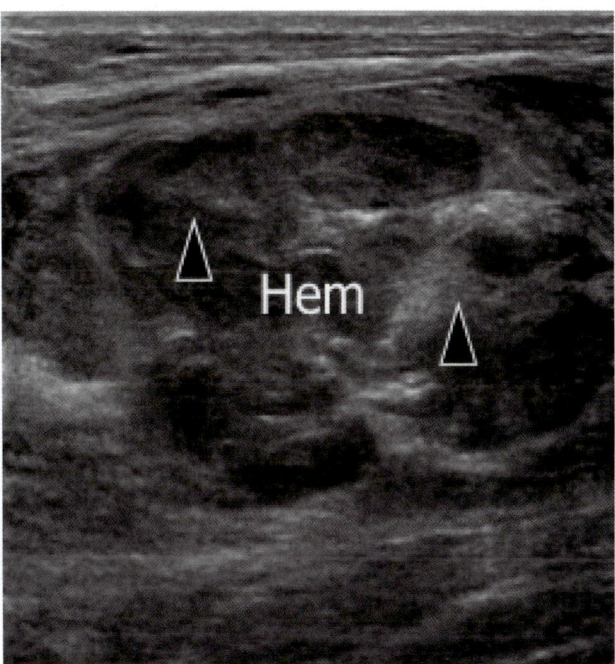

Figure 11.13.   Extrinsic muscle injuries. Axial (**A**) and longitudinal (**B**) ultrasound images of the calf show a hematoma (*Hem* in **A** and B and calipers in **A**) located inside the medial head of gastrocnemius (*GM*) muscle. Note well-defined borders (*arrow*) and internal heterogeneous appearance due to partial organization (*arrowheads*). Sol, soleus muscle.

more echogenic, show internal clots, and are not affected by local compression (**Fig. 11.13**).

Intrinsic Injuries

Intrinsic injuries are usually located at the myotendinous junction, but they may also be found inside the muscle belly.[60–62] They can be classified into four grades depending on ultrasound appearances.

Grade 1. Muscle injury without bleeding. These injuries affect only the muscle fibers without tearing the vascularized connective tissue. Therefore, there is no bleeding. Ultrasound shows an ill-defined local hyperechoic area without alteration of the muscle architecture. These subtle findings are more evident on MRI, which shows feathery hyperintense areas on T2-weighted sequences and a normal appearance on T1-weighted images. Pain relief is usually obtained after about a week.

Grade 2. Myoaponeurotic injury without hematoma. In grade 2 injuries, there are ruptures of the junctions between the muscle fascicles and the perimysium. There are also secondary changes in the internal muscle architecture and bleeding but no hematoma. Injuries are located at the insertion of the muscle fibers on the "connective skeleton," that is, the aponeurosis and tendon. Ultrasound shows an ill-defined heterogeneous area with disorganization of the muscle architecture (**Fig. 11.14**). MRI demonstrates hyperintense signal on T2- and T1-weighted images. Pain usually resolves over 3 weeks.

Grade 3. Myoaponeurotic injury with hematoma. The hallmark of grade 3 injury is the presence of a local hematoma.

The myoaponeurotic tear appears as a hematoma adjacent to an intramuscular septum, which is often difficult to detect, especially at ultrasound. In injuries at an aponeurosis, the hematoma develops along one side of the aponeurotic septum.[61,62] This is by far the most common type of injury. Examples include the proximal myotendinous junction of rectus femoris, the distal insertion of the long head of biceps femoris, the MHG (**Fig. 11.15**), the proximal septum of adductor longus, and the myotendinous junction of semimembranosus.[59] About 90%

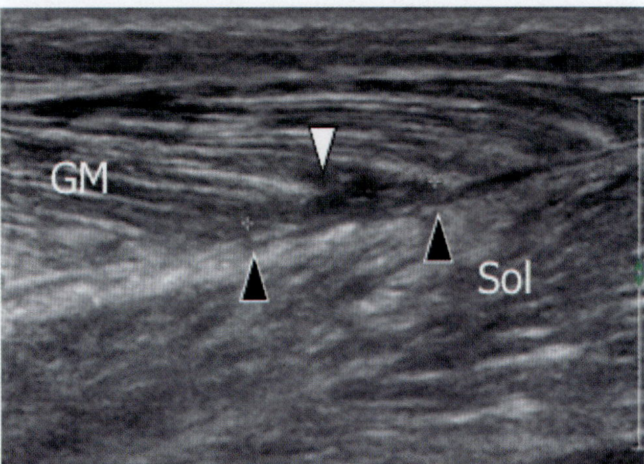

Figure 11.14.   Intrinsic muscle injuries. Grade 2. Longitudinal ultrasound image of the distal medial head of gastrocnemius (*GM*) muscle shows an ill-defined heterogeneous area (*black arrowheads*) associated with interruption of the muscle fibroadipose septa (*white arrowhead and calipers*). Note absence of a local hematoma. Sol, soleus muscle.

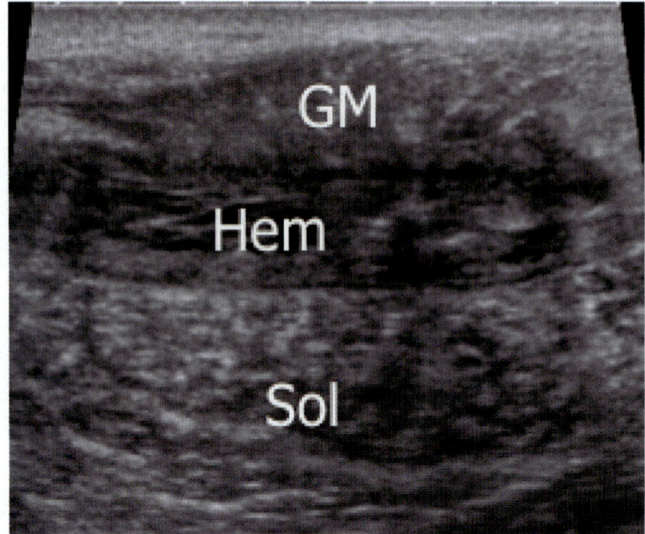

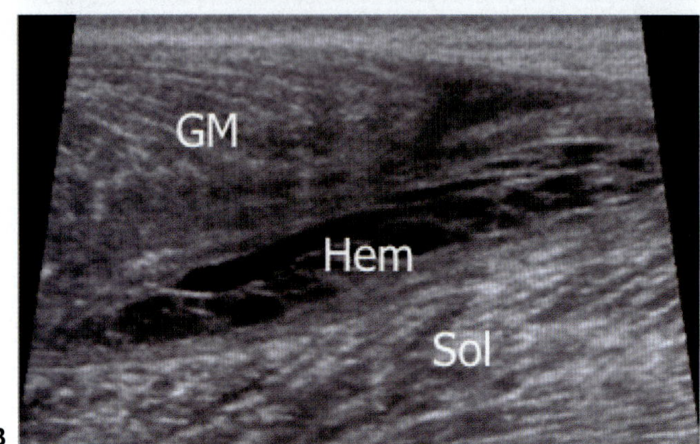

Figure 11.15.   Intrinsic muscle injuries. Grade 3. Axial (**A**) and longitudinal (**B**) ultrasound images of the calf show a distal grade 3 myoaponeurotic injury of the medial head of gastrocnemius (*GM*) muscle. Note the hematoma (*Hem*) located between the soleus and the GM. Sol, soleus muscle.

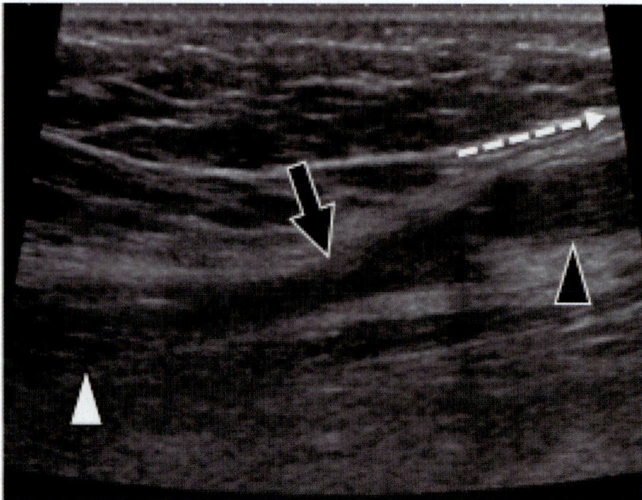

Figure 11.16.   Intrinsic muscle injuries. Grade 4. Longitudinal ultrasound image of the posterior aspect of the thigh shows a grade 4 injury of the conjoint tendon of the hamstring muscles. The proximal (*white arrowhead*) and retracted distal (*black arrowhead*) stumps are separated by an anechoic hematoma (*arrow*). Note retraction of the distal stump (*broken arrow*).

of such injuries occur in the lower limbs; the other 10% are mainly located on the biceps and brachialis muscles, and the muscles of the abdominal wall. Both ultrasound and MRI show the local hematoma. The ultrasound appearances of hematomas vary over time. Hematomas initially contain hypoechoic fluid, then solidify and become hyperechoic over the next few days, before liquefying again after 3 to 4 days and developing an anechoic center and echogenic periphery. Healing then occurs as centripetal filling-in over weeks or months, depending on the size of the hematoma. Hematomas may gradually enlarge and should be monitored by serial examination in case drainage becomes appropriate. The distinction between hematoma and reactive edema is not always easy, especially with MRI. With this type of injury, sports activity should be stopped for about 4 to 6 weeks.

Grade 4. Muscle tear. Grade 4 injury consists of a complete tear and retraction of the muscle. These injuries are observed mainly at the inferior portion of the rectus femoris or the conjoint tendon of the hamstring muscles but can also affect the long head of biceps femoris and the MHG. Both ultrasound and MRI show a defect in and proximal retraction of the muscle. The proximal stump can be surrounded by local hematoma, resulting in the typical "bell clapper" appearance (**Fig. 11.16**). Dynamic ultrasound examination during muscle contraction can help in detecting the retraction. Bleeding can extend along fascial planes and into and along the subcutaneous tissues, which explains why bruising is located distal to the site of the muscle injury. This injury usually requires 2 to 3 months of rest from sports activities.

Tip:
Dynamic ultrasound examination during muscle contraction confirms whether a muscle tear is complete and shows the extent of muscle retraction.

The size of the injury and the degree of healing are important elements for deciding when activities can be resumed as recovery time is proportionate to injury severity. Recurrent tears are frequent, especially in serious injuries or in patients with a previous injury.[63–72] Proximal injuries have a poorer prognosis.[72,73] To prevent recurrence and guide treatment, relationships between the size of the injury and the duration of rest have been proposed, especially using MRI.[73–76] At ultrasound, the presence of regular contours of the injury and the disappearance of central hyperemia on color Doppler are the two factors that confirm the healing process. Nevertheless, it is important to recognize that ultrasound findings must be correlated with clinical data before physical activity is resumed. Ultrasound can assess different post-traumatic lesions such as chronic tears, muscle fibrosis, calcification, myositis ossificans, and muscle hernias.[77,78]

Complications of Muscle Injury

Chronic Muscle Tears

Chronic muscle tears usually involve rectus femoris and present as painless soft tissue masses a few months after trauma. Often the trauma is forgotten or the causal link unrecognized. Ultrasound shows the defect in the muscle. The proximal muscle is slightly retracted and has an oval inferior margin that retracts and becomes rounder as the muscle contracts, explaining the typical clinical presentation of a mass that enlarges when the muscle contracts. Fluid may be present in the gap and along fascial planes even in chronic tears. Secondary fatty infiltration of muscle results in a hyperechoic appearance, and there may be compensatory hypertrophy of adjacent muscles.

Muscle Fibrosis and Scarring

Muscle fibrosis can cause chronic pain and slow recovery. At ultrasound, fibrosis appears as ill-defined linear, irregular, hyperechoic bands or spiculated areas. Muscle contraction does not alter their morphology, but dense scarring may result in tethering, and adjacent normal muscle may bulge when the muscle contracts. At MRI, fibrosis has low signal intensity on both T1- and T2-weighted sequences.[78]

Muscle Calcification

Muscle calcifications appear as hyperechoic structures with posterior shadowing **(Fig. 11.17)**. They are usually secondary to direct trauma. They are generally of low density and not easily detected on X-rays. Surrounding hyperemia at color or power Doppler confirms that the calcification is still active and contraindicates a return to sporting activities.

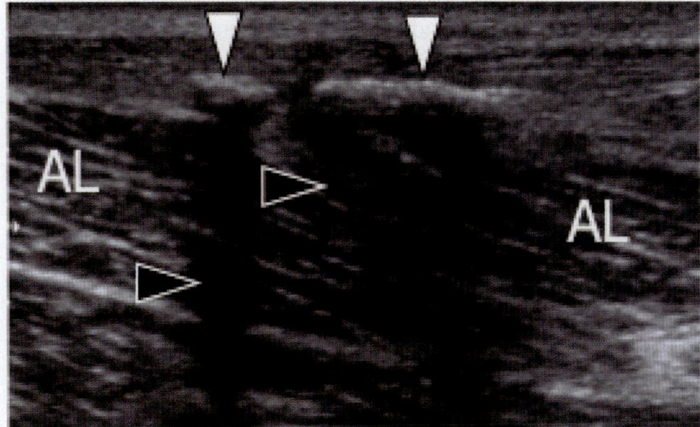

Figure 11.17. Muscle calcifications. Longitudinal ultrasound image of the proximal adductor longus (*AL*) muscle shows two hyperechoic foci of calcification (*white arrowheads*) in the superficial muscle. Note posterior shadowing (*black arrowheads*).

Myositis Ossificans

Myositis ossificans is an inflammatory pseudotumor consisting of heterotopic ossification of striated muscle. In 60% to 75% of cases it is a consequence of muscle trauma or microtrauma. Clinically, it presents as a painful mass accompanied by local signs of inflammation, which may suggest a sarcoma or an abscess. The acute phase lasts a few weeks and is followed by the chronic phase that lasts several months, during which swelling and pain decrease. In the initial phase, X-rays may be normal or show a mass in the soft tissues and periosteal reaction in the adjacent bone. After 2 to 6 weeks, flocculated calcifications appear at the periphery of the mass and may suggest the presence of a sarcoma. The juxta-diaphyseal location of the calcification suggests myositis ossificans rather than sarcoma in which calcifications are usually juxta-metaphyseal or periarticular. After several weeks, the calcifications increase in size and density and form a well-defined bony mass, often with a peripheral "eggshell" appearance. There is always a radiolucent area between the calcified mass and the adjacent bone, which helps to distinguish myositis ossificans from parosteal osteosarcoma. Eventually, the mass becomes more calcified and gradually decreases in volume. CT allows early and accurate detection of the calcifications. The MRI appearance is specific in the acute phase: The mass has intermediate or high T1 and high T2 signal, is surrounded by extensive edema (in contrast to the well-defined perilesional edema of sarcomas), and shows contrast enhancement after gadolinium injection. In the subacute and chronic phases, a line of peripheral hypointense signal on all sequences due to calcification is the most specific sign. Ultrasound shows a heterogeneous mass of variable echogenicity **(Fig. 11.18)**.[78] Longitudinal sonograms show normal muscle fibers penetrating the lesion. Ultrasound is useful in the initial phase to detect the small peripheral calcifications that MRI cannot show. Calcifications are hyperechoic and lamellar on ultrasound and extend in the same direction as the muscle fibers. With color Doppler, hyperemia gradually regresses over time. Ultrasound should be repeated to monitor the decrease in volume of the mass, the increase in density of the calcifications, and the decrease in hyperemia with Doppler.

Muscle Hernia

Muscle hernias usually present as painless small masses due to defects in the muscle fascia[79] that may result from trauma or congenital weakness where vessels penetrate the fascia. Hernias may be permanent or transient, and the latter may account for negative results obtained from imaging. On MRI, the mass has the same signal as the underlying muscle, but there may be focal hyperintense signal on T2. Ultrasound is the examination of choice as some hernias can only be seen during dynamic examination. Optimal examination technique must be deployed.

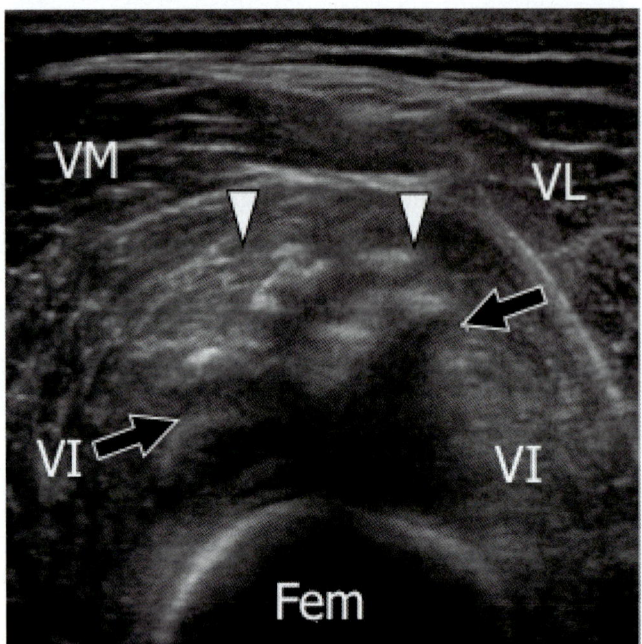

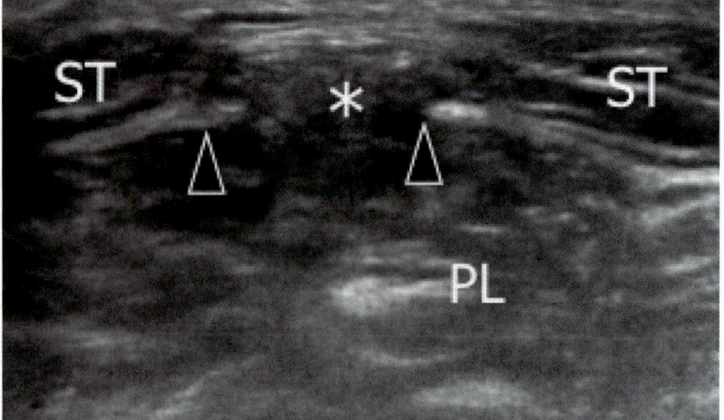

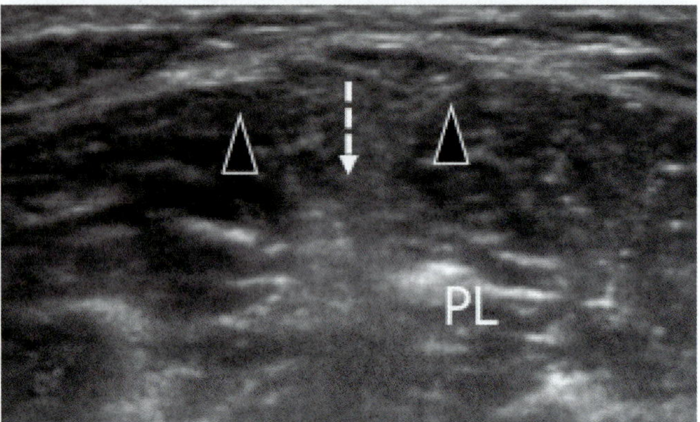

Figure 11.18.   Myositis ossificans. Axial ultrasound image of the anterior thigh shows a heterogeneous mass of increased echogenicity (*arrows*) in the vastus intermedius muscle (*VI*). The mass contains hyperechoic peripheral calcifications (*white arrowheads*). Fem, femur; VM, vastus medialis muscle; VL, vastus lateralis muscle.

Figure 11.19.   Muscle hernia. Axial ultrasound images obtained over the peroneus longus muscle (*PL*) before (**A**) and after (**B**) local compression through the transducer. In (**A**), note the muscle herniation (*asterisk*) through a defect in the hyperechoic fascia (*arrowheads*). In (**B**), pressure with the transducer effaces (*broken arrow*) the hernia. ST, subcutaneous tissues.

Large amounts of gel and light pressure on the skin with the transducer are necessary. Heavy transducer pressure should be avoided as this may reduce the hernia and result in a false-negative examination. The squatting position can be used for easier detection of herniation of anterolateral leg muscles, but examination with the patient standing or contracting the muscle or after exercise may help. Ultrasound shows focal interruption of the hyperechoic fascia and extrusion of muscle through the tear (**Fig. 11.19**). The herniated and adjacent muscle may appear slightly hypoechoic.

> **Tip:**
> If you cannot see a muscle hernia, remember that some are seen only during dynamic examination, for example, squatting, contracting the muscle, or standing. Minimize transducer pressure to avoid reducing the hernia.

Specific Locations

Adductors

The adductor muscles originate from the inferior face of the pubis and are located in the medial compartment of the thigh. In addition to hip adduction, they have a secondary role of rotation and/or flexion of the thigh.[80] They comprise gracilis, pectineus, and the three adductors (brevis, longus, and magnus) and have variable sizes and distal insertions.

The long, ribbon-like *gracilis muscle* originates from a flattened tendon at the anteroinferior aspect of the pubis. Its proximal myotendinous junction is located at the junction of the proximal and middle thirds.[81,82] The gracilis covers the adductor longus and magnus muscles and terminates in a distal tendon, which, together with the semitendinosus and sartorius tendons, forms the pes anserinus complex that inserts on the proximal medial surface of the tibia.

The *pectineus muscle* originates from the pectineal line of the pubis and inserts into the upper third of the linea aspera of the femur. Together with the obturator externus muscle, it forms the roof of the medial compartment. It is a hip flexor, and adducts and medially rotates the thigh.[83]

There are three adductor muscles, from superficial to deep: adductor longus, adductor brevis, and adductor magnus. The *adductor longus muscle* originates from a short thin tendon and from muscle fibers inserted directly on to the surface of the pubis below the public tubercle.[84] It is a bipennate muscle consisting of a central coronal aponeurosis that gives insertion to a small anterior and a large posterior muscle component. The two components merge to form the body of the muscle that inserts into the middle third of the linea aspera, between the anterior vastus medialis and the posterior adductor magnus.

The *adductor brevis muscle* originates on the anterior surface of the pubis between gracilis medially, obturator externus laterally, adductor longus superiorly, and adductor magnus inferiorly.[85,86] The muscle belly adheres to the tendon of gracilis, is covered by the adductor longus muscle, and terminates on the middle third of the linea aspera of the femur.

The *adductor magnus muscle* originates in the inferior part of the ischiopubic ramus and the ischial tuberosity. It consists of two or three main components. The two oblique medial components insert into the linea aspera of the femur between the lesser trochanter and the superior part of the medial femoral condyle. The long vertical medial component, arising from the ischial tuberosity, terminates in a strong tendon that inserts into the adductor tubercle of the femur.

For examination of the adductor muscles, the patient first lies supine with the hip flexed and abducted and the knee flexed to study the anterior and medial portions of the muscles. Then, in the prone position, assessment of the posterior part of the compartment is obtained. Flexion of the hip decreases artifacts generated by the gluteal fold.[80] Ultrasound allows easy assessment of the proximal adductor muscles, while their distal parts, with the exception of gracilis, are more difficult to examine.

Microtraumatic injuries at the origin of the adductor muscles, particularly the adductor longus, result from excessive repetitive force on the enthesis, mainly in sports requiring frequent changes of direction such as football or rugby. Ultrasound can hardly detect the resulting enthesopathy. Correlation with clinical examination, local hypervascularization at color Doppler, and comparison with the opposite side[87] can increase the diagnostic confidence. Nevertheless, only MRI can provide a definite diagnosis[88] by showing hyperintensity of the enthesis in fat-saturated T2-weighted and gadolinium-enhanced T1-weighted images.

Acute injuries affect mainly the myoaponeurotic junction and follow powerful eccentric contractions most commonly in football, rugby, and ice hockey.[89] The adductor longus is most often affected due to the superficial position of its myotendinous junction. In myoaponeurotic tears, ultrasound shows fluid close to the proximal tendon, and the central aponeurosis can have a blurred appearance **(Fig. 11.20)**. Adjacent muscle fibers show local disorganization associated with hemorrhagic infiltration. The proximal tendon must also be assessed to exclude an associated tendino-periosteal avulsion. In more severe trauma, the underlying adductor brevis can also be affected. True intramuscular tears are rare and occur in high kinetic energy accidents. They present at ultrasound as heterogeneous hematoma, focal interruption of muscle fibers, or

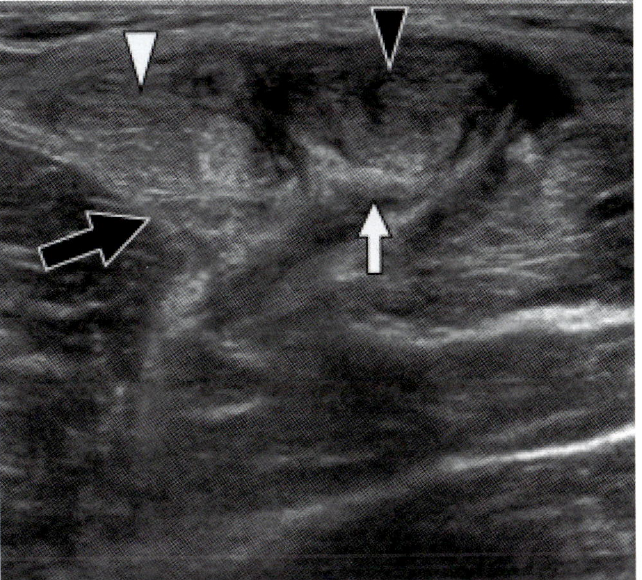

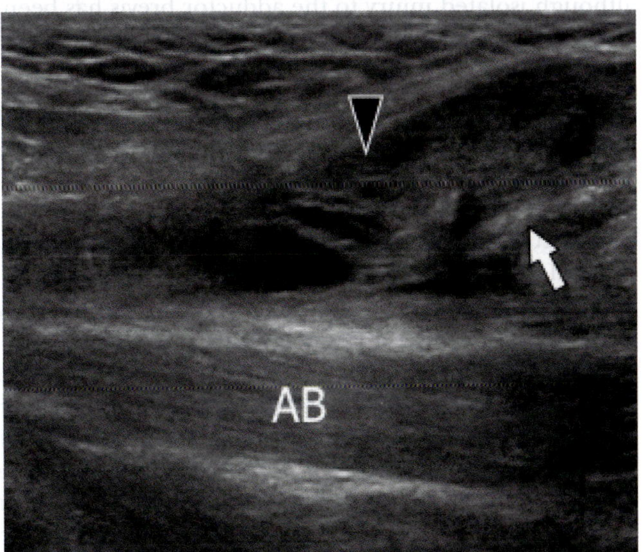

Figure 11.20. Adductor longus (AL) muscle tear. Axial **(A)** and longitudinal **(B)** ultrasound images of the proximal AL muscle (*black arrow*) show a myoaponeurotic partial tear affecting the posterior aspect of the muscle (*black arrowhead*). The ruptured muscle is occupied by hematoma. Note the torn central aponeurosis (*white arrow*). In **(A)** note the normal anterior muscle (*white arrowhead*). AB, adductor brevis muscle.

even as a "bell clapper" image. A large ecchymosis is almost always present.[90] Adductor distal avulsion syndrome has also been described in relation to the posteromedial face of the femoral diaphysis with related periostitis.[91]

The gracilis is the second most affected muscle in this group.[89] Isolated injuries are rare and well tolerated. They are located in the posterior part of the muscle at the junction of the proximal and middle thirds. They are usually partial tears[92] presenting at ultrasound as focal hyperechoic disorganization of the muscle architecture associated with minimal fluid **(Fig. 11.21)**.

Three grades of tears affect the central aponeurosis.[99,100] In grade 1, the muscle belly is of normal size with an irregular hyperechoic area (blood infiltration) surrounding the central aponeurosis, sometimes extending along the entire central aponeurosis. In grade 2, the muscle belly becomes swollen and rounded. A large area of hypoechoic and hyperechoic zones (blood infiltration and hematoma) surrounds the central aponeurosis **(Fig. 11.23)**, which may be surrounded by a hyperechoic halo (blood infiltration), giving a "bull's eye" appearance. In grade 3, there is complete disruption of muscle fibers from the central aponeurosis, which is surrounded by a hypoechoic or anechoic hematoma, often globular in appearance due to the absence of muscle fibers. The central aponeurosis may also be interrupted. Whatever the grade, the peripheral muscle remains intact. In chronic injuries, there is usually an irregular hyperechoic, or sometimes hypoechoic, area surrounding the central aponeurosis with posterior acoustic shadowing due to scar tissue. The central aponeurosis may be thickened in the absence of normal muscle tension. Dynamic ultrasound shows dysfunction of the RF during contraction (walking, running, and kicking) secondary to central myoaponeurotic chronic tears.[110] During contraction, the central aponeurosis appears stiff and fibrotic and is responsible for an abnormal tension on the superficial aponeurosis, resulting in a "heart-shape" deformation at the muscle in axial images. This can lead to chronic pain in sporting activities.[98,110] MRI is rarely necessary for acute tears but shows ill-defined hyperintense signal on T2-weighted images surrounding the central aponeurosis in grade 1 injuries. In grade 2, there is a hyperintense fluid collection due to hematoma. In grade 3, the tear is complete and the central aponeurosis crosses a collection of blood. MRI can be informative in chronic tears and shows a hypointense central scar masking the central aponeurosis on T1- and T2-weighted images. Enhancement of the scar after intravenous contrast gives a "bull's eye" appearance.[94,98,99,111] Adjacent muscles may be atrophied and show fatty infiltration[145].

Distal myoaponeurotic and distal myotendinous tears are clinically evident and easily confirmed by ultrasound,[100,112] which shows a peripheral and distal hyperechoic fusiform area due to blood infiltration deep to the aponeurosis. In more severe tears, a hypo/anechoic fusiform hematoma is present **(Fig. 11.24)**. Long-axis scans show the degree of retraction, and small tears can be detected with loss of the acute angle normally formed by the distal muscle fibers and the deep aponeurosis. In complete tears, the muscle belly is retracted and torn muscle creates a "bell clapper" appearance in the hematoma-filled defect. The deep distal aponeurosis is often thickened and irregular due to the absence of muscle tension and, in larger tears, may be interrupted. The distal tear has a better prognosis than the central tear, whatever the size of the lesion with the exception of complete tears.[111] In the chronic phase, there is usually fatty atrophy **(Fig. 11.25)**. MRI provides no additional information in acute and chronic tears.

Distal tendon tears, when isolated, correspond to partial tears of the quadriceps tendon. They can be identified with ultrasound and do not generally require MRI.[112] The superficial tendinous laminae is discontinuous, and the gap is filled by hypoechoic hematoma.

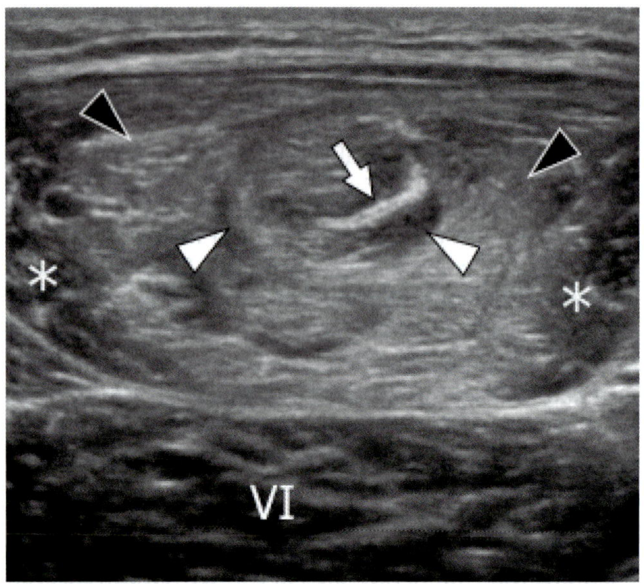

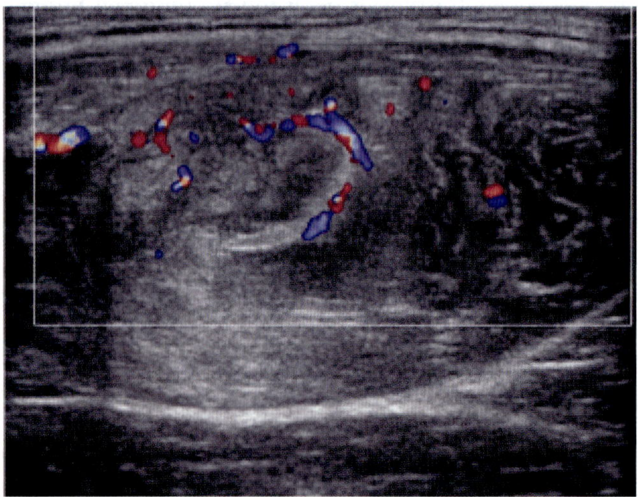

Figure 11.23.   Rectus femoris muscle central myoaponeurotic tear. Axial **(A)** and axial color Doppler **(B)** ultrasound images of the RF muscle show the hyperechoic central aponeurosis (*white arrow*) surrounded by an irregular area with mixed appearance due to tear and hematoma (*white arrowheads*). More peripherally, a hyperechoic area due to blood infiltration is evident (*black arrowheads*). Note the normal peripheral muscle (*asterisks*). In **(B)**, color Doppler shows local hyperemia. VI, vastus intermedius muscle.

Hamstrings

Anatomy.[63,86,113] The conjoint tendon of semitendinosus and biceps femoris and the tendon of semimembranosus

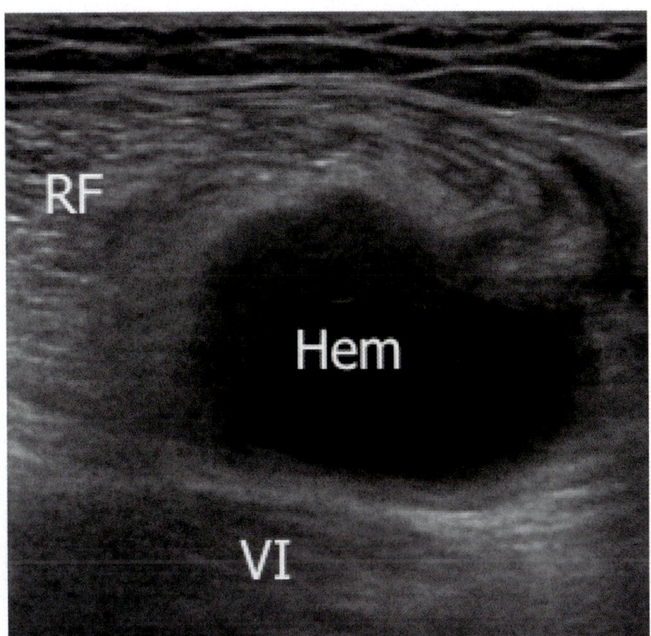

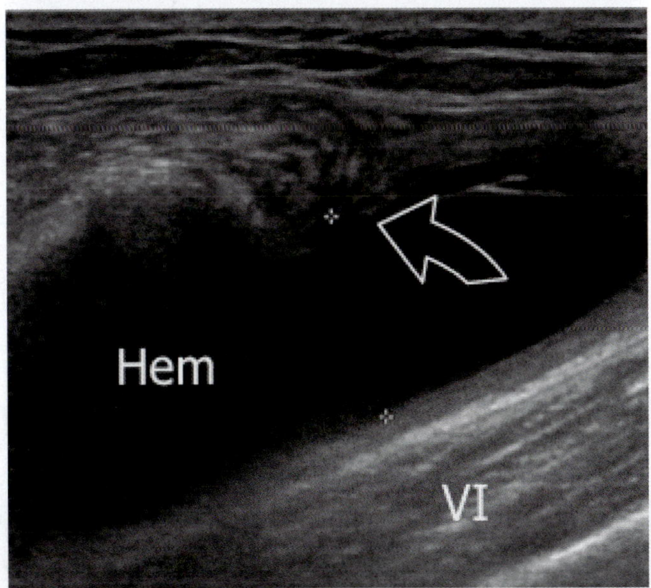

Figure 11.24. Acute RF muscle distal myoaponeurotic tear. Axial (**A**) and longitudinal (**B**) ultrasound images of the distal rectus femoris muscle (RF) show a partial tear affecting the medial portion of the distal myoaponeurotic junction. In (**B**) the muscle is retracted proximally (*curved arrow*). A large hematoma (*Hem and calipers*) is evident as a hypoechoic collection. VI, vastus intermedius muscle.

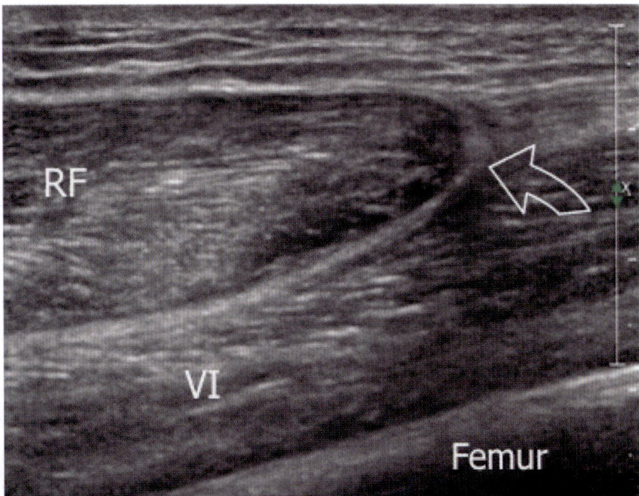

Figure 11.25. Chronic RF muscle distal myoaponeurotic tear. Longitudinal ultrasound image of the distal rectus femoris muscle (*RF*) during muscle contraction shows the retracted (*curved arrow*) muscle that presents a rounded appearance. Note absence of local hematoma. VI, vastus intermedius muscle.

originate on the posterolateral aspect of the ischial tuberosity. The conjoint tendon is more superficial and lateral than the semimembranosus tendon and passes across the deep surface of gluteus maximus. The semitendinosus muscle develops on the medial side of the conjoint tendon, close to its upper insertion. The muscle fibers of the long head of biceps femoris arise a few centimeters lower, on the lateral side of the conjoint tendon. The conjoint tendon continues in the mid thigh as a central aponeurosis. The sciatic nerve is deep to this aponeurosis, and the long head of biceps femoris is lateral. The tendon of semimembranosus originates from a large flat aponeurosis in the upper thigh between the hamstring muscles and the adductor muscles. The muscle fibers of semimembranosus originate from this aponeurosis in the distal thigh, the proximal fibers medially and the distal fibers laterally. This large myotendinous junction has an oblique orientation and can extend over 20 to 40 cm.

The sizes of hamstring muscles vary depending on the level in the thigh. *Cranially*, the semitendinosus muscle is the largest and presents with an internal sigmoid aponeurotic septum, dividing it into lateral and medial portions. In the *middle third* of the thigh, the three muscles are approximately the same size, and the short head of biceps femoris arises from the posterolateral cortex of the femoral shaft and then runs distally to join the long head. In the *lower third* of the thigh, the semitendinosus muscle becomes smaller and continues as a long thin tendon posterior to the semimembranosus muscle, which is the largest muscle at this level; and laterally, the long head of biceps femoris thins as it runs to join the superficial aponeurosis of the short head.

Ultrasound anatomy. Ultrasound is performed with the patient prone. Axial images are best. Comparison with the opposite side may help.

Tip:
If the patient is prone, flexion of the hip can help to decrease artifacts generated by the gluteal fold.

The hyperechoic ischial tuberosity is the main landmark for the conjoint and semimembranosus tendons.

In the upper thigh, the so-called hyperechoic triangle of Cohen must be identified.[113] It is defined by the conjoint tendon superficially, the sciatic nerve laterally, and the semimembranosus tendon medially. At this level, the belly of the semitendinosus is already evident and is located medial to the conjoint tendon. The fibers of the long head of the biceps femoris emerge laterally from the conjoint tendon and increase in size distally. The upper part of the semimembranosus muscle arises medially and presents as a typical triangular shape on axial images.[113] It rapidly increases in size into the mid thigh.

> **Tip:**
> If you have difficulty identifying the conjoint and semimembranosus tendons near the ischial tuberosity, identify the triangle of Cohen. The conjoint tendon is superficial, the semimembranosus tendon is medial, and the lateral part of the triangle corresponds to the sciatic nerve.

In the lower third of the thigh, the best ultrasound landmark is the myotendinous junction of the semitendinosus tendon posterior to the semimembranosus muscle. The tendon has the typical appearance of a "cherry on the cake".[113]

> **Tip:**
> In the lower third of the thigh, the semitendinosus tendon is posterior to the semimembranosus muscle and appears on axial sonograms as a "cherry on the cake." The semitendinosus tendon corresponds to the cherry, and the semimembranosus muscle to the cake.

Laterally, the insertion of the long head of the biceps femoris on the superficial aponeurosis of the short head is easily found by scanning the muscle from bottom to top.[114] This arrangement is similar to the attachment of the medial gastrocnemius muscle to the soleus and is characteristic.

Hamstring muscle injuries. These injuries are among the most common muscle injuries, especially in sports requiring fast running (sprinting, football, rugby).[63,115–120] Hamstring muscles are at risk of tearing because they cross two joints[46,63,72] and consequently are more subject to eccentric strains during simultaneous stretching and contraction. The biceps femoris is the most commonly injured hamstring muscle.[46,118,120,121] Other risk factors include the relative weakness of the hamstring muscles compared to the quadriceps muscle,[122] leg length discrepancy, and anomalies in pelvic–spinal balance.[123]

Proximal myotendinous injuries affect the muscle fibers inserting into the strong conjoint tendon of the biceps/semitendinosus or the fibers of the semimembranosus muscle inserting into the large aponeurosis. In myotendinous tears of the conjoint tendon, ultrasound generally detects heterogeneous areas (grade 2) between the tendon

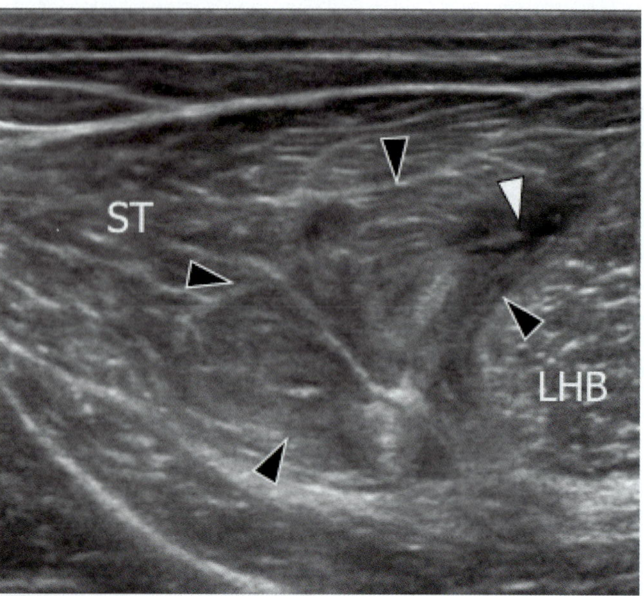

Figure 11.26. Acute semitendinosus muscle tear. Axial ultrasound image of the proximal semitendinosus muscle (*ST*) shows a partial tear affecting the lateral portion of the muscle (*black arrowheads*). A small hematoma (*white arrowhead*) is evident as a hypoechoic collection. LHB, long head of the biceps muscle.

and the proximal semitendinosus muscle fibers. Dynamic ultrasound imaging during muscle contraction can differentiate between small hypoechoic hematomas (grade 3) **(Fig. 11.26)** and muscle tears (grade 4) **(Fig. 11.27)**. The tear can be restricted to one muscle or affect both semitendinosus and biceps. Differentiation between myotendinous and true tendon tears can be difficult at ultrasound and requires MRI for optimal assessment. Myotendinous tears of semimembranosus are common in dancers[73] and are usually located at the superior myotendinous junctions. However, they can extend distally to involve lower myotendinous junctions **(Fig. 11.28)**.

In the muscle belly, small tears usually involve the central connective septa, whereas more serious injuries are commonly located at the insertion of the muscle fibers on the peripheral fascia. In small central tears, every internal septum must be examined to avoid missing a local hypoechoic area that suggests an injury. Local pressure with the transducer can help in detecting small tears. Peripheral avulsions are also difficult to detect, especially when small. Any thickening of the fascia must be considered abnormal. In doubtful cases, contralateral examination at the same level can help. The most common injury is at the level of the frontal connective septum located within the long head of the biceps. Isolated injuries to the semitendinosus sigmoid septum do occur but are rare and usually benign. Compared with MRI, ultrasound seems to be more sensitive in detecting peripheral injuries, whereas MRI seems better for tendon injuries.[49] Ultrasound can help to follow healing since it allows precise morphological analysis and can assess decreasing

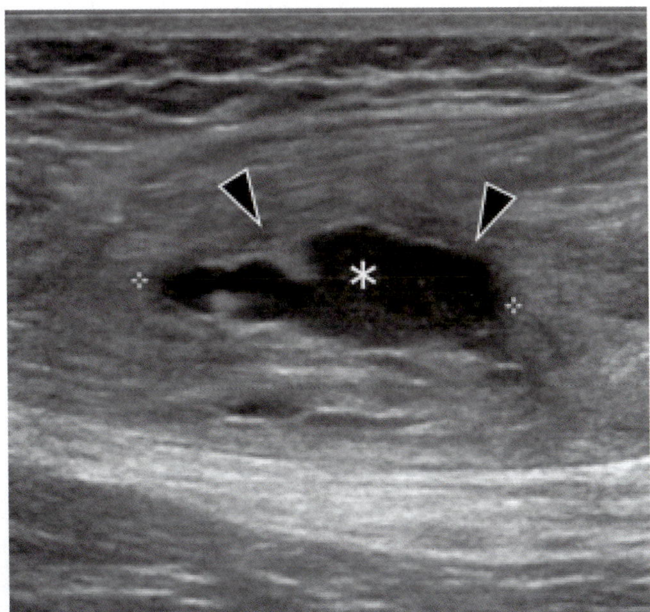

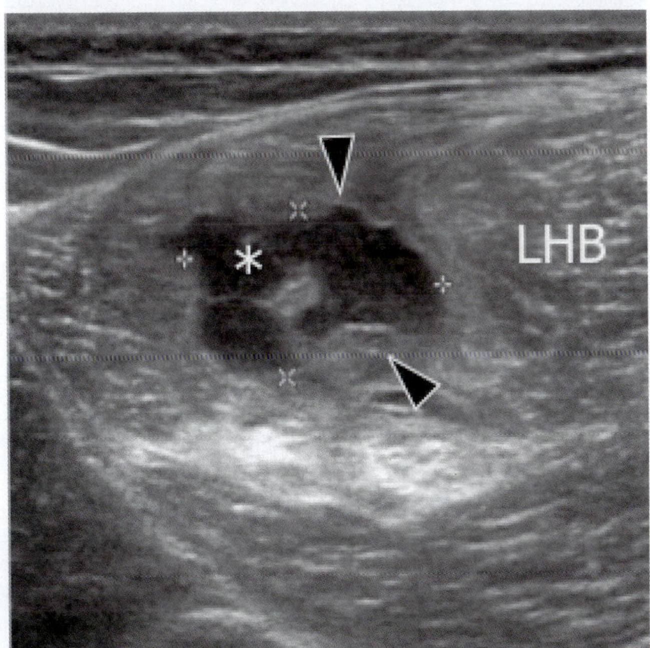

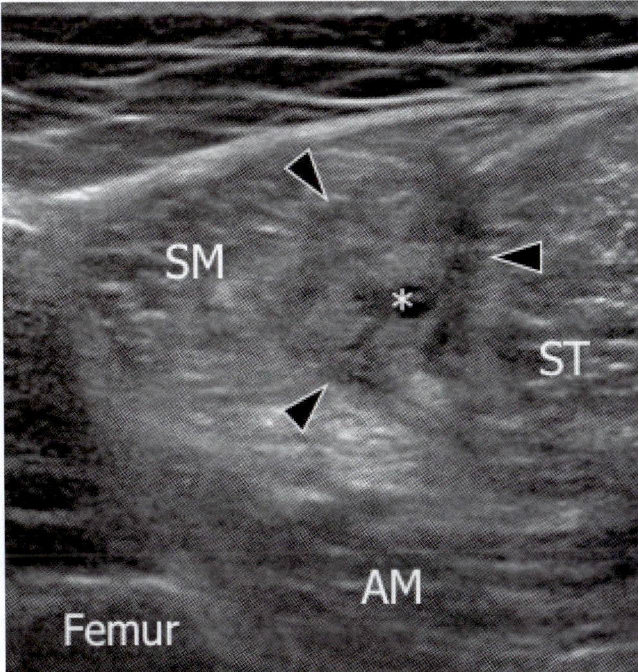

Figure 11.28. Acute semimembranosus muscle tear. Axial ultrasound image of the proximal semimembranosus muscle shows a partial tear (*black arrowheads*) located in the lateral part of the muscle. A small hematoma (*asterisks*) is evident as a hypoechoic collection. ST, semitendinosus muscle; AM, adductor muscles.

Figure 11.27. Acute semitendinosus muscle tear. Longitudinal (**A**) and axial (**B**) ultrasound images of the proximal semitendinosus muscle show a partial tear (*black arrowheads*). A large hematoma (*asterisks*) is evident as a hypoechoic collection. LHB, long head of the biceps muscle.

hyperemia with color Doppler. Complete healing appears as a local hyperechoic area. The relationship of the fibrotic area to the sciatic nerve must be evaluated to rule out nerve adhesions. At MRI, the morphological criteria of healing are not clearly established. A return to sports is possible even if there are still abnormalities on MRI.[118]

The most frequent distal injury occurs in the long head of the biceps femoris muscle at its insertion on to the aponeurosis of the short head. All grades of injury can be found, from subtle minimal tears to complete avulsion, and there is sometimes an associated interaponeurotic hematoma between the two biceps heads. Images resemble the more frequently seen tennis leg images (see below). Unlike MRI, ultrasound can assess dynamic muscle contraction and provide easy comparison with the opposite side (**Figs. 11.29, 11.30**).

Tennis Leg

Rupture of the distal myotendinous junction of the medial head of gastrocnemius (MHG), known as "tennis leg" (TL), is a common injury affecting mostly middle-aged patients ("weekend warriors"), resulting from sports injuries or relatively trivial trauma.[124–132]

Basic anatomy, technique of ultrasound examination, and ultrasound anatomy. The triceps surae is a powerful muscle located in the posterior calf. It has deep and superficial layers. The deep layer is the soleus muscle, which originates from the posterior aspects of the tibia and fibula. The superficial layer is composed of the MHG and lateral head of gastrocnemius (LHG), which originate from the supracondylar femur and the posterior knee joint capsule. The MHG is larger and descends lower than the LHG. The muscles fibers run distally and obliquely to converge on separate soleal and gastrocnemius aponeuroses, which are separated by an interaponeurotic space filled by loose connective tissue that allows gliding between the two muscles during muscle

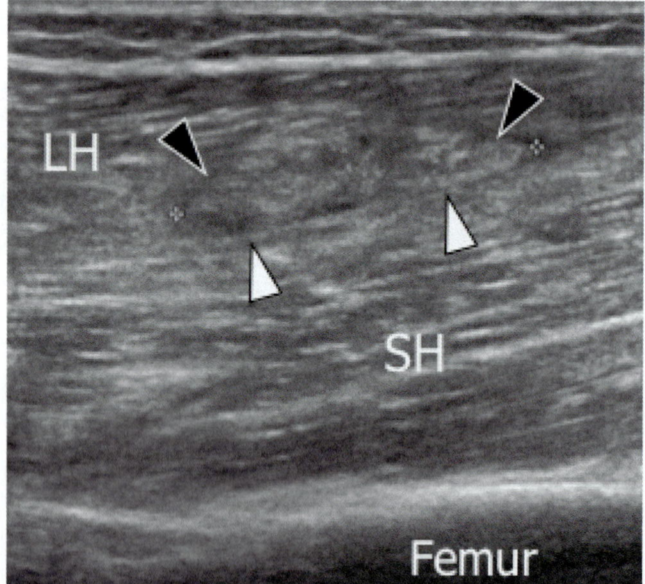

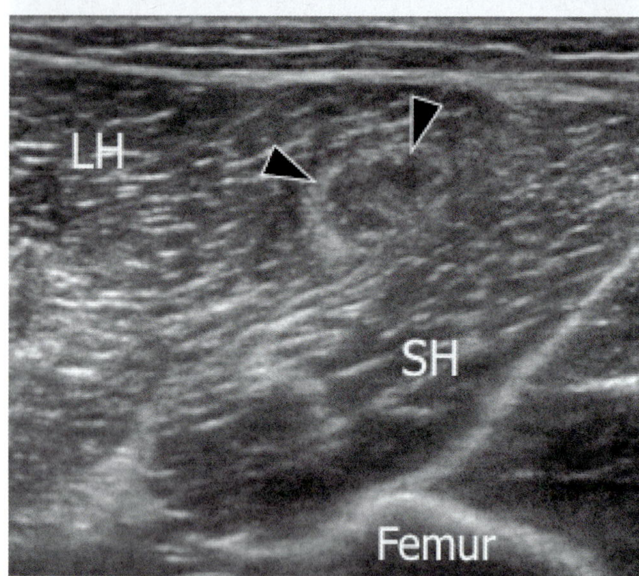

Figure 11.29.   Acute long head of the biceps muscle tear. Longitudinal **(A)** and axial **(B)** ultrasound images of the distal myotendinous junction of the long head of the biceps muscle (*LH*) show a small avulsion with local loss of the normal internal muscle architecture (*black arrowheads*). The short head of the muscle (*SH*) including its posterior aponeurosis (*white arrowheads*) is normal.

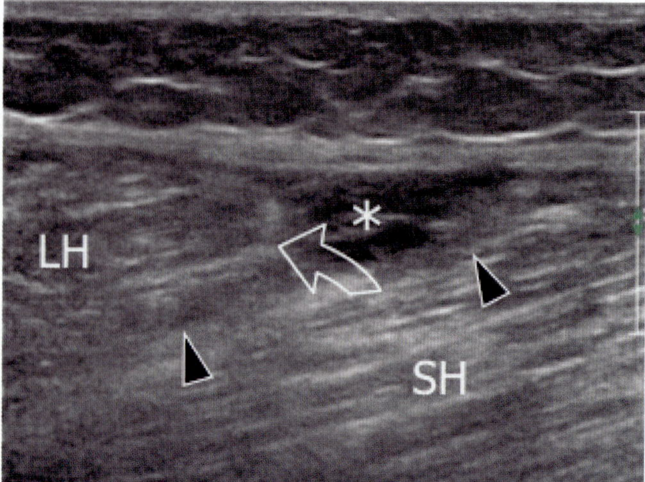

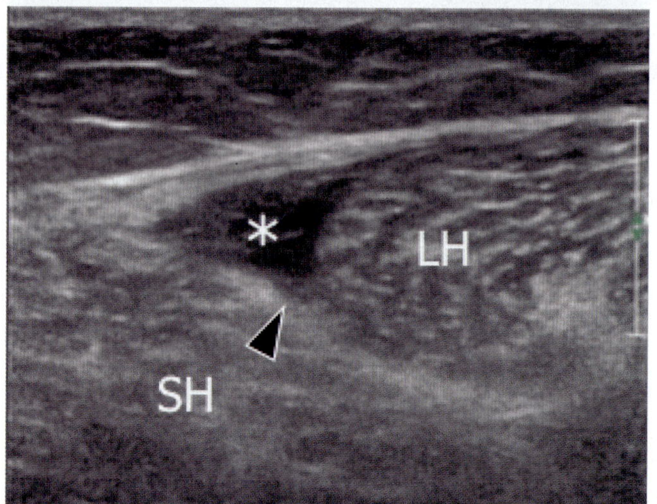

Figure 11.30.   Acute long head of the biceps muscle tear. Longitudinal **(A)** and axial **(B)** ultrasound images of the distal myotendinous junction of the long head of the biceps muscle (*LH*) show a partial avulsion of the lateral part of the junction (*black arrowheads*). The muscle is retracted proximally (*curved arrow*). A well-defined hematoma (*asterisks*) is evident. The short head of the muscle (*SH*) is normal.

contraction. Both aponeuroses thicken distally and coalesce to form the Achilles tendon. The small plantaris muscle originates medial to the LHG origin and continues distally as a long, slender tendon deep to MHG, then medial to the Achilles tendon.[128] It inserts on the posterior tuberosity of the calcaneum or fuses with the distal Achilles tendon.

The patient is examined prone with the knees held in 30 degrees of flexion[124] by placing a small pillow under the legs. This reduces stretching and decreases discomfort. Longitudinal and transverse sonograms are obtained from proximal to distal. The MHG and LHG have a regular parallel organization of muscle fibers and fibroadipose septa, while the soleus muscle has a more irregular internal arrangement. At the musculotendinous junctions, the fibroadipose septa insert into the distal aponeuroses. Accurate scanning of the anterior part of the distal myotendinous junction of the MHG is important since most small tears are located in this area. In the lower calf, the aponeuroses of gastrocnemius and soleus merge to form the Achilles tendon. The soleus muscle extends more distally than the gastrocnemius, and some of its fibers attach to the deep aspect of the Achilles tendon. The small plantaris muscle lies medial to the most cranial part of the LHG. Its long tendon may be appreciated as a thin hyperechoic structure running between the soleus and the MHG. Muscle vessels are easily evaluated with color Doppler. Firm probe pressure can focus the examination on the point of maximal tenderness, and scanning during cautious active and passive dorsiflexion of the foot helps to detect small and subtle injuries.

Triceps muscle tears. The MHG is frequently involved since it crosses two joints and has a high percentage of Type II muscle fibers. Injuries occur during active plantar flexion of the foot and simultaneous extension of the knee, causing simultaneous active contraction and passive stretching of the gastrocnemius.[129–130] Clinical findings include diffuse swelling, localized sharp pain, and local tenderness. The Achilles tendon is unaffected. Although the clinical findings are believed to be quite characteristic of TL, it is frequently misdiagnosed as tendo Achilles rupture, deep vein thrombosis (DVT), thrombophlebitis, or ruptured Baker's cyst.[127,130,132]

The ultrasound appearances depend on the size of the tear.[124,126,127] Axial sonograms are useful in differentiating partial from complete lesions. Muscle fiber retraction is more evident on sagittal sonograms. Small tears examined within a few hours of trauma may be difficult to detect in the absence of a hypo/anechoic blood collection, but careful evaluation shows that the muscle fibers and septa do not reach the aponeurosis. Dynamic studies with increased probe pressure or plantar/dorsiflexion of the foot may help. Small tears usually affect the most anteromedial portion of the medial head, and the aponeurosis is normal **(Fig. 11.31)**. In more severe partial lesions, ultrasound shows cranial displacement of a portion of the muscle associated with rupture of the anterior distal aponeurosis **(Fig. 11.32)**. The distal portion of the injured medial head assumes a heterogeneous hypo/hyperechoic appearance due to rupture of muscle fibers and hemorrhage. The appearance of the hematoma depends on the age of the injury, varying from a fusiform heterogeneous area to an anechoic collection located just distal to the tear or extending cranially in the interaponeurotic space.

Small tears are generally treated with rest and ice, whereas larger lesions usually require pharmacological

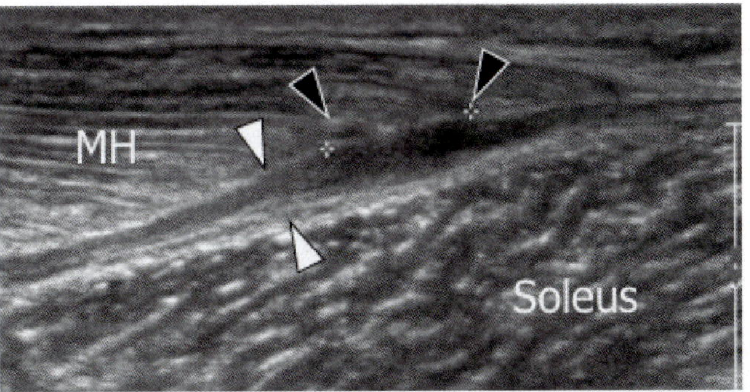
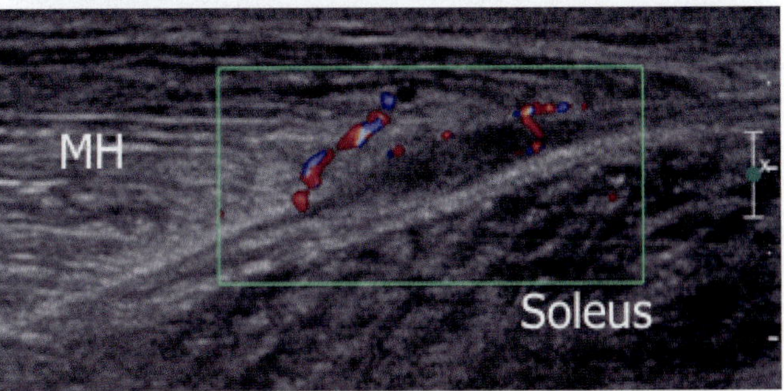

Figure 11.31.   Tennis leg. Small tear. Longitudinal gray scale **(A)** and color Doppler **(B)** ultrasound images of the distal MHG muscle (*MH*) show a small avulsion of the myotendinous junction (*black arrowheads*). The muscle does not show any significant retraction. A thin hematoma (*white arrowheads*) lies between the aponeurosis of gastrocnemius and normal soleus muscle. Color Doppler shows local hyperemia.

therapy and prolonged immobilization. Aspiration of the hematoma is followed by recurrence unless a compressive bandage is applied. Many clinicians do not perform routine drainage because of the risk of infection, and restrict the procedure to high-level sportsmen to reduce the period of inactivity. Follow-up examinations show healing starting from the periphery of the hematoma and gradually proceeding toward the center while the amount of central fluid decreases. When healing is

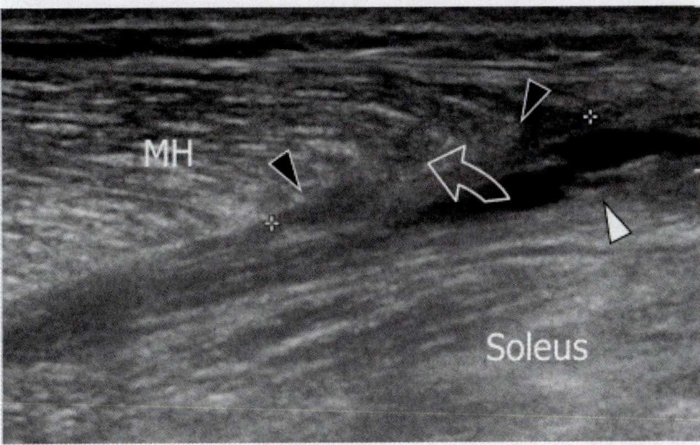

Figure 11.32.   Tennis leg. Large tear. Longitudinal gray scale ultrasound image of the distal MHG muscle (*MH*) shows a large avulsion of the myotendinous junction (*black arrowheads*). The muscle is retracted proximally (*curved arrow*). A large hematoma (*white arrowheads*) lies between the torn gastrocnemius and normal soleus muscle.

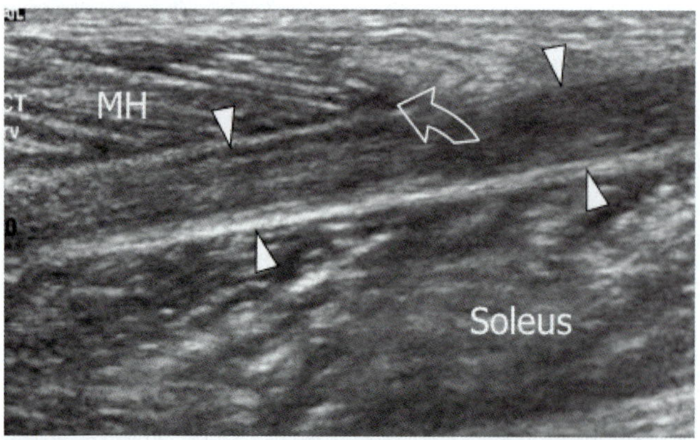

Figure 11.33.   Tennis leg. Old tear. Longitudinal gray scale ultrasound image of the distal MHG muscle (*MH*) shows a fibrotic area (*white arrowheads*) located between the retracted muscle and the normal soleus muscle. The *curved arrow* points to a small gastrocnemius tear.

complete, ultrasound shows a hyperechoic area interposed between the medial head and the soleus muscle resulting from fibrous transformation of the hematoma **(Fig. 11.33)**. Complete tears of the MHG are rare.

Differential diagnosis and complications. Clinically, TL must be differentiated from a ruptured Baker's cyst, DVT, and tears of the plantaris or soleus muscles or tendo Achilles, which can all be diagnosed with ultrasound. Ultrasound shows fluid extending in the soft tissues distal to a ruptured Baker's cyst. In popliteal vein thrombosis, hypoechoic thrombus fills the vein, which is incompressible **(Fig. 11.34)**. A proportion of patients with TL have thrombus limited to the veins of the gastrocnemius,[124,127] usually extending over 10 cm but only rarely affecting the popliteal vein. Most clinicians prefer to anticoagulate these patients to prevent pulmonary thromboembolism.

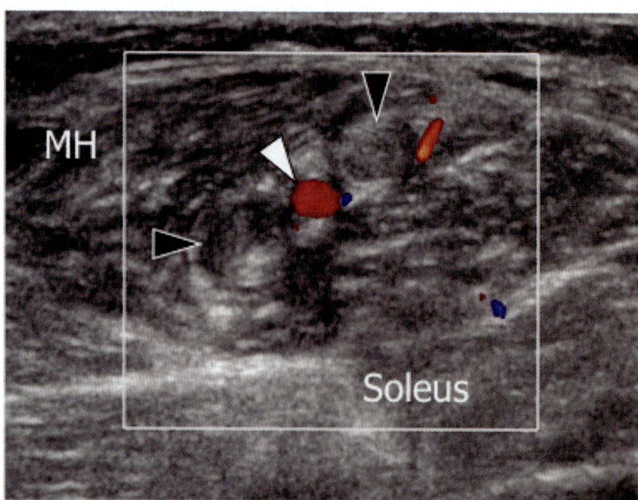

Figure 11.34.   Tennis leg. Vein thrombosis. Axial color Doppler ultrasound image of the MHG muscle (*MH*) in a patient with tennis leg. Image shows hypoechoic thrombus in two intramuscular veins (*black arrowheads*). The adjacent artery is normal (*white arrowhead*).

Small tears of the soleus muscle seem to be more frequent than previously reported. Ultrasound of soleus is difficult because of the depth of the muscle, and lower frequency transducers are required. MRI may be necessary in competitive sportsmen. Tears of the plantaris muscle or tendon are rare, and many patients previously diagnosed as having plantaris tendon tears probably had MHG tears with hematoma in the interaponeurotic space. Achilles tendon rupture is easily diagnosed by ultrasound and is discussed in Chapter 8.

> **Tip:**
> Remember, ruptured Baker's cyst, DVT, and tears of the plantaris, soleus, or Achilles tendons may mimic TL symptoms, and all can be diagnosed with sonography.

Ultrasound-guided Local Injections in Muscle Trauma

Ultrasound is a safe, cheap, and dynamic way to guide interventional procedures in muscle trauma.[133] Interventions should be performed after discussion with the appropriate clinician and require informed patient consent. Contraindications include systemic or local infection and coagulation disorders.

A routine ultrasound examination must precede every interventional procedure. The patient is usually supine to reduce the risk of vasovagal reactions. Once the target of the procedure is identified, the optimum puncture site and needle path are defined, commonly the shortest route that avoids vessels and nerves.

Interventions should be sterile procedures with appropriate skin sterilization. Sterile gloves and sterile gel are commonly used. Skin anesthesia is provided when necessary by local injection of lidocaine.

Needle visualization is optimized if the ultrasound beam is perpendicular to the long axis of the needle. Long needles help to achieve this because of the shallow angle of inclination.

Hematoma drainage. Hematoma drainage may shorten the recovery time and reduce local pain and the incidence of local fibrotic changes, although there is no firm evidence for these benefits.[118,134] Only compressible hypo/anechoic hematomas should be drained. Signs of organization such as heterogeneous echogenicity and/or absence of compressibility contraindicate aspiration. Once the shortest and safest needle path is chosen, the needle tip is directed at the center of the hematoma and blood aspirated under ultrasound control. A large bore needle (17G to 19G) of adequate length must be used. As much blood as possible must be aspirated. After complete evacuation, a compressive band is applied to reduce the risk of rebleeding.

Guided injections. Steroid injections are rarely used in muscle trauma because of possible atrophy of the muscle and adjacent structures and impaired collagen tensile strength,[135] and are probably best restricted to the treatment of painful fibrotic scars.[136,137]

Growth factor injections are frequently used in musculoskeletal diseases. Different factors can be used (e.g., TGF-beta, IGF1, BFGF, PDGF, EGF, and VEGF). They induce mesenchymal cell proliferation and differentiation, fibroblastic and endothelial cell proliferation, collagen synthesis, and angiogenesis. Platelets contain different growth factors that are liberated after platelet activation in tissue cicatrization.[138,139] Local injections of "platelet-rich plasma (*PRP*)" increase local levels of growth factors and may help the healing process.[140] Platelet-rich plasma, obtained with centrifugation, contains 94% platelets (6% in normal blood) and only 6% red blood cells, providing a high platelet concentration (1 million platelets/microliter) for subsequent therapeutic actions. There is no consensus on the amount of PRP to be injected or the number of injections.[47] In tendon disorders, injections of PRP may be more effective than autologous whole blood[141] or steroids.[142] In animal model studies, PRP allows faster healing of muscle lesions.[143] However, further scientific investigations are required to study the safety and the efficacy of this treatment.[144]

Muscle Atrophy

Complete muscle or tendon tears are usually accompanied by muscle atrophy and fatty infiltration. Recognition of atrophy and fatty infiltration is important because they are associated with poor functional outcomes after surgical reconstruction. Although differences in muscle measurements can be attributed to the dominance of the patient (muscles of the dominant side are usually larger), muscle atrophy can be estimated by comparing the cross section of a muscle to the same muscle on the opposite side. Muscle echogenicity increases, and internal echostructure becomes ill-defined and disorganized in fatty infiltration. The echogenicity of a muscle can be assessed by comparing it to an adjacent muscle, for example, by comparing infraspinatus with the adjacent trapezius muscle. For the rotator cuff, sonography has shown an accuracy that is comparable to MRI in evaluating muscle atrophy and fatty infiltration.[145] There are no studies that have evaluated the diagnostic performance of sonography in identifying and grading muscle atrophy and fatty infiltration of other muscles. Denervation also results in fatty infiltration. Occasionally, fatty infiltration presents with muscle swelling.

> **Tip:**
> Muscle atrophy can be estimated by comparing the cross-sectional area of a muscle to that of the same muscle on the opposite side. Muscle echogenicity can be evaluated by comparing one muscle to an adjacent muscle, for example, by comparing the supraspinatus with adjacent trapezius muscle.

Compartment Syndrome

Acute compartment syndrome is defined as a condition in which increased pressure within a confined fascial space leads to a reduction of local tissue perfusion. The most frequent cause of acute compartment syndrome is fracture of the tibial diaphysis. Other causes include soft tissue trauma, fractures, and reperfusion after acute arterial occlusion. Acute compartment syndrome must be diagnosed early as irreversible muscle damage occurs rapidly, and immediate fasciotomy of the affected compartment is required to prevent extensive myonecrosis. Clinical findings are highly variable and include severe pain, pain with stretching, paresthesia, paralysis, pallor, or pulselessness. The diagnosis usually relies on clinical findings and direct compartment pressure measurement. Pressure studies should not be delayed for imaging. In the early stages, ultrasound can show diffuse bulging of the fascia and an abnormal muscle echostructure with loss of the fascicular pattern. Later, ultrasound shows progressive loss of the fascicular pattern. Patchy or diffuse hyperechoicity of the muscle suggests infarction and rhabdomyolysis. Contrast-enhanced ultrasound may have a role in the diagnosis of acute compartment syndrome, but further studies are required to establish if this is the case.

Chronic exertional compartment syndrome is defined as exercise-induced reversible ischemia caused by increased pressure within a confined fascial space that leads to swelling and ischemic pain. It is often recurrent and associated with repetitive physical activity. The differential diagnosis includes stress fracture, shin splints, and popliteal artery entrapment. The anterolateral compartment of the leg is most often involved in chronic compartment syndrome. Pain usually occurs at a certain exertional level and typically disappears with rest. Rarely, if an athlete continues to compete through pain, a chronic exertional compartment syndrome can convert to an irreversible acute compartment syndrome. The exact reason why there is an increase in intramuscular pressure during exercise remains unknown. As in the acute compartment syndrome, the diagnosis of the chronic exertional compartment syndrome is largely based on clinical findings and measurement of intracompartmental pressure (rest and postexercise). Sonographic muscle changes are very subtle and are not sufficiently reliable for diagnosis.

Infection

Ultrasound is often employed to distinguish cellulitis from deeper muscle infection. Cellulitis results in swelling and diffusely increased echogenicity of the skin and subcutaneous tissues. A cobblestone appearance is due to the contrast between echogenic fat lobules and hypoechoic fluid in interlobular septa. The underlying muscles appear normal.

Conditions that increase the risk of muscle infection include diabetes, rheumatoid arthritis, malignancy and debilitation, osteomyelitis, trauma, autoimmune disease, and immune-suppression, but increasingly pyomyositis is being seen in patients with no predisposing factors. Pyomyositis results in a hard, painful swollen muscle that appears diffusely echogenic on ultrasound. Muscle abscesses are well defined and thick-walled, and there may be surrounding hyperemia. Pus in abscesses is frequently thick and echogenic. There may be overlying cellulitis.

Necrotizing fasciitis (NF) is a rapidly spreading, life-threatening infection of the soft tissues that spreads along the superficial and deep fascial planes. Streptococci are the most frequent pathogens. Clostridial infections are rarely responsible. NF is often associated with open wounds. Risk factors, as for pyomyositis, include immunosuppression, underlying chronic disease, and diabetes mellitus. Patients usually present with severe pain that is typically disproportionate to clinical findings. Subcutaneous emphysema is a very specific sign of NF, but is not always present. Early surgery (fasciotomy and debridement) and aggressive antibiotic treatment are essential.

Early sonographic findings of NF are similar to cellulitis with swelling and increased echogenicity of the subcutaneous tissues. Color or power Doppler may show local hyperemia. NF distinguishes itself by extensive and deep involvement. Fluid and gas (manifesting as hyperechoic foci with posterior acoustic shadowing) spread along fascial planes. Ultrasound is normal in a minority of cases.

CONCLUSION

Ultrasound is an excellent method of assessing muscles and performing image-guided interventions. Real-time examination during muscle contraction/relaxation can help to identify subtle injuries.

REFERENCES

1. Zamorani MP, Valle M. Muscles and tendons. In: Bianchi S, Martinoli C, eds. *Ultrasound of Musculoskeletal System.* Berlin, Germany: Springer-Verlag; 2007:45–98.
2. Peetrons P. Ultrasound of muscles. *Eur Radiol.* 2002;12(1):35–43.
3. Brasseur JL, Tardieu M. Pathologie musculaire et aponévrotique. In: JL Brasseur, ed. *Echographie du système locomoteur.* Paris, France: Masson; 1999:25–39.
4. Courthaliac C, Lhoste-Trouilloud A, Peetrons P. Sonography of muscles [in French]. *J Radiol.* 2005;86(12, pt 2):1859–1867.
5. Woodhouse JB, McNally EG. Ultrasound of skeletal muscle injury: an update. *Semin Ultrasound CT MR.* 2011;32(2):91–100.
6. Entrekin RR, Porter BA, Sillesen HH, et al. Real-time spatial compound imaging: application to breast, vascular, and musculoskeletal ultrasound. *Semin Ultrasound CT MR.* 2001;22(1):50–64.
7. Barberie JE, Wong AD, Cooperberg PL, et al. Extended field-of-view sonography in musculoskeletal disorders. *AJR Am J Roentgenol.* 1998;171(3):751–757.
8. Brasseur JL, Morvan G, Godoc B. Dynamic ultrasonography [in French]. *J Radiol.* 2005;86(12, pt 2):1904–1910.
9. Rifi M, Londero A, Mezghani S, et al. Accessory soleus muscle: a report of two cases and review of the literature [in French]. *J Radiol.* 2010;91(12, pt 1):1277–1279.
10. Martinoli C, Perez MM, Padua L, et al. Muscle variants of the upper and lower limb (with anatomical correlation). *Semin Musculoskelet Radiol.* 2010;14(2):106–121.
11. Sookur PA, Naraghi AM, Bleakney RR, et al. Accessory muscles: anatomy, symptoms, and radiologic evaluation. *Radiographics.* 2008;28(2):481–499.
12. Christodoulou A, Terzidis I, Natsis K, et al. Soleus accessorius, an anomalous muscle in a young athlete: case report and analysis of the literature. *Br J Sports Med.* 2004;38(6):E38.
13. Cheung Y, Rosenberg ZS. MR imaging of the accessory muscles around the ankle. *Magn Reson Imaging Clin North Am.* 2001;9(3):465–473.
14. Trono M, Tueche S, Quintart C, et al. Peroneus quartus muscle: a case report and review of the literature. *Foot Ankle Int.* 1999;20(10):659–662.
15. Brodie JT, Dormans JP, Gregg JR, et al. Accessory soleus muscle. A report of 4 cases and review of literature. *Clin Orthop Relat Res.* 1997;(337):180–186.
16. Yu JS, Resnick D. MR imaging of the accessory soleus muscle appearance in six patients and a review of the literature. *Skeletal Radiol.* 1994;23(7):525–528.
17. Paul MA, Imanse J, Golding RP, et al. Accessory soleus muscle mimicking a soft tissue tumor. A report of 2 patients. *Acta Orthop Scand.* 1991; 62(6):609–611.
18. Stewart JD. Compression and entrapment neuropathies. In: Dyck PJ, Thomas PK, eds. *Peripheral Neuropathy.* 3rd ed. Philadelphia, PA: WB Saunders; 1993:1354–1379.
19. Touborg-Jensen A. Carpal-tunnel syndrome caused by an abnormal distribution of the lumbrical muscles. Case report. *Scand J Plast Reconstr Surg.* 1970;4(1):72–74.
20. Kinoshita M, Okuda R, Yasuda T, et al. Tarsal tunnel syndrome in athletes. *Am J Sports Med.* 2006;34(8):1307–1312.
21. Sammarco GJ, Stephens MM. Tarsal tunnel syndrome caused by flexor digitorum accessorius longus. A case report. *J Bone Joint Surg Am.* 1990;72(3):453–454.
22. Pla ME, Dillingham TR, Spellman NT, et al. Painful legs and moving toes associates with tarsal tunnel syndrome and accessory soleus muscle. *Mov Disord.* 1996;11(1):82–86.
23. Patel N, Harvie P, Ostlere SJ. Ultrasound of accessory muscles at the Guyon canal. Paper presented at: 9th Annual Meeting of the Session European Society of Musculoskeletal Radiology; October, 2002; Valencia, Spain. 156.
24. Ogawa K, Takahashi M, Yoshida A. Aberrant muscle anterior to the shoulder joint: its clinical relevance. *J Shoulder Elbow Surg.* 1999;8(1):46–48.
25. Husarik DB, Saupe N, Pfirrmann CW, et al. Elbow nerves: MR findings in 60 asymptomatic subjects—normal anatomy, variants, and pitfalls. *Radiology.* 2009;252(1):148–156.
26. O'Hara JJ, Stone JH. Ulnar nerve compression at the elbow caused by a prominent medial head of the triceps and an anconeus epitrochlearis muscle. *J Hand Surg Br.* 1996;21(1):133–135.
27. Zeiss J, Guilliam-Haidet L. MR demonstration of anomalous muscles about the volar aspect of the wrist and forearm. *Clin Imaging.* 1996;20(3):219–221.
28. Bergman RA, Thompson SA, Afifi A, et al. *Compendium of Human Anatomic Variation.* Baltimore, MD: Urban and Schwarzemberg; 1988:23.
29. Gama C. Extensor digitorum brevis manus: a report on 38 cases and a review of the literature. *J Hand Surg Am.* 1983;8(5, pt 1):578–582.
30. Chason DP, Schultz SM, Fleckenstein JL. Tensor fasciae suralis: depiction on MR images. *AJR Am J Roentgenol.* 1995;165(5):1220–1221.
31. Somayaji SN, Vincent R, Bairy KL. An anomalous muscle in the region of the popliteal fossa: case report. *J Anat.* 1998;192(pt 2):307–308.

32. Montet X, Sandoz A, Mauget D, et al. Sonographic and MRI appearance of tensor fasciae suralis muscle, an uncommon cause of popliteal swelling. *Skeletal Radiol.* 2002;31(9):536–538.

33. Bianchi S, Abdelwahab IF, Oliveri M, et al. Sonographic diagnosis of accessory soleus muscle mimicking a soft tissue tumor. *J Ultrasound Med.* 1995;14(9):707–709.

34. Kouvalchouk JF, Fisher M. Les muscles accessoires au niveau de la cheville. Mise au point. *J Traumatol Sport.* 1998;15:101–106.

35. Grasso A, Dini P, Allegra M. An accessory musculus soleus (symptomatic and asymptomatic). The CT findings [in Italian]. *Radiol Med.* 1992;84(1–2):22–25.

36. Peterson DA, Stinson W, Lairmore JR. The long accessory flexor muscle: an anatomic study. *Foot ankle Int.* 1995;16(10):637–640.

37. Sobel M, Levy ME, Bohne WH. Congenital variations of the peroneus quartus muscle: an anatomic study. *Foot Ankle.* 1990;11(2):81–89.

38. Sobel M, Geppert MJ, Olson EJ, et al. The dynamic of peroneus brevis tendon splits: a proposed mechanism, technique of diagnosis, and classification of injury. *Foot ankle.* 1992;13(7):413–422.

39. Chepuri NB, Jacobson JA, Fessell DP, et al. Sonographic appearance of the peroneus quartus muscle: correlation with MR imaging appearance in seven patients. *Radiology.* 2001;218(2):415–419.

40. Cheung YY, Rosemberg ZS, Ramsinghani R, et al. Peroneus quartus muscle: MR imaging features. *Radiology.* 1997;202(3):745–750.

41. Diaz GC, van Holsbeeck M, Jacobson JA. Longitudinal split of the peroneus longus and peroneus brevis tendons with disruption of the superior peroneal retinaculum, *J Ultrasound Med.* 1998;17(8):525–529.

42. Mick CA, Lynch F. Reconstruction of the peroneal retinaculum using the peroneus quartus. A case report. *J Bone Joint Surg Am.* 1987; 69(2):296–297.

43. Järvinen TA, Järvinen TL, Kääriäinen M, et al. Muscle injuries: biology and treatment. *Am J sports Med.* 2005;33(5):745–764.

44. Noonan TJ, Garrett WE Jr. Injuries at the myotendinous junction. *Clin Sports Med.* 1992;11(4):783–806.

45. Verrall GM, Slavotinek JP, Barnes PG, et al. Clinical risk factors for hamstring muscle strain injury: a prospective study with correlation of injury by magnetic resonance imaging. *Br J Sports Med.* 2001;35(6):435–439.

46. Slavotinek JP, Verrall GM, Fon GT. Hamstring injury in athletes: using MR imaging measurements to compare extent of muscle injury with amount of time lost from competition. *AJR Am J Roentgenol.* 2002;179(6):1621–1628.

47. Linklater JM, Hamilton B, Carmichael J, et al. Hamstring injuries: anatomy, imaging, and intervention. *Semin Musculoskelet Radiol.* 2010;14(2):131–161.

48. Carrillon Y, Cohen M. Imaging findings of muscle traumas in sports medicine [in French]. *J Radiol.* 2007;88(1, pt 2):129–142.

49. Connell DA, Schneider-Kolsky ME, Hoving JL, et al. Longitudinal study comparing sonographic and MRI assessments of acute and healing hamstring injuries. *AJR Am J Roentgenol.* 2004;183(4):975–984.

50. Koulouris G, Connell D. Hamstring muscle complex: an imaging review. *Radiographics.* 2005;25(3):571–586.

51. Gulick DT, Kimura IF. Delayed onset muscle soreness: what is it and how do we treat it? *J Sport Rehab.* 1996;5(17):234–243.

52. MacIntyre DL, Reid WD, McKenzie DC. Delayed muscle soreness. The inflammatory response to muscle injury and its clinical implications. *Sports Med.* 1995;20(1):24–40.

53. Cheung K, Hume P, Maxwell L. Delayed onset muscle soreness: treatment strategies and performance factors. *Sports Med.* 2002;33(2):145–164.

54. Shellock FG, Fukunaga T, Mink JH, et al. Exertional muscle injury: evaluation of concentric versus eccentric actions with serial MR imaging. *Radiology.* 1991;179(3):659–664.

55. Fleckenstein JL, Wetherall PT, Parkey RW, et al. Sports-related muscle injuries: evaluation with MR imaging. *Radiology.* 1989;172(3):793–798.

56. Dierking JK, Bemben MG, Bemben DA, et al. Validity of diagnostic ultrasound as a measure of delayed onset muscle soreness. *J Orthop Sports Phys Ther.* 2000;30(3):116–122.

57. Lee JC, Healy J. Sonography of lower limb muscle injury. *AJR Am J Roentgenol.* 2004;182(2):341–351.

58. Brasseur JL, Bach G, Renoux J, et al. Classification des lésions musculaires; de quoi parle-t-on? In: Sans N, Lhoste-Trouilloud A, Cohen M, et al, eds. *L'imagerie en Traumatologie Sportive.* Montpellier, France: Sauramps Médical; 2010:145–168.

59. Kouvalchouk JF, Durey A, Saddier P, et al. Pathologie traumatique du muscle strié chez le sportif. Editions Techniques. Encyl Méd Chir (Paris), Appareil Locomoteur, 15140; A10: 1992, 6p.

60. Berquist Th. *Imaging of Sports Injuries.* Gaithersburg, MD: Aspen Press; 1992.

61. Brasseur JL, Tardieu M, Lazennec JY. L'écho-anatomie des lésions musculaires aiguës et chroniques. *Feuillets de Radiologie.* 1999;39(3):181–191.

62. Brasseur JL. Echographie des lésions musculaires traumatiques. *Le Rhumatologue.* 2008;65:8–10.

63. Beltran L, Ghazikhanian V, Padron M, et al. The proximal hamstring muscle-tendon-bone unit: a review of the normal anatomy, biomechanics, and pathophysiology. *Eur J Radiol.* 2012;81(12): 3772–3779.

64. Garrett WE Jr. Muscle strain injuries: clinical and basic aspects. *Med Sci Sports Exerc.* 1990;22(4):436–443.

65. Noonan TJ, Garrett WE Jr. Muscle Strain injury. diagnosis and treatment. *J Am Acad Orthop Surg.* 1999;7(4):262–269.

66. Folinais D, Thelen P, Delin C. Lesions musculaires du soleus -Imagerie normale et pathologique- Réflexions sur le mécanisme physiopathologiques des désinsertions musculo-aponévrotiques. In: Brasseur JL, Zeitoun-Eiss D, Renoux J, eds. *Actualités en échographie de l'appareil locomoteur (Tome 4).* Montpellier, France: Sauramps Médical; 2007:47–74.

67. Verrall GM, Slavotinek JP, Barnes PG, et al. Diagnostic and prognostic value of clinical findings in 83 athletes with posterior thigh injury: comparison of clinical findings with magnetic resonance imaging documentation of hamstring muscle strain. *Am J Sports Med.* 2003;31(6):969–973.

68. Koulouris G, Connell DA, Brukner P, et al. Magnetic resonance imaging parameters for assessing risk of recurrent hamstring injuries in elite athletes. *Am J Sports Med.* 2007;35(9):1500–1506.

69. Silder A, Reeder SB, Thelen DG. The influence of prior hamstring injury on lengthening muscle tissue mechanics. *J Biomech.* 2010;43(12):2254–2260.

70. Heiderscheit BC, Sherry MA, Silder A, et al. Hamstring strain injuries: recommendations for diagnosis, rehabilitation, and injury prevention. *J Orthop Sports Phys Ther.* 2010;40(2):67–81.

71. Orchard J, Best TM, Verrall GM. Return to play following muscle strains. *Clin J Sport Med.* 2005;15(6):436–441.

72. Askling CM, Tengvar M, Saartok T, et al. Proximal hamstring strains of stretching type in different sports: injury situations, clinical and magnetic resonance imaging characteristics, and return to sport. *Am J Sports Med.* 2008;36(9):1799–1804.

73. Askling CM, Tengvar M, Saartok T, et al. Acute first-time hamstring strains during high-speed running: a longitudinal study including clinical and magnetic resonance imaging findings. *Am J Sports Med.* 2007;35(2):197–206.

74. Slavotinek JP. Muscle injury: the role of imaging in prognostic assignment and monitoring of muscle repair. *Semin Musculoskelet Radiol.* 2010;14(2):194–200.

75. Renoux J, Mercy G, Zeitoun-Eiss D, et al. Valeur pronostique de l'échographie dans les lésions musculaires post-traumatiques. In: Brasseur JL, Zeitoun-Eiss D, Bach G, eds. *Actualités en*

échographie de l'appareil locomoteur (tome 8). Montpellier, France: Sauramps Médical; 2011.

76. Koulouris G, Ting AYI, Jhamb A, et al. Magnetic resonance imaging findings of injuries to the calf muscle complex. *Skeletal Radiol.* 2007;36(10):921–927.

77. Daenen B, Montesanti J, Houben G. Echographie dans la myosite ossifiante. In: Brasseur JL, Zeitoun-Eiss D, Bach G, eds. *Actualités en échographie de l'appareil locomoteur (tome 7)*. Montpellier, France: Sauramps Médical; 2011.

78. Blankenbaker DG, Tiute MJ. Temporal changes of muscle injury. *Semin Musculoskeletal Radiol.* 2010;14(2):176–193.

79. Beggs I. Sonography of muscle hernias. *AJR Am J Roentgenol.* 2003;180(2):395–399.

80. Courthaliac Ch, Weilbacher H. Echo-anatomie des adducteurs de la cuisse et aspects pathologiques. *Actualités en Échographie de l'Appareil Locomoteur*. Montpellier, France: Sauramps Médical Paris; 2004.

81. Pedret C, Balius R, Barceló P, et al. Isolated tears of the gracilis muscle. *Am J Sports Med.* 2011;39(5):1077–1080.

82. Zeitoun-Eiss D, Godoc B, Renoux J, et al. Echographie des pubalgies. *Actualités en Échographie de l'Appareil Locomoteur 4*. Montpellier, France: Sauramps Médical Paris; 2007.

83. Segard J. Le muscle pectiné. Mémoire pour le certificat d'anatomie, d'imagerie et de morphogénèse 2002–2003; Université de Nantes.

84. Strauss EJ, Campbell K, Bosco JA. Analysis of the cross-sectional area of the adductor longus tendon: a descriptive anatomic study. *Am J Sports Med.* 2007;35(6):996–999.

85. Davis JA, Stringer MD, Woodley SJ. New insights into the proximal tendons of adductor longus, adductor brevis and gracilis. *Br J Sports Med.* 2012;46(12):871–876.

86. Bianchi S, Martinoli C. Thigh (Chapter 13). In: Bianchi S, Martinoli C, eds. *Ultrasound of the Musculoskeletal System.* Berlin, Heidelberg: Springer-Verlag; 2007:555–636.

87. Peetrons P. Les pubalgies. Approche par l'échographie. *Bassin et Hanche Getroa-Gel opus 34*. Montpellier, France: Sauramps Médical Paris; 2007.

88. Robinson P, Barron DA, Parsons W, et al. Adductor-related groin pain in athletes: correlation of MR imaging with clinical findings. *Skeletal Radiol.* 2004;33(8):451–457.

89. Nicholas SJ, Tyler TF. Adductor muscle strains in sport. *Sports Med.* 2002;32(5):339–344.

90. Charnock BL, Lewis CL, Garrett WE Jr, et al. Adductor longus mechanics during the maximal effort soccer kick. *Sports Biomech.* 2009;8(3):223–234.

91. Weaver JS, Jacobson JA, Jamadar DA, et al. Sonographic findings of adductor insertion avulsion syndrome with magnetic resonance imaging correlation. *J Ultrasound Med.* 2003;22(4):403–407.

92. Wong LLS. Imaging of muscle injuries. *J HK Coll Radiol.* 2005;8:191–201.

93. Attarian DE. Isolated acute hip adductor brevis strain. *J South Orthop Assoc.* 2000;9(3):213–215.

94. Hasselman CT, Best TM, Hughes C IV, et al. An explanation for various rectus femoris strain injuries using previously undescribed muscle architecture. *Am J Sports Med.* 1995;23(4):493–499.

95. Kamina P. *Anatomie Clinique. Tome 1: Anatomie Générale, Membres.* 4th ed. Paris, France: Maloine; 2009.

96. Ouellette H, Thomas BJ, Nelson E, et al. MR imaging of rectus femoris origin injuries. *Skeletal Radiol.* 2006;35(9):665–672.

97. Bordalo-Rodrigues M, Rosenberg ZS. MR imaging of the proximal rectus femoris musculotendinous unit. *Magn Reson Imaging Clin North Am.* 2005;13(4):717–725.

98. Hughes C IV, Hasselman CT, Best TM, et al. Incomplete, intrasubstance strain injuries of the rectus femoris muscle. *Am J Sports Med.* 1995;23(4):500–506.

99. Bianchi S, Martinoli C, Waser NP, et al. Central aponeurosis tears of the rectus femoris: sonographic findings. *Skeletal Radiol.* 2002;31(10):581–586.

100. Bianchi S, Martinoli C. *Ultrasound of the Musculoskeletal System.* Berlin, Germany: Springer-Verlag;2007.

101. Speer KP, Lohnes J, Garrett WE Jr. Radiographic imaging of muscle strain injury. *Am J Sports Med.* 1993;21(1):89–95.

102. Garrett WE Jr. Muscle strain injuries. *Am J Sports Med.* 1996;24(suppl 6):2–8.

103. Cotten A. Imagerie musculosquelettique. *Pathologies Locorégionales.* Masson, Paris: Issy-les-Moulineaux; 2008.

104. Brasseur JL, Tardieu M. Echographie du système locomoteur. *Imagerie médicale diagnostic.* Masson, Paris: Elsevier; 2002.

105. Courthaliac C, Brun JP, Vidalin H, et al. Les lésions musculaires des membres inférieurs chez le sportif de haut niveau: aspect échographique corrélé à l'IRM. *Feuillets de Radiologie.* 2003;43:528–539.

106. Temple HT, Kuklo TR, Sweet DE, et al. Rectus femoris muscle tear appearing as a pseudotumor. *Am J Sports Med.* 1998;26(4):544–548.

107. Rask MR, Lattig GJ. Traumatic fibrosis of the rectus femoris muscle. Report of five cases and treatment. *JAMA.* 1972;221(3):268–269.

108. Ryan AJ. Quadriceps strain, rupture and charley horse. *Med Sci Sports Exerc.* 1969;1:106–111.

109. Douis H, Gillett M, James SL. Imaging in the diagnosis, prognostication, and management of lower limb muscle injury. *Semin Musculoskelet Radiol.* 2011:15(1):27–41.

110. Bordet B, Borne J, Luciani JF, et al. Echographie du muscle en mouvement droit fémoral et vaste intermédiaire. L'imagerie en traumatologie du sport. *Getroa-Gel Opus 37.* Montpellier, France: Sauramps medical; 2010.

111. Cross TM, Gibbs N, Houang MT, et al. Acute quadriceps muscle strains: magnetic resonance imaging features and prognosis. *Am J Sports Med.* 2004;32(3):710–719.

112. Bianchi S, Zwass A, Abdelwahab IF, et al. Diagnosis of tears of the quadriceps tendon of the knee: value of sonography. *AJR Am J Roentgenol.* 1994;162(5):1137–1140.

113. Cohen M, Morvan G, Brasseur JL. Les ischiojambiers. *Gel-Contact.* 2002;9:4–16.

114. Brasseur JL, Renoux J, Glatard AS, et al. Echographie du tendon distal du biceps femoral. In: Brasseur JL, Zeitoun-Eiss D, Bach G, eds. *Actualités en échographie de l'appareil locomoteur (tome 7).* Montpellier, France: Sauramps Médical; 2010:235–249.

115. Davis KW. Imaging of the hamstrings. *Semin Musculoskelet Radiol.* 2008;12(1):28–41.

116. Counsel P, Breidahl W. Muscle injuries of the lower leg. *Semin Musculoskelet Radiol.* 2010;14(2):162–175.

117. Boutin RD, Fritz RC, Steinbach LS. Imaging of sports-related muscle injuries. *Radiol Clin North Am.* 2002;40(2):333–362.

118. Koulouris G, Connell D. Imaging of hamstring injuries: therapeutic implications. *Eur Radiol.* 2006;16(7):1478–1487.

119. Armfield DR, Kim DH, Towers JD, et al. Sports-related muscle injury in the lower extremity. *Clin Sports Med.* 2006;25(4):803–842.

120. De Smet AA, Best TM. MR imaging of the distribution and location of acute hamstring injuries in athletes. *AJR Am J Roentgenol.* 2000;174(2):393–399.

121. Silder A, Heiderscheit BC, Thelen DG, et al. MR observations of long-term musculotendon remodeling following a hamstring strain injury. *Skeletal Radiol.* 2008;37(12):1101–1119.

122. Orchard J, Marsden J, Lord S, et al. Preseason hamstring muscle weakness associated with hamstring muscle injury in Australian footballers. *Am J Sports Med.* 1997;25(1):81–85.

123. Orchard JW. Intrinsic and extrinsic risk factors for muscle strains in Australian football. *Am J Sports Med.* 2001;29(3):300–303.

124. Bianchi S, Martinoli C, Abdelwahab IF, et al. Sonographic evaluation of tears of the gastrocnemius medial head ("tennis leg"). *J Ultrasound Med.* 1998;17(3):157–162.

125. Weishaupt D, Schweitzer ME, Morrison WB. Injuries to the distal gastrocnemius muscle: MR findings. *J Comput Assist Tomogr.* 2001;25(5):677–682.

126. Dessl A, Bodner G, Springer P, et al. Ruptures of the medial gastrocnemius muscle: diagnosis with high resolution ultrasound [in German]. *Ultraschall Med.* 1998;19(5):230–233.

127. Delgado GJ, Chung CB, Lektrakul N, et al. Tennis leg: clinical US study of 141 patients and anatomic investigation of four cadavers with MR imaging and US. *Radiology.* 2002;224(1):112–119.

128. Helms CA, Fritz RC, Garvin GJ. Plantaris muscle injury: evaluation with MR imaging. *Radiology.* 1995;195(1):201–203.

129. Shields CL Jr, Redix L, Brewster CE. Acute tears of the medial head of the gastrocnemius. *Foot Ankle.* 1985;5(4):186–190.

130. Miller WA. Rupture of the musculotendinous juncture of the medial head gastrocnemius muscle. *Am J Sports Med.* 1977;5(5):191–193.

131. Millar AP. Strains of the posterior calf musculature ("tennis leg"). *Am J Sports Med.* 1979;7(3):172–174.

132. Liu SH, Chen WS. Medial gastrocnemius hematoma mimicking deep vein thrombosis: report of a case. *Taiwan Yi Xue Hui Za Zhi.* 1989;88(6):624–627.

133. Cohen M, Jacob D. Ultrasound guided interventional radiology [in French]. *J Radiol.* 2007;88(9, pt 2):1223–1229.

134. Sofka CM, Collins AJ, Adler RS. Use of ultrasonographic guidance in interventional musculoskeletal procedures: a review from a single institution. *J Ultrasound Med.* 2001; 20(1):21–26.

135. Harraldsson BT, Langberg H, Aagaard P, et al. Corticosteroids reduce the tensile strength of isolated collagen fascicles. *Am J Sports Med.* 2006;34(12):1992–1997.

136. Levine WN, Bergfeld JA, Tessendorf W, et al. Intramuscular corticosteroid injection for hamstring injuries. A 13-year experience in the National Football League. *Am J Sports Med.* 2000;28(3):297–300.

137. Beiner JM, Jokl P, Cholewicki J, et al. The effect of anabolic steroids and corticosteroids on healing of muscle contusion injury. *Am J Sports Med.* 1999;27(1):2–9.

138. Lee KS, Wilson JJ, Rabago DP, et al. Musculoskeletal applications of platelet-rich plasma: fad or future? *AJR Am J Roentgenol.* 2011;196(3):628–636.

139. Menetrey J, Kasemkijwattana C, Day CS, et al. Growth factors improve muscle healing in vivo. *J Bone Joint Surg Br.* 2000;82(1):131–137.

140. Harris NL, Huffer WE, von Stade E, et al. The effect of platelet-rich plasma on normal soft tissues in the rabbit. *J Bone Joint Surg Am.* 2012;94(9):786–793.

141. Thanasas C, Papadimitriou G, Charalambidis C, et al. Platelet-rich plasma versus autologous whole blood for the treatment of chronic lateral elbow epicondylitis: a randomized controlled clinical trial. *Am J Sports Med.* 2011;39(10):2130–2134.

142. Gosens T, Peerbooms JC, van Laar W, et al. Ongoing positive effect of platelet-rich plasma versus corticosteroid injection in lateral epicondylitis: a double-blind randomized controlled trial with 2-year follow-up. *Am J Sports Med.* 2011;39(6):1200–1208.

143. Hammond JW, Hinton RY, Curl LA, et al. Use of autologous platelet-rich plasma to treat muscle strain injuries. *Am J Sports Med.* 2009;37(6):1135–1142.

144. Hamilton BH, Best TM. Platelet-enriched plasma and muscle strain injuries: challenges imposed by the burden of proof. *Clin J Sport Med.* 2011;21(1):31–36.

145. Strobel K, Hodler J, Meyer DC, et al. Fatty atrophy of supraspinatus and infraspinatus muscles: accuracy of US. *Radiology.* 2005;237(2):584–589.

CHAPTER

12

Nerves

Carlo Martinoli
Alberto Tagliafico
Ian Beggs

INTRODUCTION

Clinical assessment, supplemented by neurophysiological testing, remains fundamental to the diagnosis of peripheral nerve lesions, and can be supplemented by imaging. Radiographs and computed tomography (CT) are of limited value, although CT shows bony or osteophytic encroachment on fibro-osseous tunnels. Magnetic resonance (MR) imaging and ultrasound are both capable of demonstrating peripheral nerves. Conventional MR imaging is widely available. Specialized techniques such as MR neurography, including diffusion tensor imaging,[1,2] are particularly useful centrally and in deep nerves that are inaccessible to ultrasound, but are not widely available. Ultrasound is ideally suited for assessment of peripheral nerves. Although it is widely available, relatively cheap, assesses long segments of nerves quickly, and permits dynamic examination,[2] careful technique and good anatomical knowledge are essential.

ANATOMY AND ULTRASOUND TECHNIQUE

Peripheral nerves are composed of myelinated and non-myelinated axons that are bathed in endoneurial fluid. Axons are grouped together in fascicles that are surrounded by perineurium consisting of perineurial cells and collagen. Fascicles are embedded in connective tissue, the interfascicular epineurium, which contains vessels and elastic fibers. The outer layers of epineurium envelop the fascicles and form the nerve sheath or epineurial epineurium.[3] The size and number of fascicles vary between and within nerves.

Ultrasound scans of peripheral nerves correlate well with nerve structure (**Fig. 12.1**). Long-axis scans show narrow, elongated structures (**Fig. 1.16**) with a fascicular appearance due to alternating hypoechoic and hyperechoic bands. In short-axis scans, nerves exhibit a stippled, honeycomb-like appearance (**Fig. 12.1**) due to small hypoechoic rounded foci embedded in a hyperechoic background. The hypoechoic areas correspond to fascicles. The echogenic tissue is due to epineurium.[4] The outer boundaries of nerves are usually undefined

due to the similar hyperechoic appearances of the outer epineurium and the surrounding perineural fat.

In general, nerves are soft and flexible. They may change shape from oval to round, depending on the width of the anatomic passageways within which they run and the echogenicity of the perineural structures that lie in contact with them. Nerves are mobile. Light transducer pressure or patient movement may cause a nerve to slide over the surface of an artery, tendon, or muscle. Compared to tendons, nerves are less echogenic and less susceptible to anisotropy and the ultrasound beam does not have to be perpendicular to assess them.[4] Nerves move less than tendons. Alternating flexion and extension of the fingers, for example, show long excursions of the flexor tendons at the wrist but relatively short excursions of the median nerve. Where nerves cross narrow osteofibrous tunnels around joints, they may assume a more homogeneous hypoechoic appearance due to tighter packing of fascicles, and the outer epineurium may be slightly thickened.

Careful scanning technique based on precise knowledge of nerve position and analysis of anatomic relationships is necessary. A high-frequency (center frequency >10 MHz) linear array broadband transducer and copious gel are required. Ultrasound is initially best performed by scanning a nerve in short axis. Bony landmarks and structures such as tendons and vessels are easily identified, and help to locate the nerve. Vessels are particularly useful landmarks, but not all nerves run alongside a vessel—the median nerve at the wrist and the sciatic nerve being prominent examples. Once the nerve is identified, the transducer is swept repeatedly proximally and distally, using an "elevator" technique, to examine long segments of nerve rapidly, looking for alterations in size, shape, and texture of the nerve and abnormalities in adjacent structures. The transducer is then rotated through 90 degrees and the nerve is examined in its long axis; this is particularly useful when looking for alterations in nerve caliber. Dynamic examination may show alterations in nerve position and shape as muscles contract or joints move. Although nerves can be displayed in the limbs due to their superficial position and absence of intervening bone, not all nerves can be shown with ultrasound. Cranial nerves; nerve roots exiting the

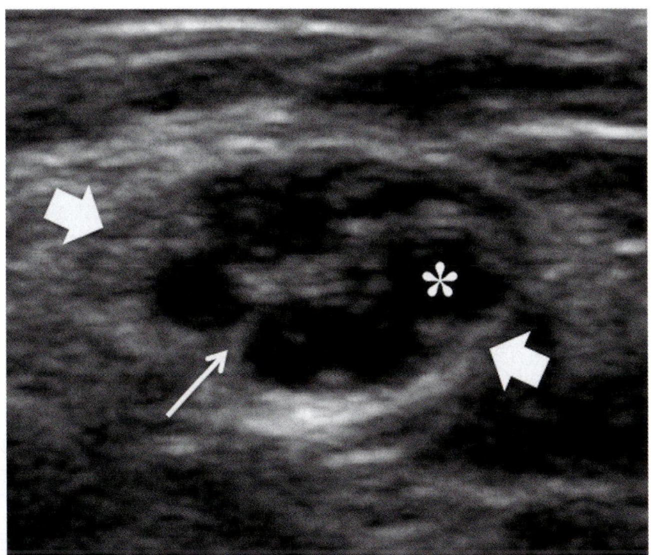

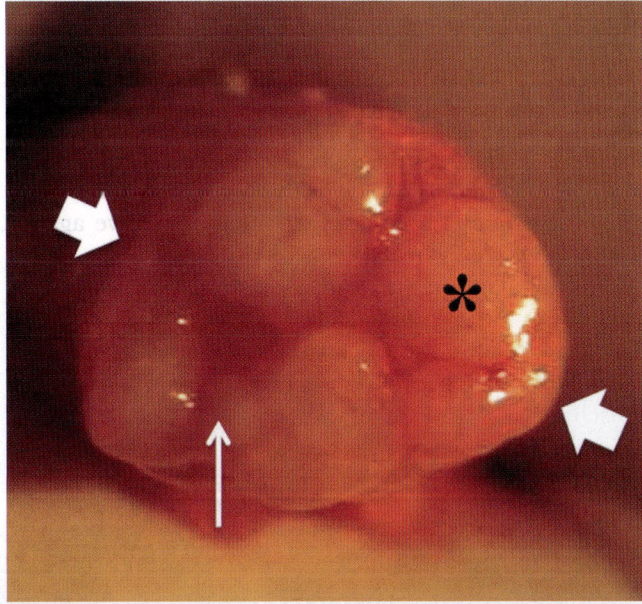

Figure 12.1. Ultrasound appearance of normal nerves. **A:** Transverse 17.5 MHz ultrasound image of ulnar nerve at the middle third of arm. The nerve (*large arrows*) is composed of rounded hypoechoic areas (*asterisk*) in a hyperechoic background (*narrow arrow*). **B:** Transverse histologic section of ulnar nerve. The cross-sectional appearance of nerve fascicles (*asterisk*) correlates well with the hypoechoic rounded areas seen in (**B**).

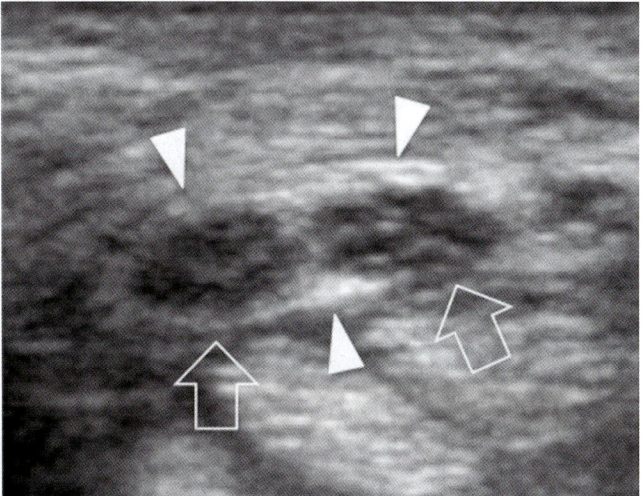

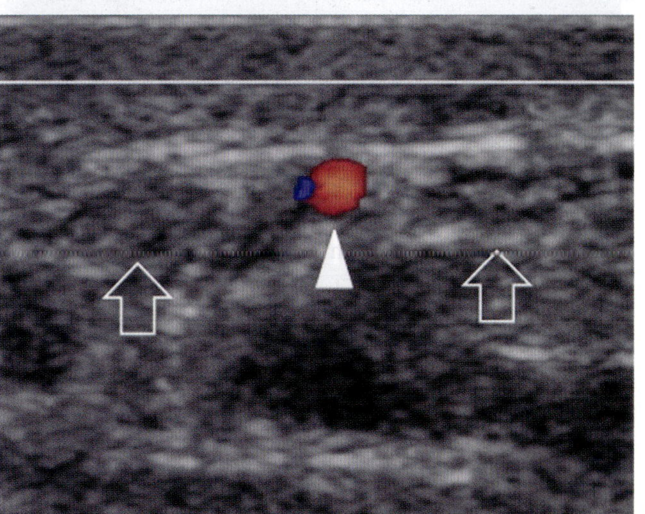

Figure 12.2. Median nerve variants. **A:** Bifid median nerve. Transverse 17.5 MHz ultrasound image of the ventral wrist reveals that the median nerve is composed of two groups of fascicles (*arrows*) enveloped in a common epineurium (*arrowheads*). **B:** Persistent median artery of the forearm. Transverse color Doppler image demonstrates the median artery (*arrowhead*) between the two groups of fascicles (*arrows*) of a bifid median nerve.

dorsal, lumbar, and sacral spine; the sympathetic chains; and the splanchnic nerves in the abdomen cannot be visualized because they are deep or obscured by interposed bony structures or bowel.

ANATOMICAL VARIANTS

Most anatomical variants affecting peripheral nerves are not of clinical significance but some variants may result in symptoms or be important for surgical planning. The most frequently encountered variant is the bifid median nerve at the wrist, with or without a persistent median artery.[5–7] In the bifid median nerve, two bundles of fascicles enter the carpal tunnel side by side (**Fig. 12.2A**). The persistent median artery is an accessory artery that arises from the ulnar artery at the proximal forearm and accompanies the median nerve along its course throughout the forearm and carpal tunnel. It can be associated with a bifid or normal nerve (**Fig. 12.2B**).

Nerves may also have an anomalous course, for example, at the brachial plexus level when the C5 and/or C6 roots do not cross between the scalenus anterior and medius but penetrate the anterior scalene. The anomalous course of the C5 root in front of the anterior scalene muscle occurs in 3% to 3.2% of cases (**Fig. 12.3**).[8]

Extrinsic abnormalities along the course of a nerve may predispose to nerve compression. The supracondylar

COMPRESSIVE NEUROPATHIES

Entrapment neuropathies are usually the result of chronic or dynamic compression of nerves in fibro-osseous or fibromuscular tunnels. Tunnels have rigid walls and accessory muscles, ganglia, osteophytes and other space-occupying lesions elevate pressure in the tunnel and compress the nerve. Compression at other sites, for example, by scarring, is less common. Chronic compression results in ischemia, Wallerian degeneration, and fibrosis of the nerve and motor and sensory disturbances. Identifying the site of the lesion depends on precise anatomical knowledge. Neurophysiological studies are often helpful but have a significant false-negative rate. Magnetic resonance imaging can show entrapment and downstream effects such as denervation changes in muscle.[17–19] Although possibly less sensitive to denervation changes than MR imaging, ultrasound has high spatial resolution and can provide excellent detail of tunnels and their contents, including nerve morphology.

On the basis of ultrasound assessment, nerve compressive syndromes can be grouped into three main classes.

Class-1 includes large nerves (e.g., median, ulnar, peroneal, and tibial) that are easily imaged by ultrasound at the compression site using conventional transducers (probe frequency up to 13 MHz). Assessment is based on pattern recognition and, for the carpal and cubital tunnels, nerve cross-sectional area (CSA) with diagnostic performance nearly equivalent to MR imaging.

Class-2 includes small (caliber <2 mm) nerves (e.g., posterior and anterior interosseous, musculocutaneous, sural, and distal divisional branches of large nerves) that require high-end equipment and higher frequency probes (up to 18 MHz). The diagnosis relies exclusively on pattern recognition because the nerves are too small for CSA measurements. There is no objective evidence comparing the performance of ultrasound and MR imaging in depicting pathology of these nerves, but in our opinion, ultrasound with an appropriate transducer in experienced hands often seems to be superior to MR imaging. Compared with MR imaging, the main advantage of ultrasound is its ability to distinguish distal nerves from vessels. The frequent absence of denervation changes, because many distal nerve branches are purely sensory, is a major disadvantage of MR imaging.

Class-3 includes small (e.g., inferior calcaneal) and large (e.g., femoral and sciatic in their intrapelvic course) nerves that are poorly visible or nondetectable with ultrasound due to a deep course or intervening bone. Although these nerves cannot be directly imaged, ultrasound can suggest a nerve problem by showing denervation changes in muscles such as loss of bulk and increased echogenicity. Ultrasound is not as accurate as MR imaging in differentiating early denervation changes of intramuscular extracellular edema from fatty atrophy.[20]

Regardless of the entrapment site, the ultrasound signs of compressive neuropathy are characteristic. The nerve appears flattened at the compression point and swollen proximally.[21] The transition between flattened and swollen segments is abrupt (notch sign). Ultrasound accurately identifies the exact level of compression based on these features. Intraneural edema and venous congestion lead to nerve enlargement in the early phases of compression.[22] The increased water content correlates with axon loss (axonotmesis),[23] and there is a positive correlation between the nerve CSA and the severity of electromyography (EMG) findings.[24] Nerve echotexture may appear uniformly hypoechoic with loss of the fascicular pattern due to swelling of the fascicles and reduced echogenicity of the epineurium. These changes are more profound in severe long-standing compression.[21] Occasionally, intraneural hyperemia can be appreciated at Doppler imaging.[21,25] At the carpal tunnel this seems to correlate with disease severity and to be a good predictor of median nerve entrapment.[25,26] Irreversible intraneural fibrosis may occur in long-standing compression. In contrast to early disease, nerves with fibrotic changes tend to remain swollen after decompressive surgery and tend to show poor functional improvement.[27]

In nerve entrapment syndromes, the measurement that has to be taken is the CSA for *class-1* nerves or the maximum cross-sectional diameter for *class-2* nerves. The CSA should be calculated where the nerve is maximally enlarged and the histopathologic changes are most severe, either by the indirect method using calipers and application of the ellipse formula (transverse diameter $\times$ anteroposterior diameter $\times$ $\pi/4$), or the direct method, based on manual tracing and automated calculation of the area.[28,29] Both methods have high reproducibility and short learning periods.[30] The CSA measurement should be obtained from the outer margin of hypoechoic fascicles. The echogenic rim surrounding the fascicles due to the outer epineurial sheath has to be excluded because it may not be clearly distinguishable from the external perineural fat.[29] Probe position can affect the variability of CSA measurements: The ultrasound beam should always be directed perpendicular to the long axis of the nerve (even if the nerve assumes a curved or oblique course). Optimal probe orientation for measurements can be defined dynamically by tilting the probe over the nerve or inducing slight changes in the joint position. When setting cutoff values for nerve CSA, gender, weight, body mass index, and race should be taken into account as possible confounders.[31]

Several sites of nerve entrapment are amenable to ultrasound examination in the upper and lower extremities. The most common conditions are described below using a regional approach.

Shoulder

The suprascapular nerve is a purely motor nerve arising from the upper trunk of the brachial plexus (C5–C6). It descends through the suprascapular foramen to the supraspinous fossa and the spinoglenoid notch. Suprascapular neuropathy leads to chronic shoulder pain and weakness. It may be secondary to constriction of the nerve at the suprascapular or spinoglenoid notches by stretching injuries, ligament abnormalities, overuse, or space-occupying lesions. When the nerve is trapped in the supraspinous fossa, the supraspinatus and infraspinatus muscles may undergo denervation changes; when it is compressed at the spinoglenoid notch, denervation is limited to infraspinatus. Paralabral cysts are the leading cause of suprascapular nerve compression[32,33] and are usually associated with tears of the posterior glenoid labrum (from 8 to 11 o'clock positions). The cyst extends into the spinoglenoid and/or suprascapular notches deep to the muscles bellies, and may cause muscle denervation **(Fig. 12.7)**. Large cysts (>3 cm) are most often associated with compressive neuropathy. Paralabral cysts are round or oval hypoechoic lesions with well-defined margins. They are relatively fixed in location and shape during arm movements. Due to their deep location, even large cysts may be missed during standard ultrasound examination of the rotator cuff. The continuity of the cyst with a defect in the posterior labrum may be revealed with ultrasound. Percutaneous needle aspiration to decompress the nerve can be attempted under ultrasound guidance.[34]

The axillary nerve originates from the posterior cord of the brachial plexus (C5–C6) near the coracoid. It proceeds along the inferolateral border of the subscapularis muscle to curve inferior to the glenohumeral joint capsule and pass to the posterior aspect of the arm with the posterior circumflex artery through the quadrilateral space.[35] The axillary nerve has two terminal branches, anterior and posterior. The anterior branch innervates the anterior part of deltoid, the posterior supplies teres minor and the posterior deltoid. Ultrasound detection of the axillary nerve is challenging due to its small size and deep course. With arm elevation, the axillary neurovascular bundle can be imaged as it runs across the quadrilateral space close to the inferior aspect of the glenohumeral joint. Axillary neuropathy is caused by stretching injuries or stenosis of the quadrilateral space by fractures, fibrous bands, or inferior (from 9 to 7 o'clock positions) paraglenoid cysts.[36] Teres minor atrophy can be assessed by comparing the size of the muscle with the adjacent infraspinatus **(Fig. 12.8)**. Atrophy of deltoid is confirmed by reduced thickness relative to the opposite side.[37] Ultrasound is able to demonstrate paralabral cysts extending from the inferior aspect of the glenoid in association with a tear of the inferior labrum.

Elbow

At the medial elbow, the ulnar nerve courses in the condylar groove, a space delimited by the olecranon and the medial epicondyle and bridged by the cubital tunnel retinaculum (Osborne fascia). The nerve then enters the proper cubital tunnel, a narrow passage between the

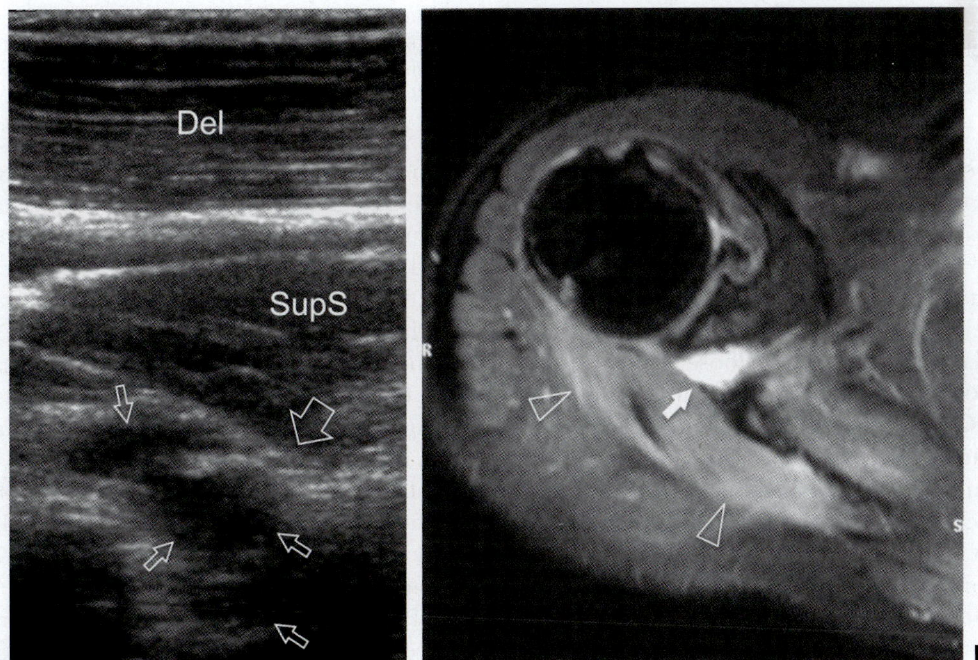

Figure 12.7. Suprascapular nerve entrapment. **A:** Coronal 12.5 MHz ultrasound image obtained over the supraspinous fossa shows a lobulated ganglion cyst (*small arrows*) close to the suprascapular nerve (*large arrow*). The cyst lies on the floor of the fossa deep to the deltoid (*Del*) and supraspinatus (*SupS*) muscles. **B:** Transverse fat-suppressed TSE T2w MR shows the ganglion (*arrow*) and diffusely increased signal in the infraspinatus muscle (*arrowheads*) due to denervation.

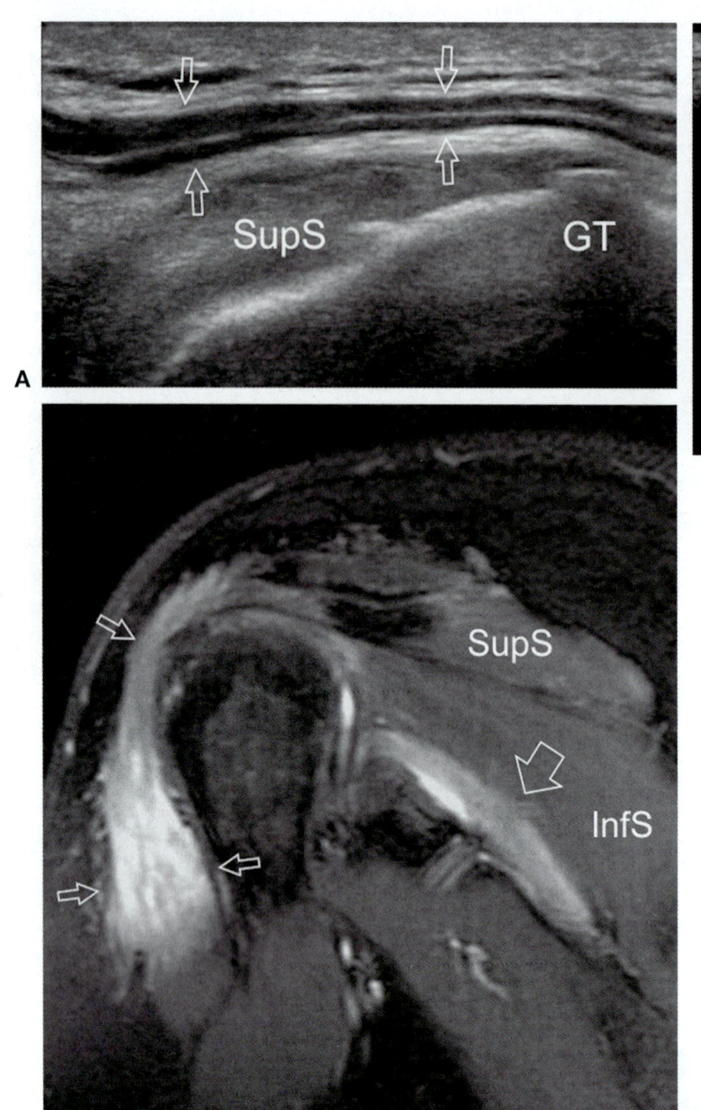

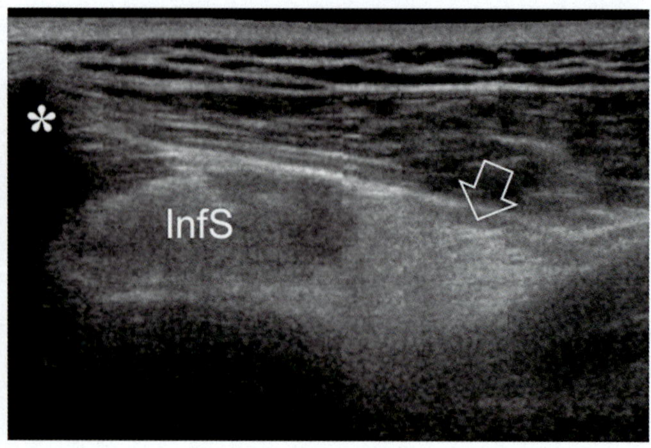

Figure 12.8.   Axillary nerve entrapment. **A:** Longitudinal 12.5 MHz ultrasound image of the supraspinatus tendon (*SupS*) shows marked atrophy of the deltoid muscle (*arrows*). GT, greater tuberosity. **B:** Sagittal extended field of view 12.5 MHz ultrasound image obtained over the posterior fossa demonstrates loss of bulk and increased echogenicity of the teres minor muscle (*arrow*), consistent with fatty atrophy, whereas the infraspinatus (*InfS*) is preserved. Note the spine of the scapula (*asterisk*). **C:** Oblique sagittal STIR MR reveals intramuscular edema with increased signal intensity in the deltoid (*small arrows*) and teres minor (*large arrow*).

ulnar and humeral heads of the flexor carpi ulnaris covered by the arcuate ligament, a distal expansion of the Osborne fascia. Ulnar nerve compression may occur at the condylar groove (proximal tunnel) or at the edge of the arcuate ligament (distal tunnel) due to bony abnormalities (e.g., cubitus valgus, deformities from previous fractures, medial osteophytes, and loose bodies), thickening of the floor of the tunnel (the joint capsule and the posterior band of the medial collateral ligament), and space-occupying masses (ganglia and accessory muscles, i.e., anconeus epitrochlearis). In early or mild cases, the clinical diagnosis of cubital tunnel syndrome may be difficult, and electrophysiology has a low sensitivity, ranging from 37% to 86%.[38] In cubital tunnel syndrome, ulnar nerve CSA >10 mm^2 is generally accepted as abnormal with sensitivity as high as 95% to 100%,[39] but there is poor correlation between ulnar nerve size and electrophysiology. Ultrasound demonstrates a fusiform hypoechoic swelling of the ulnar nerve with loss

of the fascicular pattern.[40] Ultrasound examination during elbow flexion should always be obtained to identify dynamic nerve impingement (e.g., prominent medial head of triceps) **(Fig. 12.9)**.

Anterior to the lateral epicondyle, the radial nerve gives off the posterior interosseous nerve that pierces supinator between the superficial and deep heads (radial tunnel) to reach the posterior compartment of the forearm. At the proximal edge of supinator, the nerve is bridged by a fibrous arch, the arcade of Fröhse, which joins the brachialis and brachioradialis muscles, the medial edge of the extensor carpi radialis brevis and the superficial belly of the supinator muscle. Ultrasound shows the posterior interosseous nerve as it pierces the supinator muscle. Posterior interosseous neuropathy may be caused by nerve compression at the arcade of Fröhse as a result of fibrous bands, fan-shaped recurrent radial vessels (leash of Henry), or tightness of the passage within the supinator. The main ultrasound patterns include impingement

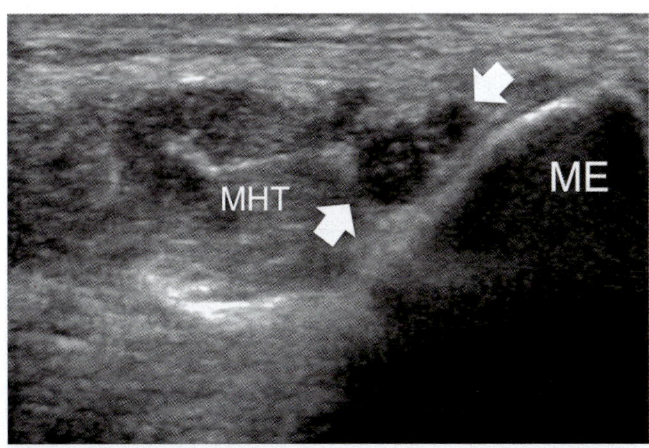

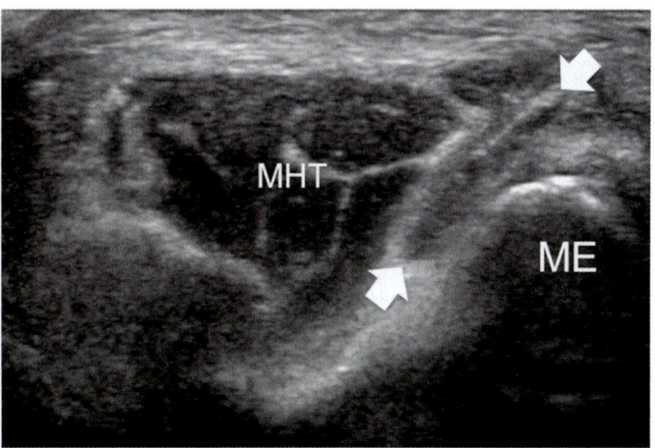

Figure 12.9.   Cubital tunnel syndrome. Transverse 12.5 MHz ultrasound images over the condylar groove during extension (**A**) and full flexion (**B**) of the elbow. With elbow flexion, the prominent medial head of triceps (*MHT*) compresses the ulnar nerve (*arrows*) dynamically against the medial epicondyle (*ME*) causing marked flattening of the nerve.

of the nerve against the fibrous arcade or fusiform nerve swelling in the middle of the tunnel[41,42] (**Fig. 12.10**). This latter location of nerve abnormality may be related to either compression (fibrous bands) or stretching trauma.

The anterior interosseous nerve is a motor branch of the median nerve that descends the forearm along the anterior surface of the interosseous membrane to supply the flexor pollicis longus, part of the flexor digitorum profundus (for the index and middle finger), and the pronator quadratus. Anterior interosseous neuropathy (Kiloh-Nevin syndrome) presents with an impaired pinch grip and may occur either above the elbow, when the nerve is still part of the median nerve, by a supracondylar bony spur and ligament of Struthers, or in the forearm at the point where the median and anterior interosseous nerves pass deep to the tendinous bridge connecting the

humeroulnar and radial heads of the flexor digitorum superficialis muscle. The anterior interosseous nerve may be compressed by fibrous bands arising from the pronator teres or the flexor digitorum superficialis and anomalous muscles in the forearm (i.e., Gantzer muscle). In general, ultrasound examination of the anterior interosseous nerve is inconclusive in the absence of a mass because it is so small and deep. Besides direct nerve assessment, ultrasound may suggest the diagnosis due to loss of bulk and the hyperechoic pattern of the innervated muscles (**Fig. 12.11**). [43,44]

Tip:

- Entrapment neuropathies are characterized by focal nerve enlargement at or near the site of compression, typically recorded as an increase in CSA.
- Ultrasound can identify a wide spectrum of causes of entrapment neuropathy in the upper extremity.
- The nerves of the upper extremity may be affected by compression or entrapment at specific anatomic locations (i.e., paraglenoid for the suprascapular nerve, quadrilateral space for the axillary nerve, cubital and Guyon tunnels for the ulnar nerve, and the supinator area for the posterior interosseous nerve).

Wrist

Carpal tunnel syndrome (CTS) is common (estimated prevalence 50 per 1,000 individuals per year). There is no gold standard for the diagnosis of CTS. Many physicians rely on the clinical presentation of pain at the wrist radiating into thumb, index, and middle fingers, with numbness and tingling, nocturnal wakening, thenar atrophy, Tinel sign, and Phalen sign. Others rely on electrodiagnostic (EDX) testing, but nerve conduction studies and EMG have an estimated sensitivity ranging from 85% to 98%. Finally, some institutions consider

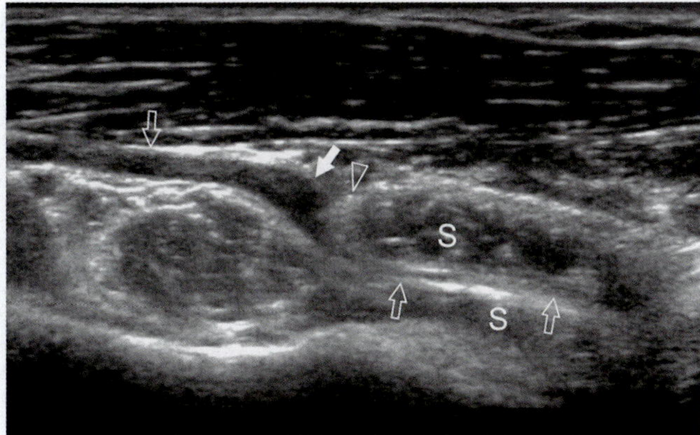

Figure 12.10.   Posterior interosseous neuropathy. Long-axis 12.5 MHz ultrasound image over the anterolateral elbow reveals fusiform swelling (*white arrow*) of the posterior interosseous nerve (*void arrow pointing down*) in front of a thickened arcade of Frohse (*arrowhead*). More distally, the nerve returns to normal (*void arrows pointing up*) as it runs within the supinator tunnel, between the superficial and deep bellies of supinator (*S*).

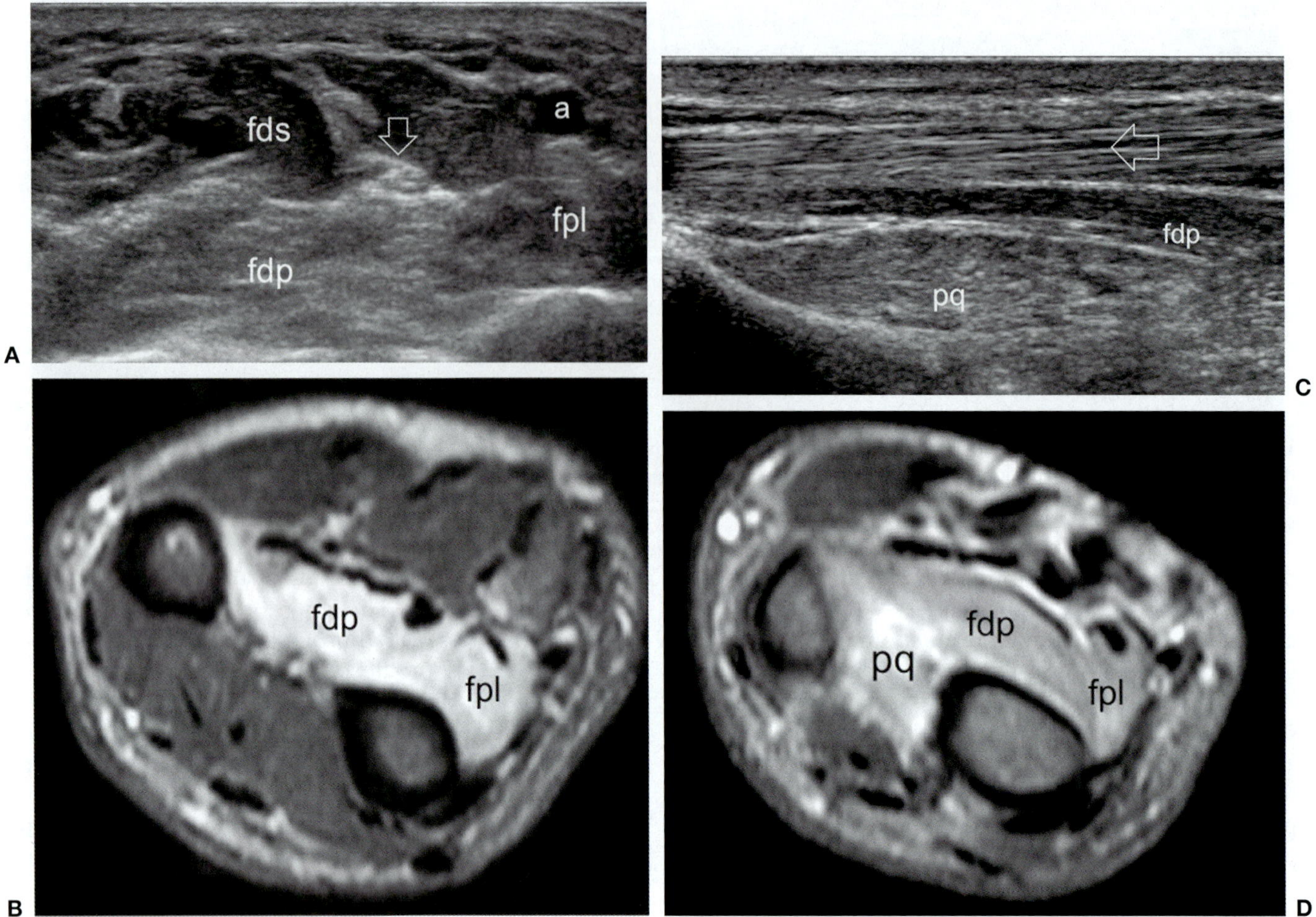

Figure 12.11. Anterior interosseous neuropathy. Transverse 12.5 MHz ultrasound image **(A)** of the mid forearm and corresponding fat-suppressed TSE T2w MR image **(B)** reveals loss of bulk and diffusely increased echogenicity and T2-signal in the flexor digitorum profundus (*fdp*) and flexor pollicis longus (*fpl*) muscles but not in the flexor digitorum superficialis (*fds*) muscle. Note the median nerve (*arrow*) and the ulnar artery (*a*) in **A**. Sagittal 12.5 MHz ultrasound image **(C)** of the distal forearm and fat-suppressed TSE T2w MR **(D)** demonstrate similar denervation changes in the pronator quadratus muscle (*pq*). Note the flexor digitorum tendons (*arrow* in **C**). Surgery confirmed anterior interosseous nerve entrapment by fibrous band soon after its origin from the median nerve.

treatment response (i.e., carpal tunnel injection, splinting, and surgical release) as a diagnostic feature of value. With such uncertainty regarding the gold standard, ultrasound provides direct depiction of size and morphologic abnormalities of the median nerve[45] and is able to rule out anatomic variants (e.g., bifid nerve and persistent median artery) and space-occupying masses (e.g., ganglion cysts, accessory muscles, and flexor tenosynovitis). Besides assessing nerve size, ultrasound shows echotextural abnormalities, volar bulging of the flexor retinaculum, flattening of the median nerve in the distal carpal tunnel, and reduced passive sliding of the nerve during flexor tendon gliding **(Fig. 12.12)**. Although CSA is the most accurate and reliable measure of nerve size, there is no consensus on the optimal threshold value for diagnosing median nerve compression. Diagnostic cutoff values range from 9 to 13 mm^2. Most studies choose >10 or 11 mm^2 at the carpal tunnel inlet.[46] Instead of

absolute cutoff values, a wrist-to-forearm ratio of median nerve CSA has been recently introduced.[47] The CSA is determined at the level of the distal wrist crease and 12 cm proximally in the forearm. An upper normal limit of wrist-to-forearm ratio of 1.4 has 100% sensitivity for detecting CTS with no false positives.[47] Others have proposed the pronator quadratus muscle as the level for the second CSA measurement. A difference (ΔCSA) between the largest CSA of the median nerve at the level of the carpal tunnel and the proximal third of the pronator quadratus is then calculated.[48] A ΔCSA threshold of 2 mm^2 has sensitivity and specificity as high as 99% and 100%, respectively for CTS.[48] The same method can be used by combining the CSAs of the radial and ulnar branches of a bifid median nerve.[49] Comparison with the opposite side has been suggested as an alternative for objective assessment of nerve size.[31] This seems particularly promising in mild initial entrapment, when electrophysiology

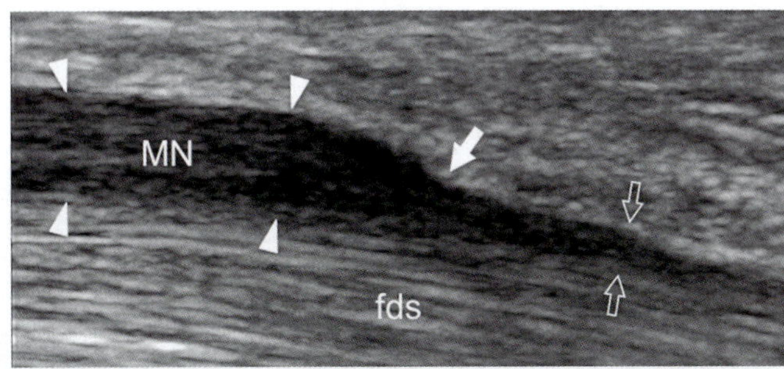

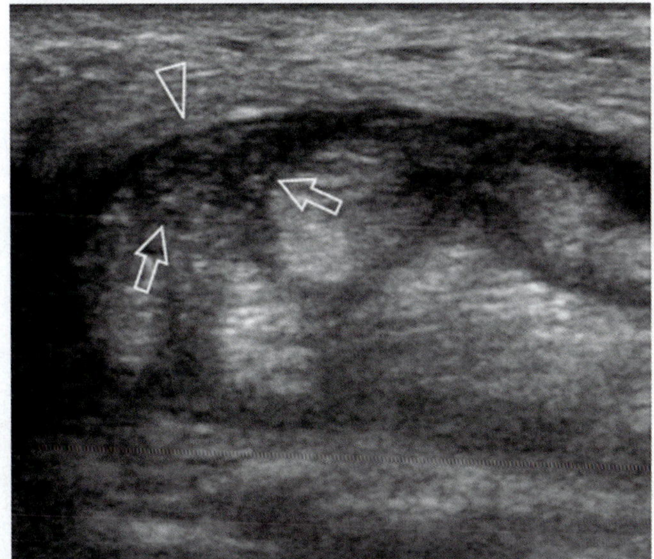

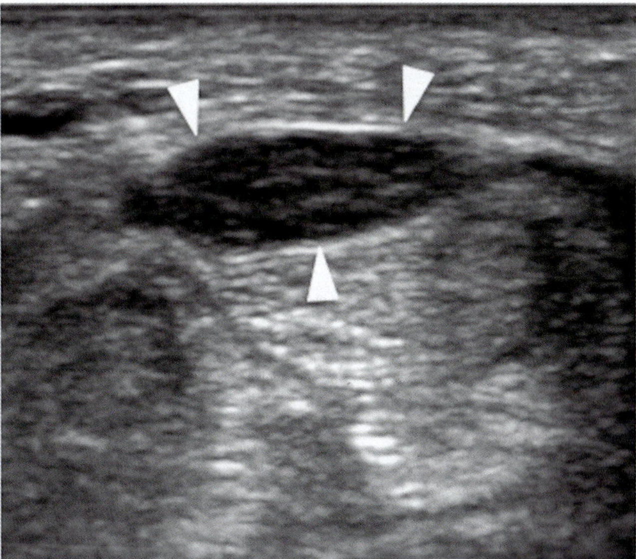

Figure 12.12. Carpal tunnel syndrome. **A:** Longitudinal 17–5 MHz ultrasound image of the wrist shows abrupt flattening (*void arrows*) of the median nerve (*MN*) in the carpal tunnel and swelling (*white arrowheads*) of the nerve proximal to the compression point (*white arrow*). fds, flexor digitorum superficialis tendons. **B, C:** Correlative transverse 12.5 MHz ultrasound images obtained (**B**) at the distal radius and (**C**) within the carpal tunnel reveal a sudden change in the cross-sectional area of the median nerve (*arrowheads* in **B**, *arrows* in **C**) at the point where the nerve goes deep to the transverse carpal ligament (*void arrowhead*).

is positive but the CSA is within or at the limits of normal. A difference in the CSA between sides might increase the examiner's confidence that mild compression exists.

There is increasing interest in the potential value of ultrasound as an indicator of disease severity. Moderate correlations between CSA and electrophysiologic severity exist, but do not reach the level of clinical significance.[50,51] The lack of a stronger correlation may be due to the duration of disease and patient age.[52] Emerging roles for nerve ultrasound in CTS include prognosis, selection of treatment options, and monitoring response to treatments. For example, a low median nerve CSA is more likely to respond to steroid injection into the carpal tunnel than a very thick nerve.[53] In patients with persistent symptoms after decompressive surgery, ultrasound can demonstrate incomplete resection of the flexor retinaculum, scar tissue around the nerve, or injury of the palmar cutaneous branch **(Fig. 12.13)**.[54,55] Much remains to be learned about nerve ultrasound in CTS, but ultrasound is already changing the approach to diagnosis and treatment, although its role has yet to be established.

Guyon canal is a rare site of ulnar nerve entrapment **(Fig. 12.14)**. Causes include space-occupying lesions such as pisotriquetral ganglia, ulnar artery pseudoaneurysms, and accessory muscles (i.e., AADM).[21] Compression may

involve the ulnar nerve prior to its bifurcation (zone-1) or be limited to one of its divisional branches, the superficial sensory (zone-2) or the deep motor (zone-3). The ulnar nerve is easily identified in Guyon canal between the pisiform and ulnar artery using short-axis planes. Moving the transducer distally, the superficial branch can be found superficial to the hamate hook, while the deep motor branch courses along the medial side of the hamate. External compression, either acute or repetitive (cyclist palsy), may cause nerve injury by squeezing it against the hamate hook. This type of injury may also cause occlusion of the ulnar artery (hypothenar hammer syndrome).

Tip:
- In CTS, the CSA of the median nerve is increased at the proximal edge of the retinaculum and the nerve is flattened within the distal tunnel.
- There is no consensus on what is an abnormal CSA measurement of the median nerve: proposed absolute threshold value is approximately 10 to 10.5 mm^2.
- To reduce the impact of intersubject and internerve variability, comparison between the CSA of the median nerve obtained at the carpal tunnel and more proximally seems a promising alterative.

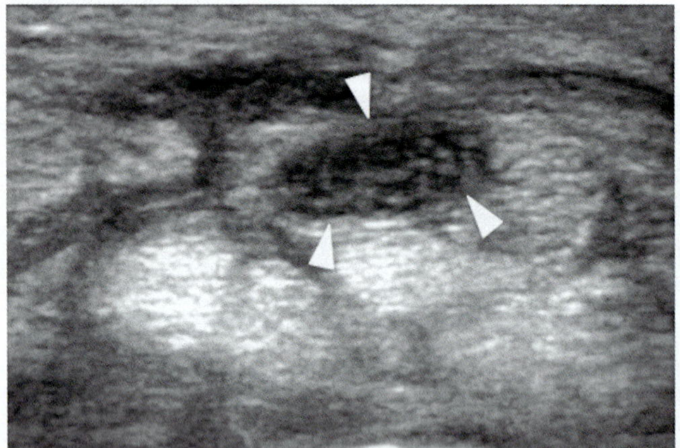

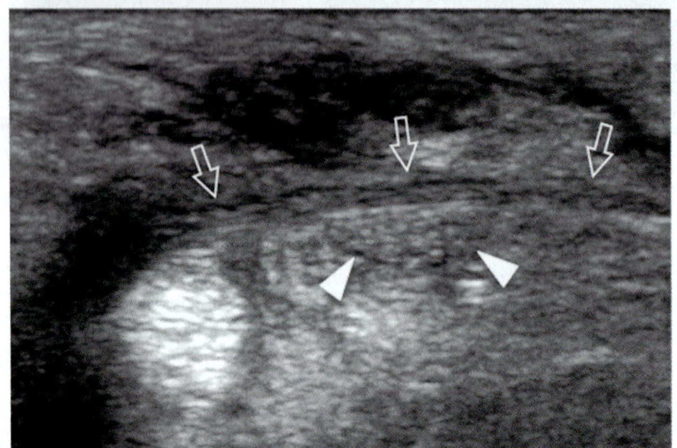

Figure 12.13. Complication after carpal tunnel release. **A, B:** Transverse 12.5 MHz ultrasound images obtained **(A)** at the proximal (scaphoid-pisiform level) and **(B)** distal (trapezium-hamate level) carpal tunnel in a patient complaining of persistent symptoms after surgery. At the proximal tunnel, the retinaculum is sectioned but the median nerve (*arrowheads*) remains thickened and hypoechoic. More distally, the nerve is narrower as a result of persistent compression by the intact distal retinaculum (*arrows*). This finding suggests incomplete sectioning of the flexor retinaculum. The patient was operated on again with good clinical results.

Hip

The main entrapment neuropathies about the hip amenable to ultrasound examination involve the lateral femoral cutaneous nerve and the femoral nerve.

The lateral femoral cutaneous nerve is a purely sensory nerve arising from L2–L3. It descends in the pelvis alongside the iliopsoas and enters the thigh deep to the inguinal ligament or through a split in the ligament close to the anterior superior iliac spine. It then divides into terminal branches to the anterolateral thigh. Lateral femoral cutaneous neuropathy (meralgia paresthetica) is caused by entrapment where the nerve crosses the inguinal ligament, and consists of numbness and sensory disturbance in the anterolateral thigh. The main ultrasound signs are fusiform nerve swelling, usually proximal to the ligament **(Fig. 12.15)**.[56–58] Short-axis scans may help to show changes in nerve shape and size across the ligament.

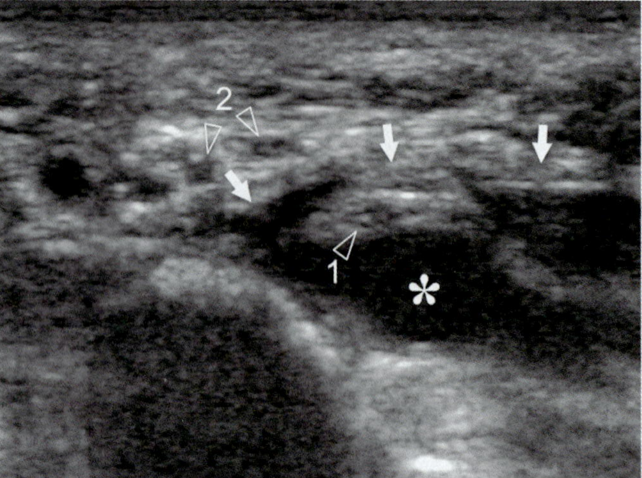

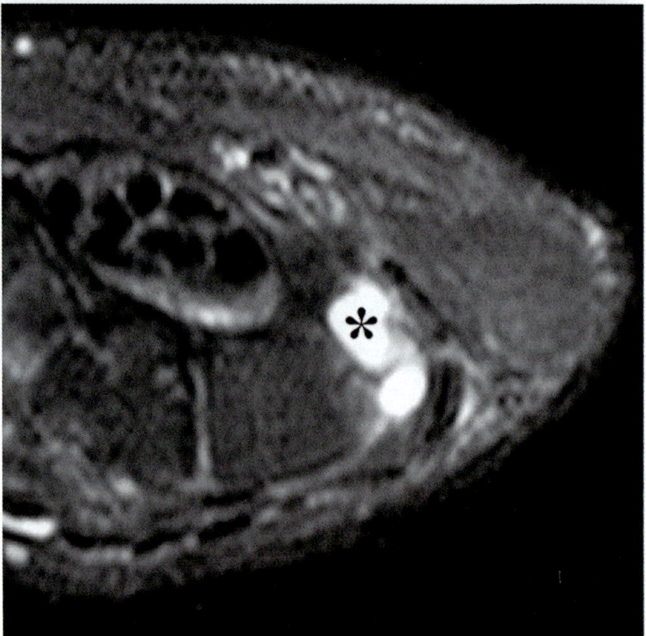

Figure 12.14. Guyon tunnel syndrome. **A:** Transverse 17.5 MHz ultrasound image shows the divisional branches of the ulnar nerve in the area of the hamate hook. The pisohamate ligament (*arrows*) separates the deep motor (*void arrowhead 1*) from the two superficial sensory (*void arrowheads 2*) branches of the ulnar nerve. A ganglion cyst (*asterisk*) compresses the motor branch against the ligament in zone 3. Corresponding axial fat-suppressed TSE T2w MR image **(B)** demonstrates the ganglion (*asterisk*).

The femoral nerve is the largest branch of the lumbar plexus and arises from L2–L4. It descends within the psoas muscle and passes distally in a groove between the psoas and iliacus muscles, behind the iliacus fascia. It exits the pelvis deep to the inguinal ligament in a rigid osteofibrous tunnel (lacuna musculorum), accompanied by the distal myotendinous junction of the iliopsoas and separated from the femoral artery and vein (lacuna vasorum). Its divisional branches supply the pectineus, sartorius, and quadriceps femoris muscles and give rise to the saphenous nerve. The femoral and the saphenous nerves

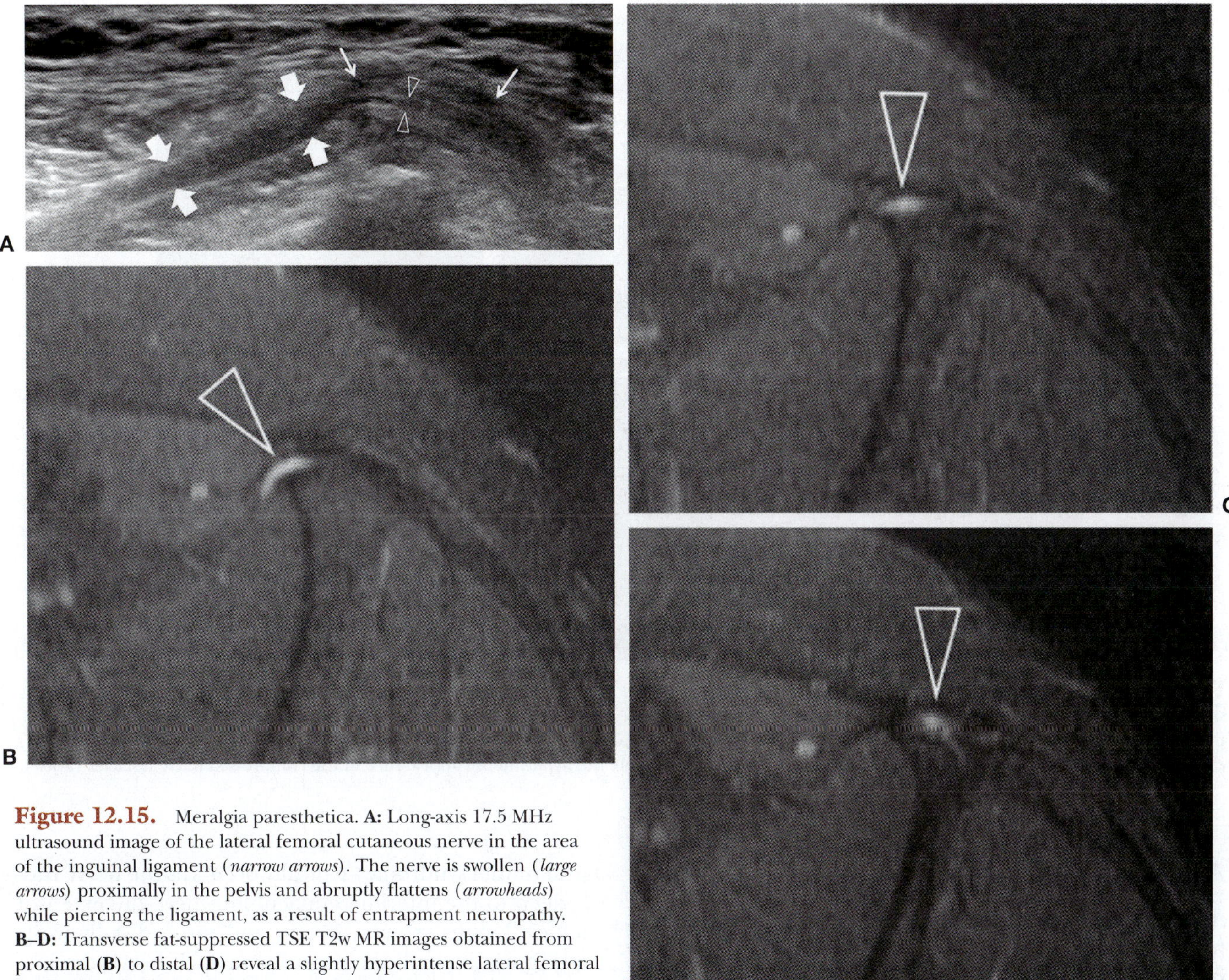

Figure 12.15. Meralgia paresthetica. **A:** Long-axis 17.5 MHz ultrasound image of the lateral femoral cutaneous nerve in the area of the inguinal ligament (*narrow arrows*). The nerve is swollen (*large arrows*) proximally in the pelvis and abruptly flattens (*arrowheads*) while piercing the ligament, as a result of entrapment neuropathy. **B–D:** Transverse fat-suppressed TSE T2w MR images obtained from proximal (**B**) to distal (**D**) reveal a slightly hyperintense lateral femoral cutaneous nerve (*arrowhead*) approaching and then crossing the inguinal ligament.

provide sensory supply to the skin of the thigh and the medial lower leg. Ultrasound depiction of the femoral nerve proximal to the inguinal ligament is difficult owing to its deep location and interposed bowel. Lower frequency transducers may identify the fat plane in the psoas where the femoral nerve runs, but are unable to depict the nerve adequately. In the infra-inguinal area, the femoral nerve exhibits a large CSA (average 22.7 mm^2)[59] but it dissolves suddenly in the groin as it divides into multiple branches of <1 mm in size. Femoral nerve entrapment deep to the inguinal ligament may be secondary to masses (e.g., acetabular ganglia and giant iliopsoas bursitis) in the confined space of the lacuna musculorum.

Knee

The common peroneal nerve branches from the sciatic nerve and descends posteromedial to the biceps femoris, moving superficially to wind round the fibular neck and give off the superficial and deep peroneal branches. The fibular area is a restricted space between the bone and the fascia and is a common site for peroneal nerve entrapment. Peroneal neuropathy may be structural; for example, it may be caused by a thick arch of the peroneus longus aponeurosis that fits tightly around the nerve inducing a state of chronic irritation, or may have a postural, dynamic, idiopathic origin, such as pressure on the nerve exerted at the fibular neck during sleeping or habitual leg crossing. Other causes of nerve compression include space-occupying lesions (e.g., superior tibiofibular ganglia—see section on Nerve Tumors and Tumorlike Lesions p 288 and pp 206–207), fractures, osteophytes, tight casts around the knee, and iatrogenic causes. A compressed peroneal nerve may appear focally enlarged at the point where it runs in close proximity to the fibula or, more cranially, in the distal popliteal fossa (**Fig. 12.16**).[60] Often, fascicular abnormalities involve one of the divisional branches only (typically the deep peroneal).

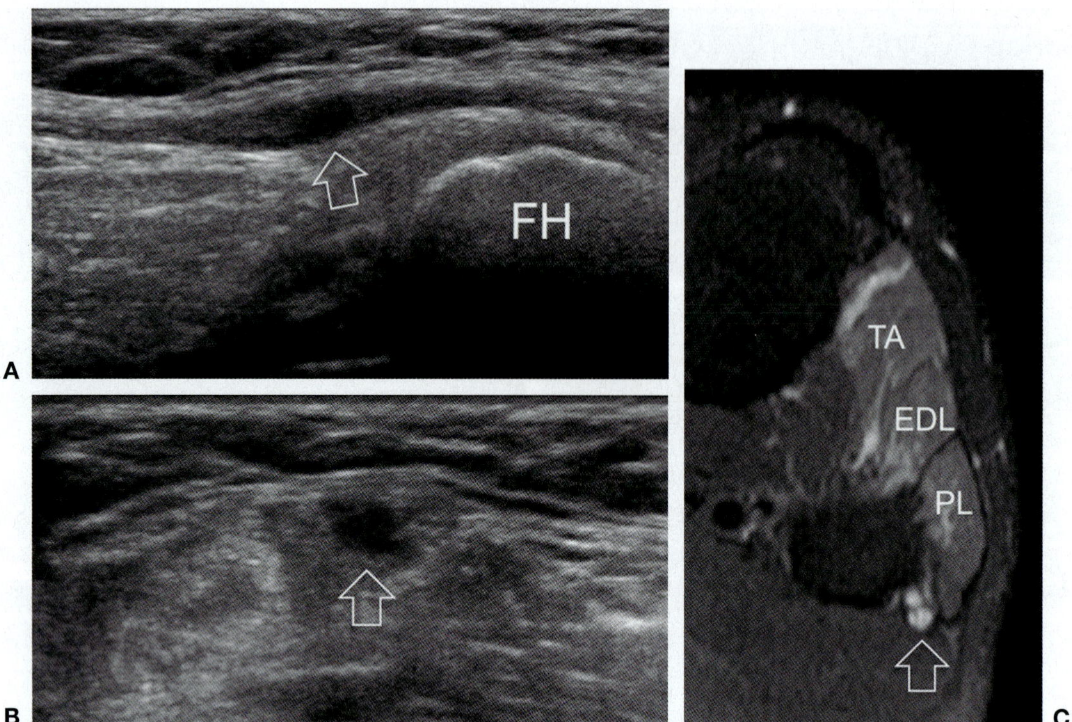

Figure 12.16.   Peroneal neuropathy at the fibular head. **A:** Long- and **(B)** short-axis 17.5 MHz ultrasound images over the posterolateral knee show fusiform hypoechoic swelling (*arrow*) of the common peroneal nerve in proximity to the fibular head (FH), as a result of entrapment neuropathy. **C:** Correlative transverse fat-suppressed TSE T2w MR image reveals denervation signs with increased T2-signal in the tibialis anterior (*TA*), extensor digitorum longus (*EDL*), and peroneus longus (*PL*) muscles. Note the hyperintense appearance of the compressed nerve fascicles (*arrow*).

Ankle and Foot

At the medial ankle, the tibial nerve traverses the tarsal tunnel, an osteofibrous passageway that extends from the posteromedial ankle to the medial heel. In or just cranial to the tarsal tunnel, the tibial nerve splits into the medial and lateral plantar nerves. Tarsal tunnel syndrome is often insidious and manifests with paresthesia or burning pain on the plantar aspect of the foot. Depending on the compression site and the nerve branch involved, symptoms can be focal, localized to the medial plantar aspect of the heel, or radiate up to the tunnel or down into the toes. The main detectable causes of tarsal tunnel syndrome include bone and joint disorders (e.g., spurs, deltoid ligament sprains, or talocalcaneal coalition), soft tissue masses (e.g., ganglion cysts, flexor hallucis longus tenosynovitis, and accessory muscles), and congenital varus or valgus deformities of the foot. The ultrasound diagnosis of tibial neuropathy relies on detection of a soft tissue mass or bone abnormality impinging on the nerve in the tunnel[61,62] as, despite its compression, the tibial nerve frequently looks normal **(Fig. 12.17)**.

On the anterior ankle, the deep peroneal nerve runs alongside the anterior tibial artery. After giving off a motor branch to the extensor brevis muscles, it continues distally, deep to the extensor retinaculum and dorsal to the talonavicular joint, to provide sensory supply to the first webspace. Deep peroneal neuropathy (anterior tarsal tunnel syndrome) typically occurs as the nerve travels deep to the inferior retinaculum where the extensor hallucis longus crosses over it, and more distally while passing underneath the extensor hallucis brevis tendon. Midtarsal osteophytes can be also implicated in nerve impingement.

The other divisional branch of the peroneal nerve, the superficial peroneal nerve, descends in the lateral leg

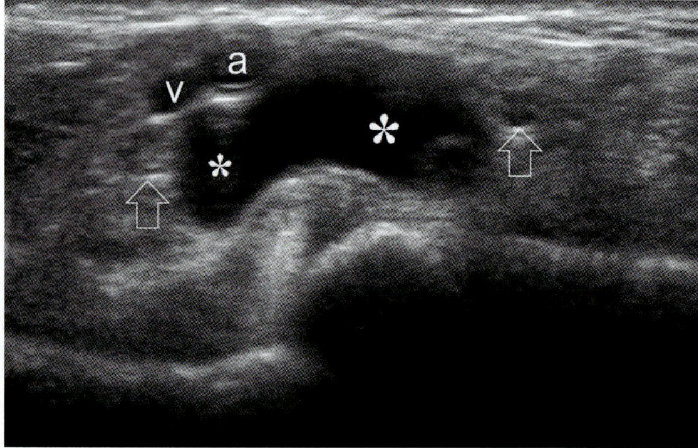

Figure 12.17.   Tarsal tunnel syndrome. Short-axis 17.5 MHz ultrasound image of the distal tarsal tunnel demonstrates a ganglion cyst (*asterisks*) arising from the subtalar joint. The ganglion extends into the neurovascular bundle displacing and compressing the lateral and medial plantar nerves (*arrows*). Note the posterior tibial artery (*a*) and vein (*v*).

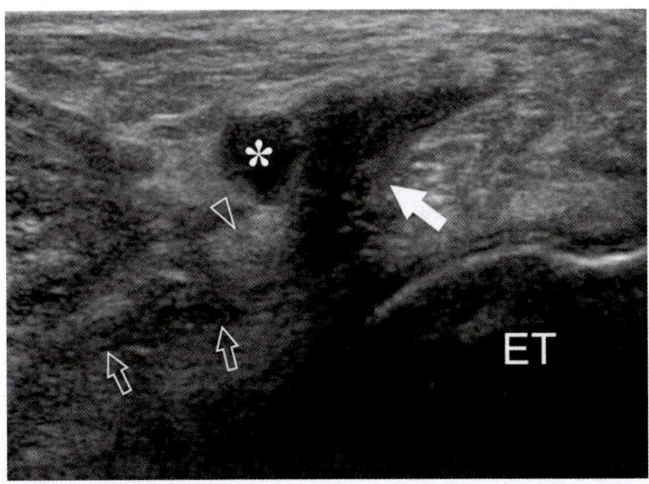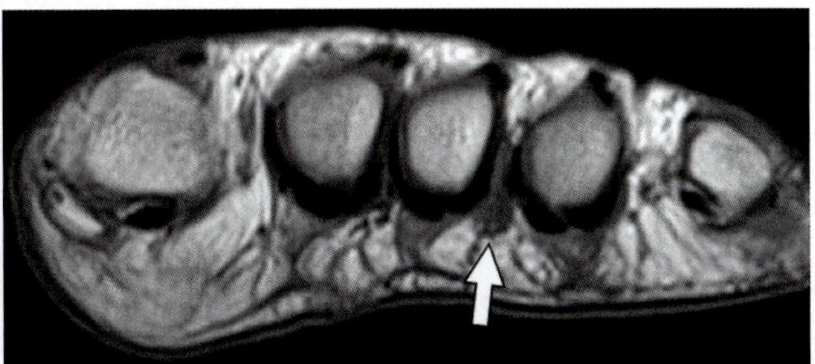

Figure 12.18. Morton neuroma. **A:** Longitudinal 12.5 MHz ultrasound image of the third webspace obtained with a dorsal approach while pressing with the thumb (*ET*) from the plantar aspect of the foot shows the interdigital nerve (*void arrows*) as it passes underneath the intermetatarsal ligament (*arrowhead*) before deflecting dorsally and continuing in a fusiform hypoechoic Morton neuroma (*white arrow*). A fluid-filled intermetatarsal bursa (*asterisk*) is dorsal to the neuroma. **B:** Correlative axial TSE T1w MR image confirms the presence of a small neuroma (*arrow*) in the third webspace.

between the peroneus longus and the extensor digitorum longus muscles. It traverses the deep (crural) fascia approximately 10 to 12.5 cm above the tip of the lateral malleolus to move into the subcutaneous tissue[63] and splits into the intermediate and medial dorsal cutaneous nerves that provide sensation over the dorsal aspect of the ankle. Superficial peroneal neuropathy may be encountered in patients with a history of inversion ankle sprains or plantar flexion injuries that result in persistent sensory disturbances along the nerve distribution.[64] This is related to a tension mechanism at the point where the nerve pierces the deep fascia. Ultrasound reveals fascial thickening and fusiform hypoechoic swelling of either the superficial peroneal nerve or one of its divisional branches at the fascial opening.

In the forefoot, the interdigital nerves course along the plantar surface of the intermetatarsal ligament before dividing into the proper digital nerves. Chronic impingement and microtrauma against the distal edge of this ligament is believed to generate a painful plantar mass that is commonly known as Morton neuroma. The second and third webspaces are usually involved. Ultrasound is accurate[65] and comparable with MR imaging,[66] although it has been suggested that imaging is inaccurate and unnecessary.[67] Ultrasound has sensitivities as high as 85% to 98%.[65,68–70] Morton neuroma appears as a round or spindle-shaped hypoechoic mass **(Fig. 12.18)**. In some cases, it may show mixed echotexture due to the coexistence of an enlarged intermetatarsal bursa.[70] The accuracy of ultrasound examination depends on a careful scanning technique based on three different approaches: plantar static, plantar dynamic (sonographic Mulder sign), and dorsal. Recently, ultrasound-guided absolute ethyl alcohol injection has been proposed as a minimally invasive technique to treat Morton neuromas.[71,72] Long-term results indicate that this procedure is very effective with >90% partial or complete response rate after four sessions of treatment.[72]

Tip:
- The role of ultrasound in imaging nerves about the hip is limited due to problems of ultrasound access. Ultrasound may be only informative in lateral femoral cutaneous and femoral neuropathies.
- MRI is the imaging modality of choice for the intrapelvic obturator, pudendal, gluteal, and sciatic nerves.
- Ultrasound is effective in diagnosing common peroneal nerve entrapment at the fibular head/neck.
- Ultrasound findings in tarsal tunnel syndrome may be inconspicuous. Detection of focal abnormalities in the tibial nerve may be encountered in case of chronic long-standing disease or direct nerve impingement.
- Ultrasound is the first-line investigation for Morton neuroma.

POLYNEUROPATHIES

Inherited Disorders

Charcot–Marie–Tooth (CMT) disease (hereditary motor and sensory neuropathy [HMSN] or peroneal muscular atrophy), encompasses a heterogeneous group of inherited disorders of the peripheral nervous system characterized by progressive distal weakness, reduced or absent deep tendon reflexes, peroneal muscle atrophy, pes cavus, and mild sensory loss.[73] Charcot–Marie–Tooth disease includes demyelinating (CMT-1) and axonal (CMT-2) forms. Demyelinating CMT is defined by widespread slowing of conduction velocities on electrophysiology and affects all peripheral nerves. Schwann cell hypertrophy due to attempted remyelination causes "onion bulb" formation.[74] The nerves may be palpable and ultrasound reveals markedly enlarged nerves with retained fascicular echotexture.[75,76] Axonal forms (CMT-2) are more heterogeneous and show only mild enlargement of nerves.[75] Marked, generalized nerve enlargement typifies CMT-1A.

Hereditary neuropathy with liability to pressure palsies (HNPP) is another congenital disorder in which segmental demyelination and tomaculous (sausage-shaped) myelin sheath swelling is responsible for multifocal nerve enlargement following trivial trauma.[77,78] Ultrasound shows fusiform nerve and fascicular swellings (tomacula) within osteofibrous tunnels and along the course of nerves.[77,78]

Immune-Mediated Polyneuropathies

Immune-mediated (disimmune) polyneuropathies include acute inflammatory demyelinating polyradiculoneuropathy (AIDP or Guillain-Barré syndrome), chronic inflammatory demyelinating polyradiculoneuropathy (CIDP), and multifocal motor neuropathy (MMN), which respond to corticosteroids, plasmapheresis, and IV immunoglobulins in combination with immunosuppressant drugs. Early recognition and treatment prior to the onset of axonal loss is critical. Early diagnosis is not straightforward and the disorder often remains unrecognized.[79,80]

CIDP is a chronic, immune-mediated disease that causes weakness, sensory loss, and possible muscle atrophy. It is caused by demyelination of peripheral nerves, often involving the nerve roots, with onion bulb formation. When severe or progressive, secondary axonal loss may occur. Ultrasound demonstrates marked segmental swelling of the affected nerve and focal swelling at sites where conduction blocks are identified at electrophysiology.[81] Fascicles may appear individually swollen with alternating thickened and thinned segments[82,83] **(Fig. 12.19)**. Nerve enlargement in CIDP occurs late and ultrasound is unlikely to be useful for the early diagnosis.

Guillain-Barré syndrome (AIDP) is an acute polyneuropathy characterized by ascending paralysis, weakness in the hands and feet migrating toward the trunk, and

sensory abnormalities due to an autoimmune attack to the myelin. It may be life-threatening if the respiratory muscles and the autonomic nervous system are involved. In mild cases (80%), axons are spared and recovery is rapid if remyelination occurs. In severe forms with axonal damage (20%), recovery depends on the regeneration process. Treatment with IV immunoglobulin and plasmapheresis within the first week of illness is effective. Cerebrospinal fluid analysis and electrophysiology may be initially negative. Initial experience suggests that ultrasound is able to detect nerve enlargement early in the disease when electrophysiologic abnormalities are still minor.[76] Focal variation in nerve/fascicle thickness can be detected along the nerve.[84] One single fascicle may be affected, surrounded by normal ones. Ultrasound shows reduced swelling during treatment before any neurophysiological improvement.[84]

MMN is much less common than either AIDP or CIDP. It is a pure motor neuropathy causing weakness of muscles, cramping, and fasciculations. Wrist drop with gradual loss of finger extension and foot drop are common signs. The diagnosis is based on detection of motor conduction blocks and preserved sensory responses at electrophysiology. Ultrasound can detect multifocal nerve swellings.[85]

Acromegaly

Acromegaly is associated with CTS. Nerve enlargement is diffuse and involves the main nerve trunks in the extremities, indicating a disease process that is basically unrelated to entrapment syndromes. Typically, there are no changes of the fascicular echotexture. Intraneural edema seems to be the main cause of the nerve swelling.[86–88]

Deposition Diseases

Amyloid arthropathy is a well-recognized complication of long-term hemodialysis treatment and multiple myeloma.[89] Clinically, this condition presents with symmetric polyarthritis possibly mimicking seronegative rheumatoid arthritis. It may be associated with CTS related to extensive deposition of amyloid within the tunnel, displacing the flexor tendons and compressing the median nerve.[90]

Leprosy

Leprosy (Hansen disease) is a multifaceted infectious disease caused by *Mycobacterium leprae* in which skin and peripheral nerves in the extremities are specifically involved. Although this condition is sporadically encountered in the Western world in immigrants, it is endemic in developing countries and represents the most diffuse neuropathy worldwide. Leprosy includes a wide spectrum of phenotypes.[91] Severe immunoreaction may produce episodes of acute neuritis, during which a nerve segment becomes intensely painful with

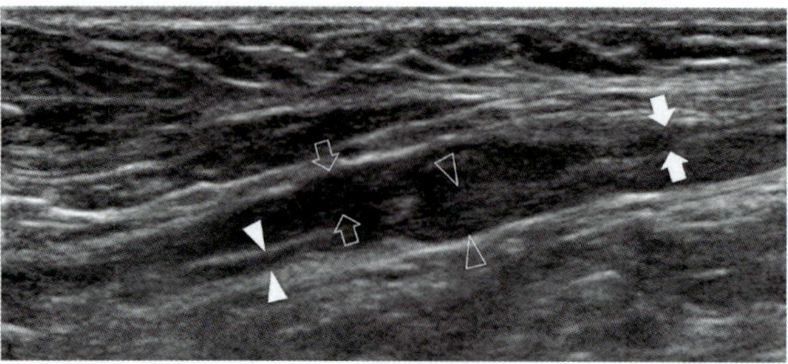

Figure 12.19. Chronic inflammatory demyelinating polyradiculoneuropathy. Long-axis 12.5 MHz ultrasound image of the common peroneal nerve in the popliteal fossa reveals segmental nerve swelling with individual fascicles (*arrows* and *arrowheads*) alternating thickened and thinned segments. Electrophysiology demonstrated a conduction block across this nerve segment.

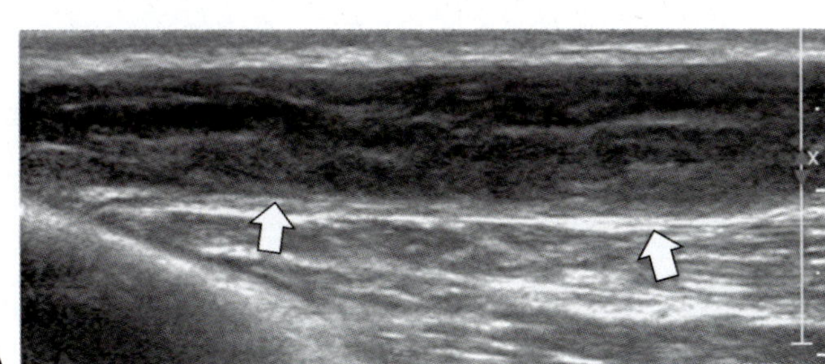

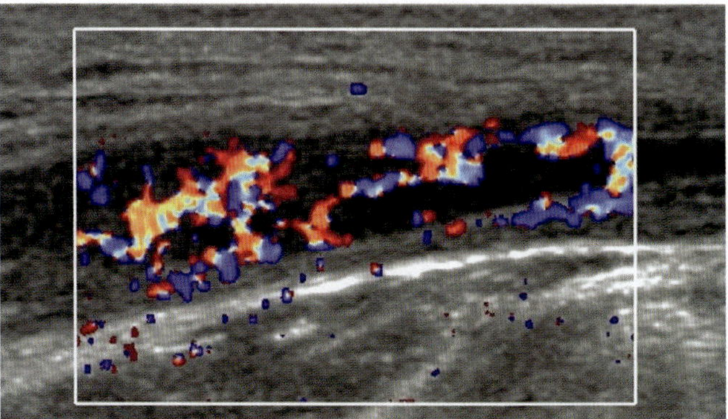

Figure 12.20. Acute neuritis in leprosy. **A:** Long-axis 17.5 MHz ultrasound image of the ulnar nerve at the elbow in a patient with borderline tuberculoid leprosy examined during the course of a reversal reaction reveals high-grade swelling of the nerve (*arrows*) with fusiform enlargement of individual fascicles. **B:** Long-axis color Doppler 12.5 MHz ultrasound image shows dramatically increased blood flow within endoneural vessels as a sign of inflammation.

rapid worsening of the histopathologic and functional damage. Ultrasound can reveal markedly swollen nerves with loss of the fascicular echotexture and thickened epineurium **(Fig. 12.20A)**.[92,93] Abnormal nerves are often found within or in proximity to osteofibrous tunnels, the cubital tunnel most commonly.[94] These changes are better appreciated in patients who have had repeated episodes of acute neuritis.[92,95] The onset of acute neuritic phases may be predicted by detection of intense intraneural hyperemia at Doppler imaging (nerve inferno), a sign suggesting rapid progression of nerve damage and the need for immediate immunosuppressive therapy with corticosteroids **(Fig. 12.20B)**.[92] Recently, ultrasound-guided needle biopsy has been suggested as a promising alternative to open nerve biopsy for diagnosis.[96]

> **Tip:**
> - Patients with Charcot–Marie–Tooth disease, HNPP, dysimmune neuropathies, amyloid deposition disease, acromegaly, and leprosy may exhibit hypertrophied nerves with preserved fascicular echotexture.
> - In CIDP, ultrasound can demonstrate segmental enlargement of the affected nerve with marked focal swelling at sites of conduction blocks. Fascicles may alternate thickened and thinned segments.
> - In leprosy, detection of intense intraneural hyperemia at Doppler imaging (nerve inferno) may predict the onset of acute neuritic phases.

NERVE INJURIES

Penetrating trauma, stretching, and contusion are the main mechanisms in nerve injuries. Nerve injuries are classified based on three main types of nerve fiber injury: neuropraxia, axonotmesis, and neurotmesis.[97] Neuropraxia, the mildest type, is characterized by the physiologic block of nerve conduction without morphological damage. Recovery is complete in days to weeks. Axonotmesis involves disruption of the axon and its

myelin cover, but preservation of the connective tissue framework of the nerve. Axonal regeneration occurs and recovery is usually possible without surgical treatment. Neurotmesis is partial or total disruption of the nerve, including fascicles and epineurium, and requires surgical repair. Sunderland classified nerve injuries as Class-1, neuropraxia; Class-2, mild axonotmesis; Class-3, severe axonotmesis (i.e., axon disruption with intact perineurium and epineurium); Class-4, severe axonotmesis (i.e., axon disruption with only epineurium remaining intact); and Class-5, neurotmesis (i.e., complete nerve transection).[98] Ultrasound is unable to detect nerve abnormalities in Class-1 and Class-2 injuries. Swelling of the nerve with fairly preserved fascicular pattern is usually encountered in Class-3 and may be confirmed by comparison with the opposite side. In Class-4 injuries, the nerve may exhibit loss of the fascicular pattern and an irregular caliber. Some fascicles may assume a fluid-filled appearance as a result of axon disruption. Focal thinning of the nerve may reflect significant damage with severe axon loss. Regeneration is often blocked by scar tissue and the process of reinnervation is partially successful. In Class-5, the nerve bed is empty due to retraction of the nerve ends. Distinguishing severe axonotmesis from neurotmesis may not be straightforward with ultrasound.

Penetrating Injuries

In penetrating wounds, the nerve may be partially or completely transected. At the nerve ends, regenerating Schwann cells, severed axons, proliferating fibroblasts, and new axonal sprouts grow in many directions to fill the gap between the torn fascicles and form a mass of disorganized repair tissues.[99] In complete tears, blunted stump (terminal) neuromas develop as small oval masses in continuity with the edges of the transected nerve **(Fig. 12.21)**. Stump neuromas appear hypoechoic at ultrasound, hyperintense on fluid-sensitive MR imaging, and slightly larger than the undamaged nerve. Most neuromas have well-defined margins but their borders may be irregular

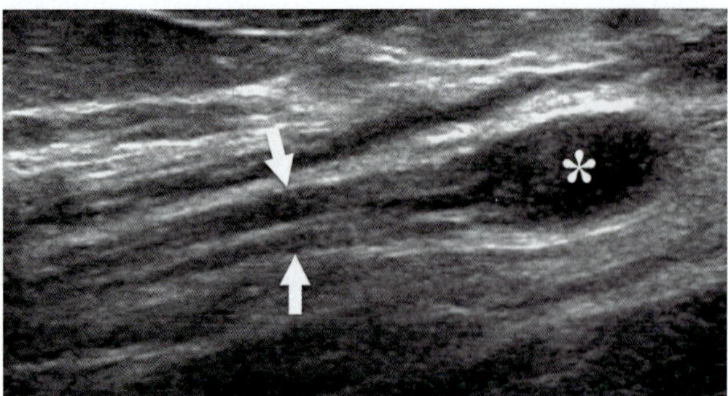

Figure 12.21. Stump neuroma of the tibial nerve following a penetrating injury. Long-axis 12.5 MHz ultrasound image over the medial aspect of the leg demonstrates the tibial nerve (*arrows*) ending in a terminal neuroma (*asterisk*). The neuroma appears as a hypoechoic bulbous-like mass in continuity with the fascicles of the proximal nerve end.

or poorly defined when they are attached to the surrounding tissues by adhesions or scar tissue.[100] Detection of terminal neuromas may help to identify nerve injury, especially if the nerve is very small in size,[54] and map the location of the nerve ends, which may be displaced and retracted away from the site of injury. If nerve ends are close together, fibrous tissue may encase them, mimicking a partial tear. In partial nerve transection, ultrasound is able to estimate the proportions of injured and preserved fascicles **(Fig. 12.22)**. A spindle neuroma may develop in continuity with the injured nerve tissue. Both ultrasound and MR imaging are intrinsically unable to assess the status of the fascicles within the neuroma or predict functional outcome and recovery time. The neuroma may encase both resected and preserved fascicles producing a homogeneous focal nerve swelling. In many instances, the neuroma develops from the superficial torn fascicles, whereas the unaffected deep fascicles continue their normal course alongside the fibrotic mass. The role of imaging is to provide information about the status of the injured nerve to help decide if early surgical treatment is needed, particularly for minor nerve lesions without axonal damage or nerve impingement by fracture fragments, orthopedic hardware, or fibrous encasement. Ultrasound has high negative predictive value in excluding structural nerve damage. Surgical repair after nerve injury includes excision of the neuroma; therefore, measurement of the gap should include the end-to-end distance of the gap and the neuroma length. The measurement should start at the base of the neuroma where the CSA is normal and the fascicular echotexture is preserved. A recent surgical development is to implant coil-reinforced hydrogel tubes between the nerve ends to impose directionality to the regenerating nerve axons and reduce the incidence of neuromas.[101] Regenerating nerve fibers grow from the proximal nerve end, through the graft, into the distal nerve segment.[102] In these cases, the surgeon needs to

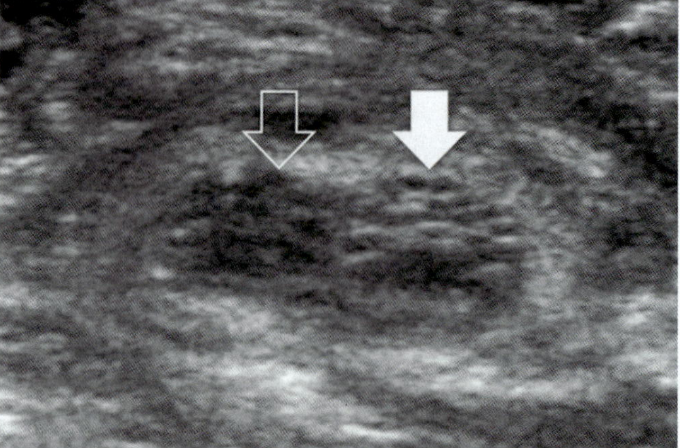

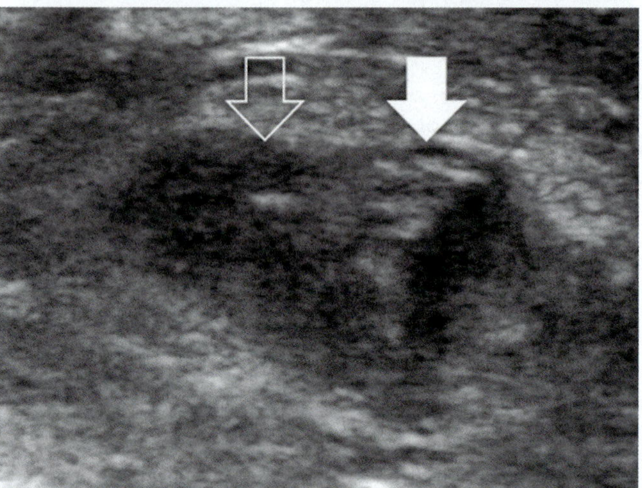

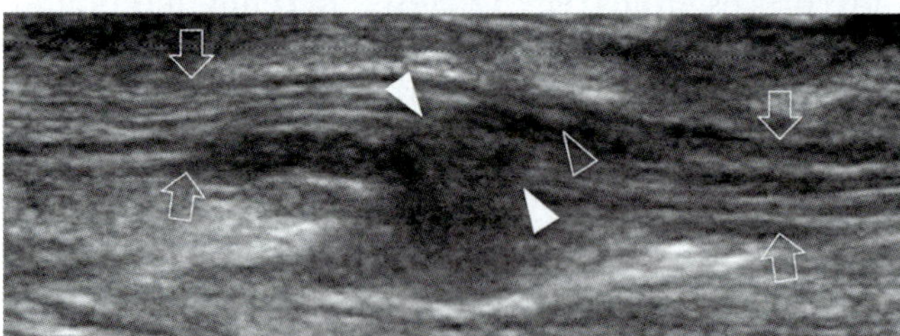

Figure 12.22. Partial sciatic nerve tear by penetrating injury. **A:** Proximal and **(B)** distal 12.5 MHz ultrasound images of the sciatic nerve in the mid-thigh demonstrate echotextural abnormalities affecting the lateral fascicles (*void arrow*). Note that the medial fascicles (*solid arrow*) are preserved and continuous. **C:** Long-axis 12.5 MHz ultrasound image of the nerve (*void arrows*) confirms that damage is partial, affecting some fascicles (*white arrowheads*), while other fascicles are preserved (*void arrowhead*).

know the end-to-end distance free of neuromas and the cross-sectional diameter of the nerve at the injury site to implant a tube of appropriate size.

Stretching Injuries

Nerve-stretching trauma typically occurs following sprain or strain injuries. In complete nerve laceration, ultrasound reveals discontinuity of the nerve bundle, interruption of the fascicles, and sometimes a wavy course of the nerve ends as a result of retraction.[103] In acute injuries, ultrasound is better than MR imaging in assessing the position of the nerve ends because edema and hemorrhage lead to diffuse high-intensity signal on MR imaging and impair nerve end detection. In significant trauma without laceration, a fusiform hypoechoic swelling with loss of the fascicular echotexture can develop reflecting a spindle neuroma with fibrosis internal to a nondisrupted nerve trunk.[104] The neuroma may involve only one or a few fascicles, and nerve CSA appears fairly normal or slightly enlarged. Nerve traction injuries commonly occur at the brachial plexus level following traffic accidents.[105] The common peroneal nerve may be stretched during high-grade knee sprains, dislocation, or fractures.[106] The oblique course and presence of fixation points (i.e., sciatic bifurcation proximally and peroneal tunnel distally) make the nerve particularly vulnerable. Stretching injuries also occur where nerves pierce fascial planes. Following ankle inversion sprains, the superficial peroneal nerve or its divisional branches, the medial, and intermediate dorsal cutaneous nerves, may be stretched at the mid-distal third of the leg forming a fusiform neuroma at the point where they cross, and are tethered to the crural fascia.[63] In minor stretching injuries (burners and stingers), ultrasound is usually normal. Symptoms include an electric shock sensation in the extremities and a feeling of burning or numbness in the nerve distribution lasting a few seconds or minutes.

Contusion Trauma

Contusion trauma most often occurs where nerves run closely apposed to bony surfaces and are vulnerable to external pressure. Most injuries are reversible and do not need imaging. Repeated minor contusion may cause abnormalities that are amenable to ultrasound examination, for example, at the deep peroneal nerve on the anterior aspect of the ankle and the dorsal midfoot.[107] Osteophytes on the dorsal aspect of the talonavicular, naviculocuneiform, or cuneiform–metatarsal joints may predispose to deep peroneal neuropathy. Nerve contusions are also reported in the axillary, spinal accessory, long thoracic, and peroneal nerves in contact sports, such as rugby and martial arts.[107] At the wrist, contusion injuries of the divisional branches of the ulnar nerve around the hamate hook may be encountered in cyclists (cyclist's palsy) as a result of chronic external pressure by ill-fitting or worn gloves, not changing hand position often enough, or body weight improperly distributed on the handlebars. Nerve contusion leads to segmental fusiform thickening of the nerve, which becomes hypoechoic with swollen fascicles and a thickened epineurium. Similar findings occur in ulnar nerve instability at the cubital tunnel.

The Postoperative Nerve

Iatrogenic trauma includes nerve stretching or compression, direct needle trauma, and chemical irritation.[108] Postoperative changes include short-lasting intraneural edema and hyperemia and possible formation of perineural hematoma or scar that needs to be distinguished from incomplete surgical repair with persistent transection of nerve bundles or neuroma development. In partial nerve discontinuity, surgical decompression of the nerve and its sheath is currently used to repair the interrupted nerve fascicles or remove intraneural scar but may damage preserved fascicles or result in formation of a new scar close to the nerve surface.

In complete nerve transection, reconstruction depends on the length of the gap between the nerve ends after removal of irreversibly damaged tissue and terminal neuromas. If the gap is short, an "end-to-end" anastomosis is enough to restore continuity. A nerve graft is required when the gap is >5 mm. Superficial sensory nerves, such as the sural or the medial brachial and antebrachial cutaneous nerves, can be harvested to create the graft. More than one segment of graft can be implanted in parallel if the damaged nerve is larger than the graft. Tiny sutures in the outer and interfascicular epineurium are used for the anastomosis and appear as intraneural hyperechoic spots with comet tail artefact. Ultrasound shows nerve continuity at the site of anastomosis and perineural hematoma. A mild, fusiform increase in nerve CSA at the site of anastomosis is normal but prominent; irregular bulging may indicate inadequate fusion of the nerve edges and postsurgical neuroma formation.[103] Anastomosis failure may be secondary to excessive tension on the nerve edges, or infection. Ultrasound may show the size, extent, and location of postsurgical scar and neuromas.[108] If fibrosis encases the nerve and compresses the fascicles, the nerve may become indistinguishable from the surrounding fibrosis. Long-axis scans may demonstrate nerve continuity within the scar better than short-axis images. The nerve may be distorted and pinched at its periphery by the scar with reactive focal swelling related to edema and venous congestion.

Tip:
- Ultrasound accurately identifies nerve injury in an acute setting, when local soft tissue edema and hemorrhage may make MR imaging difficult.
- Ultrasound reliably shows complete nerve transection and the size of the gap between nerve ends preoperatively.
- In partial nerve tears, ultrasound can demonstrate a fusiform neuroma at the site of injury and measure the proportions of involved and preserved fascicles.
- Ultrasound can show nerve status after surgical repair.

BRACHIAL PLEXOPATHIES

The brachial plexus has a complex anatomy with many nerves involved and interconnecting. Within the spinal canal, anterior (motor) and posterior (sensory) nerve rootlets exit the spinal cord and merge at the dorsal root ganglion at the level of neural foramina. Each ganglion gives off a large ventral and a small dorsal branch that include motor and sensory fibers. The plexus is formed by the ventral branches of C5, C6, C7, C8, and T1. These roots extend from the neural foramina down to the interscalene triangle. At the external border of the interscalene triangle, the roots unite to form three trunks: The roots of C5 and C6 join to form the upper trunk, the root of C7 continues as the middle trunk, and in the lower neck, the roots of C8 and T1 form the lower trunk. In the supraclavicular region, each trunk divides into anterior and posterior divisions that innervate the flexor and extensor muscles of the upper extremity, respectively. Crossing deep to the clavicle, the divisions join in various combinations to form the three cords. The lateral cord is formed by the anterior division of the upper and middle trunks, the medial cord by the anterior division of the lower trunk, and the posterior cord by the posterior divisions of all the trunks. Distal to the pectoralis minor muscle, the cords continue as the peripheral nerves of the upper limb: The axillary and radial nerves originate from the posterior cord, the musculocutaneous nerve from the lateral cord, the median nerve from the medial and lateral cords, and the ulnar nerve from the medial cord. Clinically, relevant spaces along the course of brachial plexus nerves are: (1) the interscalene triangle, (2) the costoclavicular space, and (3) the retropectoralis minor space (subcoracoid tunnel).

Scanning Technique

Ultrasound is an effective way to depict normal brachial plexus nerves.[109–111] The ultrasound examination is based on detecting landmarks in the neck, including bones (roots), muscles (trunks), and vessels (divisions and cords). As the roots exit the neural foramina, they slide between the anterior and posterior tubercles of the transverse processes of the cervical vertebrae. Because the posterior tubercle of C7 is absent, ultrasound is able to establish the level of nerve roots.[112] At the interscalene triangle, roots are aligned between the anterior and middle scalene muscles. In this space, the most superficial fascicles belong to C5 and the deepest to C8. The ability of ultrasound to recognize the exact level of the roots in the paravertebral area also leads to confident identification of trunks simply by following the nerves back to their foramina. In the supraclavicular area, the divisions and initial parts of the cords can be found alongside the posterior aspect of the subclavian artery, over the first

rib and the apical pleura. More distally, the costoclavicular space is blind to ultrasound examination due to the interposition of the clavicle and lack of an acoustic window. In the retropectoralis minor space, the nerve cords continue their course around the axillary artery.[110]

Traumatic Plexopathies

Closed brachial plexus injuries are relatively infrequent. They affect 5% of high-velocity motor vehicle accidents, primarily motorcycle accidents, and result in debilitating, often devastating, consequences in a relatively young patient group.[113] As a result of the mechanism and severity of trauma, brachial plexus injuries are either complete (i.e., C5-T1 are involved) or incomplete. Incomplete lesions are subdivided into upper (i.e., C5, C6 ± C7) and lower (C8, T1 ± C7). Injuries are also classified as preganglionic (intraspinal nerve root avulsions) or postganglionic (extraforaminal), which are treated differently.[114,115] Early assessment of the extent and severity of injury is essential for treatment planning.[115] Preganglionic injuries cannot be repaired and have a poor outcome, resulting in a flail arm.[116] Preganglionic injuries are shown by MR imaging and myelographic techniques. If a preganglionic injury has been excluded, early assessment of the extent and severity of the injury outside the spine is essential for guiding treatment. Electrophysiology often yields ambiguous findings in assessing postganglionic nerve injuries. Imaging is therefore critical, and may provide early categorization of pathology and define surgical candidates before a clear clinical picture has emerged, by identifying the site of injury, how many and which nerves are involved, the severity of involvement, and the position of retracted nerve ends. In the acute phase, the information provided by ultrasound seems very specific, possibly more detailed than provided by MR imaging, in distinguishing interrupted nerves from adjacent areas of hemorrhage and edema.[105,117–119] Ultrasound seems particularly effective in the supraclavicular region, which is difficult to examine with MR imaging **(Fig. 12.23)**. Overall, a combined approach is suggested using MR imaging to examine the spine and foramina, and ultrasound to assess the nerves in the neck.[117]

Neurogenic Thoracic Outlet Syndrome

Nerve involvement in thoracic outlet syndrome is often associated with arterial disease, possibly as a result of neurovascular compression at the interscalene triangle and the costoclavicular space.[120] The clinical diagnosis is not straightforward because symptoms are vague and nonspecific. Ultrasound is usually unable to evaluate nerve changes about the costoclavicular space due to problems of access of the ultrasound beam. In patients with supernumerary cervical ribs, dynamic ultrasound

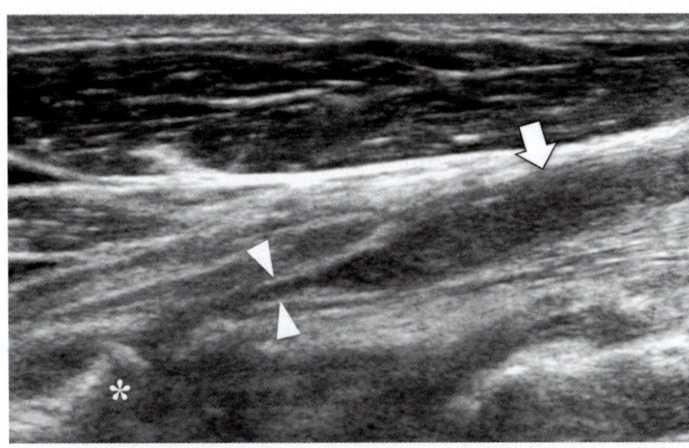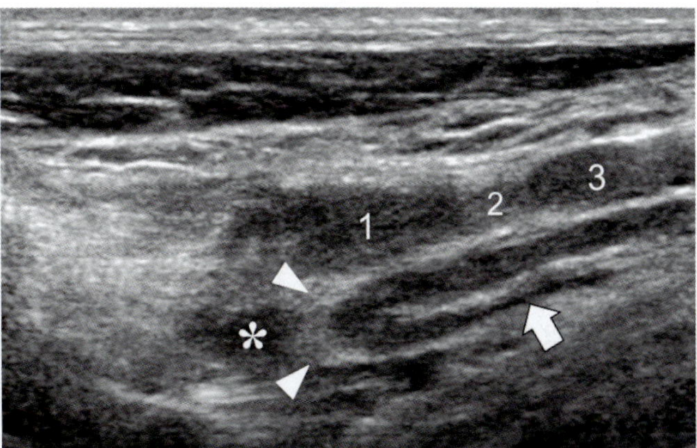

A　　　　　　　　　　　　　　　　　　　　　　　　　　　　　　　　　**B**

Figure 12.23.　Brachial plexus injury. **A:** Long-axis ultrasound image over the course of the C5 nerve root in the paravertebral region shows an avulsed and retracted root (*arrow*). Close to the spine (*asterisk*), the nerve bed (*arrowheads*) appears empty. **B:** Long-axis ultrasound images over the C6 and C7 nerve roots in the paravertebral region reveals wavy and irregular contour and less-defined fascicular echotexture of C6 with thickened (*1,3*) and thinned (*2*) segments reflecting stretching injury (axonotmesis). The C7 root (*arrow*) is torn and exhibits a blunted end (*arrowheads*) with some hematoma (*asterisk*) filling the nerve bed proximally.

may reveal tight contact and impingement of the nerve divisions with the tip of the cervical rib while performing stress manoeuvres.

Parsonage–Turner Syndrome

Although ultrasound is able to reveal denervation signs by showing loss of bulk and hyperechoic appearances of shoulder girdle muscles, MR imaging is more reliable and provides a more comprehensive view than ultrasound of the complex pattern of muscle involvement in Parsonage–Turner syndrome (brachial neuritis).

Tumors and Postradiation Imaging

Brachial plexus tumors include metastatic disease and neurogenic primary tumors. In metastatic disease, ultrasound may reveal a well-defined solid mass with irregular margins and hypoechoic echotexture encasing nerves with an abrupt nerve-to-tumor interface.[105] Alternatively, the neoplasm may cause segmental thickening and a hypoechoic appearance of the involved nerves without a clear mass effect. Satellite lymph nodes are often associated. Distinguishing metastatic plexopathy from postradiation injury is not easy with ultrasound. In radiation fibrosis, the nerve thickening is more uniform and some faint fascicular pattern is preserved.[105] However, this finding is far from specific. Primary neurogenic tumors of the brachial plexus include schwannomas and neurofibromas.

Tip:
- Careful scanning technique based on anatomical landmarks is required to image brachial plexus nerves with ultrasound.

- Outside the spinal canal, ultrasound is an excellent alternative to MR imaging to determine the presence of a lesion, establish the site and the level of nerve involvement, and confirm or exclude major nerve injuries.

NERVE TUMORS AND TUMORLIKE LESIONS

Neurogenic Histotypes (Schwannoma and Neurofibroma)

Most peripheral nerve sheath tumors (PNSTs) are benign. They may present with nerve pain and have a positive Tinel sign (tingling on tapping) but many present as asymptomatic masses. The two most common benign nerve tumors are schwannoma (neurilemmoma or neurinoma) and neurofibroma, which derive from the Schwann cell.[121] They may occur as isolated lesions or in association with Neurofibromatosis Type 1 (NF1), typically neurofibromas. Histologically, nerve sheath tumors are distinguished by the presence of Antoni A (cellular) and Antoni B (myxoid) areas, intense and uniform immunostaining with S100, and encapsulation in neurilemomas but not neurofibromas. Neurilemomas usually shell out easily at surgery without permanent nerve damage, whereas removal of a neurofibroma may require resection of the nerve.

Ultrasound diagnosis relies on detection of a soft tissue mass in continuity with a nerve at its proximal and/or distal pole.[122,123] This feature is virtually pathognomonic of PNSTs but may not be obvious in tumors arising from small or distal nerve branches, and in these cases nerve tumors cannot be differentiated from other soft tissue masses. A rim of fat, the "split-fat" sign, suggests an origin in the intermuscular space surrounding the neurovascular bundle and may result in triangular echogenic caps at the proximal and distal poles of the mass.

Differential features have been described between schwannomas and neurofibromas, but ultrasound cannot reliably distinguish between the two.[124] Schwannomas typically appear spherical. The nerve lies at the periphery of the mass.[123,125] as the tumor develops from an individual fascicle that remains in-axis with the bulk of the mass, whereas uninvolved fascicles are splayed about the neoplasm **(Fig. 12.24)**. Large masses may contain calcified foci and internal degenerative cystic changes ("ancient schwannomas"). Neurofibromas are intimately associated with the parent nerve and develop in fusiform fashion. They are slowly growing, painless, and may exhibit a "target sign," a hyperechoic fibrous center surrounded by a peripheral hypoechoic rim of myxomatous tissue.[126]

Three types of neurofibromas are classically described: localized, diffuse, and plexiform. The localized variety, described above, is the most common, and accounts for approximately 90% of all neurofibromas.[121,125] All three types of neurofibromas can be associated with type-1 neurofibromatosis (NF-1) (Recklinghausen disease). Diffuse neurofibromas present as a plaque-like elevation of the skin with regional thickening of the subcutaneous tissue. They usually occur in the head and neck but occasionally peripherally, including the ankle. They are often associated with NF1. Ultrasound shows diffuse echogenic infiltration of the subcutaneous and deep fat that envelops

structures such as nerves, tendons, and vessels.[127,128] and may result in localized tissue overgrowth. Masses are hyperemic and contain hypoechoic tubular structures that are probably due to neural tissue.

Plexiform neurofibromas are virtually pathognomonic of NF1. They often resemble a "bag of worms" and affect a large segment of nerve. Adjacent bone and soft tissue hypertrophy may be present. Ultrasound shows a lobulated mass or lobulated enlargement of a nerve with a heterogeneous appearance due to interspersed areas of nodular increased and reduced echogenicity **(Fig. 12.25)**.[129,130] Because they are so extensive, diffuse and plexiform neurofibromas are best imaged by MR imaging.

Malignant peripheral nerve sheath tumors (MPNSTs) are rare. About 20% to 50% of patients with MPNSTs

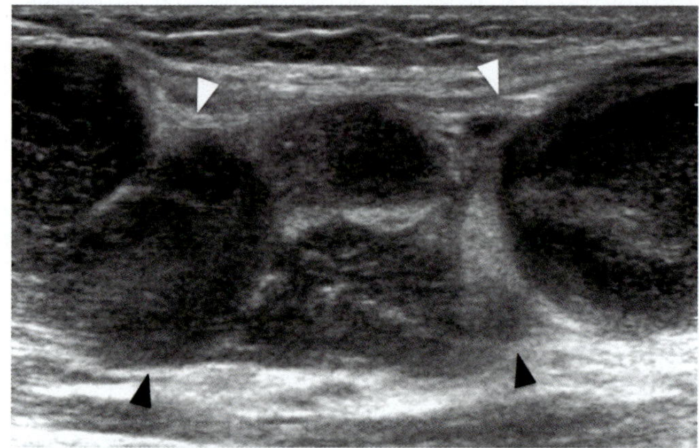

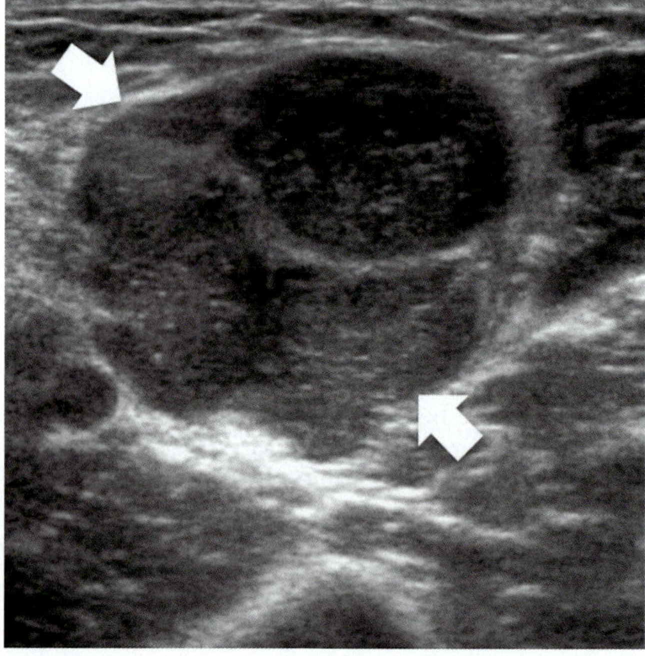

Figure 12.25.   Plexiform neurofibromas of the ulnar nerve in a patient with type-1 neurofibromatosis. **A:** Long- and **(B)** short-axis 17.5 MHz ultrasound images demonstrate striking nerve enlargement (*arrows*) by multiple neurofibromas disposed in series along the nerve axis (*arrowheads*).

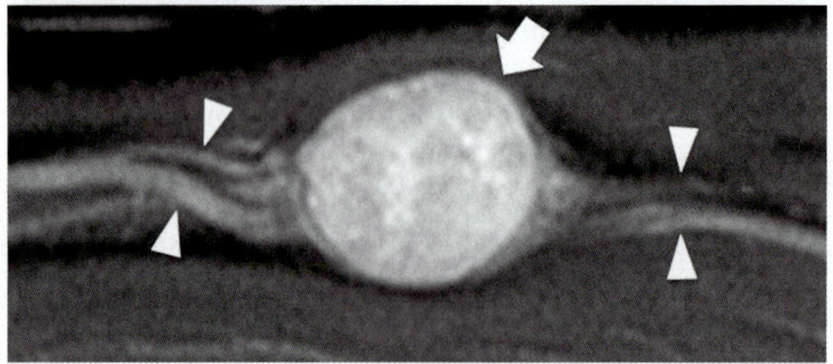

Figure 12.24.   Schwannoma of the median nerve in the proximal arm. **A:** Longitudinal 12.5 MHz ultrasound image with **(B)** correlative fat-suppressed fast T2-weighted MR image depicts the tumor as an eccentric hypoechoic mass (*arrow*) in continuity with the parent nerve (*arrowheads*). The tumor develops from one fascicle (*1*) and splays others (*2*).

have NF1, and the risk of malignant transformation in NF1 has been estimated to be as high as 29%.[125,131] Other cancer-prone genetic syndromes and irradiation are also associated with MPNST. Enlargement of a mass, new pain, or sensory or motor symptoms in a patient with NF1 should suggest malignant transformation. Ultrasound shows a nonspecific soft tissue mass. The relationship of the mass to a nerve is not always obvious, particularly in large tumors.[121] MPNSTs tend to be larger (>5 cm) than benign forms and often present as inhomogeneous hypoechoic masses with calcifications and areas of internal bleeding and necrosis. Intratumoral fluid–fluid levels from hemorrhage may be observed but are nonspecific and may be also encountered in ancient schwannomas. In contrast to benign PNSTs, malignant forms may have indistinct margins as a result of their infiltrative growth. An intratumor anarchic vascular architecture at Doppler imaging with corkscrew-like neovessels and low-resistance patterns related to arteriovenous shunting can be often found.[126] Despite these differences, ultrasound frequently cannot distinguish between benign and malignant PNSTs.[129]

Among rare neurogenic histotypes, the intraneural perineurioma is a benign neoplasm composed exclusively of whorled perineurial cells growing at the boundaries of fascicles. It preferentially involves young people and is located most commonly in the sciatic nerve and its branches. Its ultrasound appearance is nonspecific, presenting as an elongated fusiform swelling with preserved fascicular pattern.[132]

Non-Neurogenic Masses

Occasionally, other non-neural masses may originate in or infiltrate or adhere to a nerve. They include lipomatous lesions, paragangliomas, hemangiomas, lymphomas, extrinsic soft tissue neoplasms, and ganglion cysts.[126,133]

Fibrolipomatous hamartoma is a developmental disorder related to accumulation of mature fat and fibroblasts in the epineurium that often presents at birth or during early childhood. Fibrolipomatous hamartoma has a predilection for the median nerve, although other upper limb nerves are frequently involved[134] and lower extremity nerves occasionally. It may be associated with local gigantism of the hand or foot related to bony overgrowth, fat proliferation in the soft tissues, and nerve-territory-oriented macrodactyly, a condition known as "macrodystrophia lipomatosa." Ultrasound shows hypoechoic tubular structures due to thickened, fibrotic neural elements separated by echogenic fat.[121,134,135]

Intraneural ganglia most frequently involve the common peroneal nerve. The ganglion cyst extends from the proximal tibiofibular joint along the articular branch of the nerve into the common peroneal nerve or sometimes the tibial or sciatic nerves **(Fig. 12.26)**. Patients present with pain, paresthesia, foot drop, or swelling.[136–141]

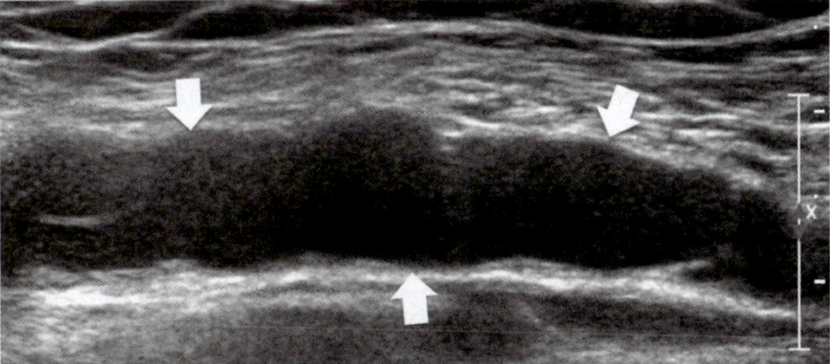

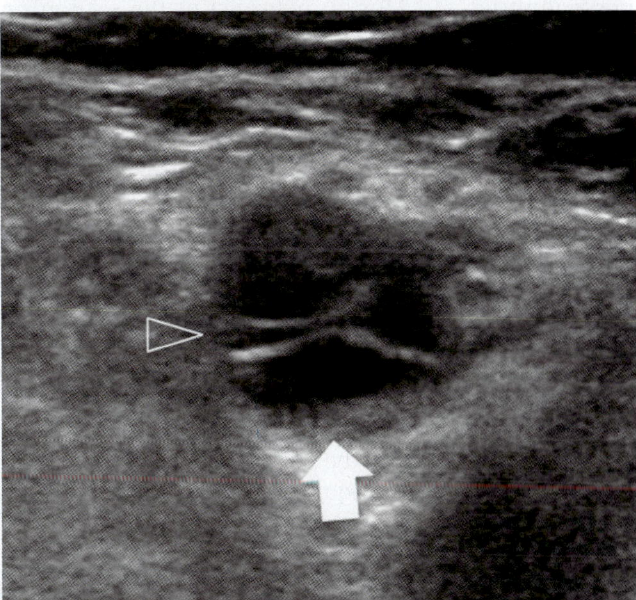

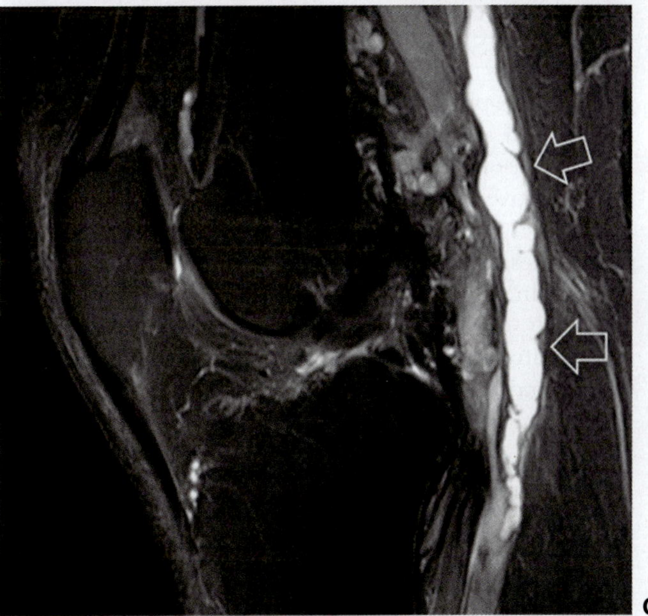

Figure 12.26.   Intraneural ganglion of the tibial nerve. **A:** Long- and **(B)** short-axis 17.5 MHz ultrasound images of the tibial nerve in the popliteal fossa with **(C)** sagittal fat-suppressed T2w MR imaging correlation reveal a swollen fluid-filled tibial nerve (*arrows*) reflecting intraneural involvement by a large ganglion cyst that expands cranially within the nerve substance from the level of the tibiofibular joint. Some residual atrophic fascicles (*arrowhead* in **B**) are demonstrated within the nerve.

Ultrasound shows an elongated, lobulated, anechoic mass on the anterolateral aspect of the fibular neck. There may be denervation changes including muscle atrophy and increased echogenicity due to fatty infiltration in the anterior compartment. Intraneural ganglia do not have a fibrous capsule or a synovial lining and must be differentiated from the more common extraneural (intramuscular) ganglia.[142]

Traumatic neuromas are discussed in the section on nerve injuiries and Morton neuroma in the section on compressive neuropathies.

Tip:
- Nerve tumors are connected with the nerve of origin at their poles. This is the only feature of value to distinguish them from other soft tissue masses.
- Although some differential features are described between schwannomas and neurofibromas, the characterization of nerve masses cannot be accomplished with ultrasound alone.
- Ultrasound may be limited, for example, in deep-seated nerve tumors, such as intra-abdominal or paraspinal tumors, due to problems of ultrasound access; in huge masses that distort the local anatomy and obscure landmarks; and in malignant forms, when the neoplasm has spread into muscles, fascial planes, and bone. In these cases, MR imaging provides better tumor assessment.

CONCLUSION

With developing experience, an increasing number of nerves and related pathologic conditions are identified with ultrasound. High-resolution ultrasound provides cost-effective, accurate, morphologic information regarding a variety of nerve abnormalities, including entrapment syndromes, injuries, polyneuropathies, and neurogenic masses. In many of these conditions, ultrasound can significantly enhance clinical decision making regarding conservative or surgical treatment. In clinical practice, ultrasound can be considered an ideal complement of clinical and electrophysiologic testing for the diagnostic workup of patients with peripheral neuropathies.

REFERENCES

1. Jambawalikar S, Baum J, Button T, et al. Diffusion tensor imaging of peripheral nerves. *Skeletal Radiol.* 2010;39(11):1073–1079.
2. Kermarrec E, Demondion X, Khalil C, et al. Ultrasound and magnetic resonance imaging of the peripheral nerves: current techniques, promising directions, and open issues. *Semin Musculoskelet Radiol.* 2010;14(5):463–472.
3. Stewart JD. Peripheral nerve fascicles: anatomy and clinical relevance. *Muscle Nerve.* 2003;28(5):525–541.
4. Silvestri E, Martinoli C, Derchi LE, et al. Echotexture of peripheral nerves: correlation between ultrasound and histologic findings and criteria to differentiate tendons. *Radiology.* 1995; 197(1):291–296.
5. Propeck T, Quinn TJ, Jacobson JA, et al. Sonography and MR imaging of bifid median nerve with anatomic and histologic correlation. *AJR Am J Roentgenol.* 2000;175(6):1721–1725.
6. Iannicelli E, Chianta GA, Salvini V, et al. Evaluation of bifid median nerve with sonography and MR imaging. *J Ultrasound Med.* 2000;19(7):481–485.
7. Gassner EM, Schocke M, Peer S, et al. Persistent median artery in the carpal tunnel: color Doppler ultrasonographic findings. *J Ultrasound Med.* 2002;21(4):455–461.
8. Natsis K, Totlis T, Tsikaras P, et al. Variations of the course of the upper trunk of the brachial plexus and their clinical significance for the thoracic outlet syndrome: a study on 93 cadavers. *Am Surg.* 2006;72(2):188–192.
9. Loukas M, Louis RG Jr, Kwiatkowska M. Chondroepitrochlearis muscle, a case report and a suggested revision of the current nomenclature. *Surg Radiol Anat.* 2005;27(4):354–356.
10. Masear VR, Hill JJ Jr, Cohen SM. Ulnar compression neuropathy secondary to the anconeus epitrochlearis muscle. *J Hand Surg Am.* 1988;13(5):720–724.
11. Degreef I, De Smet L. Anterior interosseous nerve paralysis due to Gantzer's muscle. *Acta Orthop Belg.* 2004;70(5): 482–484.
12. Schuurman AH, van Gils AP. Reversed palmaris longus muscle on MRI, report of four cases. *Eur Radiol.* 2000;10(8):1242–1244.
13. Pirola E, Hébert-Blouin MN, Amador N, et al. Palmaris profundus: one name, several subtypes, and shared potential for nerve compression. *Clin Anat.* 2009;22(6):643–648.
14. Harvie P, Patel N, Ostlere SJ. Ulnar nerve compression at Guyon's canal by an anomalous abductor digiti minimi muscle: the role of ultrasound in clinical diagnosis. *Hand Surg.* 2003;8(2):271–275.
15. Sammarco GJ, Stephens MM. Tarsal tunnel syndrome caused by flexor digitorum accessorius longus. A case report. *J Bone Joint Surg Am.* 1990;72(3):453–454.
16. Jacobson JA, Jebson PJL, Jeffers AW, et al. Ulnar nerve dislocation and snapping triceps syndrome: diagnosis with dynamic sonography—report of three cases. *Radiology.* 2001; 220(3):601–605.
17. Spratt JD, Stanley AJ, Grainger AJ, et al. The role of diagnostic radiology in compressive and entrapment neuropathies. *Eur Radiol.* 2002;12(9):2352–2364.
18. Andreisek G, Burg D, Studer A, et al. Upper extremity peripheral neuropathies: role and impact of MR imaging on patient management. *Eur Radiol.* 2008;18(9):1953–1961.
19. Subhawong TK, Wang KC, Thawait SK, et al. High resolution imaging of tunnels by magnetic resonance neurography. *Skeletal Radiol.* 2012;41(1):15–31.
20. Küllmer K, Sievers KW, Reimers CD, et al. Changes of sonographic, magnetic resonance tomographic, electromyographic, and histopathologic findings within a 2-month denervation period of examinations after experimental muscle denervation. *Arch Orthop Trauma Surg.* 1998;117(4–5):228–234.
21. Martinoli C, Bianchi S, Gandolfo N, et al. Ultrasound of nerve entrapments in osteofibrous tunnels of the upper and lower limbs. *Radiographics.* 2000;20 Spec No:S199–S213.
22. Sugimoto H, Miyaji N, Ohsawa T. Carpal tunnel syndrome: evaluation of median nerve circulation with dynamic contrast-enhanced MR imaging. *Radiology.* 1994;190(2):459–466.
23. Powell HC, Myers RR. Pathology of experimental nerve compression. *Lab Invest.* 55(1):91–100.
24. Ziswiler HR, Reichenbach S, Vögelin E, et al. Diagnostic value of sonography in patients with suspected carpal tunnel syndrome: a prospective study. *Arthritis Rheum.* 2005;52(1):304–311.
25. Ghasemi-Esfe AR, Khalilzadeh O, Vaziri-Bozorg SM, et al. Color and power Doppler Ultrasound for diagnosing carpal

tunnel syndrome and determining its severity: a quantitative image processing method. *Radiology.* 2011;261(2):499–506.

26. Mallouhi A, Pültzl P, Trieb T, et al. Predictors of carpal tunnel syndrome: accuracy of gray-scale and color Doppler sonography. *AJR Am J Roentgenol.* 2006;186(5):1240–1245.

27. Mondelli M, Filippou G, Aretini A, et al. Ultrasonography before and after surgery in carpal tunnel syndrome and relationship with clinical and electrophysiological findings. A new outcome predictor? *Scand J Rheumatol.* 2008;37(3):219–224.

28. Duncan I, Sullivan P, Lomas F. Sonography in the diagnosis of carpal tunnel syndrome. *AJR Am J Roentgenol.* 1999;173(3):681–684.

29. Yesildag A, Kutluhan S, Sengul N, et al. The role of ultrasonographic measurements of the median nerve in the diagnosis of carpal tunnel syndrome. *Clin Radiol.* 2004;59:910–915.

30. Alemán L, Berná JD, Reus M, et al. Reproducibility of sonographic measurements of the median nerve. *J Ultrasound Med.* 2008;27(2):193–197.

31. Thoirs K, Williams MA, Phillips M. Ultrasonographic measurements of the ulnar nerve at the elbow: role of confounders. *J Ultrasound Med.* 2008;27(5):737–743.

32. Tung GA, Entzian D, Stern JB, et al. MR imaging and MR arthrography of paraglenoid labral cysts. *AJR Am J Roentgenol.* 2000;174(6):1707–1715.

33. Martinoli C, Bianchi S, Prato N, et al. Ultrasound of the shoulder: non-rotator cuff disorders. *Radiographics.* 2003;23(2):381–401.

34. Hashimoto BE, Hayes AS, Ager JD. Sonographic diagnosis and treatment of ganglion cysts causing suprascapular nerve entrapment. *J Ultrasound Med.* 1994;13(9):671–674.

35. Loomer R, Graham B. Anatomy of the axillary nerve and its relation to inferior capsular shift. *Clin Orthop Relat Res.* 1989;(243):100–105.

36. Chautems RC, Glauser T, Waeber-Fey MC, et al. Quadrilateral space syndrome: case report and review of the literature. *Ann Vasc Surg.* 2000;14(6):673–676.

37. Brestas PS, Tsouroulas M, Nikolakopoulou Z, et al. Ultrasound findings of teres minor denervation in suspected quadrilateral space syndrome. *J Clin Ultrasound.* 2006;34(7):343–347.

38. Campbell WW. Guidelines in electrodiagnostic medicine. Practice parameter for electrodiagnostic studies in ulnar neuropathy at the elbow. *Muscle Nerve Suppl.* 1999;8(suppl):171–205.

39. Yoon JS, Walker FO, Cartwright MS. Ultrasonographic swelling ratio in the diagnosis of ulnar neuropathy at the elbow. *Muscle Nerve.* 2008;38(4):1231–1235.

40. Okamoto M, Abe M, Shirai H, et al. Diagnostic ultrasonography of the ulnar nerve in cubital tunnel syndrome. *J Hand Surg Br.* 2000;25(5):499–502.

41. Bodner G, Harpf C, Meirer R, et al. Ultrasonographic appearance of supinator syndrome. *J Ultrasound Med.* 2002;21(11):1289–1293.

42. Chien AJ, Jamadar DA, Jacobson JA, et al. Sonography and MR imaging of posterior interosseous nerve syndrome with surgical correlation. *AJR Am J Roentgenol.* 2003;181(1):219–221.

43. Hide IG, Grainger AJ, Naisby GP, et al. Sonographic findings in the anterior interosseous nerve syndrome. *J Clin Ultrasound.* 1999;27(8):459–464.

44. Martinoli C, Bianchi S, Pugliese F, et al. Sonography of entrapment neuropathies in the upper limb (wrist excluded). *J Clin Ultrasound.* 2004;32(9):438–450.

45. Buchberger W, Judmaier W, Birbamer G, et al. Carpal tunnel syndrome: diagnosis with high-resolution sonography. *AJR Am J Roentgenol.* 1992;159(4):793–798.

46. Hobson-Webb LD, Padua L, Martinoli C. Ultrasonography in the diagnosis of peripheral nerve disease. *Expert Opin Med Diagn.* 2012;6(5):457–471.

47. Hobson-Webb LD, Massey JM, Juel VC, et al. The ultrasonographic wrist-to-forearm median nerve area ratio in carpal tunnel syndrome. *Clin Neurophysiol.* 2008;119(6):1353–1357.

48. Klauser AS, Halpern EJ, De Zordo T, et al. Carpal tunnel syndrome assessment with Ultrasound: value of additional cross-sectional area measurements of the median nerve in patients versus healthy volunteers. *Radiology.* 2009;250(1):171–177.

49. Klauser AS, Halpern EJ, Faschingbauer R, et al. Bifid median nerve in carpal tunnel syndrome: assessment with Ultrasound cross-sectional area measurement. *Radiology.* 2011;259(3):808–815.

50. Moran L, Perez M, Esteban A, et al. Sonographic measurement of cross-sectional area of the median nerve in the diagnosis of carpal tunnel syndrome: correlation with nerve conduction studies. *J Clin Ultrasound.* 2009;37(3):125–131.

51. Karadağ YS, Karadağ O, Çiçekli E, et al. Severity of carpal tunnel syndrome assessed with high frequency ultrasonography. *Rheumatol Int.* 2010;30(6):761–765.

52. Miwa T, Miwa H. Ultrasonography of carpal tunnel syndrome: clinical significance and limitations in elderly patients. *Intern Med.* 2011;50(19):2157–2161.

53. Meys V, Thissen S, Rozeman S, et al. Prognostic factors in carpal tunnel syndrome treated with a corticosteroid injection. *Muscle Nerve.* 2011;44(5):763–768.

54. Tagliafico A, Pugliese F, Bianchi S, et al. High-resolution sonography of the palmar cutaneous branch of the median nerve. *AJR Am J Roentgenol.* 2008;191(1):107–114.

55. Kim JY, Yoon JS, Kim SJ, et al. Carpal tunnel syndrome: clinical, electrophysiological and ultrasonographic ratio after surgery. *Muscle Nerve.* 2012;45(2):183–188.

56. Damarey B, Demondion X, Boutry N, et al. Sonographic assessment of the lateral femoral cutaneous nerve. *J Clin Ultrasound.* 2009;37(2):89–95.

57. Tagliafico A, Serafini G, Lacelli F, et al. Ultrasound-guided treatment of meralgia paresthetica (lateral femoral cutaneous neuropathy): technical description and results of treatment in 20 consecutive patients. *J Ultrasound Med.* 2011;30(10):1341–1346.

58. Aravindakannan T, Wilder-Smith EP. High resolution ultrasonography in the assessment of meralgia paresthetica. *Muscle Nerve.* 2012;45(3):434–435.

59. Gruber H, Peer S, Kovacs P, et al. The ultrasonographic appearance of the femoral nerve and cases of iatrogenic impairment. *J Ultrasound Med.* 2003;22(2):163–172.

60. Peer S, Kovacs P, Harpf C, et al. High-resolution sonography of lower extremity peripheral nerves: anatomic correlation and spectrum of disease. *J Ultrasound Med.* 2002;21(3):315–322.

61. Nagaoka M, Matsuzaki H. Ultrasonography in tarsal tunnel syndrome. *J Ultrasound Med.* 2005;24(8):1035–1040.

62. Vijayan J, Therimadasamy AK, Teoh HL, et al. Sonography as an aid to neurophysiological studies in diagnosis tarsal tunnel syndrome. *Am J Phys Med Rehabil.* 2009;88(6):500–501.

63. Canella C, Demondion X, Guillin R, et al. Anatomic study of the superficial peroneal nerve using sonography. *AJR Am J Roentgenol.* 2009;193(1):174–179.

64. Johnston EC, Howell SJ. Tension neuropathy of the superficial peroneal nerve: associated conditions and results of release. *Foot Ankle Int.* 1999;20(9):576–582.

65. Oliver TB, Beggs I. Ultrasound in the assessment of metatarsalgia: a surgical and histological correlation. *Clin Radiol.* 1998;53(4):287–289.

66. Lee MJ, Kim S, Huh YM, et al. Morton neuroma: evaluated with ultrasonography and MR imaging. *Korean J Radiol.* 2007;8(2):148–155.

67. Sharp RJ, Wade CM, Hennessy MS, et al. The role of MRI and ultrasound imaging in Morton's neuroma and the effect of size of lesion on symptoms. *J Bone Joint Surg Br.* 2003; 85(7):999–1005.

68. Redd RA, Peters VJ, Emery SF, et al. Morton neuroma: sonographic evaluation. *Radiology.* 1989;171(2):415–417.

69. Pollak RA, Bellacosa RA, Dornbluth NC, et al. Sonographic analysis of Morton's neuroma. *J Foot Surg.* 1992;31(6):534–537.

70. Quinn TJ, Jacobson JA, Craig JG, et al. Sonography of Morton's neuromas. *AJR Am J Roentgenol.* 2000;174(6):1723–1728.

71. Fanucci E, Masala S, Fabiano S, et al. Treatment of intermetatarsal Morton's neuroma with alcohol injection under Ultrasound guide: 10-month follow-up. *Eur Radiol.* 2004;14(3):514–518.

72. Hughes RJ, Ali K, Jones H, et al. Treatment of Morton's neuroma with alcohol injection under sonographic guidance: follow-up of 101 cases. *AJR Am J Roentgenol.* 2007;188(6):1535–1539.

73. Dyck RJ, Chance P, Lebo R, et al. Hereditary motor and sensory neuropathies. In: Dyck PJ, Thomas PK, eds. *Peripheral Neuropathy.* 3rd ed. Philadelphia, PA: Saunders; 1993:1094–1136.

74. Sereda M, Griffiths I, Pühlhofer A, et al. A transgenic rat model of Charcot-Marie-Tooth disease. *Neuron.* 1996;16(5):1049–1060.

75. Martinoli C, Schenone A, Bianchi S, et al. Sonography of median nerve in Charcot-Marie-Tooth disease. *AJR Am J Roentgenol.* 2002;178(6):1553–1556.

76. Zaidman CM, Al-Lozi M, Pestronk A. Peripheral nerve size in normals and patients with polyneuropathy: an ultrasound study. *Muscle Nerve.* 2009;40(6):960–966.

77. Beekman R, Visser LH. Sonographic detection of diffuse peripheral nerve enlargement in hereditary neuropathy with liability to pressure palsies. *J Clin Ultrasound.* 2002;30(7):433–436.

78. Hooper DR, Lawson W, Smith L, et al. Sonographic features in hereditary neuropathy with liability to pressure palsies. *Muscle Nerve.* 2011;44(6):862–867.

79. De Sousa EA, Chin RL, Sander HW, et al. Demyelinating findings in typical and atypical chronic inflammatory demyelinating polyneuropathy: sensitivity and specificity. *J Clin Neuromuscul Dis.* 2009;10(4):163–169.

80. Magda P, Latov N, Brannagan TH III, et al. Comparison of electrodiagnostic abnormalities and criteria in a cohort of patients with chronic inflammatory demyelinating polyneuropathy. *Arch Neurol.* 2003;60(12):1755–1759.

81. Granata G, Pazzaglia C, Calandro P, et al. Ultrasound visualization of nerve morphological alteration at the site of conduction block. *Muscle Nerve.* 2009;40(6):1068–1070.

82. Taniguchi N, Itoh K, Wang Y, et al. Sonographic detection of diffuse peripheral nerve hypertrophy in chronic inflammatory demyelinating polyradiculoneuropathy. *J Clin Ultrasound.* 2000;28(9):488–491.

83. Matsuoka N, Kohriyama T, Ochi K, et al. Detection of cervical nerve root hypertrophy by ultrasonography in chronic inflammatory demyelinating polyradiculoneuropathy. *J Neurol Sci.* 2004;219(12):15–21.

84. Almeida V, Mariotti P, Veltri S, et al. Nerve ultrasound follow-up in a child with Guillain-Barré syndrome. *Muscle Nerve.* 2012;46(2):270–275.

85. Beekman R, van den Berg LH, Franssen H, et al. Ultrasonography shows extensive nerve enlargements in multifocal motor neuropathy. *Neurology.* 2005;65(2):305–307.

86. Tagliafico A, Resmini E, Nizzo R, et al. Ultrasound measurement of median and ulnar nerve cross-sectional area in acromegaly. *J Clin Endocrinol Metab.* 2008;93(3):905–909.

87. Tagliafico A, Resmini E, Nizzo R, et al. The pathology of the ulnar nerve in acromegaly. *Eur J Endocrinol.* 2008;159(4):369–373.

88. Resmini E, Tagliafico A, Nizzo R, et al. Ultrasound of peripheral nerves in acromegaly: changes at 1-year follow-up. *Clin Endocrinol (Oxf).* 2009;71(2):220–225.

89. Cobby MJ, Adler RS, Swartz R, et al. Dialysis-related amyloid arthropathy: MR findings in four patients. *AJR Am J Roentgenol.* 1991;157(5):1023–1027.

90. Ferrara MA, Marcelis S. Ultrasound examination of the wrist. *J Belge Radiol.* 1997;80(2):78–80.

91. Ridley DS, Jopling WH. Classification of leprosy according to immunity: a five group system. *Int J Lepr Other Micobact Dis.* 1966;34(3):255–273.

92. Martinoli C, Derchi LE, Bertolotto M, et al. Ultrasound and MR imaging of peripheral nerves in leprosy. *Skeletal Radiol.* 2000;29(3):142–150.

93. Visser LH, Jain S, Lokesh B, et al. Morphological changes of the epineurium in leprosy: a new finding detected with high-resolution sonography. *Muscle Nerve.* 2012;46(1):38–41.

94. Bathala L, Kumar K, Pathapati R, et al. Ulnar neuropathy in Hansen disease: clinical, high-resolution ultrasound and electrophysiologic correlations. *J Clin Neurophysiol.* 2012; 29(2):190–193.

95. Fornage BD, Nerot C. Sonographic diagnosis of tuberculoid leprosy. *J Ultrasound Med.* 1987;6(2):105–107.

96. Lolge SJ, Morani AC, Chaubal NG, et al. Sonographically guided nerve biopsy. *J Ultrasound Med.* 2005;24(10): 1427–1430.

97. Seddon H. Surgical disorders of the peripheral nerve. In: Sunderland S, ed. *Nerves and Nerve Injury.* Edinburgh, NY: Churchill Livingstone; 1978:823–824.

98. Sunderland S. *Nerve Injuries and their Repair: A Critical Appraisal.* Edinburgh, NY: Churchill Livingstone; 1991.

99. Chiou HJ, Chou YH, Chiou SY, et al. Peripheral nerve lesions: role of high-resolution Ultrasound. *Radiographics.* 2003;23(6):e15.

100. Bodner G, Buchberger W, Schocke M, et al. Radial nerve palsy associated with humeral shaft fracture: evaluation with Ultrasound—initial experience. *Radiology.* 2001;219(3):811–816.

101. Battiston B, Geuna S, Ferrero M, et al. Nerve repair by means of tubulization: literature review and personal clinical experience comparing biological and synthetic conduits for sensory nerve repair. *Microsurgery.* 2005;25(4):258–267.

102. Belkas JS, Munro CA, Shoichetb MS, et al. Peripheral nerve regeneration through a synthetic hydrogel nerve tube. *Restor Neurol Neurosci.* 2006;23(1):19–29.

103. Peer S, Bodner G, Mairer R, et al. Examination of postoperative peripheral nerve lesions with high-resolution sonography. *AJR Am J Roentgenol.* 2001;177(2):415–419.

104. Martinoli C, Bianchi S. In: Bianchi S, Martinoli C, eds. *Ultrasound of the Musculoskeletal System.* Berlin, Germany: Springer-Verlag; 2007:637–744.

105. Graif M, Martinoli C, Rockind S, et al. Sonographic evaluation of brachial plexus pathology. *Eur Radiol.* 2004;14(2): 193–200.

106. Gruber H, Peer S, Meirer R, et al. Peroneal nerve palsy associated with knee luxation: evaluation by sonography–initial experiences. *AJR Am J Roentgenol.* 2005;185(5):1119–1125.

107. Toth C. Peripheral nerve injuries attributable to sport and recreation. *Phys Med Rehabil Clin North Am.* 2009;20(1):77–100.

108. Peer S, Harpf C, Willeit J, et al. Sonographic evaluation of primary peripheral nerve repair. *J Ultrasound Med.* 2003; 22(12):1317–1322.

109. Sheppard DG, Iyer RB, Fenstermacher MJ. Brachial plexus: demonstration at Ultrasound. *Radiology.* 1998;208(2):402–406.

110. Demondion X, Herbinet P, Boutry N, et al. Sonographic mapping of the normal brachial plexus. *AJNR Am J Neuroradiol.* 2003;24(7):1303–1309.

111. Cash CJC, Sardesai AM, Berman LH, et al. Spatial mapping of the brachial plexus using three-dimensional ultrasound. *Br J Radiol.* 2005;78(936):1086–1094.

112. Martinoli C, Bianchi S, Santacroce E, et al. Brachial plexus sonography: a technique for assessing the root level. *AJR Am J Roentgenol.* 2002;179(3):699–702.

113. Songcharoen P. Management of brachial plexus injury in adults. *Scand J Surg.* 2008;97(4):317–323.

114. Birch R. Brachial plexus injuries. *Current Orthopaedics.* 1987;1:316–323.

115. Tavakkolizadeh A, Saifuddin A, Birch R. Imaging of adult brachial plexus traction injuries. *J Hand Surg Br.* 2001; 26(3):183–191.

116. Schenker M, Birch R. Diagnosis of the level of intradural rupture of the rootlets in transaction lesions of the brachial plexus. *J Bone Joint Surg Br.* 2001;83(6):916–920.

117. Gruber H, Glodny B, Galiano K, et al. High-resolution ultrasound of the supraclavicular brachial plexus—can it improve therapeutic decisions in patients with plexus trauma? *Eur Radiol.* 2007;17(6):1611–1620.

118. Haber HP, Sinis N, Haerle M, et al. Sonography of brachial plexus traction injuries. *AJR Am J Roentgenol.* 2006; 186(6):1787–1791.

119. Tagliafico A, Succio G, Serafini G, et al. Diagnostic performance of ultrasound in patients with suspected brachial plexus lesions in adults: a multicenter retrospective study with MRI, surgical findings and clinical follow-up as reference standard. *Skeletal Radiol.* 2013;42(3):371–376.

120. Wittenberg KH, Adkins MC. MR imaging of nontraumatic brachial plexopathies: frequency and spectrum of findings. *Radiographics.* 2000;20(4):1023–1032.

121. Murphey MD, Smith WS, Smith SE, et al. From the archives of the AFIP. Imaging of musculoskeletal neurogenic tumors: radiologic-pathologic correlation. *Radiographics.* 1999;19(5): 1253–1280.

122. Beggs I. Sonographic appearances of nerve tumors. *J Clin Ultrasound.* 1999;27(7):363–368.

123. Lin J, Martel W. Cross-sectional imaging of peripheral nerve sheath tumors: characteristic signs on CT, MR imaging, and sonography. *AJR Am J Roentgenol.* 2001;176(1):75–82.

124. Tsai WC, Chiou HJ, Chou YH, et al. Differentiation between schwannomas and neurofibromas in the extremities and superficial body: the role of high-resolution and color Doppler ultrasonography. *J Ultrasound Med.* 2008;27(2):161–166.

125. Abreu E, Aubert S, Wavreille G, et al. Peripheral tumor and tumor-like neurogenic lesions. *Eur J Radiol.* 2013;82(1):38–50.

126. Gruber H, Glodny B, Bendix N, et al. High-resolution ultrasound of peripheral neurogenic tumors. *Eur Radiol.* 2007;17(11):2880–2888.

127. Beggs I, Gilmour HM, Davie RM. Diffuse neurofibroma of the ankle. *Clin Radiol.* 1998;53(10):755–759.

128. Chen W, Jia JW, Wang JR. Soft tissue diffuse neurofibromas: sonographic findings. *J Ultrasound Med.* 2007;26(4):513–518.

129. Reynolds DL Jr, Jacobson JA, Inampudi P, et al. Sonographic characteristics of peripheral nerve sheath tumors. *AJR Am J Roentgenol.* 2004;182(3):741–744.

130. Lin J, Jacobson JA, Hayes CW. Sonographic target sign in neurofibromas. *J Ultrasound Med.* 1999;18(7):513–517.

131. Evans DG, Huson SM, Birch JM. Malignant peripheral nerve sheath tumors in inherited disease. *Clin Sarcoma Res.* 2012;2(1):17.

132. Mauermann ML, Amrami KK, Kuntz NL, et al. Longitudinal study of intraneural perineurioma—a benign, focal hypertrophic neuropathy of youth. *Brain.* 2009;132(pt 8): 2265–2276.

133. Châtillon CE, Guiot MC, Jacques L. Lipomatous, vascular and chondromatous benign tumors of the peripheral nerves: representative cases and review of the literature. *Neurosurg Focus.* 2007;22(6):1–8.

134. Toms AP, Anastakis D, Bleakney RR, et al. Lipofibromatous hamartoma of the upper extremity: a review of the radiologic findings for 15 patients. *AJR Am J Roentgenol.* 2006;186(3):805–811.

135. Chen P, Massengill A, Maklad N, et al. Nerve territory-oriented macrodactyly: unusual cause of carpal tunnel syndrome. *J Ultrasound Med.* 1996;15(9):661–664.

136. Spinner RJ, Atkinson JL, Tiel RL. Peroneal intraneural ganglia: the importance of the articular branch. A unifying theory. *J Neurosurg.* 2003;99(2):330–343.

137. Spinner RJ, Amrami KK, Rock MG. The use of MR arthrography to document an occult joint communication in a recurrent peroneal intraneural ganglion. *Skeletal Radiol.* 2006;35(3):172–179.

138. Spinner RJ, Mokhtarzadeh A, Schiefer TK, et al. The clinico-anatomic explanation for tibial intraneural ganglion cysts arising from the superior tibiofibular joint. *Skeletal Radiol.* 2007;36(4):281–292.

139. Spinner RJ, Desy NM, Amrami KK. Sequential tibial and peroneal intraneural ganglia arising from the superior tibiofibular joint. *Skeletal Radiol.* 2008;37(1):79–84.

140. Spinner RJ, Luthra G, Desy NM, et al. The clock face guide to peroneal intraneural ganglia: critical "times" and sites for accurate diagnosis. *Skeletal Radiol.* 2008;37(12):1091–1099.

141. Young NP, Sorenson EJ, Spinner RJ, et al. Clinical and electrodiagnostic correlates of peroneal intraneural ganglia. *Neurology.* 2009;72(5):447–452.

142. Bianchi S, Abdelwahab IF, Kenan S, et al. Intramuscular ganglia arising from the superior tibiofibular joint: CT and MR evaluation. *Skeletal Radiol.* 1995;24(4):253–256.

CHAPTER

13

Pediatrics

David Wilson
Gina Allen

INTRODUCTION

The principal advantages of ultrasound in the examination of children are that it is noninvasive, does not use ionizing radiation, and can be used when motion artifact might degrade alternative imaging techniques in a restless child. Also, the examiner can obtain the clinical history at first hand from the family and child.

EXAMINATION TECHNIQUE

At the outset, it is wise to introduce the child to the equipment, preferably demonstrating its use with the ultrasound jelly on another person, either the examiner or the parent. Involving the child in the process and perhaps allowing them to hold the probe usually helps to obtain cooperation. It helps to show and explain the images on the screen as well as explaining at each stage what movements and positions are required.

High-frequency transducers with a linear array are most often used for musculoskeletal examinations in children. Small footprint "hockey stick" probes are particularly useful provided that they achieve the same near-field resolution as conventional-shaped probes. Typical frequency ranges are from 5 to 20 MHz, the most useful probes being in the center of this range.

If an interventional procedure is considered likely, informed consent should be obtained from the parent. This is best done in advance. Prior to procedures we ask children under 16 years if they assent to the procedure, as they are under the age of consent. Almost invariably, children agree. As soon as they do, it is important to undertake the procedure with minimal delay. Clear instructions should be given, including warnings that there will be some pain. In practice, if the injection is performed within 30 to 40 seconds of the warning, cooperation usually results. It is wise to ask the parent to sit alongside the child to avoid the risk of the parent experiencing a vasovagal episode.

If it is likely that an aspiration will be undertaken, local anesthetic cream can be applied prior to the procedure.[1,2] This takes at least 1 hour to work, ideally 90 minutes. Anesthetic creams are principally based on lignocaine or other short-acting local anesthetics. They should be applied on the area of the intended puncture and placed under an occlusive dressing. Drawbacks include the time to take effect and the occasional skin reaction. Anesthetic injections hurt as much as, if not more than, the puncture for aspiration or injection, and the experienced operator is less likely to cause discomfort when not using local anesthetic injection.

Examination techniques and interpretation in children are identical to those in adults but with the added difficulty that unossified epiphyses and metaphyses show hypoechoic areas that may mimic fluid in the eyes of the unwary. If there is doubt, gentle pressure or comparison with the opposite side will clarify.

In general, examination of children is easier than in adults as children are normally thinner and have better defined tissue planes.

> **Tip:**
> - Local anesthetic gel should be applied at least 90 minutes before injection.
> - Unossified bone is hypoechoic.

DEVELOPMENTAL DYSPLASIA OF THE HIP

Developmental dysplasia of the hip (DDH) affects approximately one to three per thousand live births, although these figures do not include lesser degrees of dysplasia, which may present as premature adult osteoarthritis. It is possible that the incidence of hip dysplasia is ten to twenty times higher than the recorded incidence.

Factors that increase the risk of developmental dysplasia are:

- Family history in a first degree relative
- Breech presentation
- Female gender
- Other congenital abnormalities including ankle and spinal cord defects.

Screening philosophies depend on the local health care environment. In some countries, for example, Germany and Switzerland, all children are examined using diagnostic ultrasound at birth. In others, only those at high risk undergo ultrasound.

Ultrasound examination is more sensitive to abnormalities of the hip, in particular a shallow acetabulum, than clinical examination. Twenty-three percent of children with abnormal ultrasound examinations have normal clinical examination even in the hands of the experienced practitioners.[3]

In the majority of health care systems, children are examined at birth by an experienced practitioner, and those with any abnormality detected using the Ortolani and Barlow procedures will also be examined using ultrasound.

A variety of ultrasound techniques has been proposed. The technique described by Graf is a static examination of the hips in the coronal plane.[4] The infant lies in a soft but firm trough in a lateral position with the hips flexed. The ultrasound probe is placed in a coronal plane over the acetabulum and hip. Precise coronal alignment is necessary to ensure that positioning errors do not mimic shallow or deep hips. When the plane is properly achieved, the lateral aspect of the acetabulum is seen as a linear structure. The maximum diameter of the femoral head should also be identifiable on these images.

Static images are analyzed by placing a line along the ilium and a second line along the roof of the acetabulum (Graf alpha angle). The angle described by these two lines can be measured using bespoke software on many ultrasound machines. This roof angle reflects the depth and shape of the acetabulum. A second line drawn along the labrum of the acetabulum describes the cartilage cover and is termed the beta angle. By combining these measurements, Graf creates a numeric classification.

The difficulty with the Graf technique[5] is that a roof angle of 42 degrees or greater is regarded as normal, whereas less is abnormal. As it is very difficult to reproduce angles with the precision required to classify patients accurately, the grading may vary between observers.[6] Graf described a fairly complex grading system based on the alpha and beta angles.[7] An alternative technique described by Terjesen[8] is to draw parallel lines along the ilium and at the maximum depth and maximum height of the femoral head. The three lines provide a measurement of how well the femoral head is covered or contained within the acetabulum. Coverage of >55% of the femoral head is normal; 50% or less is regarded as shallow, and <45% is very shallow **(Figs. 13.1 and 13.2)**.

The majority of practitioners assess children in the first few weeks of life when there is an opportunity to treat conservatively with double nappies and splinting. In children younger than 6 weeks with a shallow acetabulum and normally located femoral capital epiphysis, it is reasonable to wait a week or two and then reexamine the hip. In many cases, the acetabulum will have developed and acquired a normal depth. If the depth does not become normal, longer term splintage and potential orthopedic procedures may be considered. The key is to keep the child under review.

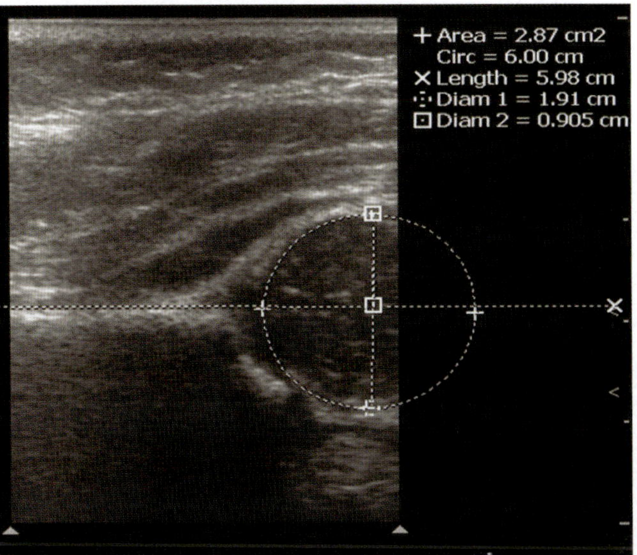

Figure 13.1. Ultrasound of a normal infant hip in the coronal plane. The ball is the femoral head and the spoon-shaped white line is the ilium and acetabulum. Measurements are placed using the Terjesen method.

Many workers add dynamic assessment.[9] Subluxation of the hip during gentle pressure on the hip in an upward and outward direction whilst examining in the coronal plane is regarded as a risk factor. If a shallow hip is clinically normal, firmly located, and cannot be subluxed, many practitioners defer more aggressive forms

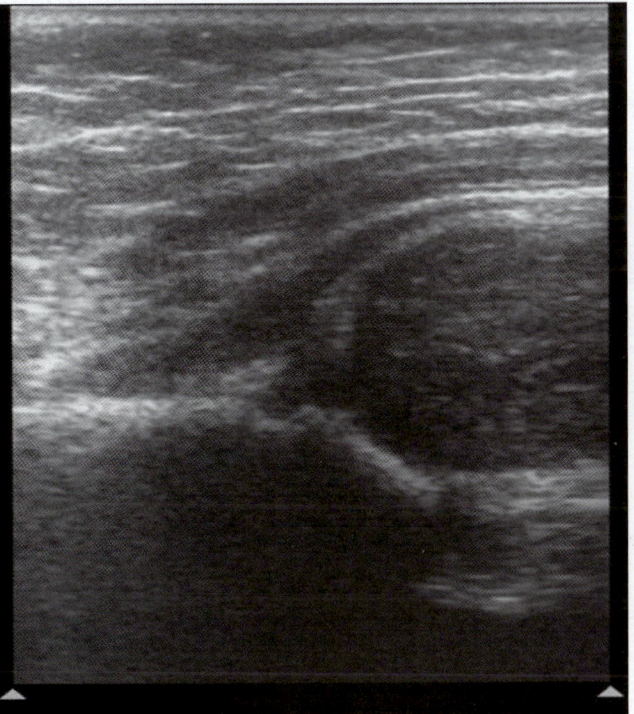

Figure 13.2. Ultrasound of a shallow hip showing mild but significant subluxation. The ball no longer sits in the socket. This worsens under dynamic load.

of treatment. If the hip is subluxable, early intervention should be considered.

Screening processes have considerably reduced the incidence of late presentation. Children normally walk by the age of 1 year, and without screening for hip dysplasia, it may only be at this stage that a dislocation is recognized. Dislocation may present later in childhood subsequent to subluxable and shallow acetabula. Therefore, dislocation at birth is not the hallmark of all children with hip dysplasia problems.

In patients where the hips are relocated surgically, the child is placed in a plaster spica to hold the hip in place. Magnetic resonance (MR) examination is useful in assessing correct relocation.

Tip:
- Ultrasound is the technique of choice in assessing for DDH.

IRRITABLE HIP

The majority of children who present with an irritable hip do so between the ages of 3 and 8 years; older children are less likely to develop an irritable hip but are more likely to suffer more serious hip disorders.

Transient Synovitis and Septic Arthritis

The commonest form of irritable hip is transient synovitis, which is of unknown etiology, although a viral origin has been suggested. Children between the ages of 4 and 8 years are most commonly affected. The typical history is of a few hours or perhaps one day of pain and irritability. The child is reluctant to walk or move the hip in any direction, is tearful, and distressed. In most cases, there is a hip joint effusion that varies from 1 to >4 mL. The pain persists while the effusion is present, but as the effusion reduces spontaneously over the next 24 to 48 hours, the pain diminishes. Analgesia is rarely of much benefit. In the past, these children were admitted to hospitals and observed and treated in traction. However, aspiration of the hip in the early stages is not only diagnostic but can rule out rarer causes of acute irritable hip such as septic arthritis or hemarthrosis. At the same time, aspiration alleviates symptoms by relieving pressure on the joint capsule.[10–12] Transient synovitis is self-limiting. It is a common disorder, and the majority of general hospitals will see several patients a week with this condition. The greatest concern is the much more serious condition of septic arthritis.

Fortunately, septic arthritis is rare, occurring in approximately 1 in every 400 to 500 patients who present with an irritable hip. Septic arthritis can destroy articular cartilage within 12 hours of onset, and therefore early diagnosis is critical. The appropriate treatment is arthrotomy, joint lavage, and intravenous antibiotics, which is more effective than treating with antibiotics alone.

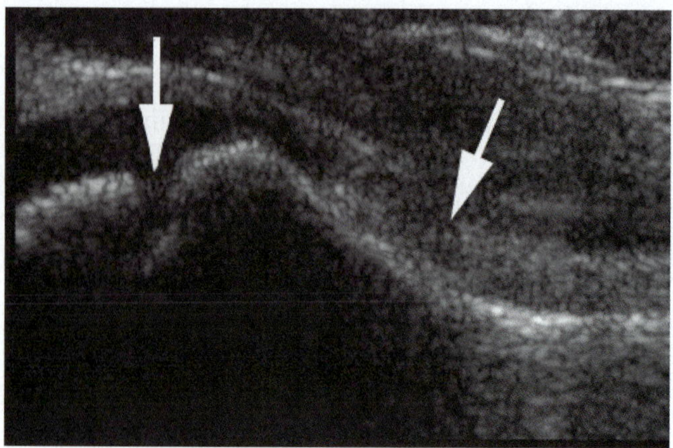

Figure 13.3. Ultrasound of the anterior aspect of the femoral neck in a 6-year-old child. The open growth plate is visible (*left arrow*). The iliofemoral ligament (*right arrow*) is closely applied to the anterior aspect of the femoral neck.

Ultrasound of transient synovitis shows an effusion that elevates the anterior capsule of the joint. Fluid pools anteriorly as the capsule here is thin. The hip is externally rotated as this gives the greatest relaxation of the anterior capsule. An ultrasound probe placed obliquely along the femoral neck best shows the effusion. Deflection of the iliofemoral ligament by >2 mm compared with the normal side is definitely abnormal (**Figs. 13.3 and 13.4**). It is probable that a difference of 1 mm is sufficient to diagnose a small effusion.[13] Septic arthritis presents with exactly the same clinical and ultrasound signs as transient synovitis. Synovial thickening may occur in transient synovitis. Some cases of septic arthritis are not associated with thickening of the synovium. Particulate debris in the joint does not discriminate between

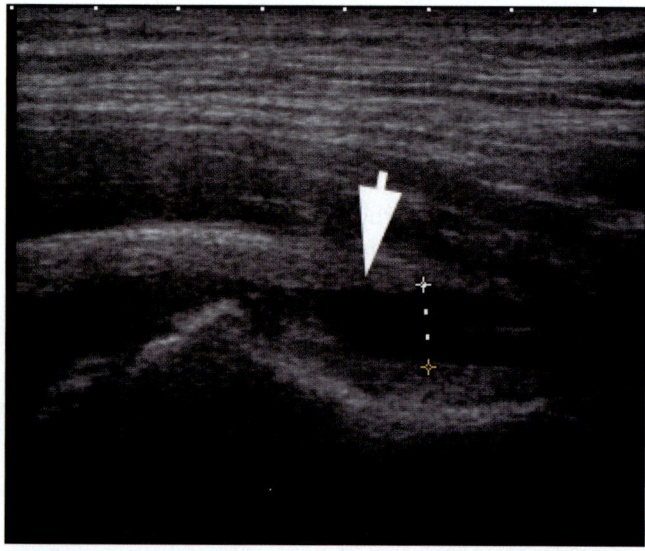

Figure 13.4. Ultrasound of the hip of a 5-year-old child with a substantial echo-free joint effusion (calipers) due to transient synovitis. The iliofemoral ligament (*arrow*) is elevated by the effusion.

infection and transudate. A hemarthrosis presents with fluid in the joint, and there may be particulate matter and debris, but this is not always the case. Ultrasound demonstration of a joint effusion determines that the hip is the problem and excludes other disorders such as muscle strain, apophyseal injury, and abdominal conditions including retrocecal appendicitis.[14] However, the presence and ultrasound appearances of joint fluid do not determine the nature of the effusion, and color Doppler examination does not assist in this discrimination.[15] Systemic manifestations of infection are rare in the early stages of septic arthritis. The majority of patients with an acute septic arthritis have normal body temperature, white count, erythrocyte sedimentation rate, and C-reactive protein. Therefore, blood tests do not help triage the children at the onset of symptoms when appropriate therapy for septic arthritis is urgently needed.[16,17]

Ultrasound-guided aspiration of the hip is simple and relatively atraumatic. It provides material for microbiological assessment, including an urgent Gram stain.

The patient should be prepared by placing a local anesthetic jelly patch on the anterior aspect of the hip for at least 1½ hours before the procedure. Informed consent should be obtained from the parents and assent from the child. The needle is placed without any further anesthetic by a direct anterior approach to the femoral neck by marking the transducer position over the fluid on sagittal and transverse scans. The needle is inserted where the scan planes intersect, and any fluid is aspirated. Attempts should be made to aspirate to dry as this will alleviate symptoms. It is exceptionally rare to find any late growth of organisms in cultures if the Gram stain is negative. The majority of patients with septic arthritis have purulent or green fluid. Those patients with septic arthritis go immediately to arthrotomy. Patients with transudates will have had their symptoms relieved and may be discharged. In the vast majority of cases, they recover without further management.[10]

Recurrent irritable hip with transudates on more than one occasion is an indication for a semi-urgent MR examination as other conditions including osteomyelitis, osteoid osteoma, and neoplasm may mimic recurrent irritable hip, and most are identifiable using MRI. At the upper end of the age spectrum, cases of Perthes disease and even slipped epiphysis may present as an irritable hip. They can be identified by additional imaging. In patients over the age of 8 years, a frog lateral radiograph should be used to exclude slipped epiphysis.

Tip:
- A normal ultrasound examination excludes septic arthritis.
- Septic arthritis may mimic transient synovitis with normal clinical and laboratory markers.
- Diagnostic aspiration to exclude sepsis is also therapeutic for transient synovitis.

Perthes Disease

Perthes disease (Legg–Calvé–Perthes disease) is of unknown etiology. It presents as pain and irritability of the hip and is commonly seen in children aged 8 to 12 years. Perthes typically presents unilaterally but may present subsequently in the opposite hip. If bilateral, changes are usually asymmetric. The conventional radiographic appearances are thickening of the medial joint space due to cartilage edema, not a joint effusion, although an effusion is present in a large proportion of patients. Conventional radiographs later in the disease process show fragmentation of the femoral head, then deformity due to remodeling.

Ultrasound shows a joint effusion in most cases. It may also show fragmentation of the femoral head, but a conventional radiograph is more sensitive in this respect. It has been suggested that the blood supply of the femoral head, largely arising from vessels around the femoral neck, can be assessed using Doppler ultrasound[18,19] and that flow around the femoral neck may be an indicator of the integrity of the blood supply to the femoral head. Children with Perthes disease show small arterial caliber and reduced flow in the brachial artery, suggesting that there is a systemic disorder of vessels.[18] The role of Doppler ultrasound in Perthes disease is yet to be defined.

Meyer dysplasia is rare and presents with bilateral and symmetrical fragmentation of the femoral head, which may mimic Perthes disease.[20] Meyer dysplasia is regarded as a normal variant, and the hips develop normally. Key to the diagnosis of Meyer dysplasia is symmetric changes and the absence of a joint effusion.

The treatment of Perthes disease is initially conservative. Attempts are made to allow the hip to remodel by limiting weight bearing, but eventually osteotomies may be necessary. Ultrasound examination can be used to assess containment of the femoral head by the acetabulum during treatment.[21,22]

Staging and assessing Perthes disease and judging its progress is probably best achieved with MR, but many cases of Perthes disease are initially examined with ultrasound.

Tip:
- Ultrasound may show epiphyseal fragmentation in Perthes disease, but MR is the sensitive test.

Slipped Upper Femoral Epiphysis

Slipped upper femoral epiphysis (SUFE) typically affects patients who are 12 to 14 years old. Prompt surgical treatment is essential to avoid complete displacement of the capital epiphysis and potentially severe long-term consequences. An acute slip should be treated urgently, whilst a chronic slip could wait for a day or two. SUFE is more common in overweight boys and rare under 10 years. The slip occurs because of excessive biomechanical load on a femoral capital epiphysis that is insufficiently strong to take the weight. The condition is rarely seen under the age of 10, and 8 years is considered to be an absolute lower limit for the disorder. Patients usually present with a short history of pain and limitation of movement and should be investigated urgently. They should be non–weight bearing until investigated and the diagnosis discounted, as even walking short distances can cause severe displacement of the epiphysis and irreversible damage to the hip.

The primary investigation is a frog lateral radiograph, which demonstrates the slip in the majority of cases. Occasionally, an ultrasound examination is performed. Over three- quarters of patients with a slipped epiphysis have a joint effusion. It is possible to detect a difference in the alignment of the femoral capital epiphysis by comparing sides, but ultrasound is less sensitive than conventional radiographs.[23] In cases of doubt, MRI should be performed as the edema in the metaphysis may be a more specific sign when there is doubt about the alignment of the epiphysis.[24]

The immediate management of a slipped epiphysis is to ensure the child is non–weight bearing. Surgical management with pin fixation prevents further slippage. Many cases of slipped epiphysis are bilateral, and both sides should always be investigated. This may result in bilateral pinning in a patient who presented with unilateral symptoms.

Tip:
- Over three-quarters of children with SUFE have a joint effusion.
- A frog lateral radiograph is the primary investigation.
- MR is the most sensitive test.

APOPHYSEAL INJURIES

An apophysis is a separate ossification center and is a site of insertion of a tendon into bone. The ultrasound appearances of apophyses have been used to assess the true age of children for forensic or legal purposes.[25,26]

Acute Avulsion

Children differ from adults in that the weakest link in the muscle–tendon–bone chain is the cartilage that attaches an apophysis to bone. An excess load results in avulsion of the apophysis, and avulsion injuries are common. They present with acute pain after trauma. As children are often involved in energetic physical exercise, it may be difficult to determine the nature of trauma. In all children who present with a localized bone or muscle pain, an avulsion injury should be considered. Typical sites include the origins of the hamstrings at the ischial tuberosity, rectus femoris at the anterior inferior iliac

spine and sartorius at the anterior superior iliac spine, and the insertions of the patellar tendon on the tibial tubercle and the abdominal muscles at the iliac crests. Conventional radiographs may show avulsion injuries, but they are often difficult to detect and commonly overlooked whilst ultrasound examination is very sensitive. Comparison with the normal side shows widening of the gap between the apophysis and the bone. Neovascularity and sometimes hematoma are present. Apophyseal injuries are treated by rest and unloading. If the child continues to exercise and load the apophysis, further avulsion and new bone formation may occur, leading to long-term disability. In some cases, MRI examination is useful and shows bone edema and asymmetry. However, in general, ultrasound is more sensitive and accurate in detecting apophyseal injury[27] (**Fig. 13.5A, B**).

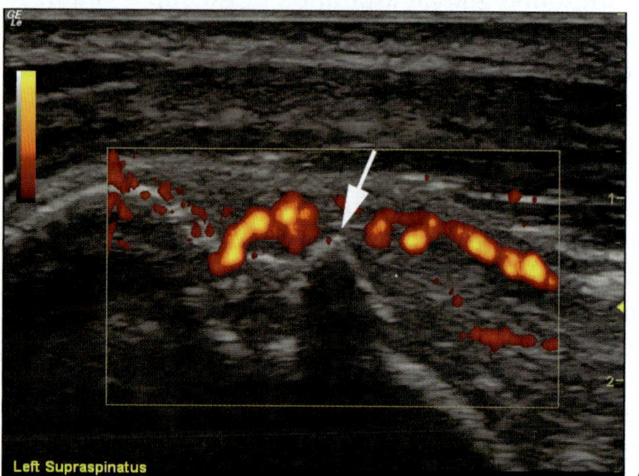

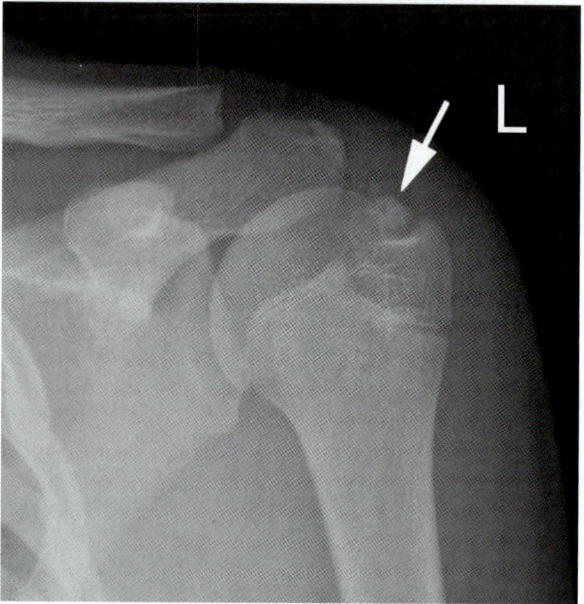

Figure 13.5. **A.** Doppler ultrasound of the left shoulder in a child with an injury that is a few days old. There is a minimally displaced avulsion (*arrow*) of the greater tuberosity of the humerus with bone fragments and a soft tissue response. **B.** Radiograph of the left shoulder confirms the fracture (*arrow*).

Chronic Apophyseal Injury

Chronic traction on an immature apophysis may lead to minor, repetitive injury without a remembered acute incident and present with pain, swelling, and dysfunction. The repair processes are associated with neovascularization, swelling, and edema in the soft tissues and bone. The apophysis may fragment, and subsequent new bone formation may in turn lead to bony deformity and a hard mass effect.

The most frequent chronic apophyseal injury is at the distal patellar tendon insertion (Osgood–Schlatter disease)[28] (**Figs. 13.6 and 13.7**), but any tendon insertion may be affected. The proximal patellar tendon (jumper's knee)and the Achilles insertion are other common locations of apophyseal injury.[29,30]

Ultrasound examination is the imaging technique of choice as all the above features will be apparent. Comparison with the opposite side is very useful, but the examiner should be aware that the changes are often bilateral.

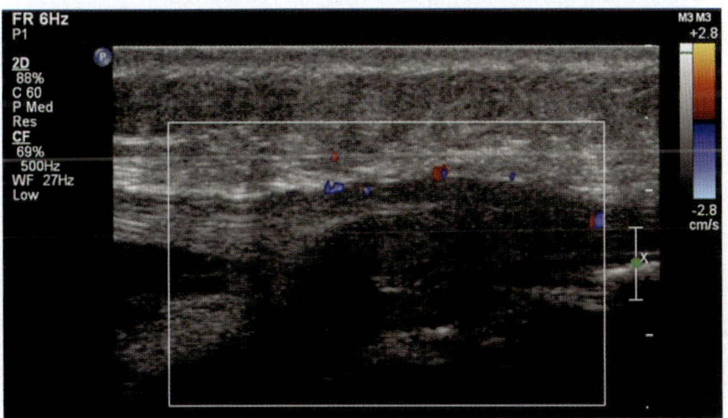

Figure 13.6. Ultrasound of the distal insertion of the patellar tendon shows thickening, apophyseal irregularity, and neovascularization in the adjacent tissues, typical of Osgood–Schlatter disease.

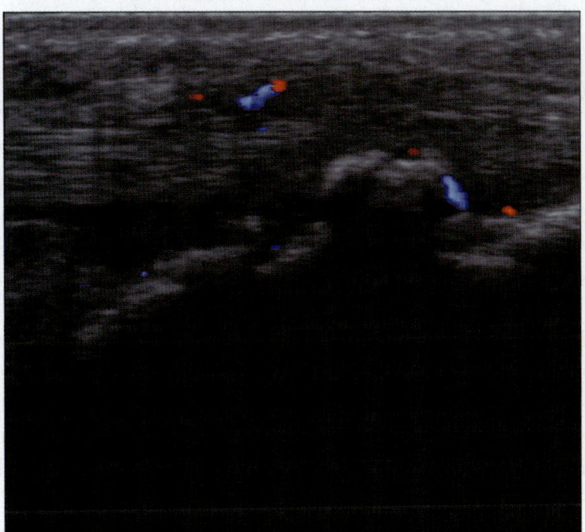

Figure 13.7. A second case of Osgood–Schlatter disease with more abundant irregular bone formation at the tibial insertion. This should not be mistaken for a bone-forming neoplasm.

Tip:
- Apophyseal avulsion may be disabling in the long term, and early treatment is important.
- Ultrasound is sensitive to avulsion injuries and has advantages over MR.

FRACTURES IN CHILDREN

Fractures in children may be detected by using ultrasound. It is a useful screening test in cases of localized limb pain. Irregularity of the cortex, defects in the bone surface, and periosteal elevation may all be observed.[31–33] Ultrasound should not be used as a substitute for conventional radiographs, and the combination of the two is often particularly sensitive for the diagnosis of occult injuries, including both acute and stress fractures (**Fig. 13.8**). In cases of suspected non-accidental injury,

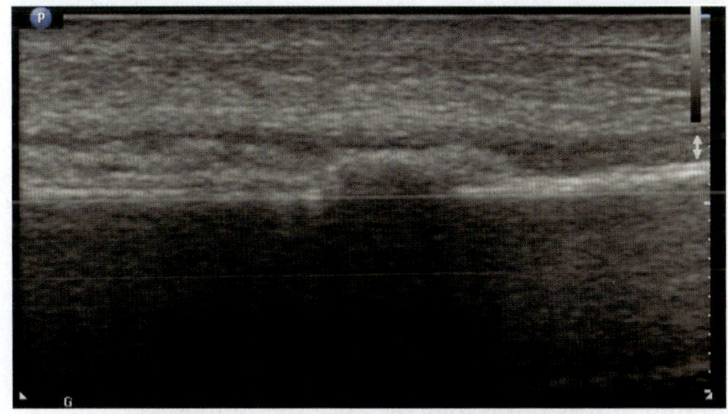

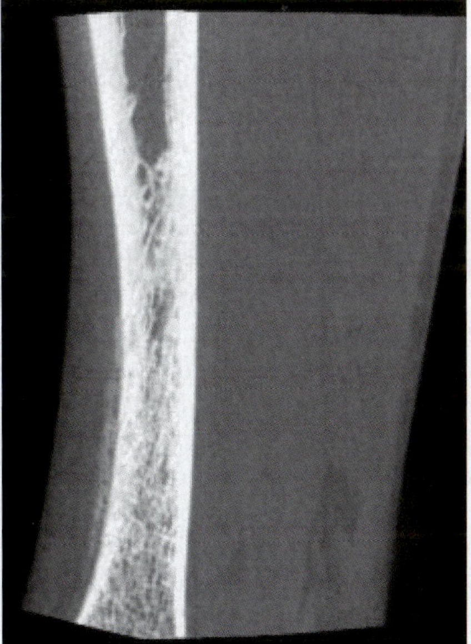

Figure 13.8. **A:** Ultrasound examination of a 12-year-old male with anterior shin pain showing periosteal reaction. **B:** Low-dose cone beam computed tomography of the tibia showing established periosteal reaction. **C:** Magnetic resonance using a FSTIR sequence demonstrates an area of bone edema deep to the periosteal reaction seen in Figures 13.8A and 13.8B confirming the diagnosis of a stress fracture.

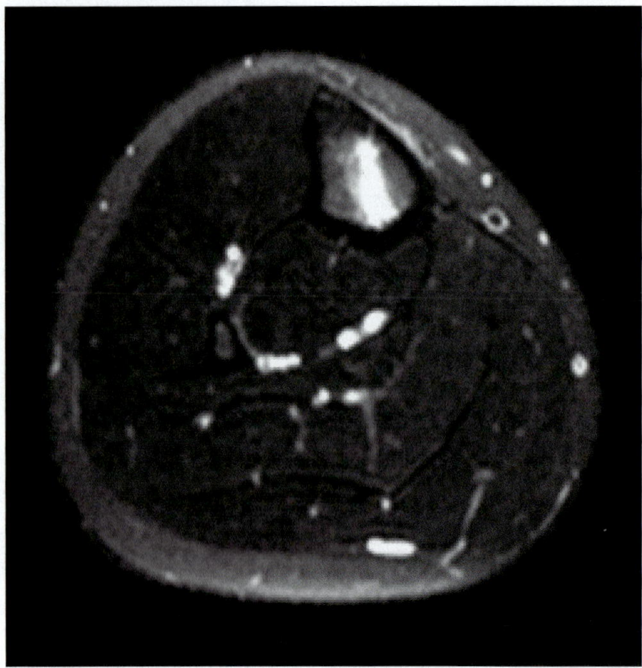

Figure 13.8. (*Continued*)

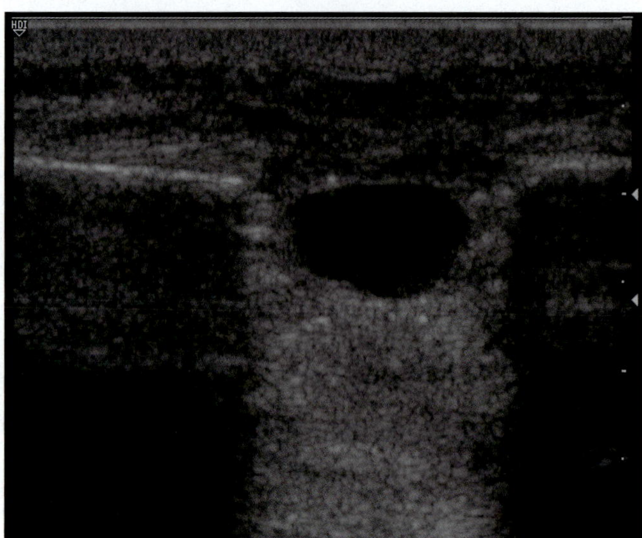

Figure 13.9. Ultrasound examination following a leg-lengthening procedure shows a cyst forming in the defect. This indicates too rapid a distraction and will inhibit healing. Aspiration of the cyst using ultrasound guidance may be considered.

particular care should be taken in observing the metaphyses as metaphyseal corner fractures are equally visible using ultrasound and conventional radiographs. Ultrasound should not be regarded as the primary imaging method for bone injuries, including suspected non-accidental injury, but it may be a useful adjunct.

> **Tip:**
> - Ultrasound will show cortical defects due to fracture.

LIMB LENGTHENING PROCEDURES

Limb lengthening procedures are undertaken in patients who have short limbs due to congenital disorders or post-traumatic premature epiphyseal fusion. The bone is osteotomized, and external frames are applied. Lengthening is undertaken by mechanically distracting the fragments of bone. For a large bone defect, a segment of bone may be dragged across the gap. The difficulty is to distract or move the bone sufficiently fast to prevent early healing and premature fusion whilst sufficiently slowly to prevent breakdown of the tissues and hemorrhagic cyst formation. Conventional radiographs only show bone formation late in the process, and the osteotomy may become "stuck" long before the bone formation is apparent. Cyst formation is not visible using conventional radiographs, but ultrasound detects early cyst formation as an echo-free cavity in the osteotomy defect **(Fig. 13.9)**. Ultrasound-guided aspiration of the cyst may accelerate new bone formation in the distraction gap. Ultrasound also

demonstrates premature ossification as reflective material bridging the defect.[34] Ultrasound monitoring is useful and many surgeons use ultrasound to judge the rate of distraction. Patients often become preoccupied by the external fixator. The area of distraction may be tender. Our experience is that it is best to ask patients to place the ultrasound probe over the defect. They know which areas are painful and become rather better at performing the ultrasound examination than the professionals.

> **Tip:**
> - Ultrasound detects cyst formation that indicates a too rapid distraction in limb lengthening procedures.
> - Ultrasound-guided aspiration may be used to treat cysts.

ACUTE ARTHROPATHIES

Acute arthropathies in children include septic arthritis (see above) and juvenile arthropathy. Juvenile arthropathy typically affects large joints initially but may extend to smaller joints. Ultrasound is an effective way of showing a joint effusion, synovial thickening, or neovascularity, and assessing the extent and pattern of involvement[35–37] **(Fig. 13.10)**. A screening examination of multiple joints provides useful information for the rheumatologist in cases of juvenile arthropathy. The detection of active synovitis provides critical information that may determine whether potent disease-modifying drugs are to be used.

Doppler signal in the synovium of a joint should be low. If there is doubt, comparison scan can be made with the pulp of the examiner's finger. Blood flow in the synovium should be less than that in the normal pulp of the finger.

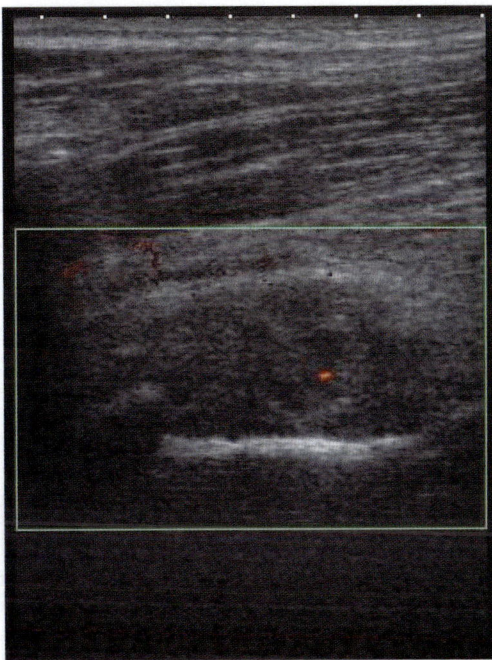

Figure 13.10. Thickened synovium in the hip in a child with an inflammatory arthropathy shows some neovascularization. There may be little clear fluid and a negative joint aspiration is common.

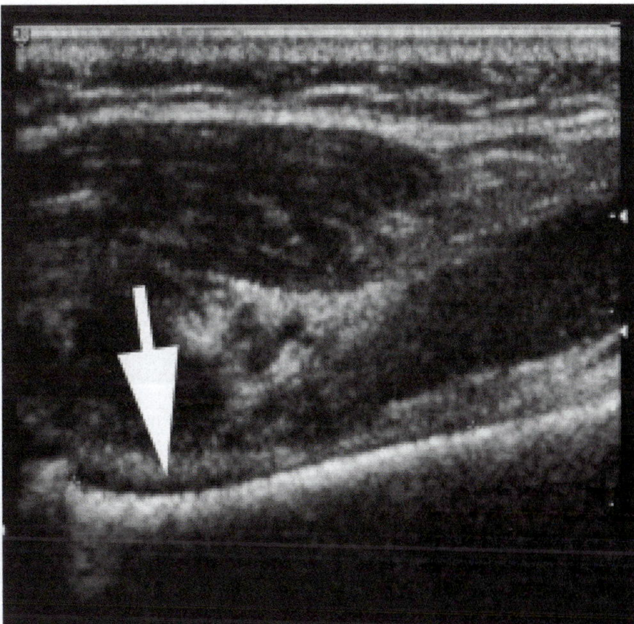

Figure 13.11. Ultrasound demonstrates a subperiosteal collection seen as a black line parallel to bone (*arrow*) in the proximal femur of a child with acute osteomyelitis.

Tip:
- Ultrasound is an effective screening test and can be used to monitor progress in juvenile arthropathy.

OSTEOMYELITIS

Osteomyelitis is uncommon but potentially serious. It is typically due to hematogenous spread. Patients present with pain, disability, restricted movement, and in the early stages may not be febrile or have elevated inflammatory markers.

Conventional radiographs in the early stages are usually normal but later show periosteal elevation, lysis, bone destruction, and eventually sclerosis. When radiographs are normal, ultrasound examination is particularly useful in detecting early periosteal elevation by a small amount of hypoechoic fluid[17] at the site of maximum tenderness. Comparison with the opposite confirms that the appearance is abnormal. In cases of doubt, MR examination may be needed but often requires sedation or a general anesthetic.

A negative ultrasound examination does not exclude osteomyelitis, and if clinical suspicion persists MR is mandatory.

Ultrasound is particularly helpful in determining the extent of disease in cases where osteomyelitis is associated with septic arthritis.[38] In particular, soft tissue infection with abscess formation is easily detected using ultrasound[39] **(Fig. 13.11).** However, MRI is the preferred method of defining the extent of non-cavitating soft tissue infection, especially when surgery is under consideration.

Tip:
- Whilst ultrasound may detect periosteal reaction, MR is the most sensitive investigation for osteomyelitis.

SKELETAL MASSES IN CHILDREN

The management of mass lesions in children is similar to that in adults. Ultrasound is an effective screening test. The nature of the mass should be determined as echogenic (solid) or echo free (fluid).

Ganglia occur in children as commonly as adults and are benign. A ganglion should contain free fluid that is compressible and does not contain particulate matter. It should have a neck or isthmus extending to the tendon or joint where the ganglion originates. If typical findings are identified, a definitive diagnosis of a ganglion can be made without recourse to further imaging. Care should be taken not to mistake solid tumors that are homogeneous in texture and have low reflectivity for cysts. This is a particular problem with neural tumors and myxoid chondrosarcoma. Comparison with known areas of fluid (vessels or the bladder) should help to avoid this pitfall.[40]

Foreign body reaction may produce a soft tissue mass. In smaller children, there is often no history of trauma.

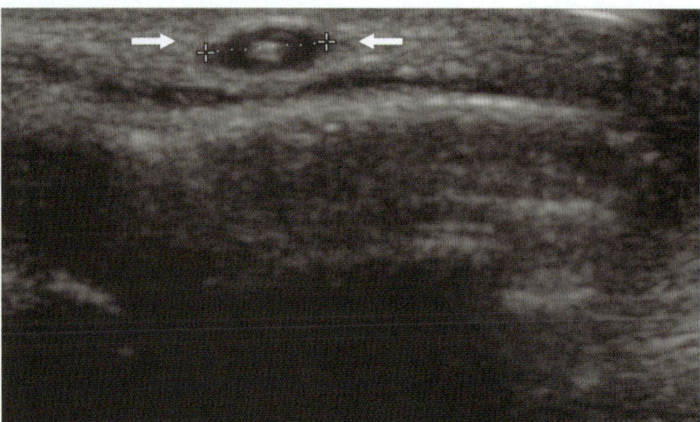

Figure 13.12.   Ultrasound examination of a foreign body next to the elbow. The echogenic lesion is surrounded by a halo of low echogenicity (*calipers and arrows*) that is part of the granulation tissue reaction. The reactive changes take a few weeks to develop and may be more obvious than the small subcutaneous piece of implanted material.

The foreign body typically produces a highly echogenic focus with distal acoustic shadowing (**Figs. 13.12 and 13.13**). There may be a halo of hypoechoic granulation tissue, but this normally takes several days to develop, and it may be worth repeating the examination after an interval of several days if the initial examination is negative. An alternative cause of an echogenic mass is calcification or ossification in myositis ossificans. Conventional radiographs may be normal in the early stages of myositis ossificans (**Fig. 13.14**), while ultrasound shows characteristic echogenic foci at the periphery of the mass several weeks before radiographic changes occur.

If there is doubt, a solid component, or particulate matter, further investigation is indicated, in the first instance by MR, although the definitive diagnosis is usually only achieved by biopsy or excision. A solid soft tissue

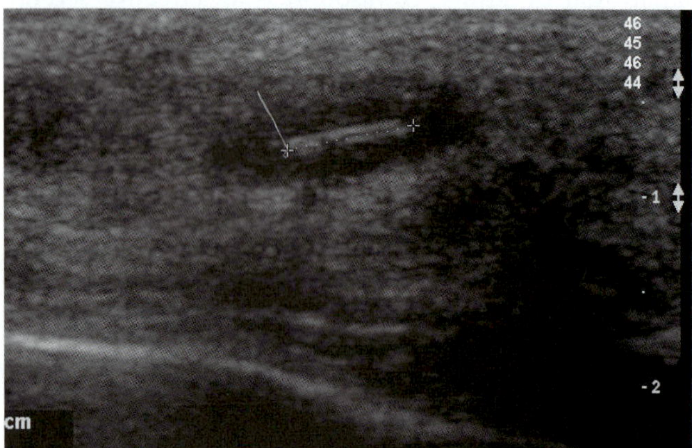

Figure 13.13.   A splinter (calipers) in the finger of a 13-year-old is clearly identified and can be marked using ultrasound guidance to aid the surgeon who removes the piece of wood.

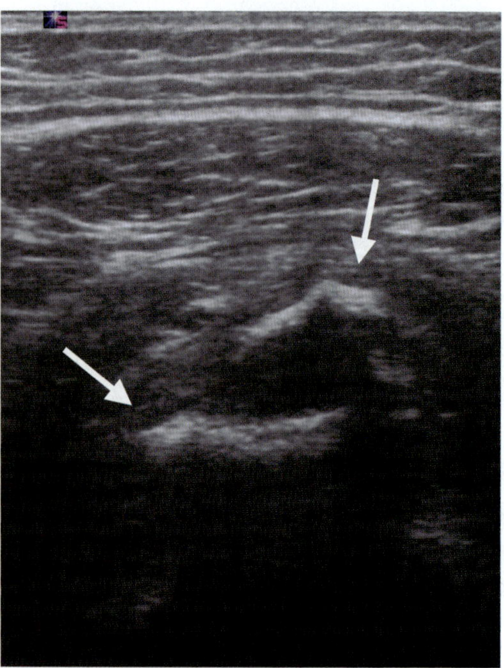

Figure 13.14.   When ossification (*arrows*) occurs in areas of previous trauma, layers of echogenic reflective material are seen. These changes occur well before conventional radiographs show a lesion and are much more obvious than the signs seen using MRI. Progressive ossification may occur if immediate changes in management are not made; hence this is an important sign to detect. Oral indomethacin and reduced activity may be considered.

mass should be considered potentially malignant and the patient referred urgently to a specialist soft tissue tumor center. Biopsy should only be performed in the specialist tumor center after adequate staging with MRI and discussion with the surgical oncologist who will provide definitive surgery to avoid inappropriate biopsy that might compromise future surgery. In children, primary soft tissue tumors are more common than secondary deposits, although conditions such as rhabdomyosarcoma or nephroblastoma may produce secondary lesions in soft tissues.

Bone tumors that extend into soft tissues may present as soft tissue lumps.[40,41] Radiographs are invaluable, but ultrasound also demonstrates the bony nature of the lesion and its soft tissue extension. An osteochondroma is a benign exostosis with a cartilage cap of low echogenicity that sits on the apex of the lesion (**Figs. 13.15A and 13.15B**). A cartilage cap >1 cm in thickness may indicate malignant transformation, and excision biopsy is indicated.

Normal variants including accessory ossicles and bifid ribs may mimic soft tissue masses, and comparison with conventional radiographs is important. Accessory muscles have normal radiographs, but ultrasound is diagnostic. The clue is the presence of normal contracting muscle fibers on dynamic examination.

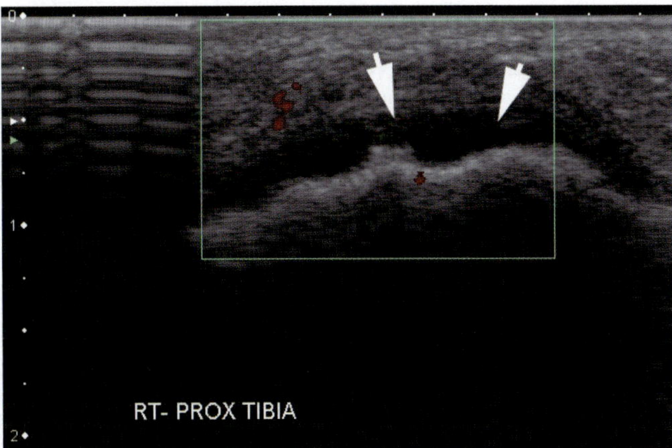

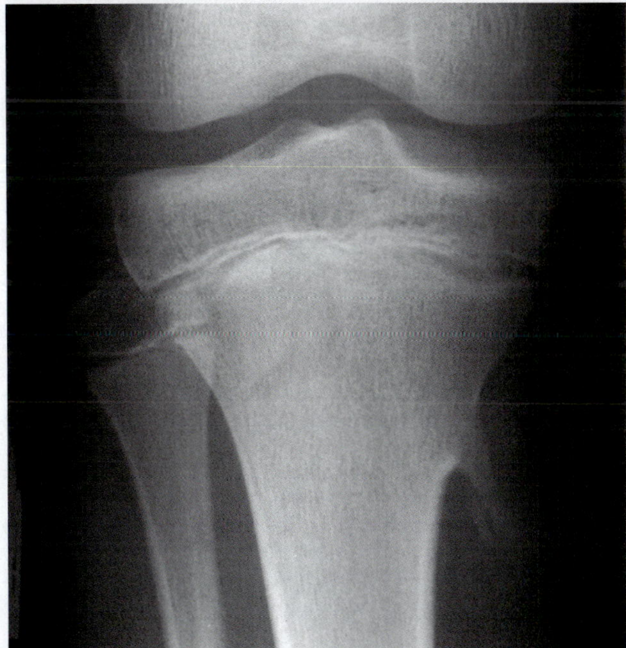

Figure 13.15. **A:** The cartilage cap of the osteochondroma as seen in Figure 13.15B is of low echogenicity (*arrows*). Ultrasound examination allows measurement, and in this case it is only a few millimeters thick and clearly benign. **B:** Although the conventional radiograph shows the lesion well, it does not define the cartilage cap seen using ultrasound.

Tip:
- Ultrasound detects soft tissue extension of bone tumors.
- Ultrasound may be used to measure cartilage caps in osteochondromas.

HEREDITARY NEUROPATHIES AND MUSCLE DISORDERS

Ultrasound examination is useful in the assessment of muscle groups for signs of atrophy, denervation, and edema. Patients with muscular dystrophies may have a typical pattern in a distribution related to the nature of the myopathy. Edema, neovascularity, and swelling are early signs. Muscle groups can be examined with ultrasound and comparisons made with adjacent areas. Arguably MRI is more specific as the size can be compared on adjacent images more easily than using ultrasound. However, in children ultrasound may be the more practical examination. Elastography allows assessment of muscle softness or stiffness, and in cases of myopathy this changes before MR appearances alter.[42]

Neuropathies may lead to denervation although the nerves themselves are rarely identifiably abnormal. Ultrasound is an effective way of examining nerves, but the neuropathy usually leads to a dysfunction of nerve rather than a morphological change, and the assessment of the muscle remains the cornerstone of diagnosis.

Tip:
- Ultrasound (with elastography) has potential for defining the extent of muscle disease.

REFERENCES

1. Huff L, Hamlin A, Wolski D, et al. Atraumatic care: EMLA cream and application of heat to facilitate peripheral venous cannulation in children. *Issues Compr Pediatr Nurs.* 2009;32(2):65–76.
2. Gursoy A, Ertugrul DT, Sahin M, et al. The analgesic efficacy of lidocaine/prilocaine (EMLA) cream during fine-needle aspiration biopsy of thyroid nodules. *Clin Endocrinol (Oxf).* 2007;66(5):691–694.
3. Zieger M, Schul RD. Ultrasonography of the infant hip. Part III: clinical application. *Pediatr Radiol.* 1987;17(3):226–232.
4. Graf R. Fundamentals of sonographic diagnosis of infant hip dysplasia. *J Pediatr Orthop.* 1984;4(6):735–740.
5. Graf R. Profile of radiologic-orthopedic requirements in pediatric hip dysplasia, coxitis and epiphyseolysis capitis femoris [in German]. *Radiologe.* 2002;42(6):467–473.
6. Dias JJ, Thomas IH, Lamont AC, et al. The reliability of ultrasonographic assessment of neonatal hips. *J Bone Joint Surg Br.* 1993;75(3):479–482.
7. Langer R. Ultrasonic investigation of the hip in newborns in the diagnosis of congenital hip dislocation: classification and results of a screening program. *Skeletal Radiol.* 1987;16(4):275–279.
8. Terjesen T. Ultrasound as the primary imaging method in the diagnosis of hip dysplasia in children aged <2 years. *J Pediatr Orthop B.* 1996;5(2):123–128.
9. Engesaeter LB, Wilson DJ, Nag D, et al. Ultrasound and congenital dislocation of the hip. The importance of dynamic assessment. *J Bone Joint Surg Br.* 1990;72(2):197–201.
10. Fink AM, Berman L, Edwards D, et al. The irritable hip: immediate ultrasound guided aspiration and prevention of hospital admission. *Arch Dis Child.* 1995;72(2):110–113.
11. Berman L, Fink AM, Wilson D, et al. Technical note: identifying and aspirating hip effusions. *Br J Radiol.* 1995;68(807):306–310.
12. Klauser AS, Tagliafico A, Allen GM, et al. Clinical indications for musculoskeletal ultrasound: a Delphi-based consensus paper of the European Society of Musculoskeletal Radiology. *Eur Radiol.* 2012;22(5):1140–1148.
13. Wilson, DJ, Green, DJ, MacLarnon, JC. Arthrosonography of the painful hip. *Clin Radiol.* 1984;35(1):17–19.

14. Eich GF, Superti-Furga A, Umbricht FS, et al. The painful hip: evaluation of criteria for clinical decision-making. *Eur J Pediatr.* 1999;158(11):923–928.

15. Strouse PJ, DiPietro MA, Adler RS. Pediatric hip effusions: evaluation with power Doppler sonography. *Radiology.* 1998; 206(3):731–735.

16. Rutz E, Brunner R. Septic arthritis of the hip—current concepts. *Hip Int.* 2009;19(suppl 6):9–12.

17. Collado P, Naredo E, Calvo C, et al. Role of power Doppler sonography in early diagnosis of osteomyelitis in children. *J Clin Ultrasound.* 2008;36(4):251–253.

18. Perry DC, Green DJ, Bruce CE, et al. Abnormalities of vascular structure and function in children with Perthes disease. *Pediatrics.* 2012;130(1):E126–E131.

19. Doria AS, Guarniero R, Molnar LJ, et al. Three-dimensional (3D) contrast-enhanced power Doppler imaging in Legg-Calvé-Perthes disease. *Pediatr Radiol.* 2000;30(12):871–874.

20. Mattace Raso M, Carbone M, Rossi E, et al. Meyer's femoral dysplasia. Description of a case [in Italian]. *Radiol Med.* 2000;99(1–2):89–90.

21. Stücker MH, Buthmann J, Meiss AL. Evaluation of hip containment in legg-calvé-perthes disease: a comparison of ultrasound and magnetic resonance imaging. *Ultraschall Med.* 2005;26(5):406–410.

22. Dimeglio A, Canavese F. Imaging in legg-calvé-perthes disease. *Orthop Clin North Am.* 2011;42(3):297–302.

23. Martinoli C, Garello I, Marchetti A, et al. Hip ultrasound. *Eur J Radiol.* 2012;81(12):3824–3831.

24. Futami T, Suzuki S, Seto Y, et al. Sequential magnetic resonance imaging in slipped capital femoral epiphysis: assessment of preslip in the contralateral hip. *J Pediatr Orthop B.* 2001;10(4):298–303.

25. Wagner UA, Diedrich V, Schmitt O. Determination of skeletal maturity by ultrasound: a preliminary report. *Skeletal Radiol.* 1995;24(6):417–420.

26. Schmidt S, Schmeling A, Zwiesigk P, et al. Sonographic evaluation of apophyseal ossification of the iliac crest in forensic age diagnostics in living individuals. *Int J Legal Med.* 2011; 125(2):271–276.

27. Lazović D, Wegner U, Peters G, et al. Ultrasound for diagnosis of apophyseal injuries. *Knee Surg Sports Traumatol Arthrosc.* 1996;3(4):234–237.

28. Mahlfeld K, Kayser R, Franke J, et al. Ultrasonography of the Osgood-Schlatter disease [in German]. *Ultraschall Med.* 2001;22(4):182–185.

29. Grechenig W, Mayr JM, Peicha G, et al. Sonoanatomy of the Achilles tendon insertion in children. *J Clin Ultrasound.* 2004;32(7):338–343.

30. Ducher G, Cook J, Spurrier D, et al. Ultrasound imaging of the patellar tendon attachment to the tibia during puberty: a 12-month follow-up in tennis players. *Scand J Med Sci Sports.* 2010;20(1):E35–E40.

31. Williamson D, Watura R, Cobby M. Ultrasound imaging of forearm fractures in children: a viable alternative? *J Accid Emerg Med.* 2000;17(1):22–24.

32. Moritz JD, Hoffmann B, Meuser SH, et al. Is ultrasound equal to X-ray in pediatric fracture diagnosis? [in German] *Rofo.* 2010;182(8):706–714.

33. Hübner U, Schlicht W, Outzen S, et al. Ultrasound in the diagnosis of fractures in children. *J Bone Joint Surg Br.* 2000;82(8): 1170–1173.

34. Maffulli N, Hughes T, Fixsen JA. Ultrasonographic monitoring of limb lengthening. *J Bone Joint Surg Br.* 1992;74(1): 130–132.

35. Filippou G, Cantarini L, Bertoldi I, et al. Ultrasonography vs. clinical examination in children with suspected arthritis. Does it make sense to use poliarticular ultrasonographic screening? *Clin Exp Rheumatol.* 2011;29(2):345–350.

36. Spannow AH, Stenboeg E, Pfeiffer-Jensen M, et al. Ultrasound and MRI measurements of joint cartilage in healthy children: a validation study. *Ultraschall Med.* 2011;32(suppl 1): 110–116.

37. Spârchez M, Fodor D, Miu N. The role of power Doppler ultrasonography in comparison with biological markers in the evaluation of disease activity in juvenile idiopathic arthritis. *Med Ultrason.* 2010;12(2):97–103.

38. Azam Q, Ahmad I, Abbas M, et al. Ultrasound and colour Doppler sonography in acute osteomyelitis in children. *Acta Orthop Belg.* 2005;71(5):590–596.

39. Chau CL, Griffith JF. Musculoskeletal infections: ultrasound appearances. *Clin Radiol.* 2005;60(2):149–159.

40. Hughes DG, Wilson DJ. Ultrasound appearances of peripheral nerve tumours. *Br J Radiol.* 1986;59(706):1041–1043.

41. Saifuddin A, Burnett SJ, Mitchell R. Pictorial review: ultrasonography of primary bone tumours. *Clin Radiol.* 1998;53(4): 239–246.

42. Drakonaki EE, Allen GM. Magnetic resonance imaging, ultrasound, and real-time ultrasound elastography of the thigh muscles in congenital muscle dystrophy. *Skeletal Radiol.* 2010;39(4):391–396.

Ultrasound-Guided Interventions

Ronald S. Adler

INTRODUCTION

The real-time nature of ultrasound makes it ideally suited to providing guidance for a variety of musculoskeletal interventions.[1–9] Continuous observation of the needle ensures accurate needle placement and appropriate distribution of the injected and/or aspirated material. Needles can be positioned close to neurovascular bundles without damaging nerves or vessels. The potential deleterious effects of not attaining proper needle placement during corticosteroid administration are well documented[10–17] and are discussed later.

The current generation of high-frequency small parts transducers allows excellent depiction of soft tissue details and articular surfaces, particularly in the hand, wrist, foot, and ankle,[18] facilitating exact needle insertion into non-distended structures, such as joints, tendon sheaths, or bursae. Injected fluid produces a contrast effect, which improves delineation of adjacent structures (e.g., labral morphology) and shows the distribution of the injected material.[19,20] The advent of newer technology that permits image registration to other modalities, such as computed tomography or magnetic resonance imaging (MRI), is expected to enhance further the role of ultrasound in performing a broad variety of interventions.[21] Ultrasound guidance to target sites of maximal tendon and/or muscle pathology has been used to administer growth factors using platelet-rich plasma (PRP) or autologous blood.[22–26] A brief discussion of these newer applications will be included. Ultrasound guidance does not involve ionizing radiation, and this is an advantage in the pediatric population and during pregnancy.

Following a discussion of sonographic technique, ultrasound-guided interventions in the musculoskeletal system will be reviewed with particular attention to injections of joints, tendon sheaths, bursae, and ganglion cysts, with an emphasis on the most commonly requested procedures. Newer applications will also be discussed, such as perineural injections/ablations and intratendinous therapy. Finally, the utility of ultrasound guidance in performing soft tissue biopsies will be discussed.

ULTRASOUND-GUIDED THERAPEUTIC INJECTIONS/ASPIRATIONS

The most common clinical indication for ultrasound-guided injections generally relates to pain that has failed to respond to conservative measures, regardless of the anatomic site. The pain may be the result of a chronic repetitive injury in the work environment, a sports-related injury, or injury from an underlying inflammatory disorder, such as rheumatoid arthritis. This chapter presents illustrative examples of the most relevant studies, without dwelling on the specific clinical entities.

TECHNICAL CONSIDERATIONS

Diagnostic examinations and subsequent therapeutic interventions are often performed using either linear or curved phased array transducers, depending on depth and local geometry. Needle selection is based on specific anatomic conditions (i.e., depth and size of the region of interest). I employ a freehand technique in which the basic principle is to ensure that the needle is visualized as a specular reflector.[7–8] This relies on orienting the needle to be perpendicular (or nearly so) to the insonating beam **(Fig. 14.1)**. The needle then becomes a specular reflector, often having a strong ringdown artifact. Needle guides are available and may be of value, but I have found that a freehand technique allows greater flexibility in adjusting needle position. Needle visualization can be enhanced by injecting a small amount of anesthetic and observing the consequent moving echoes in either grayscale or color flow imaging.[1]

Patient positioning to ensure comfort and optimal visualization of the anatomy should first be assessed. Tendons are anisotropic[27]; therefore, the transducer should be oriented to maximize tendon echogenicity to avoid misinterpretation as tendinopathy, complex fluid, or synovium. An offset may be required at the skin entry point of the needle relative to the transducer

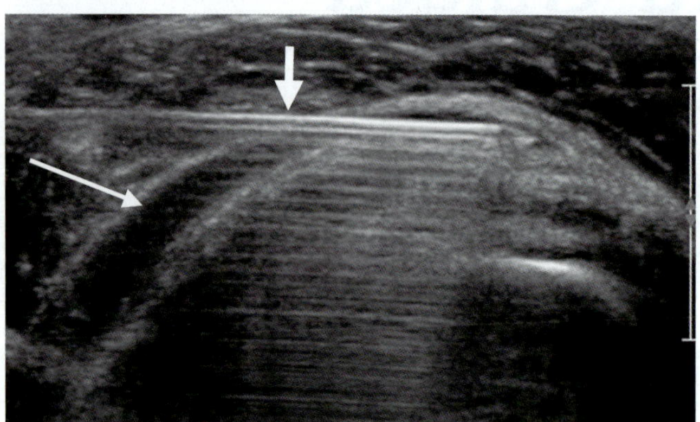

Figure 14.1.   Needle as a specular reflector. The needle (*short arrow*) has been placed in the subdeltoid bursa (*long arrow*) which is distended following an injection of long-acting steroid and local anesthetic. Note the reverberation artefact, thin echogenic lines parallel to the needle, that is typical of metallic artifact.

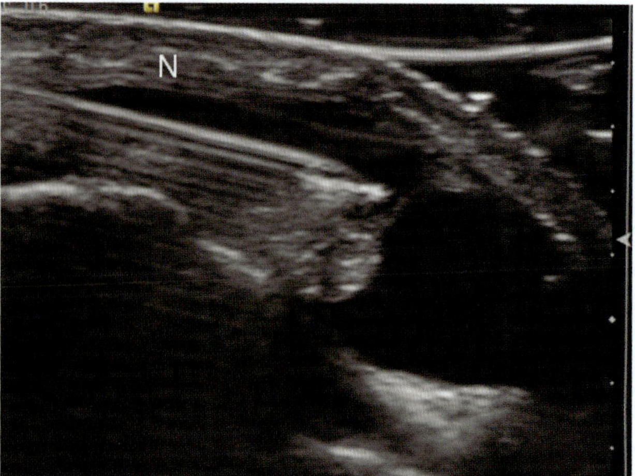

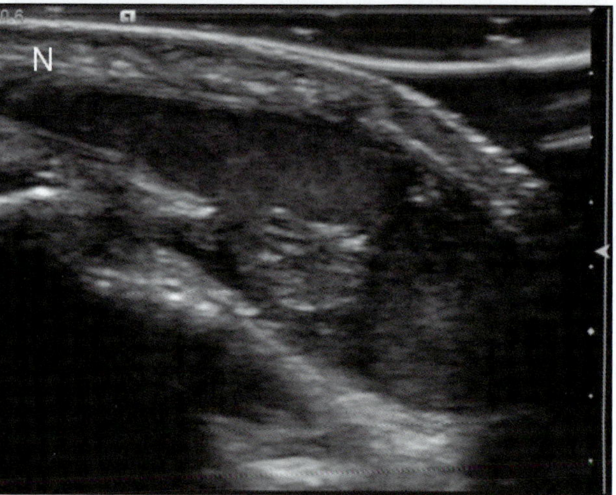

Figure 14.2.   Contrast effect: Tenosynovitis of extensor hallucis longus tendon sheath in the dorsum of the foot. **A:** Shows a 22G needle in the fluid-distended tendon sheath prior to aspiration. The needle is positioned perpendicular to the long axis of the tendon (short-axis approach). **B:** Following aspiration, the tendon sheath was injected with a therapeutic mixture consisting of triamcinolone and local anesthetic. Notice the low-level echoes produced by therapeutic mixture during the injection as a result of the differences in acoustic impedance within the injected suspension. N, needle.

to provide appropriate needle orientation. Deep structures such as deep flexor tendons of the hip are often better imaged using a curved or sector transducer, operating at center frequencies of approximately 3.5 to 7.5 MHz. Superficial, linearly oriented structures, such as tendons in the wrist or ankle, are best approached using a linear array transducer with higher center frequencies (>10 MHz). Transducers with a small footprint ("hockey stick") are particularly well suited to superficial injections. These factors should be assessed prior to skin preparation.

The immiscible nature of the steroid–anesthetic mixture may produce temporary contrast effect **(Fig. 14.2).** In vitro experiments suggest that this property is due to alterations in acoustic impedance by the scattering material formed by the suspension of steroid in an aqueous background, resulting in an approximate increase in echo intensity of 20 dB.[20] This increases the conspicuity of the delivered agent during real time and helps to define the distribution of the delivered agent during the injection.

Tip:
- Choose transducer geometry and entry site to visualize the needle as a specular reflector.
- Orient transducer to maximize tendon echogenicity (anisotropy).
- Injected corticosteroid/anesthetic suspension often displays a contrast effect, which can help localize injected mixture.

INJECTION TECHNIQUE

Sterile technique is essential. The skin is cleaned with an iodine or alcohol-based solution and may be covered with a sterile drape **(Fig. 14.3)**. The transducer is immersed in iodine-based solution and surrounded by a sterile drape or placed into a sterile probe cover. A drape can also be placed over portions of the ultrasound unit, although many radiologists keep drapes to a minimum or avoid them completely. One percent lidocaine is used for local anesthesia. Once the needle is in position, the procedure is undertaken while imaging in real time. Depending on anatomic location and personal preference, a 1.5″ blue (25G), brown (22G), or green (21G) needle, or a 22G spinal needle with a stylet is used to administer the anesthetic/corticosteroid mixture, generally consisting of long-acting anesthetic and one of the standard injectable corticosteroid derivatives. Several steroid solutions with different properties regarding duration in the soft tissues and potential untoward effects are available (see below).

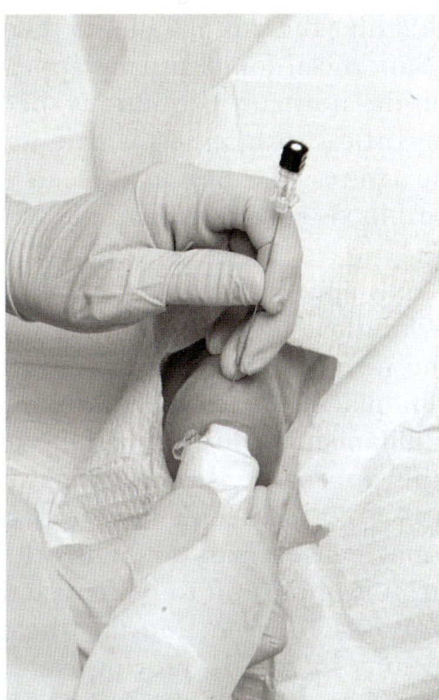

Figure 14.3.   Sterile setup during injection of the plantar fascia. The transducer is cleaned and draped as is the area of interest. The drape should be positioned to allow adequate room for placement of the transducer on the skin surface and overlying the target anatomy.

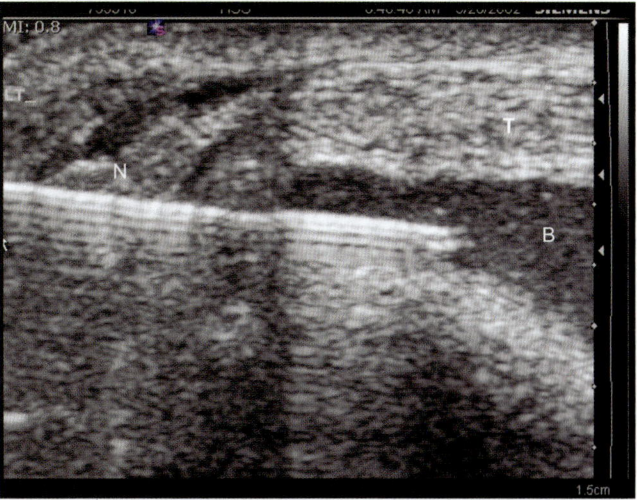

Figure 14.5.   Short-axis approach. Patient with achillodynia, during injection of the retrocalcaneal bursa. The Achilles tendon (*T*) is seen in short axis. A 25G needle (*N*) is positioned perpendicular to the Achilles tendon into the distended retrocalcaneal bursa (short-axis approach). The distended bursa (*B*) contains numerous low-level echoes due to the inherent contrast effect of the therapeutic mixture.

It is convenient to distinguish two separate approaches to performing injections, long axis and short axis, which relate to needle orientation relative to the structure to be injected. The long-axis approach refers to needle placement in the plane parallel to the structure of interest (**Fig. 14.4**). Examples include longitudinal imaging of the hip to display a hip effusion and employing this as the plane in which to direct the needle for ultrasound-guided aspiration. The short-axis approach refers to needle entry in the plane perpendicular to the long axis of a structure (**Fig. 14.5**). Examples include injecting the

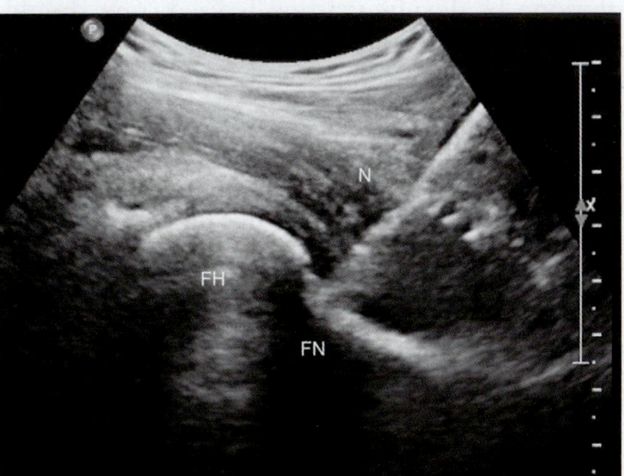

Figure 14.4.   Long-axis approach: Patient with labral tear and groin pain referred for a hip injection. **A:** Therapeutic injection of the hip is typically performed using a long-axis technique. The needle (*N*) is advanced to the femoral head–neck junction. A small injection of anesthetic may be used to confirm position. FH, femoral head; FN, femoral neck.

retrocalcaneal bursa using a lateral approach. The short-axis approach works well when performing injections/aspirations in small joints and tendon sheaths of the hand and foot. The long-axis approach appears better suited to deep joint injections, such as the hip or shoulder. It is important to recognize, however, that such approaches serve merely as guidelines and that there is no unique method that necessarily applies to any specific injection.

INJECTION MATERIALS

Most injections use long-acting corticosteroid in combination with local anesthetic in relatively small volumes. A detailed review of these agents is beyond the scope of the current chapter. Injectable steroids usually come in crystalline form, associated with a slower rate of absorption, or a soluble form, characterized by rapid absorption.[27–30] Examples of the former are triamcinolone and methylprednisolone, whereas commonly used examples of the latter are betamethasone and dexamethasone. Because of their rapid resorption, soluble preparations may be preferable in superficial structures where subcutaneous fat atrophy and/or skin depigmentation are potential complications. In the case of the crystalline agents, a reactive inflammatory response or flushing response may occur, and patients should be warned that they may experience severe pain in the 2 to 3 days following the injection. The soluble forms are not typically associated with these complications, but crystalline forms are usually preferred because they are long-acting. A painful steroid "flare" is less likely with triamcinolone than methylprednisolone, but skin depigmentation and fat atrophy are more likely with triamcinolone. Patients with diabetes should be cautioned that they may develop transient hyperglycemia that can last for 5 to10 days.

The most significant complications associated with injectable steroid use in the musculoskeletal system relate to chondrolysis (when used in weight-bearing joints), skin depigmentation, fat necrosis, and impaired healing response (when used in soft tissues). The latter has been associated with tendon, ligament, and plantar fascia rupture.[10–17] As the most commonly used mixtures contain insoluble particles, a systemic injection could theoretically result in an embolic phenomenon, and this has been implicated as a mechanism for neurological complications associated with transforaminal injections.[31] I have not encountered this as a complication when performing injections in the appendicular skeletal system.

The most commonly used anesthetics are lidocaine and bupivacaine (i.e., Marcaine).[17,31,32] They are both local injectable anesthetics, but differ in the onset and duration of action. Lidocaine has rapid onset (seconds) and short duration (1 to 2 hours). Bupivacaine becomes effective in 5 to 10 minutes and generally lasts 4 to 6 hours. Potential adverse reactions include neurotoxicity, cardiotoxicity, and allergic reactions,[30] but are rare when used in small doses under image guidance and avoiding intravascular injection. Recent studies also report that bupivacaine is associated with chondrolysis when used for intra-articular applications. This effect has only been seen during constant infusions at arthroscopy and in vitro. Chondrolysis is not likely to be an issue when used in the small volumes typically employed during injections in the musculoskeletal system, although 0.5% ropivacaine would provide a potentially safer alternative.

> **Tip:**
> - Patients should be warned that they may experience severe pain in the 2 to 3 days following the injection (flare response) with crystalline-based corticosteroid.
> - Patients with diabetes should be cautioned that they may develop a transient hyperglycemia that lasts 5 to 10 days following steroid injection.

INJECTION OF JOINTS

Injection techniques are also discussed in the appropriate anatomical chapters.

Small Joint Injections

A high-frequency linear transducer is used for hand, wrist, elbow, foot, and ankle injections.[5,6,33] A short-axis approach is often technically easier for small joints. The needle should enter the skin parallel to the plane of the joint space. Superficial joints usually appear as separations between the normally continuous specular echoes produced by cortical surfaces. As is true in other fluid-containing structures, the presence of an effusion is a helpful feature in visualizing the needle as it enters the joint.

The short-axis approach entails scanning across the joint and looking for the transition from one cortical surface to the next, marking the skin (with a surgical marker), then placing a needle into the joint using ultrasound guidance. When imaging the joint in long axis, using this approach, the needle is seen in cross section **(Fig. 14.6)**. If the needle does not appear within the joint, it may be necessary to "walk" the needle tip into the joint. It is important to recognize that the skin entry site acts as a fulcrum. Moving the needle hub proximally results in the tip moving caudally. Ideally, adjustments should require only minimal needle excursions. Needle position is confirmed by injecting a small amount of local anesthetic that should run away from the needle tip and distend the joint with fluid and echoes. If fluid pools around the needle tip, it is unlikely to be intra-articular. Small joints generally accommodate 0.5 to 1 mL; therefore it is important not to inject too much local anesthetic before the therapeutic mixture. It is convenient to employ a mixture of 1 mL (40 mg) of triamcinolone or methylprednisolone with 1 mL of long-acting anesthetic. Alternatively, the two are injected separately with a small volume of local anesthetic first to show that the needle is intra-articular, then the steroid. In this way the amount of injected corticosteroid is controlled. For small joints, 10 to 15 mg (0.5 to 0.75 mL) is usually adequate. For medium-sized joints (e.g., radiocapitellar joint), a larger volume (1 to 2 mL) of this mixture is often beneficial. When betamethasone or dexamethasone is used, one should be cognizant of dose equivalents. Betamethasone usually is distributed in multidose vials with concentrations of 6 mg/mL. Two milliliters of betamethasone has similar efficacy to 1 mL of triamcinolone or methylprednisolone. Dexamethasone is distributed in 1 mL vials (4 mg/mL), equivalent to 40 mg of either triamcinolone or methylprednisolone.

The short-axis approach works well in the metatarsophalangeal (MTP)/metacarpophalangeal and interphalangeal joints, midfoot, ankle, and elbow. Occasionally, a long-axis approach may be efficacious, as in the radiocarpal joint, lateral gutter of the ankle **(Fig. 14.7),** and dorsal midfoot when it is possible to insert the needle tip just deep to the joint capsule without having to incline the needle steeply. Ultrasound guidance helps to negotiate osteophytes and joint bodies. It allows identification of capsular outpouching, thereby affording a more convenient indirect approach into a joint than slipping a needle into a small joint space.

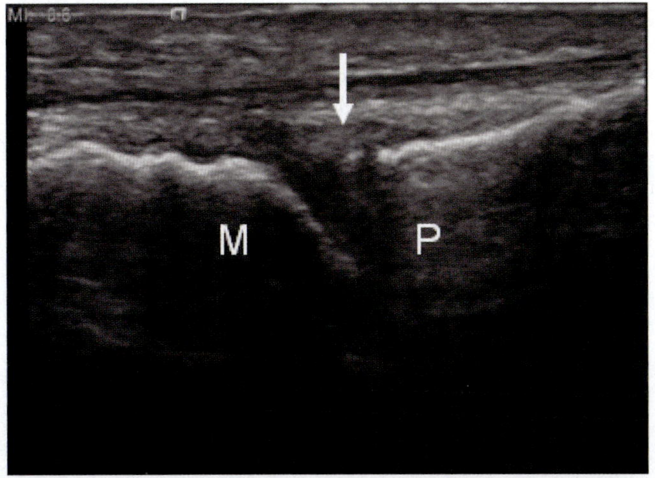

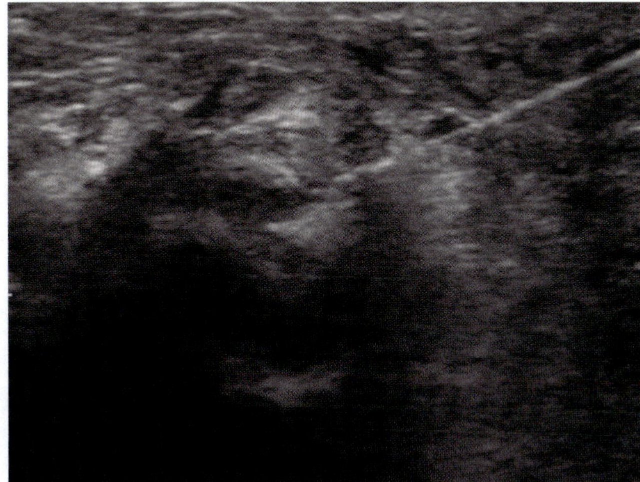

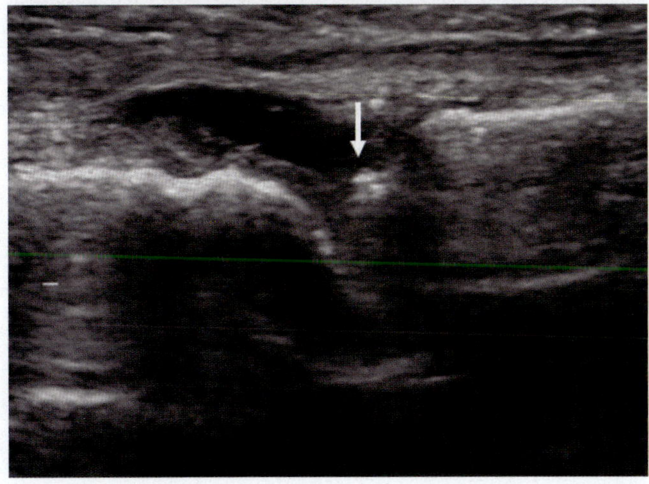

Figure 14.6.   Short-axis approach: Small joint injection. **A:** Image depicts the dorsal recess of the second MTP joint seen in long axis in a patient with metatarsalgia. A punctate echogenic focus with mild ring-down artifact (*arrow*) corresponds to a 25G 1.5″ needle seen in cross section. The metatarsal head (*M*) and proximal phalanx (*P*) are labeled. **B:** Rotating the transducer 90 degrees shows the needle in long axis in the plane of the joint. **C:** The image shows distention of the dorsal capsule during injection. The needle (*arrow*) is now more conspicuous due to the overlying intra-articular fluid.

Large Joint Injections

Shoulder

A long-axis approach and a 22G spinal needle are used when performing injections of large joints such as the shoulder or hip **(Fig. 14.8)**.[34,35] A greater volume is usually injected, typically 5 mL of the steroid/anesthetic mixture. In most cases the injectate contains 1 to 2 mL (40 to 80 mg) of triamcinolone or methylprednisolone. In the case of adhesive capsulitis, significantly larger volumes of local anesthetic (5 to 10 mL) may be added to provide additional joint distension (hydrodistention), which may promote lysis of focal adhesions. A posterior approach to the glenohumeral joint with the patient in a decubitus position, the shoulder to be injected upward, and the arm placed in cross adduction is generally used. An intermediate frequency linear or curved transducer suffices in the majority of cases. A linear transducer often results in better anatomic detail than curved arrays. The posterior recess of the glenohumeral joint is usually well seen with the patient in the decubitus position. The hypoechoic articular cartilage overlying the humeral head, echogenic posterior labrum, thin echogenic posterior capsule, and overlying infraspinatus muscle belly

are identified. I use a long-axis approach with the needle directed from superolateral toward the joint and deep to the echogenic joint capsule. Others prefer the opposite direction. A test injection with 1% lidocaine shows bright echoes filling the posterior recess or distributed along

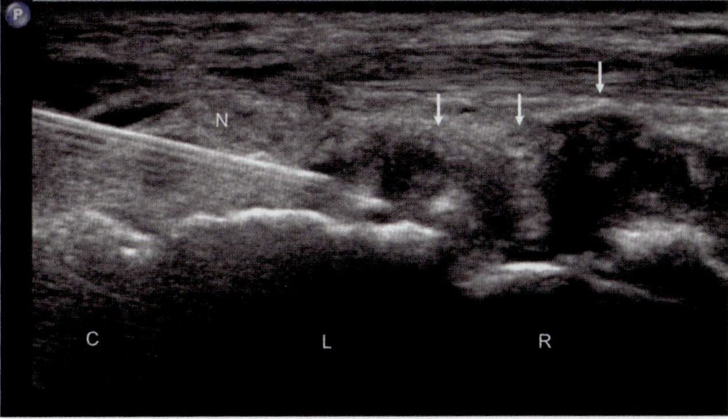

Figure 14.7.   Long-axis view of the dorsal aspect of the wrist in a patient with wrist pain and swelling and a history of pseudogout. Image shows distension of the dorsal compartment (*arrows*) by fluid and soft tissue. R, radius; L, lunate; C, capitate. With the wrist in mild palmar flexion, a 1.5″ 25G needle (*N*) is placed into the distended dorsal recess of the wrist using a long-axis approach for therapeutic injection.

the articular cartilage if the needle is intra-articular. Pooling of fluid at the needle tip indicates an extra-articular injection, and the needle should be repositioned.

Hip

The hip is also approached in long axis with the transducer placed over the proximal anterior thigh at the level of the joint **(Fig. 14.4)**, similar to the approach looking for an effusion. Ideally, the anterior capsule is imaged at the head–neck junction of the femur. In this approach, the scan plane is lateral to the neurovascular bundle. The needle is directed into the joint while maintaining its position in the scan plane of the transducer. A test injection of 1% lidocaine confirms the intra-articular needle position, and the therapeutic injection follows, using a similar mixture to the shoulder.

Fibrous Joints

Fibrous joints, such as the acromioclavicular joint, can be injected using ultrasound guidance **(Fig. 14.9)**.[34] A short-axis technique is employed similar to that in the foot. The transducer is placed sagittally on the clavicle

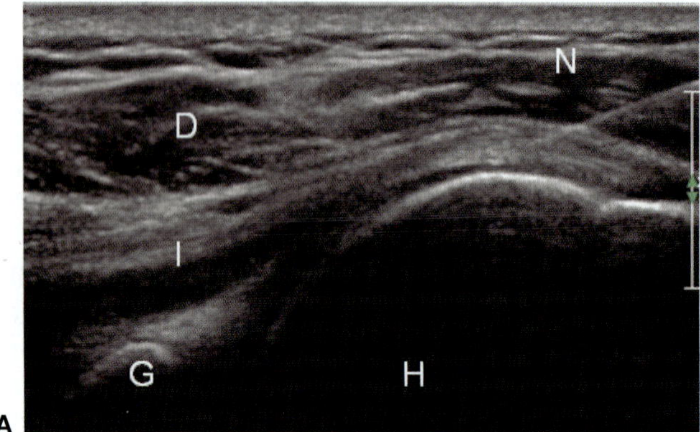

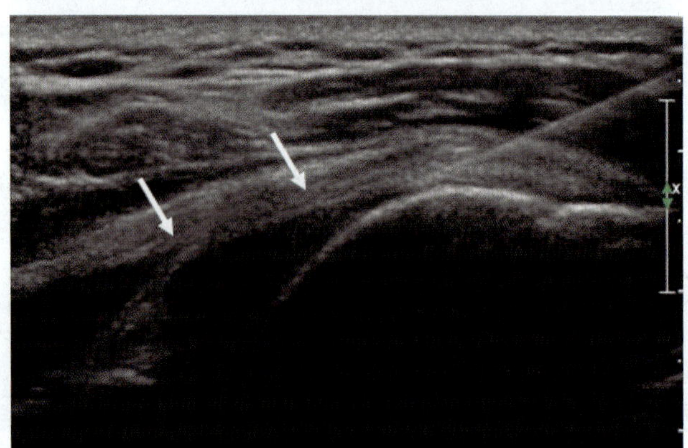

Figure 14.8.   Glenohumeral joint injection: Long-axis approach. **A:** A 25G needle (*N*) has been positioned deep to the posterior capsule during a glenohumeral joint injection. *H,* humeral head; *G,* glenoid; *I,* infraspinatus; *D,* deltoid. **B:** During the injection, there is fluid distension of the posterior recess of the joint. The posterior capsule is more conspicuous (*arrows*).

and then moved laterally until the echogenic clavicle is replaced by the hypoechoic disc of the joint. The majority of fibrous joint injections are performed using a 1.5″ hypodermic needle. The joint has a small capacity and will accept only 0.5 to 1 mL of fluid. The volume of the test injection should therefore be minimal otherwise it may not be possible to inject the full therapeutic dose of 10 to 20 mg corticosteroid. This approach is also useful in the sternoclavicular joint and pubic symphysis.

> **Tip:**
> - Most small joints of the hand and foot can be injected using a short-axis approach with 10 to 15 mg long-acting corticosteroid.
> - Shoulder and hip joints can be injected using a long-axis approach with 40 to 80 mg of long-acting corticosteroid.
> - Hydrodistention in combination with corticosteroid may be of value in adhesive capsulitis.

Superficial Peritendinous/Periarticular Injections

Peritendinous injections of anesthetic and long-acting corticosteroid are effective in tenosynovitis in the hand, foot, and ankle. The tendons are superficial and well-imaged on ultrasound. Ultrasound guidance is effective in ensuring that the injection is correctly placed. Bursae and ganglia can also be injected.

Foot and Ankle

The most commonly requested peritendinous injections in the foot and ankle are for chronic achillodynia or medial or lateral ankle pain due to posterior tibial or peroneal tendinosis/ tenosynovitis, respectively.[33] Less commonly, patients are referred to differentiate the pain of posterior impingement from stenosing tenosynovitis of the flexor hallucis longus (FHL) tendon, which may be difficult to distinguish clinically. Patients with plantar foot pain due to plantar fasciitis or forefoot pain from Morton neuroma are also frequently referred for ultrasound-guided injections.

Many patients with achillodynia have pain referable to the enthesis, with associated retrocalcaneal bursitis and Achilles tendinosis. Injection of 10 to 20 mg of methylprednisolone or triamcinolone may help to alleviate local pain and inflammation in the deep retrocalcaneal bursa. The patient is scanned prone with the ankle in mild dorsiflexion using a 10 MHz or higher frequency linear transducer. A 1.5″ hypodermic needle usually suffices using a short-axis approach. The deep retrocalcaneal bursa is usually well seen and can also be injected using a short-axis approach from the lateral aspect of the tendo Achilles. Distension of the bursa by injecting a small amount of anesthetic confirms that the needle is correctly placed, and the steroid is then injected. I have had limited success

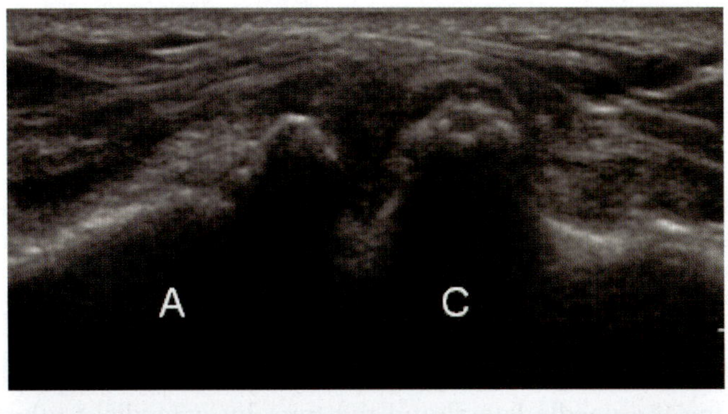

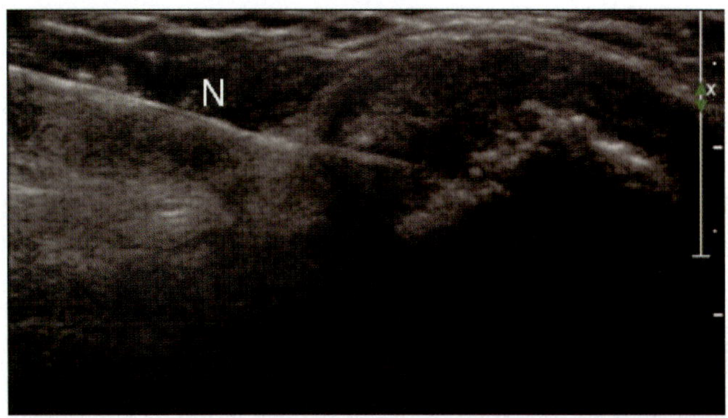

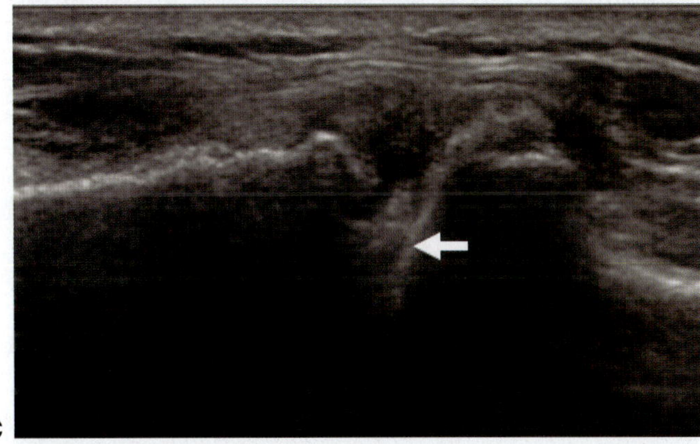

Figure 14.9.   AC joint injection. **A:** Long-axis view of the acromio-clavicular joint showing bony and capsular hypertrophic changes. *A*, acromion; *C*, clavicle. **B:** A 25G 1.5″ needle (*N*) is positioned into the joint using a short-axis technique. The needle is seen as a linear specular reflector when imaged in the plane of the joint. **C:** Following the injection and needle removal, the joint is filled with echogenic material from the therapeutic mixture (*arrow*).

in treating central Achilles tendinosis with peritendinous injections, superficial to the paratenon. It is generally taught that steroid injections into tendons are probably best avoided because of the possible risk of tendon rupture although there is no good evidence of the risk. Alternative approaches include intratendinous procedures (discussed below) such as dry needling. Intratendinous vascularity is seen in symptomatic tendinosis and may be amenable to injection of sclerosant such as polidocanol into peritendinous (but not intratendinous) vessels.[36]

Brisement using high-volume (40 to 50 mL) injections of saline or local anesthetic are said to break adhesions between the tendon and the paratenon and promote healing.[37] The needle is slipped between tendon and paratenon using a long-axis or short-axis approach, and a small test injection is made. If the needle is correctly positioned, the fluid will strip the paratenon from the tendon, and the full volume of fluid is then injected.

The posterior tibial or peroneal tendons are also approached in short axis (**Fig. 14.10**). Patients with pain in

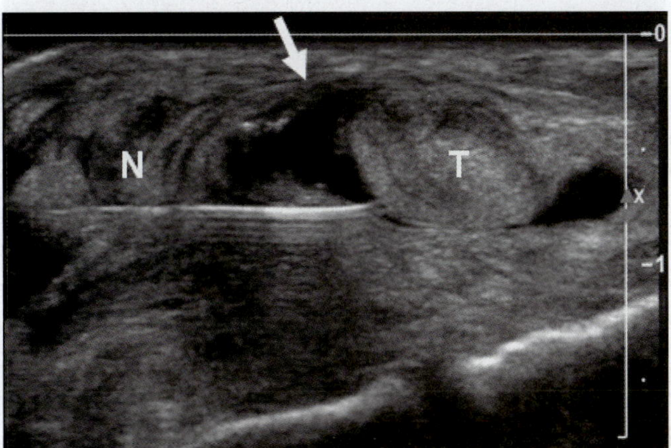

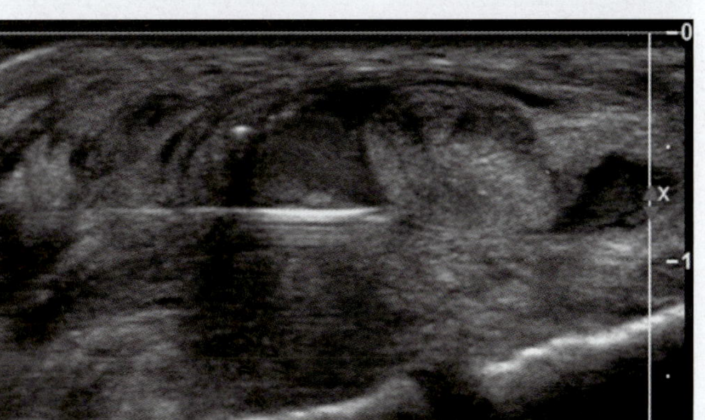

Figure 14.10.   Injection of posterior tibial tendon sheath in patient with medial ankle pain using a short-axis approach. **A:** A 1.5″ 25G needle (*N*) is positioned in the tendon sheath of the posterior tibial tendon. The tendon (*T*) is seen in cross section with a small to moderate amount of surrounding fluid (*arrow*). **B:** While observing in real time, injection of the therapeutic mixture displays a contrast effect, confirming the appropriate deposition.

these distributions benefit from injections of 10 to 20 mg of methylprednisolone or triamcinolone into the tendon sheath. Tendon sheath fluid facilitates the procedure and offers an easier target. Scanning prior to the procedure should assess the needle trajectory relative to adjacent neurovascular structures that are better seen using color or power Doppler imaging. The posterior tibial nerve is closely related to adjacent posterior tibial artery and veins, and is usually well seen proximal to its bifurcation into medial and lateral plantar branches. Fluid is frequently seen in the posterior tibial tendon sheath, in the submalleolar region. The peroneal tendons are less predictable. Power Doppler imaging in conjunction with real-time guidance can be beneficial in localizing areas of inflammation for direct injection. In stenosing tenosynovitis, the tendons may be surrounded by a thickened retinaculum, proliferative synovium, or scar tissue without fluid, and a test injection of local anesthetic to confirm position is invaluable.

The FHL tendon poses a more challenging problem due to its close relation to the neurovascular bundle of the posterior medial ankle. One helpful feature in FHL tendon sheath injections is that tendon sheath effusions tend to localize at the posterior recess of the tibiotalar joint. The neurovascular bundle is easily circumvented by placing the needle lateral and the transducer medial to the Achilles tendon **(Fig. 14.11)**.[38] This approach results in

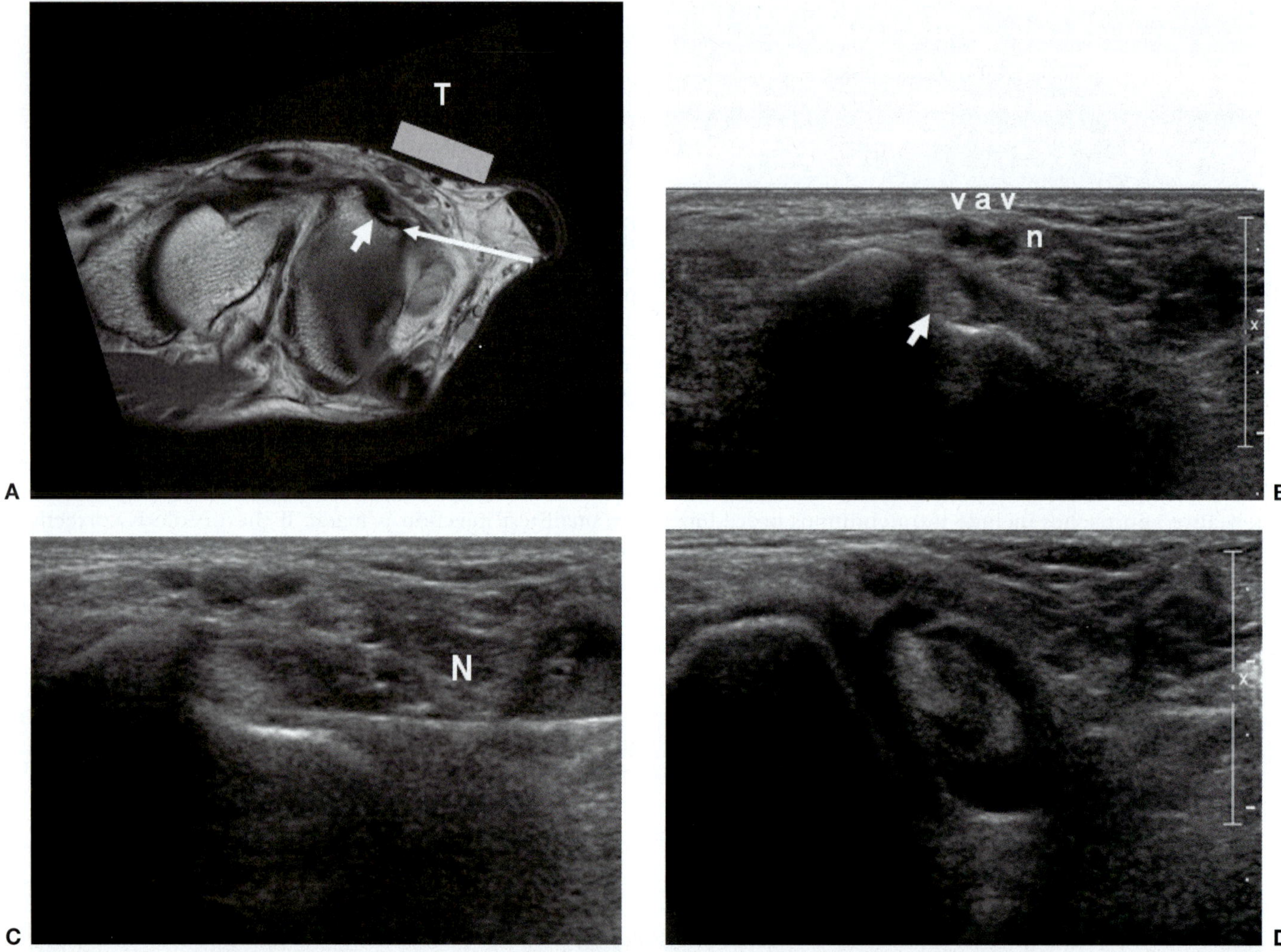

Figure 14.11.   Flexor hallucis longus injection. **A:** Proton density axial image of the ankle depicting the posterior sulcus (*short arrow*) for the FHL tendon. The tendon appears as a low signal intensity ellipse within the sulcus. The transducer (*T, box*) is positioned along the posteromedial aspect of the ankle. The needle trajectory is denoted by the long arrow. In this way the needle is well seen as a specular reflector, and the neurovascular structures overlying the tendon can be circumvented. Note that the needle enters the skin along the lateral margin of the Achilles tendon. **B:** The corresponding ultrasound anatomy. The neurovascular structures are labeled: Vein (*v*), artery (*a*), and nerve (*n*). **C:** The needle (*N*) is positioned along the deep margin of the tendon in its sulcus, and a test injection is performed to ensure distention of the tendon sheath. **D:** Postinjection image shows fluid distention of the FHL tendon sheath.

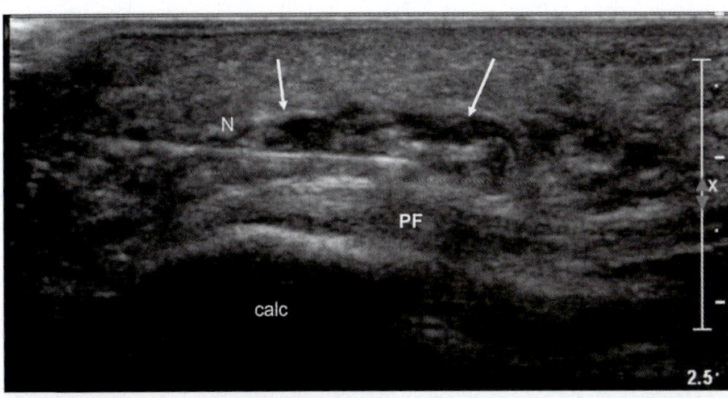

Figure 14.12. Plantar fascia injection. The proximal medial band of the plantar fascia (*PF*) is mildly thickened and inhomogeneous. A 1.5″ 25G needle (*N*) has been positioned superficial to the plantar fascia and a perifascial injection has been performed. The injected material (*arrows*) is distributed along the superficial margin of the medial band. Calc, calcaneum.

flexibility in needle placement, while maintaining the needle perpendicular to the insonating beam.

Ultrasound features of plantar fasciitis include thickening of the medial band of the plantar fascia and fat pad edema. One treatment option for severe plantar fasciitis is regional corticosteroid injection, typically performed using anatomic landmarks. Blind injections into the heel have been associated with rupture of the plantar fascia and failure of the longitudinal arch.[16] Ultrasound can be used to guide a needle along the plantar margin of the fascia avoiding direct intrafascial injection.[35,39] The plantar fascia is imaged with the patient prone and the foot mildly dorsiflexed using a long-axis approach. The transducer is centered over the medial band, which is most often implicated. A mark is placed over the posterior aspect of the heel and the needle is advanced superficial to the plantar fascia, approximately to the margin of the medial tubercle **(Fig. 14.12)**. I perform a perifascial injection using this approach, monitoring

the distribution of injected material in real time. Alternatively, a short-axis approach can be employed from the medial aspect of the heel with the patient supine. This may be less painful than the long-axis approach. The needle can be advanced both superficial and deep to the fascia (provided there is no preexisting tear) without necessarily puncturing the fascia. An advantage of this technique is that most or all of the steroid can be injected deep to the fascia, possibly reducing the risk of atrophy of the heel fat pad. Both long-axis and short-axis injections can be combined with dry needling or intrafascial injections as an alternative or supplement to corticosteroid injections.

Interdigital (Morton) neuromas, a common cause of forefoot pain especially in women, are hypoechoic masses that replace the normal hyperechoic fat in the interdigital web spaces. Occasionally, an enlarged hypoechoic interdigital nerve is identified. The second and/or third web spaces are most often involved. I generally inject Morton neuromas using a dorsal approach, while imaging the neuroma in long axis **(Fig. 14.13)**.[40] This approach is well tolerated by the majority of patients. In certain instances, plantar scanning with the foot in a "toes-up" position is preferred, such as with severe subluxation at the MTP joint. In either case, the needle is positioned directly within the neuroma and/or adjacent intermetatarsal bursa if present, and a small volume of therapeutic mixture is injected, similar to a small joint injection (i.e., 10 to 20 mg methylprednisolone or triamcinolone). The injection usually also fills the intermetatarsal bursa. The same basic approach applies for ablation therapy,[9,41,42] which is discussed in greater detail below.

Hand and Wrist

In the hand and wrist, de Quervain tenosynovitis, which involves the abductor pollicis longus and/or extensor

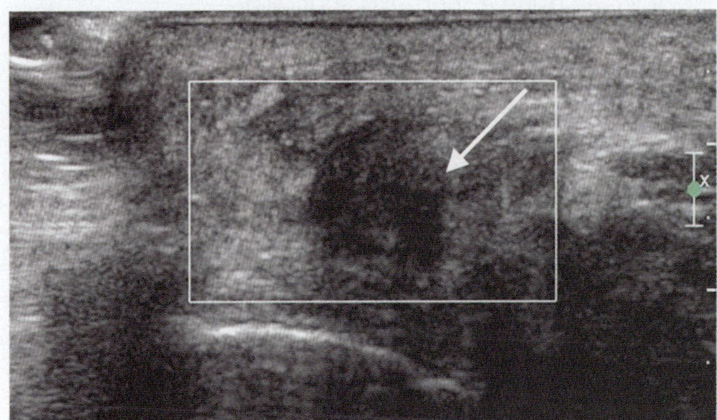
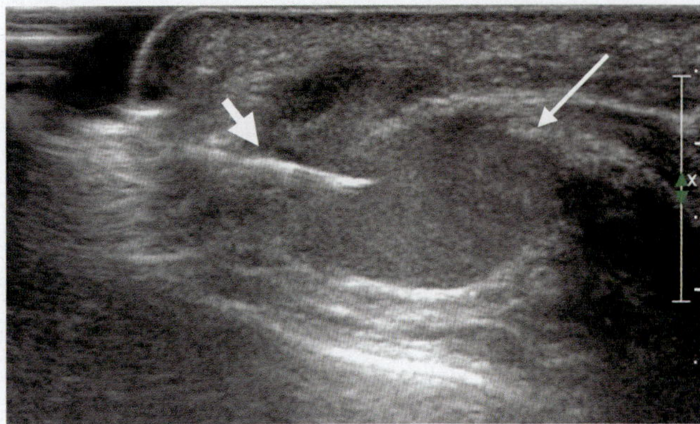

Figure 14.13. Morton neuroma. **A:** Long-axis scan of plantar aspect of foot shows hypoechoic Morton neuroma (*arrow*) between third and fourth metatarsal heads. **B:** The neuroma (*long arrow*) is now echogenic following insertion of a needle (*short* arrow) and injection of a therapeutic mixture of long-acting steroid and local anesthetic.

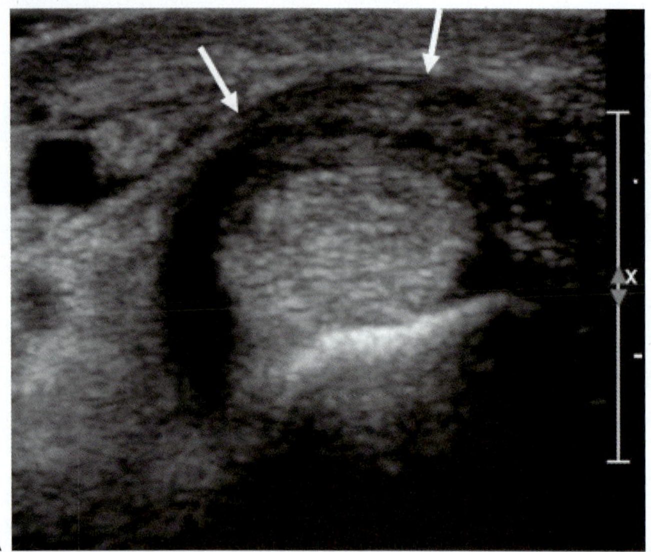

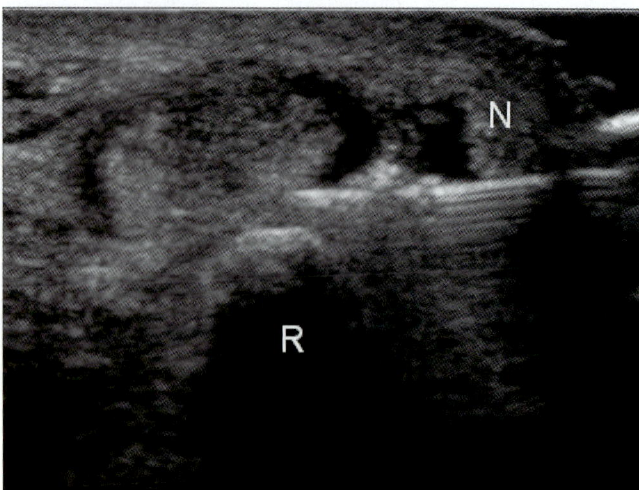

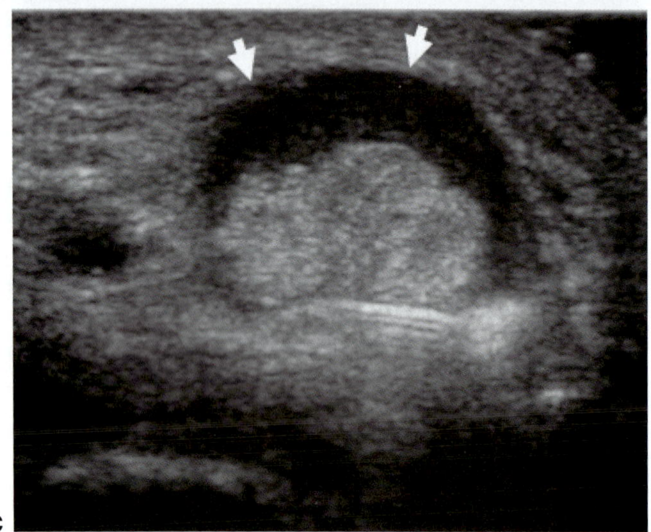

Figure 14.14.   de Quervain tendinitis. **A:** Transverse sonogram of the first dorsal compartment shows a thickened hypoechoic extensor retinaculum (*arrows*) producing a stenosing tenosynovitis **B:** Short-axis view of a 25G 1.5″ needle (*N*) deep to the abductor pollicis longus tendon, obtained at the level of the radial styloid (*R*). **C:** Short-axis view of the abductor pollicis longus tendon during injection. Fluid distends the tendon sheath (*short arrows*).

pollicis brevis tendons, may respond to steroid injections **(Fig. 14.14)**.[43] Patients with rheumatoid and psoriatic arthritis commonly experience severe tenosynovitis, which can lead to secondary tendon rupture and deformity. They may also benefit from steroid injections.[5,6] In either case, the approach is similar to superficial structures in the foot and ankle. A short-axis approach is taken in which the surrounding neurovascular structures are avoided, and the appropriate tendon sheaths are injected. A septum may divide the tendon sheath of abductor pollicis longus and extensor pollicis brevis. Care should be taken to ensure that the injected material surrounds both tendons. Occasionally, separate injections into the two compartments are needed. In the majority of cases, the amount of therapeutic mixture injected is similar to a small-to-medium-sized joint, depending on location. For cosmetic reasons, methylprednisolone may be preferred to triamcinolone, or betamethasone or dexamethasone may be preferable to crystalline preparations.

Tip:
- Superficial tendon sheaths of the hand and foot can be injected using a short-axis approach.
- Use 10 to 20 mg of long-acting corticosteroid in combination with long-acting anesthetic.
- Power Doppler in combination with grayscale imaging helps to localize sites of maximum tendon pathology.

INJECTION OF DEEP TENDONS

The most commonly requested deep tendon injections include the bicipital tendon sheath, iliopsoas tendon, gluteal tendon insertion on the greater trochanter, and hamstring tendon origin.

Biceps Tendon

Anterior shoulder pain with radiation into the arm may be secondary to bicipital tendonitis and/or tenosynovitis.

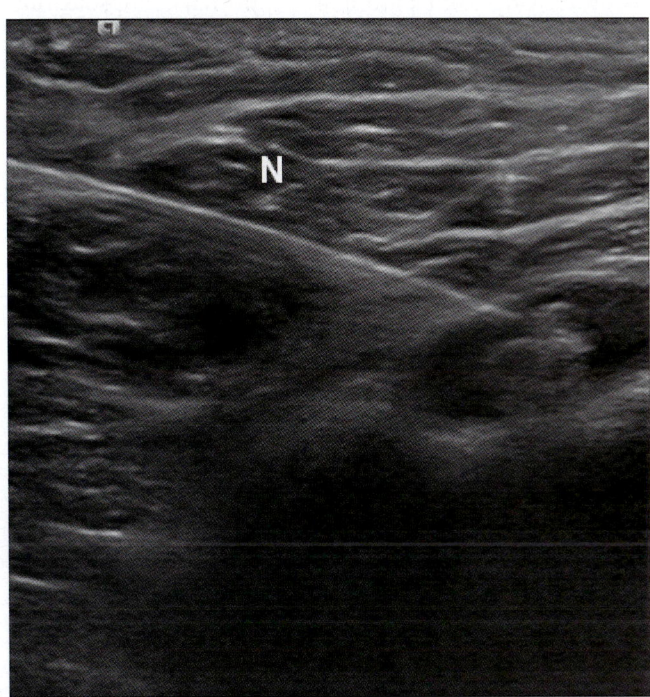
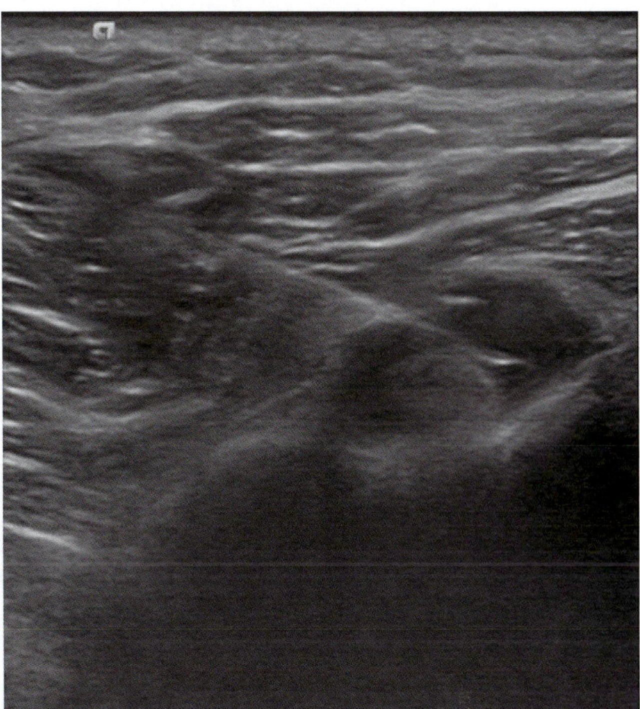

Figure 14.15. Biceps—extra-articular approach. **A:** Transverse image of the extra-articular long head of biceps tendon. A 22G spinal needle (*N*) has been advanced into the distended tendon sheath under ultrasound guidance. Note that the needle lies superficial to the tendon. **B:** The image depicts progressive distension of the tendon sheath during injection, confirming appropriate positioning.

The biceps tendon can be palpated, but its sheath, if nondistended, may offer <2-mm clearance to place a needle and is easily missed.[44] This is complicated by the caudal extension of the subacromial–subdeltoid bursa, which may overlie the bicipital tendon sheath. A blind injection could result in delivery of the therapeutic mixture into the bursa or tendon or outside the biceps tendon sheath. Ultrasound guidance ensures that the therapeutic agent is injected into the biceps tendon sheath.[34]

The patient is supine with the forearm supinated and the shoulder mildly elevated. The bicipital groove lies anteriorly. Using a linear transducer, typically 7.5 MHz, the long head of biceps is scanned in short axis and a 25G 1.5″ or 22G spinal needle is inserted laterally and guided into the tendon sheath (**Figs. 14.15 and 14.16**). If the bicipital tendon sheath contains fluid, the needle is directed into the fluid. Otherwise, the needle is directed along the superficial margin of the tendon, and a test injection of local anesthetic is used to confirm local distension of the sheath, followed by administration of long-acting corticosteroid. Fluid distension of the sheath with superficially located microbubbles helps to confirm a successful injection. Alternatively, the needle can be directed into the rotator interval, proximal to the transverse humeral ligament. This often results in reflux into the sheath as well as distension of the rotator interval. This approach requires needle placement adjacent to the biceps tendon in the rotator interval and "feeling"

for lack of resistance during a test injection with local anesthetic and can be helpful if there is no fluid in the biceps sheath.

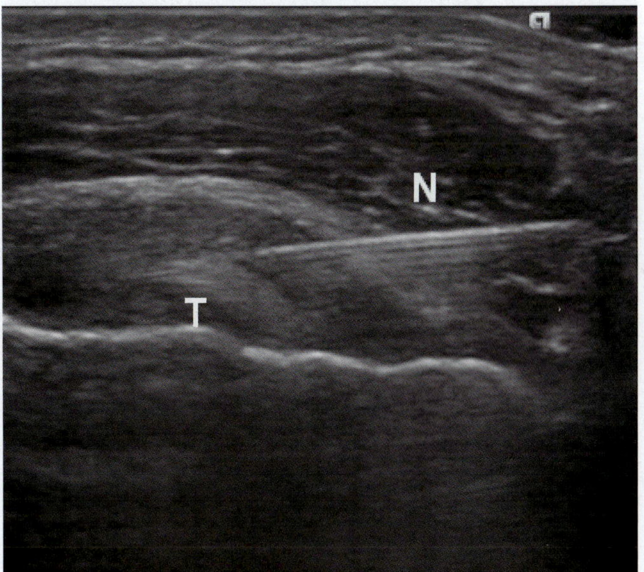

Figure 14.16. Biceps tendon–rotator interval. **A:** Transverse image of the distal intra-articular biceps tendon entering the rotator interval shows no significant effusion. A 25G 1.5″ needle (*N*) is placed adjacent to the proximal biceps tendon (*T*) under ultrasound guidance. A small test injection with local anesthetic confirms peritendinous location.

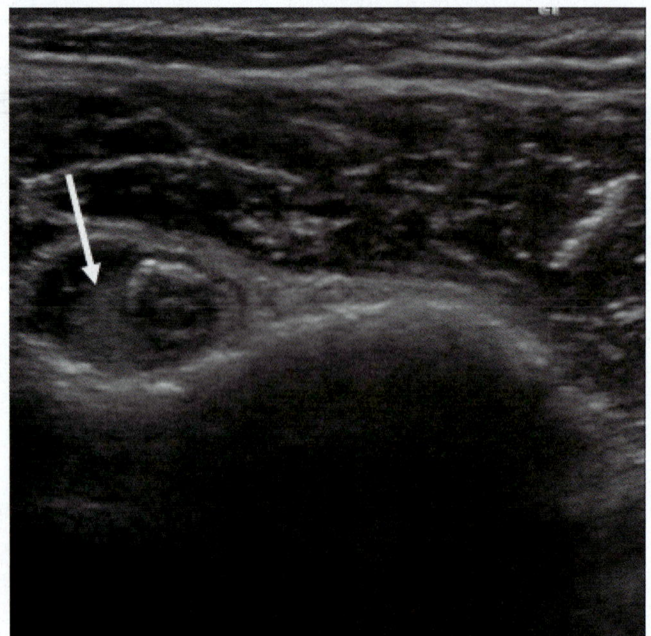

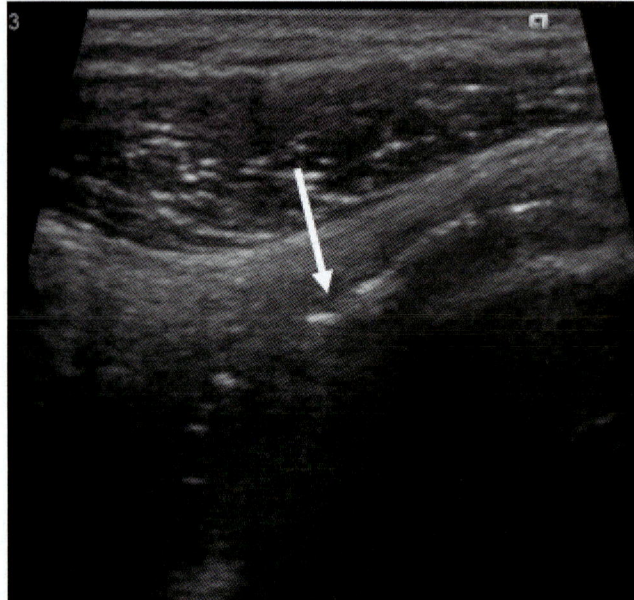

to underlying joint pathology or primary iliopsoas bursitis. Bursitis and iliopsoas tendinosis in the absence of bursitis may require injection.[45] A lower frequency transducer with curved or sector geometry is often required. The neurovascular bundle lies medial and superficial to the tendon, so it is advantageous to approach the tendon in short axis from the lateral margin of the hip using a 22G spinal needle, which is angled deeply. A small test injection to confirm needle position shows fluid and/or microbubbles distending the bursa along the axis of the tendon **(Fig. 14.17),** and 40 mg of methylprednisolone or triamcinolone are then injected.

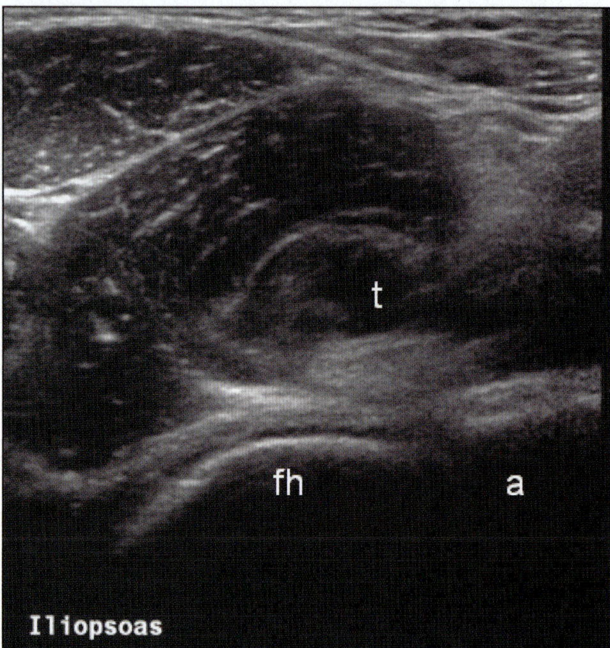

Figure 14.16. *(Continued)* **B:** In postinjection images of the extra-articular biceps, there is fluid distention of the biceps tendon sheath with the contrast effect *(arrow)* confirming retrograde flow of part of the therapeutic mixture. **C:** Transverse image of the proximal rotator interval, near the biceps anchor, shows both micro-bubbles and contrast effect from the therapeutic mixture *(arrow)*, confirming forward flow of injected material.

Iliopsoas Tendon

The iliopsoas tendon lies superficial to and along the medial margin of the anterior capsule of the hip and the iliopectineal eminence of the anterior acetabulum. It inserts on the lesser trochanter of the femur. The iliopsoas bursa frequently communicates with the hip joint and lies deep to the tendon. The bursa may be distended due

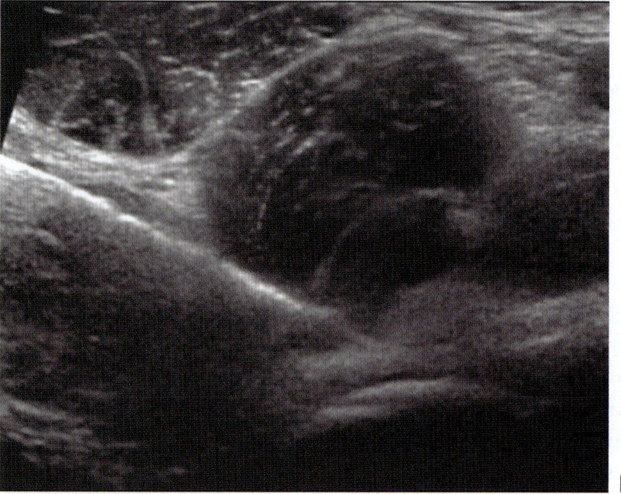

Figure 14.17. Iliopsoas bursa injection for clinically suspected iliopsoas tendinosis. **A:** Baseline image depicts the femoral head *(fh)*, iliopectineal eminence of the acetabulum *(a)*, and iliopsoas tendon *(t)*. **B:** A 22G spinal needle has been positioned deep to the tendon at the level of the capsulolabral junction.

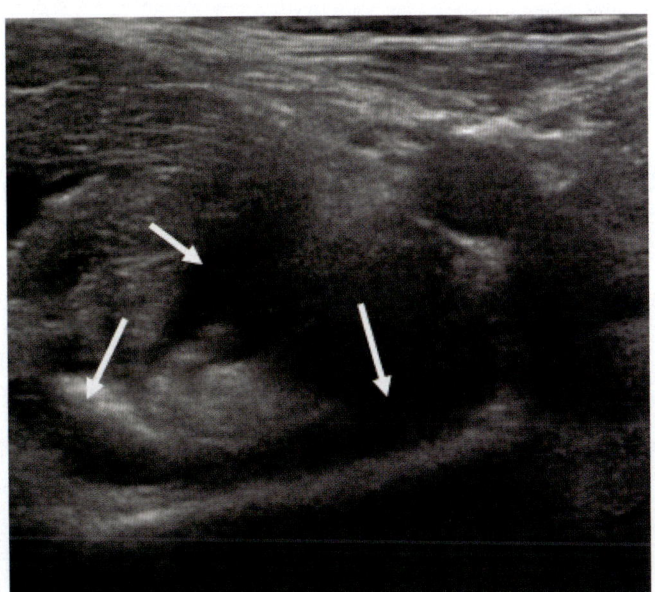

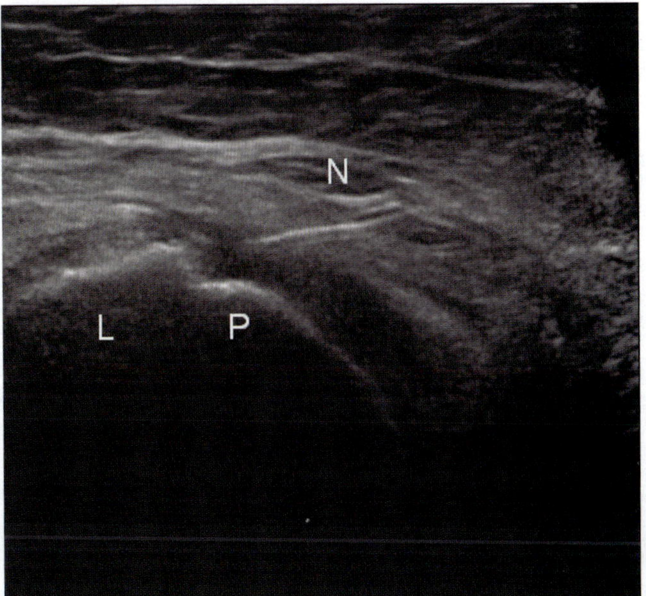

Figure 14.17. *(Continued)* **C:** During injection, fluid appears both deep and superficial to the tendon within the bursa (*arrows*). This image was obtained at a slightly more proximal location with the tendon superficial to the anterior acetabulum.

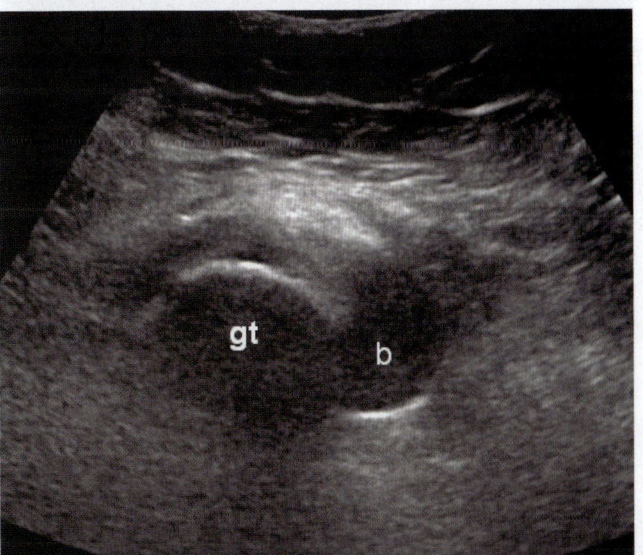

Figure 14.18. Greater trochanteric bursa injection for lateral hip pain. **A:** Short-axis image of the greater trochanter showing the lateral (*L*) and posterior (*P*) facets. A 22G spinal needle (*N*) has been positioned at the posterior facet corresponding to the expected location of the greater trochanteric bursa. The injection was performed using a 9-MHz linear transducer for guidance. **B:** Postinjection image using a 6-MHz curvilinear transducer shows distension of the bursa (*b*). The greater trochanter is labeled (*gt*). It should be noted that multiple bursae may be evident in relationship to the abductor tendon insertions, which can be individually targeted.

BURSAL AND GANGLION CYST INJECTIONS

Distended bursae provide anatomic targets for therapeutic injections. Injections are often requested for localized bursitis with or without tendon abnormality. Examples include the retrocalcaneal, iliopsoas, greater trochanteric, or ischial bursae (**Fig. 14.18**). Alternatively, bursitis or a distended synovial cyst or ganglion cyst may cause mechanical impingement of adjacent tendons and/or neurovascular structures. Cyst decompression and administration of therapeutic agent may alleviate symptoms (**Fig. 14.19**). Ultrasound guidance avoids intratendinous injections and adjacent neurovascular structures, and the needle may be redirected as necessary in a multiloculated cyst (**Fig. 14.20**).[46,47] The nature of the material aspirated is quite variable, ranging from watery fluid to viscous jelly. In the case of a complex bursa, I often indicate that there may be minimal return so that the patient has a realistic expectation that the procedure may not be successful. A synovial cyst often recurs within weeks to months, and aspiration and injection may be more palliative than therapeutic until the underlying cause (e.g., osteoarthrosis) is tackled. Ganglion/paralabral cyst fluid is often clear and highly viscous, giving rise to the particular hard nature of these cysts to palpation and a larger bore needle, in some cases an 18G hypodermic or spinal needle, may be needed. I have found it helpful to use a lavage technique similar to that employed in calcific tendinosis (below), employing either local anesthetic and/or a therapeutic corticosteroid mixture as the lavage fluid. It is important to advise the patient that the cyst may recur after several months and require either repeat aspiration or surgery. The long-term results from aspirating ganglion cysts at the wrist or doing nothing are similar.

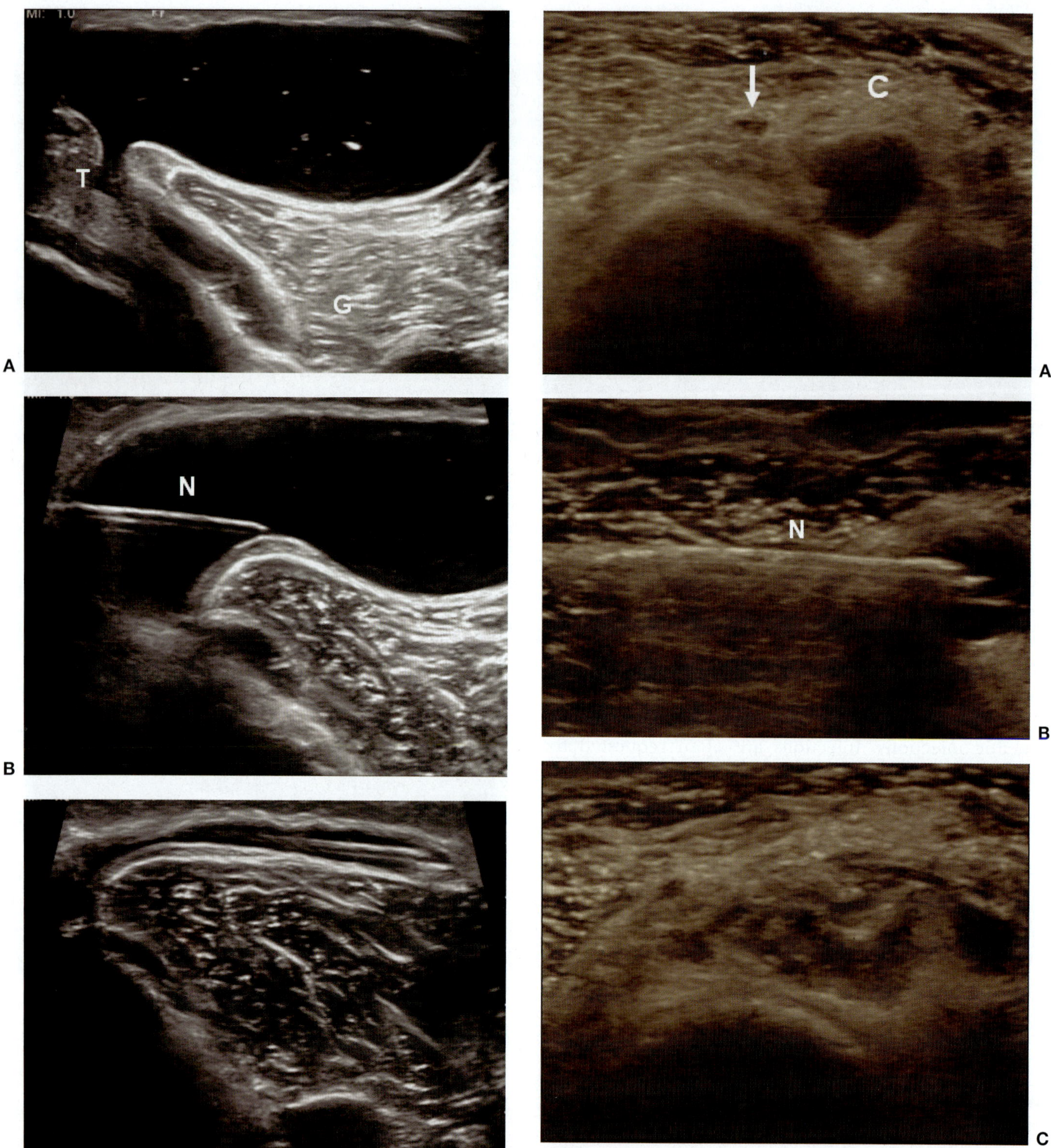

Figure 14.19.   Baker cyst. A 55-year-old female with swelling of the posterior medial aspect of the knee. **A:** A large Baker cyst is present containing low-level echoes. The characteristic location of the cyst's neck between the medial gastrocnemius (*G*) and semimembranosus tendon (*T*) is evident. **B:** An 18G spinal needle (*N*) has been placed into the cyst under ultrasound guidance. **C:** The cyst has been aspirated to near completion on the final image.

Figure 14.20.   Ganglion adjacent to nerve. **A:** Transverse colorized grayscale image of the ganglion cyst (*C*) and posterior interosseus nerve (PIN, *arrow*). **B:** A 22G spinal needle (*N*) has been placed into the cyst under ultrasound guidance. **C:** Post-aspiration image shows successful decompression of the cyst.

CALCIFIC TENDONITIS

Symptomatic intra or peritendinous deposition of calcium hydroxyapatite often appears as a nodular echogenic mass within or adjacent to the tendon and may or may not display posterior acoustic shadowing. Calcific tendonitis most often occurs in the shoulder, but may occur elsewhere in the musculoskeletal system. Ultrasound-guided fragmentation and lavage have been described[48–50] and excellent results reported. I first inject local anesthetic into the subdeltoid bursa for pain relief. An alternative approach is to inject local anesthetic around the suprascapular nerve. I currently employ a single needle technique with the needle acting as inflow for anesthetic and/or sterile saline, and also as an outflow for the resulting calcium solution (**Fig. 14.21**). It is my experience that the elasticity of the pseudocapsule encasing the calcification is sufficient to decompress the calcific mass in the majority of cases. A 10-cc syringe filled with anesthetic or sterile saline is used. Injection of small aliquots (1 to 2 cc) into the lesion resulting in distension, followed by release of pressure and subsequent

decompression back into the syringe, releases calcium from the deposit. The returning fluid often has the appearance of a "puff of smoke," as it contains progressive amounts of calcific debris. As the syringe contents become progressively cloudy, fresh syringes are employed. Following multiple lavages and extraction of the majority of the calcification, the needle is used to fenestrate the pseudocapsule and then inject anesthetic and steroid mixture (typically 40 mg triamcinolone with 1 to 2 mL of long-acting anesthetic) into the subdeltoid bursa. If the calcification is too small or fragmented to allow lavage and decompression, an effective technique is to fenestrate the calcium deposit and make a peritendinous therapeutic injection.[49] Double-needle techniques have been described using one needle to inject and the other to aspirate. (Barbotage of the rotator cuff is also discussed in Chapter 3.)

INTRATENDINOUS INJECTIONS/ PERCUTANEOUS DRY NEEDLING TECHNIQUES

Intratendinous injection therapies are thought to promote a direct healing response. These techniques date back to as early as the 1930s in the case of prolotherapy and to the 1970s in the case of autologous blood/PRP injections.[36] Ultrasound imaging is believed to ensure optimal deposition of injected material and can be used to assess the distribution of injected material and the response to therapy.

Prolotherapy has traditionally entailed the percutaneous injection of a proliferant, which is defined as any

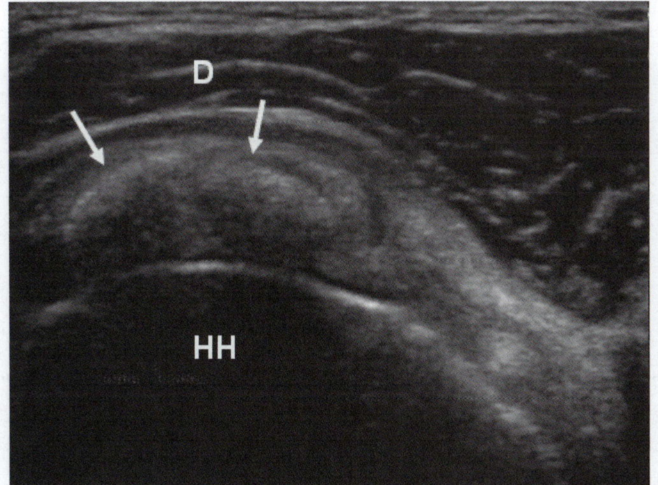

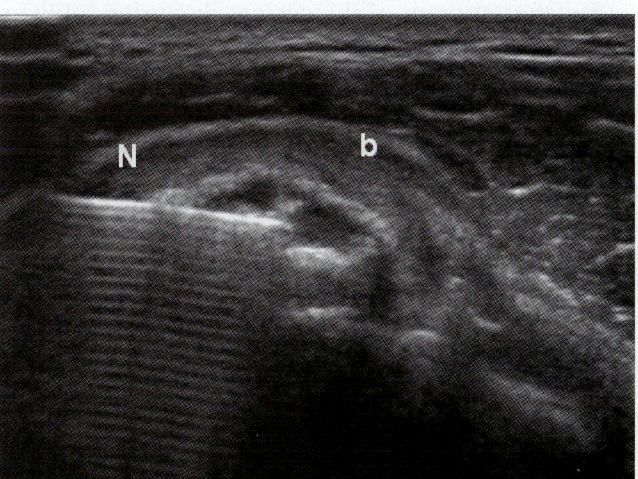

Figure 14.21.   Calcific tendinosis of the shoulder. **A:** Globular echogenic calcification (*arrows*) along the bursal surface of the supra and infraspinatus tendons seen in short axis, displays weak posterior acoustic shadowing. D, deltoid; HH, humeral head. **B:** A 20G spinal needle (*N*) is positioned centrally within the calcification and a series of lavages and re-aspirations of the calcification are performed while observing in real time. A central hypoechoic mixture within the calcification corresponds to progressively diluted contents consisting of lavage fluid and calcium hydroxyapatite. Some reflux into the adjacent subdeltoid bursa (*b*) is present.

substance capable of producing cellular proliferation and collagen formation, thereby promoting healing.[36,51–53] This has largely been confined to one of three substances: instead of, hypertonic dextrose (15% to 20%), sodium morrhuate, and phenol. It is believed that they initiate an inflammatory response that ultimately promotes hypertrophy and strengthening of tendons and ligaments, resulting in improved biomechanics and reduced pain. A variety of case series and randomized controlled studies provide limited supportive evidence, although the precise mechanisms are not well understood.[36] Dry needling (i.e., multiple needle perforations of the tendon without injection of therapeutic material) can promote a healing response, which has been postulated to relate to the presence of micro hemorrhage with the release of platelets.[54]

Autologous blood or platelet concentrates derived from autologous blood take advantage of a variety of growth factors contained within platelets that promote vascular and cellular proliferation. Platelet-rich plasma, in particular, allows for delivery of high concentrations of these growth factors to the area of injury.[55,56] Theoretically, PRP has the potential to improve tendon healing. It contains a more concentrated amount of platelets than whole blood and includes many reparative growth factors such as platelet-derived growth factor, transforming growth factor-beta, epidermal growth factor, and vascular endothelial growth factor. In a human tenocyte model, de Mos et al.[55] found that PRP accelerates the catabolic demarcation of traumatically injured tendon matrices and promotes angiogenesis and formation of fibrovascular callus. Clinical studies have suggested that autologous blood or PRP significantly improves healing in refractory tendinosis, although definitive studies showing the efficacy of either technique are still lacking.[22–24,26,56]

For the purposes of the current discussion, only injections using blood products will be discussed. Dry needling techniques have been employed successfully in patients with lateral epicondylitis refractory to other conservative measures **(Fig. 14.22).**[54] Autologous blood and PRP injections have been successfully used in the elbow and knee **(Fig. 14.22).**[22,23] The advantage of performing these procedures under ultrasound-guidance becomes evident when injecting tendons close to neurovascular structures, such as the hamstring tendon origin **(Fig. 14.23).**

Dry needling techniques entail mechanical fenestration of the tendon employing a hypodermic or spinal needle. I often use a 22G spinal needle. Ultrasound guidance permits targeting of regions of tendinosis and angiofibroblastic proliferation, thereby promoting bleeding and induction of a subsequent inflammatory cascade to produce a healing response. The addition of 5 mL of fresh autologous blood at the site of fenestration is believed to augment the release of bioactive growth factors associated with tendon healing. In my own practice, I have largely replaced dry needling with PRP injections.

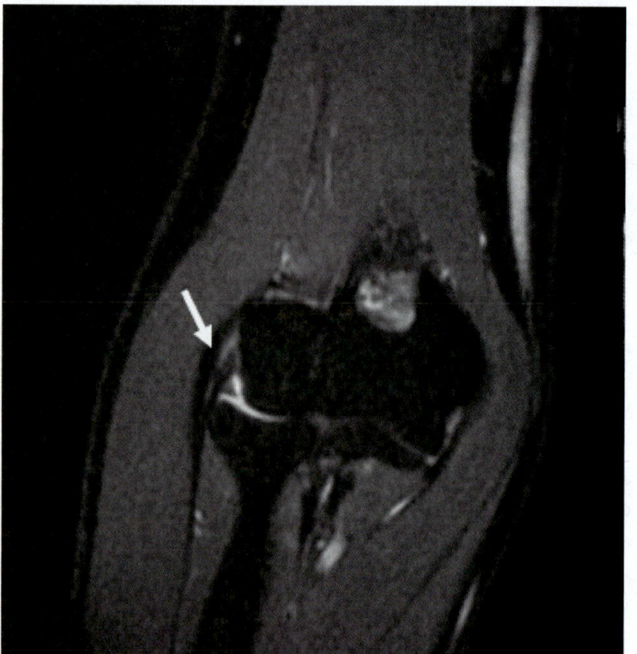

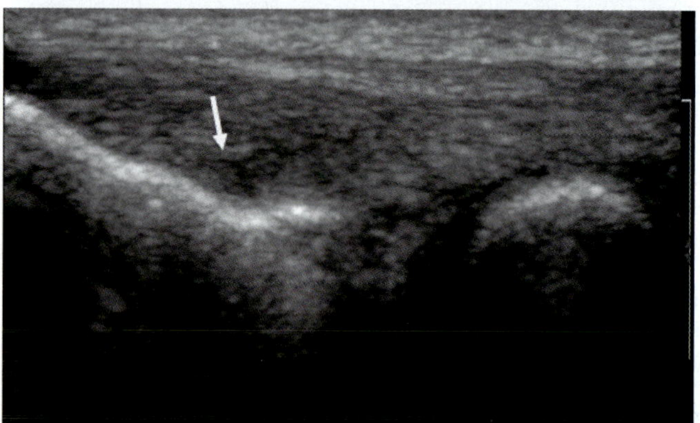

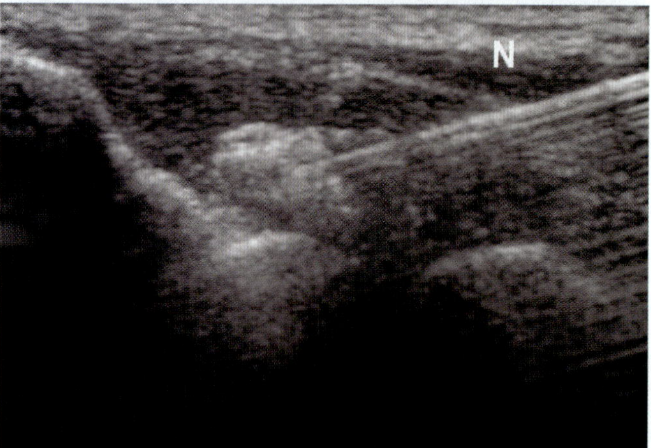

Figure 14.22. Lateral epicondylitis. **A:** Fluid-sensitive fat-suppressed coronal MR of the right elbow shows interstitial tear (*arrow*) at common extensor origin. **B:** Longitudinal sonogram of the common extensor origin shows tendinosis with suggestion of tear (*arrow*). **C:** A 22G 1.5″ needle within the tendon substance during a PRP injection. Increased echoes relate to micro-bubbles within the injected material.

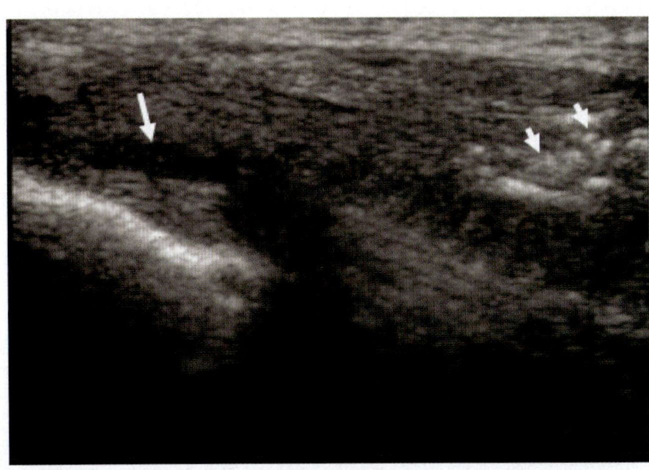

D

Figure 14.22.   *(Continued)* **D:** Following needle removal, the tear is distended with injected blood products and becomes more conspicuous (*arrow*). Micro-bubbles (*short arrows*) distally within the myotendinous junction show extent of spread of injected material.

The PRP is prepared from autologous whole blood, which is centrifuged to concentrate platelets in the plasma. A concentration of 1,000,000 platelets per μL has been suggested to be the working definition of PRP; this represents a platelet concentration five times higher than whole blood.[56] Typical volumes of injectate vary according to the specific kit employed and the area injected, but 3 to 5 mL of platelet concentrate is typical. As nonsteroidal anti-inflammatory drugs (NSAIDS) can act as platelet inhibitors, I advise patients to refrain from

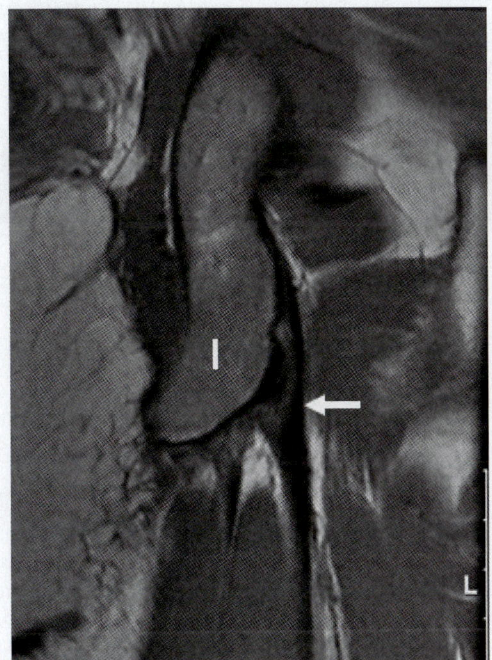

A

Figure 14.23.   Hamstring PRP injection. **A:** Marked tendinosis at the hamstring origin (*arrow*) on coronal proton density image. I, ischium.

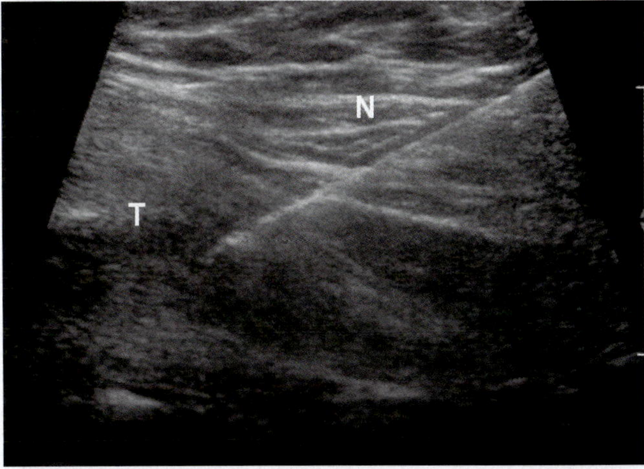

B

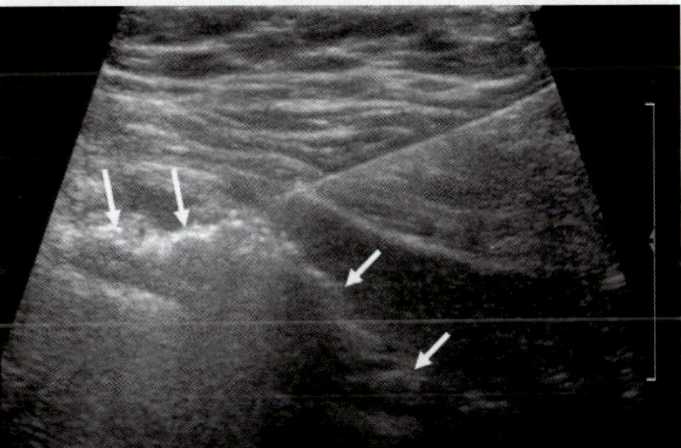

C

Figure 14.23.   *(Continued)* **B:** A 22G spinal needle (*N*) has been positioned in the hamstring tendon origin (*T*) in long axis while mechanically fenestrating the tendon. **C:** During injection of the PRP, microbubbles within the injectate distribute throughout the tendon often as far proximal as the myotendinous junction (*arrows*), providing an indirect measure of the distribution of injected material within the tendon/muscle complex.

using these agents 1 week before and 2 weeks following the procedure. It has also been suggested that PRP should be performed in combination with an appropriate strengthening program, beginning 2 to 3 weeks after the procedure. A more extensive discussion of these techniques is beyond the scope of the current chapter.

Tip:
- Intratendinous injections of PRP should be performed in combination with intratendinous fenestration to promote bleeding and initiate an inflammatory response.
- Patients should avoid NSAIDS immediately, 1 week prior to and for 2 weeks following the procedure.

PERINEURAL INJECTIONS

Ultrasound has shown promise in evaluating and treating patients with painful lesions of peripheral nerves due to compressive neuropathies, such as in carpal or cubital tunnel syndromes, or in cases of post-traumatic/postsurgical neuromas.[57–59] Injections include nerve blocks with long-acting anesthetic, therapeutic injections using an injectable steroid, or neurolytic therapy with an agent that promotes cellular death such as absolute ethanol.[60–63] A rapidly absorbed injectable steroid, such as dexamethasone, may be preferable for superficial lesion to minimize potential complications such as depigmentation or atrophy of the subcutaneous fat.

A thorough knowledge of the normal sonographic appearances of nerves and their anatomic course is a prerequisite.[64] In the case of small sensory nerves, which can be difficult to visualize, knowledge of the anatomic relationships of the nerves to adjacent anatomic compartments is of value. Nerves are best visualized in short axis as clusters of hypoechoic fascicles with echogenic septations (endoneurium), which have a surrounding echogenic epineurial sleeve. An enlarged hypoechoic nerve may indicate neuritis. A focal hypoechoic nodule may represent a neuroma.

Ultrasound allows direct targeting of the perineural soft tissue or a neuroma for injection **(Fig. 14.24)**. The nerve is best approached in short axis, usually with a 1.5″ 25G needle or occasionally a spinal needle. In the case of a perineural injection, it is helpful to position the needle in close proximity to the nerve, injecting small amounts of anesthetic until a clear-cut fluid plane outlining the epineurium is evident. When this is achieved, the therapeutic mixture can be instilled. The same procedure is employed when performing ultrasound-guided neurolytic therapy. I generally inject a mixture of long-acting anesthetic with a total of 0.5 to 1 mL of absolute ethanol for peripheral nerve lesions. Absolute ethanol may require multiple injections and produce a marked postinjection inflammatory response that can last for several days. The volume injected is variable and generally does not exceed 1 mL. Multiple small injections (0.25 to 0.5 mL) have been advocated for Morton neuromas.

When performing either radiofrequency (RF) ablations or cryoablations, it is recommended that a proximal nerve block is performed before the ablative procedure.[40,62–64] The cryo- or RF probe is placed either in the lesion or contiguous with the nerve, and a variable number of applications are performed to obtain adequate intralesional coverage **(Fig. 14.25)**. Potential complications of

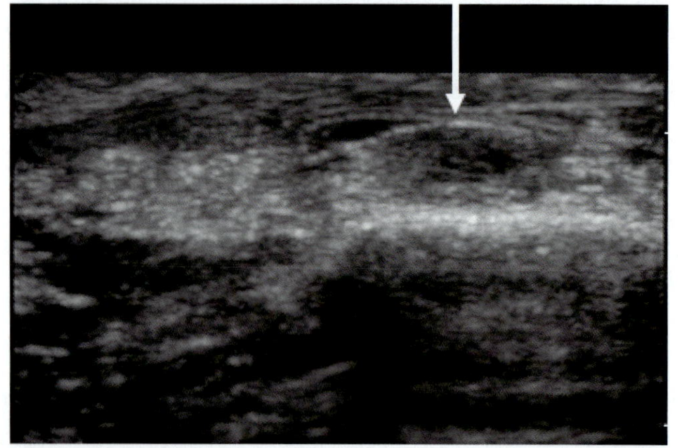

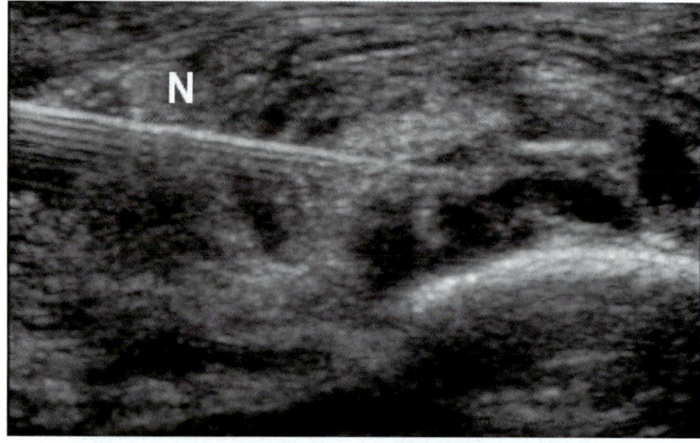

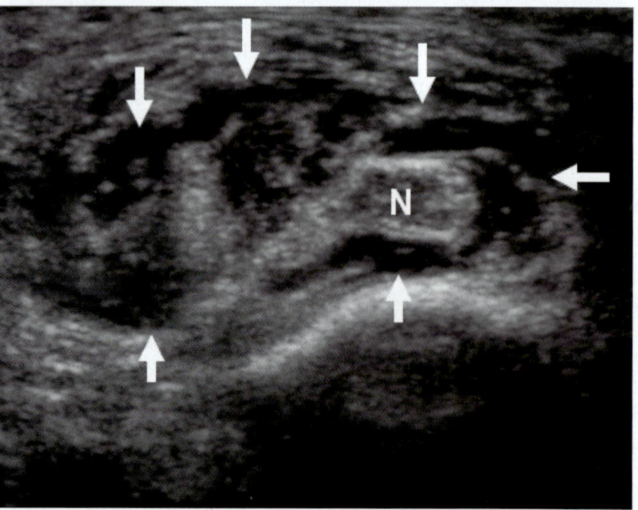

Figure 14.24. Perineural injection. **A:** Postsurgical neuritis of the superficial peroneal nerve (*arrow*) following anterior compartment release surgery. **B:** A 25G 1.5″ needle (*N*) is placed adjacent to the deep surface of the nerve under ultrasound guidance. A small test injection with local anesthetic confirms perineural distribution. **C:** The needle has been removed following perineural injection with 0.75% bupivacaine and dexamethasone. Notice the distribution of injected material (*short arrows*) circumferentially about the nerve (*N*).

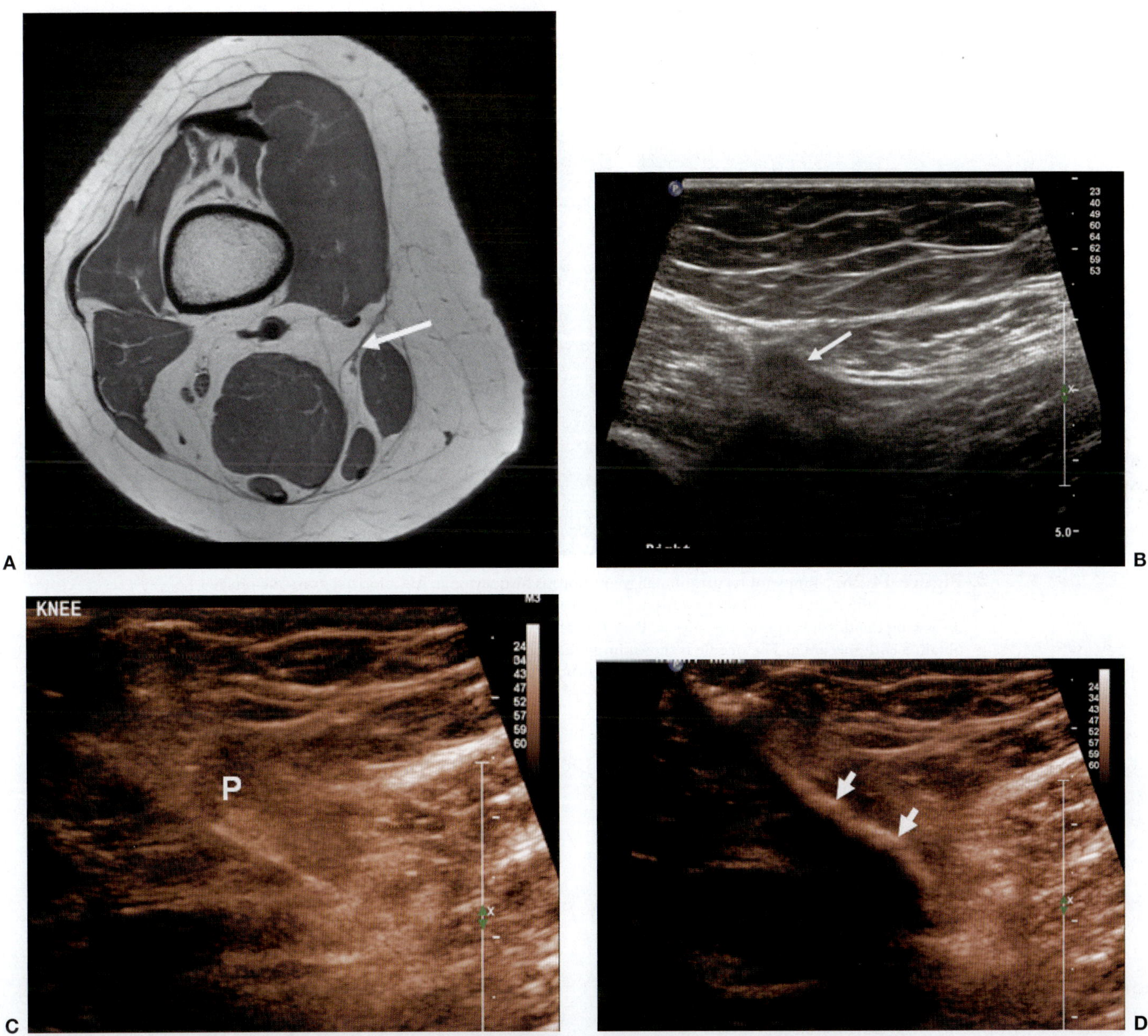

Figure 14.25. Cryoablation. A 27-year-old female with development of scar encasement of the saphenous nerve following arthroscopic surgery for meniscal repair. Patient had saphenous nerve neurectomy with development of perineural scarring at the stump site within the adductor canal. **A:** Baseline FSE axial T1 MR scan depicts linear low signal intensity scar formation involving the saphenous nerve (*arrow*). **B:** Transverse sonogram shows hypoechoic stump neuroma (*arrow*) corresponding to abnormality seen on MR. **C:** A 17G trochar tip cryoablation probe (*P*) has been positioned into the stump neuroma. **D:** Formation of an ice ball (*arrows*) at the probe tip is evident with the appearance of an irregular curvilinear reflector with dense posterior shadowing.

RF and alcohol ablation include neuritis and neuroma formation. Pulse RF is postulated to be safer than traditional RF ablation. It is efficacious for cervical radicular pain, but in lumbar facet arthropathy and trigeminal neuropathy, results are not equal to traditional RF ablation. The optimal method for performing RF ablation has not been fully elucidated.

In an animal model, controlled cryoinjury to the nerves results in total degeneration of the myelin fibers. Non-myelin fibers and vessels are less affected. Regeneration follows the injury, as the Schwann cell basal lamina is spared and provides the structure for regeneration. When the endoneurium is spared, neuroma formation does not occur. Early regeneration begins 2 weeks after

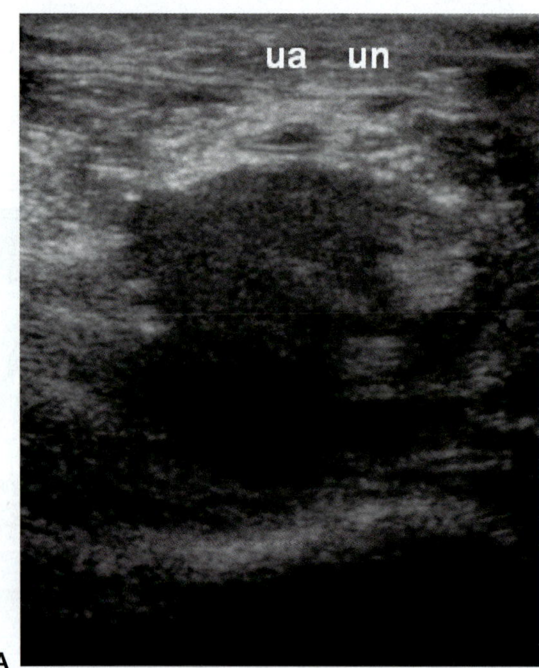

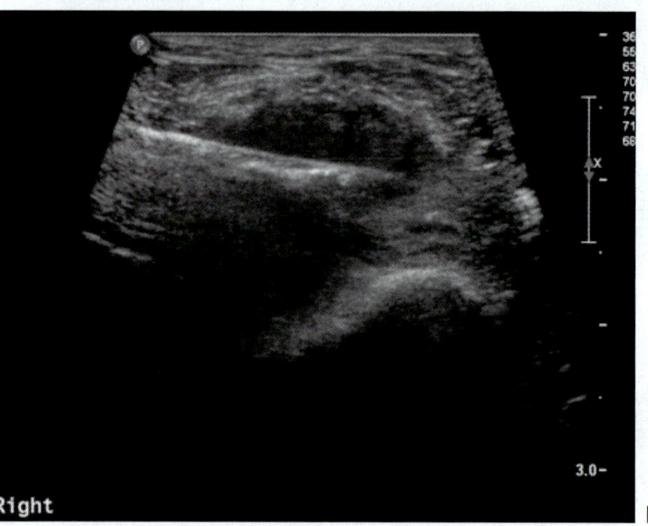

Figure 14.26. Biopsy of recurrent malignant fibrous histiocytoma. **A:** Colorized grayscale image obtained in the right forearm shows a hypoechoic mass deep to the ulnar artery (*ua*) and nerve (*un*), displacing the flexor carpi ulnaris muscle. **B:** A 12G biopsy needle (*N*) with a 2-cm throw is used to obtain a core specimen. The needle is shown immediately following specimen acquisition contained within the lesion and avoiding the neurovascular structures.

freezing. The time to total regeneration is related to the rate of axonal regrowth and the distance of the cryo-produced lesion from the end organ.[63,65,66] It is postulated that cryotherapy will have fewer negative outcomes than other methods of nerve ablation. I perform cryoablation using a 17G trocar tip catheter positioned at the lesion with a co-axial technique.[42] Once localized, the trocar is removed and replaced by a cryo-probe followed typically by two to four freeze cycles of 3-minute duration with short (<1 minute) intervening passive thaw cycles. The goal is to encompass the entire lesion with ice. The principal complication is skin necrosis, which can potentially occur for superficial lesions. This can usually be avoided by observing for ischemic changes that appear as a transient blanching of the skin.

> **Tip:**
> - Prior to perineural therapeutic injection, inject with local anesthetic to dissect a plane adjacent to epineurium.
> - Use of a co-axial technique can be of value in ablative therapy to minimize extralesional soft tissue damage.

ULTRASOUND-GUIDED SOFT TISSUE BIOPSIES

Ultrasound guidance has been advocated for percutaneous biopsies of soft tissue masses. Ultrasound-guided biopsies have high sensitivity and specificity when compared

to surgical pathology and long-term follow-up.[67,68] Soft tissue extension of a bone tumor is also amenable to percutaneous ultrasound-guided biopsy (**Figs. 14.26 and 14.27**). Biopsy of soft tissue masses should be preceded by local staging and discussion with the surgical oncologist who will perform definitive surgery. The biopsy track should be chosen to ensure that it does not compromise definitive surgery and will be excised at the time of surgery. The majority of biopsies are performed using local

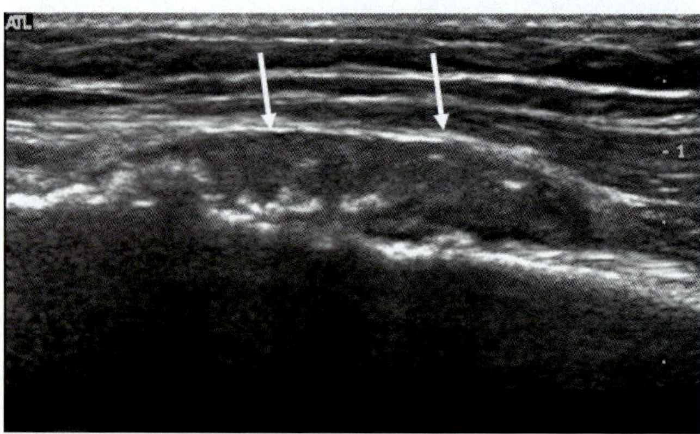

Figure 14.27. A 35-year-old pregnant female with bone tumor diagnosed on limited radiographs of the forearm. To limit radiation dose, ultrasound-guided biopsy was performed following discussion with the referring tumor surgeon. **A:** Long-axis view of the ulnar diaphysis shows displacement of the periosteum by a soft tissue mass (*arrows*). In addition to the soft tissue mass, spicules of periosteal new bone are seen in close relation to the native cortex.

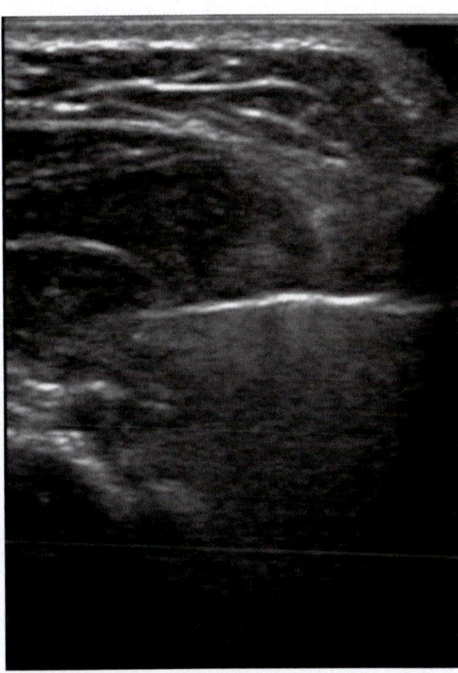

Figure 14.27. *(Continued)* **B:** Biopsy of the soft tissue component was performed using a 14G biopsy gun with a 1-cm throw. Histologic diagnosis was periosteal osteosarcoma.

anesthetic alone. Small peripheral biopsies (e.g., giant cell tumor of tendon sheath at the distal interphalangeal joint) may benefit from a proximal regional nerve block to make the procedure more comfortable for the patient, although in most cases this is not necessary. The principal advantages of ultrasound are the ability to localize potentially high-yield portions of the mass such as solid or more vascular components as well as avoiding necrotic fluid-filled areas and neurovascular structures. An automatic or semiautomatic biopsy gun with a cutting needle of at least 16G caliber is typically used **(Fig. 14.28).** The throw

of the needle must be selected to fall within the mass. Use of an introducer containing a trocar tip can be of value in minimizing trauma and minimizing the possibility of tumor seeding of the biopsy track.

SUMMARY

Ultrasound provides several distinct advantages as a guidance method for therapeutic injections. Observing and adjusting the needle position in real time ensures that therapeutic injections are delivered accurately and other structures such as neurovascular bundles are avoided. As clinical examples have shown, the current generation of ultrasound scanners provides excellent depiction of the relevant anatomy. The needle has a unique sonographic appearance and can be monitored in real time, as can the steroid–anesthetic injection. The same principles apply to ultrasound-guided aspirations and biopsies. Given these advantages, ultrasound guidance should be the method of choice to perform a large variety of guided musculoskeletal interventions.

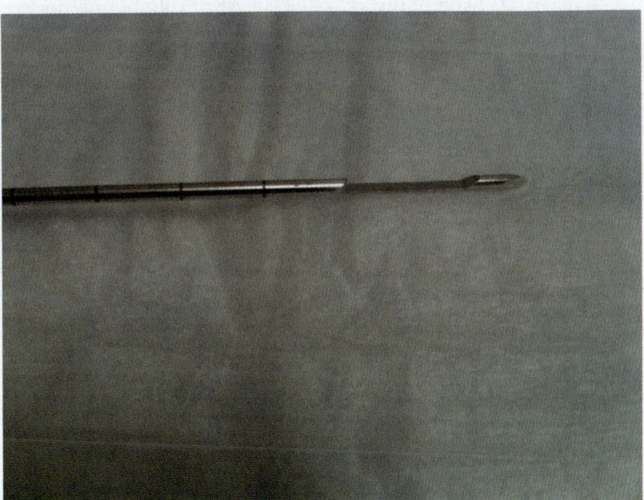

Figure 14.28. Exposure of sample surface of cutting needle from a 16G biopsy gun. Activation of the cutting cylinder results in capture of the specimen within the sample surface of the needle.

REFERENCES

1. Christensen RA, Van Sonnenberg E, Casola G, et al. Interventional ultrasound in the musculoskeletal system. *Radiol Clin North Am.* 1988;26(1):145–156.
2. Cunnane G, Brophy DP, Gibney RG, et al. Diagnosis and treatment of heel pain in chronic inflammatory arthritis using ultrasound. *Semin Arthritis Rheum.* 1996;25(6):383–389.
3. Brophy DP, Cunnane G, FitzGerald O, et al. Technical report: ultrasound guidance for injection of soft tissue lesions around the heel in chronic inflammatory arthritis. *Clin Radiol.* 1995;50(2):120–122.
4. Cardinal E, Chhem RK, Beauregard CG. Ultrasound-guided interventional procedures in the musculoskeletal system. *Radiol Clin North Am.* 1998;36(3):597–604.
5. Koski JM. Ultrasound guided injections in rheumatology. *J Rheumatol.* 2000;27(9):2131–2138.
6. Grassi W, Farina A, Filippucci E, et al. Sonographically guided procedures in rheumatology. *Semin Arthritis Rheum.* 2001;30(5):347–353.
7. Sofka CM, Collins AJ, Adler RS. Use of ultrasonographic guidance in interventional musculoskeletal procedures: a review from a single institution. *J. Ultrasound Med.* 2001;20(1):21–26.
8. Adler RS, Sofka CM. Percutaneous ultrasound-guided injections in the musculoskeletal system. *Ultrasound Q.* 2003;19(1):3–12.
9. Davidson J, Jayaraman S. Guided interventions in musculoskeletal ultrasound: what's the evidence? *Clin. Radiol.* 2011;66(2):140–152.
10. Unverferth LJ, Olix ML. The effect of local steroid injections on tendon. *J Sports Med.* 1973;1(4):31–37.
11. Ford LT, DeBender J. Tendon rupture after local steroid injection. *South Med J.* 1979;72(7):827–830.
12. Gottlieb NL, Riskin WG. Complications of local corticosteroid injections. *JAMA.* 1980;243(15):1547–1548.
13. Oxlund H, Manthorpe R. The biochemical properties of tendon and skin as influenced by long term glucocorticoid treatment and food restriction. *Biorheology.* 1982;19(5):631–646.

14. Stapczynski JS. Localized depigmentation after steroid injection of a ganglion cyst on the hand. *Ann Emerg Med.* 1991;20(7):807–809.

15. Shrier I, Matheson GO, Kohl HW III. Achilles tendonitis: are corticosteroid injections useful or harmful? *Clin J Sport Med.* 1996;6(4):245–250.

16. Kim C, Cashdollar MR, Mendicino RW, et al. Incidence of plantar fascia ruptures following corticosteroid injection. *Foot Ankle Spec.* 2010;3(6):335–337.

17. Kamath R, Strichartz G, Rosenthal D. Cartilage toxicity from local anesthetics. *Skeletal Radiol.* 2008;37(10):871–873.

18. Ahmed R, Nazarian LN. Overview of musculoskeletal sonography. *Ultrasound Q.* 2010;26(1):27–35.

19. Koski JM, Saarakkala SJ, Heikkinen JO, et al. Use of air-steroid-saline mixture as contrast medium in greyscale ultrasound imaging: experimental study and practical applications in rheumatology. *Clin Exp Rheumatol.* 2005;23(3):373–378.

20. Luchs JS, Sofka CM, Adler RS. Contrast effect of combined steroid and anesthetic injections: in vitro analysis. *J Ultrasound Med.* 2007;26(2):227–231.

21. Krücker J, Xu S, Venkatesan A. Clinical utility of real-time fusion guidance for biopsy and ablation. *J Vasc Interv Radiol.* 2011;22(4):515–524.

22. James SL, Ali K, Pocock C, et al. Ultrasound guided dry needling and autologous blood injection for patellar tendinosis. *Br J Sports Med.* 2007;41(8):518–521.

23. Connell D, Ali KE, Ahmad M, et al. Ultrasound-guided autologous blood injection for tennis elbow. *Skeletal Radiol.* 2006;35(6):371–377.

24. Mishra A, Pavelko T. Treatment of chronic elbow tendinosis with buffered platelet-rich plasma. *Am J Sports Med.* 2006;34(11):1774–1778.

25. de Vos RJ, Weir A, Van Schie HT, et al. Platelet-rich plasma injection for chronic achilles tendinopathy: a randomized controlled trial. *JAMA.* 2010; 303(2):144–149.

26. Peerbooms JC, Sluimer J, Bruijn DJ, et al. Positive effect of an autologous platelet concentrate in lateral epicondylitis in a double-blind randomized controlled trial: platelet-rich plasma versus corticosteroid injection with a 1-year follow-up. *Am J Sports Med.* 2010;38(2):255–262.

27. Bouffard JA, Eyler WR, Introcaso JH, et al. Sonography of tendons. *Ultrasound Q.* 1993;11:259–286.

28. Kannus P, Järvinen M, Niittymäki S. Long- or short-acting anesthetic with corticosteroid in local injections of overuse injuries? A prospective, randomized, double-blind study. *Int J Sports Med.* 1990;11(5):397–400.

29. Caldwell JR. Intra-articular corticosteroids. Guide to selection and indications for use. *Drugs.* 1996;52(4):507–514.

30. Curatolo M, Bogduk N. Pharmacologic pain treatment of musculoskeletal disorders: current perspectives and future prospects. *Clin J Pain.* 2001;17(1):25–32.

31. MacMahan PJ, Eustace SJ, Kavanagh EC. Injectable corticosteroids and anesthetic preparations: a review for radiologists. *Radiology.* 2009;252(3):647–661.

32. Cox B, Durieux ME, Marcus MA. Toxicity of local anesthetics. *Best Pract Res Clin Anaesthesiol.* 2003;17(1):111–136.

33. Sofka CM, Adler RS. Ultrasound-guided interventions in the foot and ankle. *Semin Musculoskeletal Radiol.* 2002;6(2):163–168.

34. Adler RS, Allen A. Percutaneous ultrasound guided injections in the shoulder. *Tech Shoulder Elbow Surg.* 2004;5(2):122–133.

35. Sofka CM, Saboeiro G, Adler RS. Ultrasound-guided adult hip injections. *J Vasc Interv Radiol.* 2005;16(8):1121–1123.

36. Rabago D, Best TM, Zgierska AE, et al. A systematic review of four injection therapies for lateral epicondylosis. *Br J Sports Med.* 2009;43(7):471–478.

37. Wijesekera NT, Calder JD, Lee JC. Imaging in the assessment and management of achilles tendinopathy and paratendinitis. *Semin Musculoskelet Radiol.* 2011;15(1):89–100.

38. Mehdizade A, Adler RS. Sonographically guided flexor hallucis longus tendon sheath injection. *J Ultrasound Med.* 2007;26(2):233–237.

39. Tsai WC, Wang CL, Tang FT, et al. Treatment of proximal plantar fasciitis with ultrasound-guided steroid injection. *Arch Phys Med Rehabil.* 2000;81(10):1416–1421.

40. Sofka CM, Adler RS, Ciavarra G, et al. Ultrasound-guided interdigital neuroma injections: short-term clinical outcomes after a single percutaneous injection–preliminary results. *HSS J.* 2007;3(1):44–49.

41. Hughes RJ, Ali K, Jones H, et al. Treatment of Morton's Neuroma with alcohol injection under sonographic guidance: follow-up of 101 cases. *AJR Am J Roentgenol.* 2007;188(6):1535–1539.

42. Friedman T, Richman D, Adler RS. Sonographically guided cryoneurolysis: preliminary experience and clinical outcomes. *J Ultrasound Med.* 2012; 31(12):2025–2034.

43. Jeyapalan K, Choudhary S. Ultrasound-guided injections of triamcinolone and bupivacaine in the management of De Quervain's disease. *Skeletal Radiol.* 2009;38(11):1099–1103.

44. Middleton WD, Reinus WR, Totty WG, et al. Ultrasound of the biceps tendon apparatus. *Radiology.* 1985;157(1):211–215.

45. Adler RS, Buly R, Ambrose R, et al. Diagnostic and therapeutic use of sonography-guided iliopsoas peritendinous injections. *AJR Am J Roentgenol.* 2005;185(4):940–943.

46. Breidahl WH, Adler RS. Ultrasound-guided injection of ganglia with corticosteroids. *Skeletal Radiol.* 1996;25(7):635–638.

47. Chiou HJ, Chou YH, Wu JJ, et al. Alternative and effective treatment of shoulder ganglion cyst: ultrasonographically guided aspiration. *J Ultrasound Med.* 1999;18(8):531–535.

48. Farin PU, Räsänen H, Jaroma H, et al. Rotator cuff calcifications: treatment with ultrasound-guided percutaneous needle aspiration and lavage. *Skeletal Radiol.* 1996;25(6):551–554.

49. Aina R, Cardinal E, Bureau NJ, et al. Calcific shoulder tendinitis: treatment with modified US-guided fine-needle technique. *Radiology.* 2001;221(2):455–461.

50. Lin JT, Adler RS, Bracilovic A, et al. Clinical outcomes of ultrasound-guided aspiration and lavage in calcific tendonitis of the shoulder. *HSS J.* 2007;3(1):99–105.

51. Jensen KT, Rabago DP, Best TM, et al. Early inflammatory response of knee ligaments to prolotherapy in a rat model. *J Ortho Res.* 2008;26(6):816–823.

52. Rabago D, Slattengren A, Zgierska AE. Prolotherapy in primary care practice. *Prim Care.* 2010;37(1):65–80.

53. Fullerton BD, Reeves KD. Ultrasonography in regenerative injection (prolotherapy) using dextrose, platelet-rich plasma, and other injectants. *Phys Med Rehabil Clin North Am.* 2010;21(3):585–605.

54. McShane JM, Nazarian LN, Harwood MI. Sonographically guided percutaneous needle tenotomy for treatment of common extensor tendinosis in the elbow. *J Ultrasound Med.* 2006;25(10):1281–1289.

55. de Mos M, van der Windt AE, Jahr H, et al. Can platelet-rich plasma enhance tendon repair? A cell culture study. *Am J Sports Med.* 2008;36(6):1171–1178.

56. Foster TE, Puskas BL, Mandelbaum BR, et al. Platelet-rich plasma: from basic science to clinical applications. *Am J Sports Med.* 2009;37(11):2259–2272.

57. Klauser AS, Faschingbauer R, Bauer T, et al. Entrapment neuropathies II: carpal tunnel syndrome. *Semin Musculoskelet Radiol.* 2010;14(5):487–500.

58. Tagliafico A, Cadoni A, Fisci E, et al. Nerves of the hand beyond the carpal tunnel. *Semin Musculoskelet Radiol.* 2012;16(2):129–136.

59. Tagliafico A, Altafini L, Garello I, et al. Traumatic neuropathies: spectrum of imaging findings and postoperative assessment. *Semin Musculoskelet Radiol.* 2010;14(5):512–522.

60. Speed CA. Injection therapies for soft tissue lesions. *Best Pract Res Clin Rheumatol.* 2007;21(2):333–347.

61. Tagliafico A, Bodner G, Rosenberg I. Peripheral nerves: ultrasound-guided interventional procedures. *Semin Musculoskelet Radiol.* 2010;14(5):559–566.

62. Sabharwal T, Katsanos K, Buy X, et al. Image-guided ablation therapy of bone tumors. *Sem Ultrasound CT MR.* 2009;30(2):78–90.

63. Chua NH, Vissers KC, Sluijter ME. Pulsed radiofrequency treatment in interventional pain management: mechanisms and potential indications—a review. *Acta Neurochir (Wien).* 2011;153(4):763–771.

64. Ramamurthy S, Walsh NE, Schoenfeld LS, et al. Evaluation of neurolytic blocks using phenol and cryogenic block in the management of chronic pain. *J Pain Symptom Manage.* 1989;4(2):72–75.

65. Fasano VA, Peirone SM, Zeme S, et al. Cryoanalgesia. Ultrastructural study on cryolytic lesion of sciatic nerve in rat and rabbit. *Acta Neurochir Suppl (Wien).* 1987;39:177–180.

66. Trescot AM. Cryoanalgesia in interventional pain management. *Pain Physician* 2003;6(3):345–360.

67. Torriani M, Etchebehere M, Amstalden E. Sonographically guided core needle biopsy of bone and soft tissue tumors. *J Ultrasound Med.* 2002;21(3):275–281.

68. Lopez JL, Del Cura JL, Zabala R. Usefulness and limitations of ultrasound-guided core biopsy in the diagnosis of musculoskeletal tumors. *APMIS.* 2005;113(5):353–360.

INDEX

Note: Page numbers followed by *f* indicate figures; those followed by *t* indicate tables.